Neurological Disorders: Clinical Biomarkers

Neurological Disorders: Clinical Biomarkers

Editor: Ernie Murphy

hayle medical

New York

Hayle Medical,
750 Third Avenue, 9th Floor,
New York, NY 10017, USA

Visit us on the World Wide Web at:
www.haylemedical.com

ISBN 978-1-64647-580-3 (Hardback)

Cataloging-in-Publication Data

Neurological disorders : clinical biomarkers / edited by Ernie Murphy.
p. cm.
Includes bibliographical references and index.
ISBN 978-1-64647-580-3
1. Nervous system--Diseases. 2. Biochemical markers. 3. Nervous system--Diseases--Diagnosis.
4. Nervous system--Diseases--Treatment. I. Murphy, Ernie.
RC346 .N483 2023
616.8--dc23

Contents

Preface

This book has been a concerted effort by a group of academicians, researchers and scientists, who have contributed their research works for the realization of the book. This book has materialized in the wake of emerging advancements and innovations in this field. Therefore, the need of the hour was to compile all the required researches and disseminate the knowledge to a broad spectrum of people comprising of students, researchers and specialists of the field.

Neurological disorders refer to the type of disorders that affect the brain, nerves and spinal cord. Such disorders may lead to a variety of symptoms that are caused by structural, electrical or biochemical abnormalities in any part of the nervous system. The signs and symptoms of neurological disorders include muscle weakness, loss of sensation, confusion, altered levels of consciousness, paralysis, poor coordination, seizures and pain. Some common types of neurological disorders are multiple sclerosis (MS), migraines, Alzheimer's disease (AD), Parkinson's disease and epilepsy. Biomarkers offer a potent and dynamic approach to study different neurological diseases and have applications in screening, observational and analytic epidemiology, randomized clinical trials, diagnosis, and prognosis of neurological disorders. This book explores all the important aspects of clinical biomarkers used in neurological disorders. It presents researches and studies performed by experts across the globe. The book is appropriate for students seeking detailed information in this area of study as well as for experts.

At the end of the preface, I would like to thank the authors for their brilliant chapters and the publisher for guiding us all-through the making of the book till its final stage. Also, I would like to thank my family for providing the support and encouragement throughout my academic career and research projects.

Editor

Preface

1

Parahippocampal Involvement in Mesial Temporal Lobe Epilepsy with Hippocampal Sclerosis: A Proof of Concept from Memory-Guided Saccades

*Silvia Colnaghi[1,2], Giorgio Beltrami[3], Guy Poloni[4], Anna Pichiecchio[4], Stefano Bastianello[4,5], Carlo Andrea Galimberti[6] and Maurizio Versino[1,5]**

[1] Laboratory of Neuro-otology and Neuro-ophtalmology, Fondazione Istituto Neurologico Nazionale Casimiro Mondino (IRCCS), Pavia, Italy, [2] Department of Public Health, Experimental and Forensic Medicine, University of Pavia, Pavia, Italy, [3] Department of Electrical, Computer and Biomedical Engineering, University of Pavia, Pavia, Italy, [4] Neuroradiology Department, Fondazione Istituto Neurologico Nazionale Casimiro Mondino (IRCCS), Pavia, Italy, [5] Department of Brain and Behavioral Sciences, University of Pavia, Pavia, Italy, [6] Epilepsy Centre, Fondazione Istituto Neurologico Nazionale Casimiro Mondino (IRCCS), Pavia, Italy

***Correspondence:**
Maurizio Versino
mversino@unipv.it

Objective: Mesial temporal lobe epilepsy with hippocampal sclerosis (MTLE-HS) may involve extrahippocampal areas of structural damage and dysfunction. The accuracy of medium-term spatial memory can be tested by memory-guided saccades (MGS) to evaluate a functional impairment of the parahippocampal cortex (PHC), while voxel-based morphometry (VBM) analysis can be used to detect a structural damage of the latter region.

Methods: MGS with 3- and 30-s memorization delays were compared between 7 patients affected by right MTLE-HS (r-MTLE-HS), 6 patients affected by left MTLE-HS, and 13 healthy controls. The same subjects underwent brain MRI for a VBM analysis. Correlation analysis was performed between the results of VBM and MGS and with patients' clinical data.

Results: Right MTLE-HS patients showed impaired accuracy of leftward MGS with a 30-s memorization delay; their gray-matter volume was reduced in the right hippocampus and inferior temporal gyrus, and bilaterally in the cerebellum. Left MTLE-HS patients had normal MGS accuracy; their gray-matter volume was reduced in the left hippocampus, in the right-inferior temporal gyrus and corpus callosus, and bilaterally in the insular cortex and in the cerebellum. The difference between right and left parahippocampal volumes correlated with MGS accuracy, while right and left hippocampal volumes did not. Hippocampal and parahippocampal volume did not correlate with clinical variables such as febrile seizures, age at disease onset, disease duration, and seizure frequency.

Conclusion: MGS abnormalities suggested the functional involvement of the right PHC in patients with r-MTLE-HS, supporting a right lateralization of spatial memory control and showing a relation between functional impairment and degree of atrophy.

Keywords: memory-guided saccade, voxel-based morphometry, spatial memory, parahippocampal cortex, mesial temporal lobe epilepsy

INTRODUCTION

Extrahippocampal areas of structural damage may be detected in mesial temporal lobe epilepsy with hippocampal sclerosis (MTLE-HS), including the parahippocampal and mesial temporal lobe cortex (1–5).

These findings have been emphasized in the MTLE-HS workshop promoted by the International League Against Epilepsy (6), when the importance of defining the site and characteristics of extrahippocampal damage was underlined. In fact, structural damage of these areas has an incidence that varies in relation with the different diagnostic methods, and the characteristics of extrahippocampal pathology in MTLE-HS (6) as well as its pathogenesis are still a matter of debate.

Here, we aimed at evaluating the consistency of neurophysiological data indicating a functional involvement of the parahippocampal cortex (PHC) with voxel-based morphometry (VBM) data.

Many brain regions have been shown to be reduced in volume in temporal lobe epilepsy (TLE) patients with respect to healthy subjects [see Ref. (7) for a review]. Temporal lobe abnormalities were mainly ipsilateral to the epileptic focus, while extratemporal and subcortical abnormalities were bilateral. This distribution of brain abnormalities in TLE patients is consistent with postmortem and fMRI imaging results. Hippocampal atrophy ipsilateral to the epileptic focus is the most common neuropathological correlate of TLE (8), and patients with right-sided epileptic focus are more likely to have bilateral hippocampal volume reduction (9).

A recent study (10) showed that history of febrile convulsions (FC), dystonic posturing, and secondary generalized tonic–clonic seizures are cardinal criteria that could be reliably helpful to distinguish TLE patients with hippocampal sclerosis from those with other TLE (i.e., patients with mesial structural lesion other than hippocampal sclerosis and MRI-negative cases), suggesting that MTLE-HS could be considered as a distinctive syndrome. When HS is detectable, patients with MTLE showed an earlier epilepsy onset, exhibited more frequently early febrile seizures (FS), and presented more ictal gestural automatisms, dystonic posturing and secondary generalized tonic–clonic seizures.

Mesial temporal lobe epilepsy with hippocampal sclerosis patients show material-specific memory impairment depending on their hemispheric language dominance. For instance, verbal memory impairment was found in left MTLE-HS (l-MTLE-HS) patients with left language dominant hemisphere, while a weaker association was found between visual memory impairment and right temporal dysfunction (11, 12) in right MTLE-HS (r-MTLE-HS) patients.

The memory-guided saccades (MGS) can be used to study cortical control of short and medium-term spatial memory in humans (13, 14). In the MGS paradigm, subjects are requested to make a volitional saccade directed toward a location in which a target was previously present.

Functional imagery, transcranial magnetic stimulation, and lesion studies have been used to obtain a spatially and temporally accurate model of the MGS cortical control in normal subjects and in patients with lesions of the temporal lobe structures (15).

In particular, it has been showed that accuracy of MGS with memorization delays from 1 to 20 s depends on the dorsolateral prefrontal cortex (DLPFC) (16), while the PHC is responsible for the accuracy of MGS with memorization delays longer than 20 s and up to a few minutes (16–19). Ploner et al. (18) exploited the MGS paradigm to test the role of the PHC for the accuracy of spatial memory in humans. They recorded the MGS with delays op to 30 s in patients that underwent resection of the right mesial temporal lobe for intractable epilepsy. Patients whose lesion was limited to the PHC made amplitude error of memory guided eye movements with 30-s delay (30 MGS) directed contralateral to the lesion side, while patient as whose resection included the perirhinal cortex but not the PHC were able to perform the MGS with no such errors. Taking into account these findings, in a previous study (20) we recorded the MGS with memorization delays of 3 (3 MGS) and 30 s in patients with r-MTLE-HS and we found a delay-dependent inaccuracy of 30 MGS contralateral to the lesion suggesting a functional impairment of the right PHC.

Here, we hypothesized that the accuracy of 30 MGS directed contralaterally to the epilepsy focus could be impaired in MTLE-HS patients with VBM signs of structural involvement of extrahippocampal brain regions, particularly of the PHC of the ipsilateral mesial temporal lobe, and that this impairment could be associated with clinical data, particularly disease duration, and seizure frequency.

MATERIALS AND METHODS

Subjects

Thirteen right-handed subjects with r-MTLE-HS (n = 7) or l-MTLE-HS (n = 6) and 13 healthy subjects underwent recording of 3 MGS and 30 MGS and brain MRI for VBM quantitative analysis.

Mesial temporal lobe epilepsy with hippocampal sclerosis patients were recruited among the outpatients consecutively referred to the Epilepsy Centre of the Neurological Institute C. Mondino of Pavia.

We excluded patients unable to participate due to difficulties in understanding the experimental procedures or in maintaining attention for a long time, those older than 60 years, those with a seizure frequency more than 2 per week, and those who modified antiepileptic treatment in the previous month or experienced an epileptic seizure in the previous 36 h. Exclusion criteria were chosen in order to avoid gray mater reduction associated with age (21) and biases in eye movement test performance possibly due to post-ictal dysfunction.

Patients' demographical and clinical data are shown in **Table 1**.

Epilepsy diagnosis was supported by clinical, electroencephalography (EEG), and MRI criteria. More in detail, conventional brain MRI showed atrophy and T2 signal increase that were limited to the hippocampal formation in each patient, and did not show parahippocampal atrophy in any of them. EEG traces, ictal symptoms, and signs suggested a mesial temporal lobe seizure onset in each patient (6).

All patients were on treatment with antiepileptic drugs with serum levels in therapeutic range.

TABLE 1 | Demographic and clinical features of patients with right (r-MTLE-HS) and left (l-MTLE-HS) mesial temporal lobe epilepsy with hippocampal sclerosis.

	Age (decade)	Age at epilepsy onset (years or months)	Disease duration (years)	FS	AED	Seizure frequency (per month)
r-MTLE-HS	6th	43 years	9	y	PHT 325 LEV 4000 CLB 20	1.5
	4th	7 months	20	n	CBZ CR 800 PHT 200 CLB 30	4.5
	6th	37 years	15	y	LTG 600 CLB 20 LEV 500	1.5
	4th	9 month	38	y	CBZ CR 1100 LTG 500	8.5
	4th	29 years	7	y	CBZ CR 800 LTG 200	3
	7th	6 month	35	n	CBZ CR 1000 LEV 3500 PHT 0.5	3
	3th	14 years	15	n	LTG 550 LEV 3000	2.5
l-MTLE-HS	5th	23 years	23	n	CLB 10 OXC 600	0.1
	5th	14 years	28	y	LTG 500 CBZ 900 LEV 550	2.5
	4th	8 years	22	y	CBZ 800 LEV 3000	0.1
	6th	20 years	34	n	CBZ 800	0.1
	6th	22 years	36	y	CBZ 800 LEV 3000	0.25
	4th	15 years	22	n	LTG 600 CBZ 400 LEV 3000	4.50

M, male; F, female; FS, febrile seizures; n, no; y, yes. AED, antiepileptic drug treatment, mg daily; CBZ, carbamazepine; LTG, lamotrigine; LEV, levetiracetam; OXC, oxcarbazepine; PHT, fenitoine; CLB, clobazam. Seizure frequency = monthly mean calculated on the basis of the seizure reported in the last year on the patient's seizure diary.

Thirteen right-handed healthy subjects (seven women and six men; mean age: 38.4 years, SD: 10.5, range: 27–60 years) age-matched with the patient group (mean age: 43.8 years, SD 11.0, range: 29–60 years) were included in the control group.

The research protocol received approval from the local Ethics Committee and all the procedures were conducted in accordance with the Declaration of Helsinki. All the subjects gave written informed consent before participating in the study.

Memory-Guided Saccades

The eye movements were calibrated and recorded monocularly from the right eye with the scleral search coil technique (22) (SKALAR system S3020: spatial resolution better than 0.1°; sampling rate 250 Hz, bandwidth 0–70 Hz).

The eye movement recording sessions, data acquisition, and analysis were the same as reported in our previous study (20).

The subjects were seated in a dark room with their head in the upright position on a chinrest. For every subject, we recorded the reflexive saccades (RS), the 3 MGS, and the 30 MGS in three separate sessions. In each session, every subject performed 18 trials in both directions (leftward and rightward saccades) for a total of 108 trials each.

In the RS paradigm, a horizontally presented lateral target with an unpredictable direction and amplitude (10°, 15°, or 20°) was lit for 2 s, while the subject was staring at a central point. The subjects were instructed to look at this light immediately after its appearance and until it disappeared. The next trial began at the central fixation point.

In the MGS paradigm, the subjects tried to memorize the location of a horizontally presented lateral target lit for 200 ms, while they were staring at the central point. The target had unpredictable direction and amplitude (10°, 15°, or 20°). After the memorization delay of 3 or 30 s, the central fixation point was switched off, which was the signal for the subject to perform a saccade toward the memorized location. The previously flashed target was shown again after 2 s and the subject had to make a corrective saccade if necessary. The next trial began at the central fixation point.

Memory-guided saccades trials with prosaccades, namely erroneous RS directed at the flashed target, were excluded from analysis. We used a custom-made program developed with LabView software (National Instruments, Austin, TX, USA) to analyze the saccades offline by identifying the beginning and the end of each saccade based on threshold velocity criteria; the difference in the eye position at these two points corresponded to the pulse amplitude. The operator positioned one additional mark that identified the final position, namely the position the eye reached after all the corrective saccades and before the reappearance of the target; the difference between the starting and final positions corresponded to the final amplitude.

We computed the following equations:

1. the saccade accuracies (SA) as

$$\text{pulseSA} = \text{pulse amplitude / target amplitude},$$
$$\text{finalSA} = \text{final amplitude / target amplitude}$$

2. the amplitude errors (E) as

$$\text{pulseE} = \ln|1 - \text{pulseSA}|,$$
$$\text{finalE} = \ln|1 - \text{finalSA}|$$

3. the amplitude error difference (ED) as

$$\text{ED} = \text{finalE} - \text{pulseE}.$$

A logarithmic transformation was needed in order to approximate a normal distribution of the values, and we used the absolute value of the $|1 - \text{SA}|$ differences to express a scatter of the MGS endpoints despite the presence of both hypometric and hypermetric saccades.

For each subject, paradigm, and saccade direction, we computed the mean value of latency, SA, *E*, and ED.

The patients were compared with the controls as a group by using repeated measure analyses of variance on all the parameters listed before. The RS and the 3- and 30-s MGS were analyzed separately. The analyses considered one intra-individual factor (saccade direction: right or left), one inter-individual factor (group: controls or patients), and their interactions.

The significance value was set at $p = 0.05$.

We used chi-square test to evaluate the occurrence of patients whose mean value exceeded the normal range, which was calculated on the control group as the mean ± 2.5 SDs.

Voxel-Based Morphometry

All the subjects' MRI were performed with the same machine (Philips Intera Gyroscan 1.5 T), using coronal T1 Gradient Echo sequences, with identical acquisition parameters [echo time (TE) 4.6 ms, repetition time (TR) = 25 ms, thickness = 1.6 mm, slice gap = 0.8 mm, matrix = 256 × 256, voxel = 0.9 mm × 0.9 mm × 0.8 mm, means = 1].

The VBM study was performed through a between-groups comparison by dividing the subjects in three groups on the basis of presence and side of the hippocampal atrophy: controls (Ctrls), r-MTLE-HS (seven subjects), and l-MTLE-HS (six subjects). The areas of reduced gray-matter volume were identified first, then a study on the hippocampal region was performed: the mean volume of the hippocampal gray matter on each side and the difference in volume between the two sides were correlated with the clinical data (age at epilepsy onset, epilepsy duration, seizure frequency, antiepileptic drugs) and the results of MGS recording.

Neuroimage processing was done by statistical parametric map (SPM) (discrete cosine transform cutoff 8 mm) and MATLAB 7.4 programs. Acquired images were normalized on a whole-brain standard template MNI 152, with masking of the hippocampal region (7). Normalized images were segmented through the standard gray and white matter (GM/WM) templates from SPM. Filter value was set at 6-mm smoothing kernel, as suggested for studying structures with dimensions comparable with the hippocampus (7).

Normalized, segmented, and smoothed images were weighted regarding confounding variables (sex, age, and total brain volume). After the described preprocessing and normalization operations, anatomical images underwent a voxel-wise statistical analysis aimed at identifying differences between the three groups.

Statistical parametric maps of the whole brain were created for several comparisons: Ctrls vs. r-MTLE-HS, Ctrls vs. l-MTLE-HS, and l-MTLE-HS vs. r-MTLE-HS. All contrasted images were created using a $p < 0.005$.

We correlated the hippocampal and parahippocampal gray-matter volumes with the clinical and MGS parameters, and compared hippocampal and parahippocampal volumes of MTLE-HS patients with and without abnormal MGS.

RESULTS

Saccades

Accuracy parameters' mean and SE values are shown in **Table 2**.

The effects of saccade direction and experimental group on all saccadic parameters are shown in **Table 3**.

The peak velocity values were significantly influenced by saccade direction being larger for rightward than for leftward saccades for all kinds of saccades, with no significant effect of group or group*direction interaction.

The latency values of RS, 3 MGS, and 30 MGS were not significantly influenced by direction, group, or group*direction interaction.

The pulseE values of both RS and 3 MGS were not significantly influenced by saccade direction, group, or group*direction interaction, whereas the pulseE of 30 MGS was significantly influenced by saccade direction being larger for rightward than for leftward saccades, with no significant effect of group or group*direction interaction.

The finalE values showed a different behavior depending on the different kinds of saccades.

For RS it proved to be smaller to the right than to the left, showing a significant direction effect with no significant effect of group and direction*group interaction. The finalE values of 3 MGS were not significantly influenced by saccade direction, group, or group*direction interaction. The finalE values of 30 MGS showed the same behavior detectable for pulseE of the same kind of saccades, since they were significantly influenced by saccade direction being larger to the right than to the left, with no significant effect of group or group*direction interaction.

TABLE 2 | Mean and SE values of rightward and leftward saccades pulse and final amplitude, natural logarithm of pulse and finalError, and error difference (ED) between final and pulse for each diagnostic group (healthy controls = Ctrls, patients with right temporal lobe epilepsy and hyoppocampal sclerosis = r-MTLE-HS, and patients with left temporal lobe epilepsy and hyoppocampal sclerosis = l-MTLE-HS) in reflexive saccades (RS), 3 s (3 MGS) and 30 s (30 MGS) memory-guided saccades.

Side	Paradigm	Group	Amplitude				Error				ED	
			Pulse		Final		Pulse		Final		Final-Pulse	
			Mean	SE	Mean	SE	Mean	SE	Mean	SE	Mean	SE
RIGHTWARD	RS	Ctrls	0.907	0.019	0.986	0.011	−2.659	0.196	−4.178	0.201	−1.519	0.177
		r-MTLE-HS	0.909	0.020	0.970	0.009	−2.346	0.165	−3.738	0.369	−1.392	0.237
		l-MTLE-HS	0.843	0.021	0.959	0.016	−2.230	0.207	−3.858	0.277	−1.628	0.204
	3 MGS	Ctrls	0.868	0.033	0.944	0.021	−2.059	0.127	−2.579	0.095	−0.520	0.137
		r-MTLE-HS	0.899	0.058	0.962	0.019	−1.875	0.170	−2.438	0.237	−0.564	0.201
		l-MTLE-HS	0.845	0.024	0.996	0.046	−2.002	0.196	−2.722	0.231	−0.721	0.321
	30 MGS	Ctrls	0.778	0.049	0.940	0.029	−1.606	0.141	−2.363	0.180	−0.756	0.121
		r-MTLE-HS	0.875	0.097	0.889	0.085	−1.610	0.236	−1.852	0.120	−0.242	0.196
		l-MTLE-HS	0.827	0.103	0.928	0.095	−1.578	0.282	−2.121	0.252	−0.543	0.266
LEFTWARD	RS	Ctrls	0.878	0.016	0.970	0.000	−2.318	0.140	−3.738	0.200	−1.420	0.163
		r-MTLE-HS	0.874	0.008	0.953	0.000	−2.180	0.000	−3.229	0.000	−1.049	0.201
		l-MTLE-HS	0.836	0.032	0.949	0.000	−2.036	0.000	−3.363	0.000	−1.328	0.158
	3 MGS	Ctrls	0.833	0.033	0.921	0.024	−1.875	0.140	−2.652	0.193	−0.777	0.156
		r-MTLE-HS	0.851	0.037	0.987	0.044	−1.835	0.201	−2.604	0.195	−0.769	0.174
		l-MTLE-HS	0.879	0.047	0.988	0.040	−1.813	0.257	−2.491	0.155	−0.678	0.244
	30 MGS	Ctrls	0.826	0.056	0.919	0.026	−1.644	0.141	−2.465	0.174	−0.821	0.131
		r-MTLE-HS	0.875	0.059	0.980	0.050	−2.092	0.338	−2.151	0.096	−0.059	0.310
		l-MTLE-HS	0.943	0.093	0.987	0.057	−1.886	0.186	−2.556	0.155	−0.671	0.207

TABLE 3 | Effects of saccade direction, diagnostic group, and direction*group interaction on saccade peak velocity, latency, pulseError, finalError, and pulseError–finalError difference in reflexive saccades (RS), and 3- and 30-s memory-guided saccades (3 MGS and 30 MGS). Bold font is used to highlight the statistically significant comparisons.

Saccade parameter	Saccade kind	Direction effect		Group effect		Direction*group interaction	
		F	p	F	p	F	p
Peak velocity	RS	**5.114**	**0.033**	0.440	0.648	2.310	0.122
	3 MGS	**8.301**	**0.008**	0.428	0.657	0.029	0.972
	30 MGS	**14.325**	**0.001**	0.937	0.406	1.169	0.329
Latency	RS	0.481	0.495	0.382	0.687	0.114	0.893
	3 MGS	1.162	0.292	0.133	0.876	0.873	0.431
	30 MGS	1.009	0.744	1.117	0.360	0.797	0.721
PulseE	RS	3.279	0.083	1.540	0.235	0.019	0.797
	3 MGS	1.554	0.225	0.208	0.814	0.341	0.715
	30 MGS	**5.691**	**0.025**	0.437	0.651	1.543	0.234
FinalE	RS	**8.456**	**0.008**	1.250	0.305	0.012	0.988
	3 MGS	**8.456**	**0.008**	0.130	0.878	0.702	0.505
	30 MGS	**7.133**	**0.013**	1.555	0.232	1.010	0.379
ED	RS	4.090	0.054	0.298	0.745	0.479	0.625
	3 MGS	0.884	0.357	0.030	0.971	0.379	0.688
	30 MGS	0.000	0.988	4.992	0.015	0.413	0.666

The ED values of both RS and 3 MGS were not significantly influenced by saccade direction, group, or group*direction interaction, whereas the ED of 30 MGS was significantly influenced by group. This effect was mainly attributed to r-MTLE-HS patients who were unable to reduce the pulseE, and hence to minimize ED, as effectively as controls for leftward saccades (Sheffè *post hoc* test: $p = 0.035$), but a similar trend was detectable in r-MTLE-HS patients for rightward saccades also.

Thereby, the results of group analyses can be summarized as follows:

- RS pulseE and ED values were independent from direction, group, and their interaction, while finalE values were smaller for rightward than for leftward saccades both in controls and in patients.
- 3 MGS pulseE, finale, and ED values were independent from direction, group, and their interaction.
- 30 MGS pulseE and finalE values were larger for rightward than for leftward saccades both in controls and in patients; moreover, patients with r-MTLE-HS showed a larger ED than controls.

We also considered the patients individually; that is, we checked if accuracy values of their saccades fell within the normal limits defined as the mean ± 2.5 SDs computed in the control group (**Figure 1**).

The pulseE was invariably normal both in the control and in the patient groups for all kind of saccades.

The finalE was abnormal in a few subjects: two subjects (1 r-MTLE-HS and 1 control) for r-RS, 1 r-MTLE-HS patient for r-3MSG, no subjects for 30 MGS: the chi-square test showed that the distribution of abnormalities did not differ between patients and controls.

The ED was abnormal only in one l-MTLE-HS patient for r-3MGS: again, the chi-square test showed that the distribution of abnormalities did not differ in the patients as compared with controls.

The main finding derives from 30 MGS that showed an abnormal ED in four r-MTLE-HS patients (all of them for

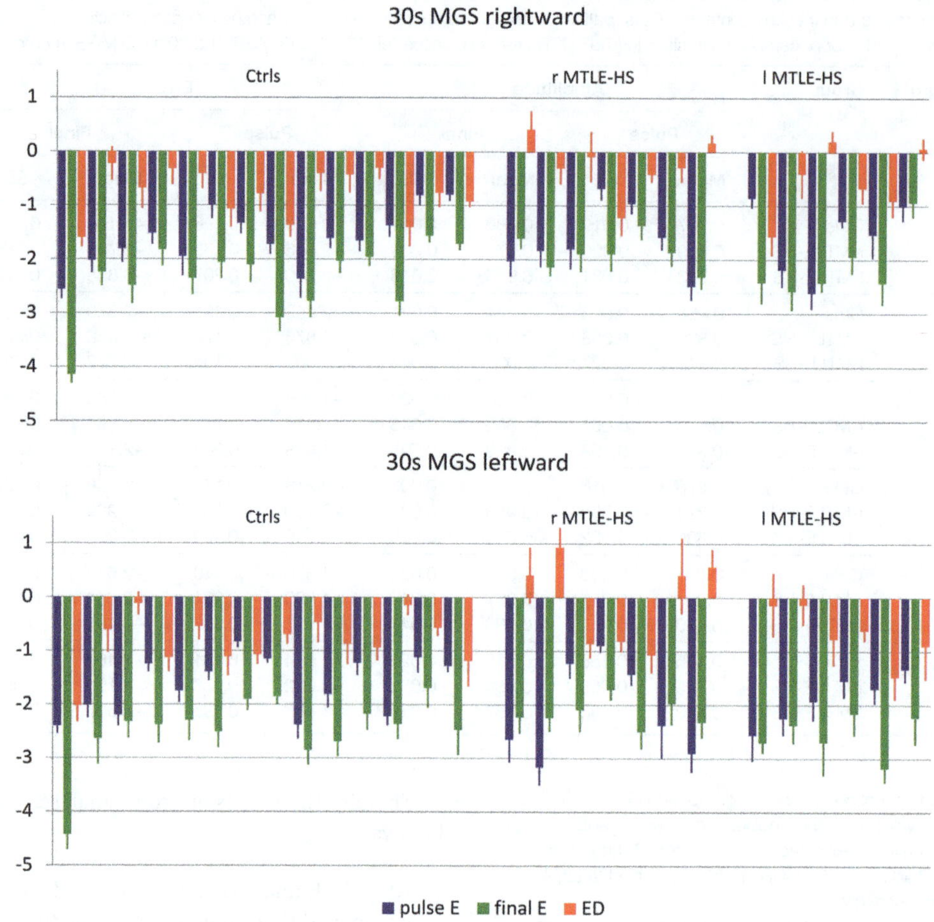

FIGURE 1 | Mean and SE values of pulseError (pulseE), finalError (finalE), and error difference between pulse and final (ED) of 30-s delay memory-guided saccades (30 MGS) directed rightward (upper panel) and leftward (lower panel) for each subject in each diagnostic group. ctrls, healthy controls; r-MTLE-HS, patients with right-sided mesial temporal lobe epilepsy with hippocampal sclerosis; l-MTLE-HS, patients with left-sided mesial temporal lobe epilepsy with hippocampal sclerosis.

leftward saccades and in one of them for rightward saccades also) and in none of the l-MTLE patients or of the controls: the higher occurrence of abnormalities in the r-MTLE-HS group proved to be statistically significant (Fisher' exact test $p = 0.003$).

Voxel-Based Morphometry

Table 4 displays the results of gray-matter changes.

Right MTLE-HS patients showed right hippocampal atrophy (**Figure 2A**) as compared with healthy controls, and when the statistical significance threshold was lowered to $p < 0.03$, contralateral hippocampal atrophy was also detected (**Figure 2B**). r-MTLE-HS patients showed relative right hippocampal atrophy as compared with l-MTLE-HS patients (**Figure 2C**).

Regions with significantly reduced gray-matter volume involved several extrahippocampal brain regions in addition to the ipsilateral hippocampus.

Compared with healthy controls, r-MTLE-HS patients had regions with significantly reduced gray-matter volume also in the right-inferior temporal gyrus, and in the ipsi- and contralateral

TABLE 4 | Regions of statistically significant difference between groups.

Relative atrophy regions in right MTLE-HS (r-MTLE-HS) subjects ($p < 0.005$)	
vs. Ctrls	**vs. left MTLE-HS (l-MTLE-HS) subjects**
Right hippocampus [26, −28, −14]	Right hippocampus [28, −26, 14]
Right-inferior temporal gyrus [54, −44, −14]	Left central sulcus [−42, 20, 12]
Cerebellum bilaterally [−18, −64, −44] [24, −62, −44]	Left precentral gyrus [−44, 32, 22]
Relative atrophy regions in l-MTLE-HS subjects ($p < 0.005$)	
vs. Ctrls	**vs. r-MTLE-HS subjects**
Left hippocampus [−32, −26, −14]	Left-inferior temporal gyrus [−54, −28, −18]
Right-inferior temporal gyrus [5, −48, −10]	Left insula [−40, 16, 10]
Right corpus callosum [8, −10, 28]	Left putamen [−20, 8, −8]
Insula bilaterally [−34, −8, 10] [28, −8, 10]	
Cerebellum bilaterally [−28, −60, −44] [26, −60, −44]	

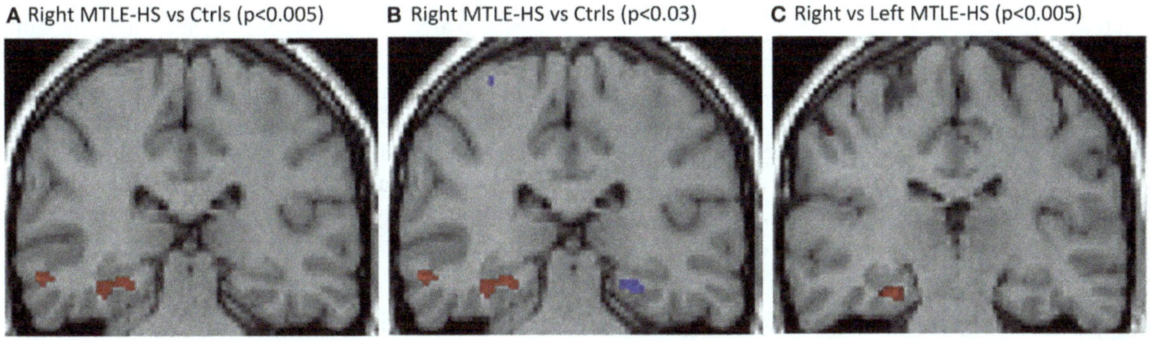

FIGURE 2 | VBM T1-weighted multiplanar images comparing **(A)** r-MTLE-HS patients vs. healthy controls, showing relative right hippocampal atrophy; **(B)** r-MTLE-HS patients vs. healthy controls with $p < 0.005$ in red and $p < 0.03$ in blue, showing bilateral relative hippocampal atrophy; **(C)** r-MTLE-HS vs. l-MTLE-HS patients, showing relative right hippocampal atrophy. SPM results are superimposed on a T1 3d image of one of the healthy subjects. l-MTLE-HS, left MTLE-HS patients; r-MTLE-HS, right MTLE-HS patients; SPM, statistical parametric map; VBM, voxel-based morphometry.

TABLE 5 | Mean and SE values of the right and left volumes and volume difference between right and left parahippocampus (PH) in controls (Ctrl), right (r MTLE-HS), and left (l MTLE-HS) MTLE-HS patients.

	Group	Mean	SE
Right PH volume	Ctrl	650.380	2.230
	r-MTLE-HS	621.000	4.170
	l-MTLE-HS	655.330	3.160
Left PH volume	Ctrl	570.850	1,600
	r-MTLE-HS	580.430	3.500
	l-MTLE-HS	551.000	3.340
Right–left PH volume difference	Ctrl	40.570	2.090
	r-MTLE-HS	104.330	3.040
	l-MTLE-HS	76.530	1.830

TABLE 6 | Mean and SE values of right and left volume and volume difference between right and left parahippocampus (PH) in MTLE-HS patients showing impaired 30 MGS ED and in MTLE-HS patients not showing impaired 30 MGS ED.

	Impaired ED in 30 MGS	*N*	Mean	SE	*t*	*p*
Right PH volume	No	9	646.560	7.370	1.596	0.186
	Yes	4	615.000	18.340		
Left PH volume	No	9	563.670	9.010	0.628	0.554
	Yes	4	574.000	13.770		
Right–left PH volume difference	No	9	82.889	11.760	2.667	0.024
	Yes	4	41.000	10.320		

cerebellum. Compared with l-MTLE-HS patients, they showed reduced gray-matter volume of the left central sulcus and the left precentral gyrus.

Left MTLE-HS patients showed relative left hippocampal atrophy as compared with healthy controls and not compared with r-MTLE-HS patients. When the statistical significance threshold was lowered to $p < 0.03$, no contralateral hippocampal atrophy was detected.

Compared with healthy controls, l-MTLE-HS patients had regions with significantly reduced gray-matter volume also in the left-inferior temporal gyrus and corpus callosus and in the ipsi- and contralateral insula and cerebellum. Compared with r-MTLE-HS patients, they showed reduced gray mater volume of the left-inferior temporal gyrus, insula, and putamen.

Correlation analysis in MTLE-HS subjects showed no significant effects. In particular, no significant correlation was found between ipsilateral H and PH gray-matter volume and 30 MGS ED, number of anti-epileptic drugs, seizure frequency, age, age at epilepsy onset, and disease duration.

MGS ED and VBM Data

The PHC volumes were invariably larger in the right than in the left hemisphere both in controls and in patients (**Table 5**).

The right and the left PHC volumes were not different in patients with and in those without abnormal 30 MGS ED values (**Table 6**). By contrast, the patients with abnormal 30 MGS ED values showed a right–left PHC volume difference smaller than those with normal 30 MGS ED, namely abnormal 30 MGS ED values are associated with smaller right PHC volumes as expected on the basis of their left PHC volume. All the four patients with abnormal 30 MGS ED belonged to the r-MTLE-HS group, and three of them showed the smallest volume difference, whereas the other one showed the largest difference and the shortest disease duration.

Finally, concerning the hippocampus, none of the volume parameters, including the right–left difference, proved to be different depending on the abnormality of 30 MGS ED.

DISCUSSION

Memory-guided saccades abnormalities together with VBM results in our study (i) suggested the functional involvement of the right PHC in patients with right MTLE-HS, (ii) supported a right lateralization of spatial memory control, and (iii) showed a relation between functional impairment and degree of atrophy.

Our results showed in detail that the saccade velocity and latency values in MTLE-HS patients were not different from controls for all kind of saccades, thus suggesting that the cortical and brainstem mechanisms to program and trigger saccades were not affected.

Moreover, MTLE-HS patients do not differ from controls for the accuracy of RS and of 3 MGS: no differences could be found for the accuracy of the first saccade (pulseE), and for the improvement that could be obtained after corrective saccades (finalE), and the capability to improve the accuracy of the first saccade (ED). The finalE of RS showed a larger accuracy for rightward than for leftward saccades, but this difference was the same in patients and in controls.

Interestingly, r-MTLE-HS patients differ from controls for the accuracy of 30 MGS. Both the patients and the controls showed a pulseE and a finalE that were smaller for leftward than for rightward saccades; that is leftward 30 MGS were more accurate both after the first and after all the corrective saccades were made; however, the r-MTLE-HS patients were less effective in improving the accuracy of the first saccade than both the controls and the l-MTLE-HS patients. This finding is supported by ED value evaluation both in the group and in the individual analyses. Concerning the group analyses, it is noteworthy that, even if it proved to be statistically significant only for the leftward direction, the mean ED values of 30 MGS from r-MTLE-HS showed a similar trend for the rightward direction also.

The individual values showed that four out of seven r-MTLE-HS patients (vs. none of l-MTLE-HS patients and controls) had an abnormally positive ED value, meaning that in these subjects the corrective saccades did not improve and even worsen the accuracy of the position reached by the first saccade. In all of these four patients, ED was abnormal for l-30 MGS; in one of them the abnormality was bilateral, and this specific r-MTLE-HS patient was the one showing the smallest PH volumes not only for the right side but also for the left side.

Memory-guided saccades results suggest the functional involvement of the right PHC in patients with r-MTLE-HS, in keeping with the results of a previous study by our group (20) and, in agreement with previous observations (19, 23), our data suggest a possible specialization of the right PHC for visual spatial memory (24–29).

Voxel-based morphometry analysis results confirmed the presence of hippocampal atrophy as detected by conventional MRI in our patients and were in accordance with the results of previous imaging studies. Furthermore, VBM analysis showed that, despite no PHC alteration detected by conventional MRI, the mean volume of the parahippocampus was smaller in patients with impaired accuracy of 30 MGS.

Many neuroimaging studies showed that MTLE-HS patients have also areas of extrahippocampal atrophy, including the PHC (30–36). The presence of extrahippocampal structural damage in MTLE-HS has been correlated with postsurgery outcome in these patients; for instance, it was demonstrated that seizures after surgery commonly arise within the spared structures of the resected temporal lobe (37, 38) and patients with extrahippocampal atrophy had a lower probability of becoming seizure free after complete hippocampal resection (39).

Thereby, MGS and VBM could be useful in presurgical evaluations aimed at deciding the extension to extrahippocampal structures of the surgical resection.

Temporal lobe atrophy is considered the result of an apoptotic mechanism due to frequent seizure recurrence (40–43) and FS are considered as a precipitating insult for the neuronal loss in MTLE-HS patients (44). Since hippocampal atrophy in MTLE-HS patients is associated with white matter fiber disconnections, an alternative hypothesis is that deafferentation from hippocampal fibers could be the major determinant of extrahippocampal atrophy (45). Clinical variables such as FS, age at seizure onset, disease duration, and seizure frequency were not correlated with MGS and VBM parameters in our patients, but these results could be biased by a relatively small sample size in our study. Repeated evaluations in MTLE-HS patients could give some information regarding the evolution over time of the cortical functional and structural damage.

AUTHOR CONTRIBUTIONS

SC and MV contributed to the conception or design of the work and made acquisition, analysis, and interpretation of data for the work. GB, AP, GP, SB, and CAG contributed to the acquisition, analysis, and interpretation of data for the work. SC, GB, AP, GP, SB, CAG, and MV drafted the manuscript, critically reviewed the manuscript for important intellectual content, approved the final version of the manuscript, and agreed to be accountable to all aspects of this work ensuring that questions related to the accuracy or integrity of any part of the work are appropriately investigated and resolved.

FUNDING

This work was supported by grants of the Italian Ministry of Health to RC2015-2017.

REFERENCES

1. Bocti C, Robitaille Y, Diadori P, Lortie A, Mercier C, Bouthillier A, et al. The pathological basis of temporal lobe epilepsy in childhood. *Neurology* (2003) 60:191–5. doi:10.1212/01.WNL.0000044055.73747.9F
2. Capizzano AA, Vermathen P, Laxer KD, Matson GB, Maudsley AA, Soher BJ, et al. Multisection proton MR spectroscopy for mesial temporal lobe epilepsy. *AJNR Am J Neuroradiol* (2002) 23:1359–68.
3. Ferreira NF, de Oliveira V, Amaral L, Mendonca R, Lima SS. Analysis of parahippocampal gyrus in 115 patients with hippocampal sclerosis. *Arq Neuropsiquiatr* (2003) 61:707–11. doi:10.1590/S0004-282X2003000500001
4. Kasper BS, Stefan H, Buchfelder M, Paulus W. Temporal lobe microdysgenesis in epilepsy versus control brains. *J Neuropathol Exp Neurol* (1999) 58:22–8. doi:10.1097/00005072-199901000-00003
5. Moran NF, Lemieux L, Kitchen ND, Fish DR, Shorvon SD. Extrahippocampal temporal lobe atrophy in temporal lobe epilepsy and

mesial temporal sclerosis. *Brain* (2001) 124:167–75. doi:10.1093/brain/124.1.167

6. Wieser HG; ILAE Commission on Neurosurgery of Epilepsy. Epilepsy, ILAE Commission Report. Mesial temporal lobe epilepsy with hippocampal sclerosis. *Epilepsia* (2004) 45:695–714. doi:10.1111/j.0013-9580.2004.09004.x
7. Keller SS, Roberts N. Voxel-based morphometry of temporal lobe epilepsy: an introduction and review of the literature. *Epilepsia* (2008) 49:741–57. doi:10.1111/j.1528-1167.2007.01485.x
8. Duncan JS. Imaging and epilepsy. *Brain* (1997) 120(Pt 2):339–77. doi:10.1093/brain/120.2.339
9. Garcia-Finana M, Denby CE, Keller SS, Wieshmann UC, Roberts N. Degree of hippocampal atrophy is related to side of seizure onset in temporal lobe epilepsy. *AJNR Am J Neuroradiol* (2006) 27:1046–52.
10. No YJ, Zavanone C, Bielle F, Nguyen-Michel VH, Samson Y, Adam C, et al. Medial temporal lobe epilepsy associated with hippocampal sclerosis is a distinctive syndrome. *J Neurol* (2017) 264:875–81. doi:10.1007/s00415-017-8441-z
11. Helmstaedter C, Pohl C, Elger CE. Relations between verbal and nonverbal memory performance: evidence of confounding effects particularly in patients with right temporal lobe epilepsy. *Cortex* (1995) 31:345–55. doi:10.1016/S0010-9452(13)80367-X
12. O'Brien CE, Bowden SC, Bardenhagen FJ, Cook MJ. Neuropsychological correlates of hippocampal and rhinal cortex volumes in patients with mesial temporal sclerosis. *Hippocampus* (2003) 13:892–904. doi:10.1002/hipo.10128
13. Colnaghi S, Beltrami G, Cortese A, Zangemeister WH, Cosi V, Versino M. Multiple memory-guided saccades: movement memory improves the accuracy of memory-guided saccades. *Prog Brain Res* (2008) 171:425–7. doi:10.1016/S0079-6123(08)00662-6
14. Leigh RJ, Kennard C. Using saccades as a research tool in the clinical neurosciences. *Brain* (2004) 127:460–77. doi:10.1093/brain/awh035
15. Pierrot-Deseilligny C, Muri RM, Rivaud-Pechoux S, Gaymard B, Ploner CJ. Cortical control of spatial memory in humans: the visuooculomotor model. *Ann Neurol* (2002) 52:10–9. doi:10.1002/ana.10273
16. Muri RM, Gaymard B, Rivaud S, Vermersch A, Hess CW, Pierrot-Deseilligny C. Hemispheric asymmetry in cortical control of memory-guided saccades. A transcranial magnetic stimulation study. *Neuropsychologia* (2000) 38:1105–11. doi:10.1016/S0028-3932(00)00030-0
17. Nyffeler T, Pierrot-Deseilligny C, Pflugshaupt T, von Wartburg R, Hess CW, Muri RM. Information processing in long delay memory-guided saccades: further insights from TMS. *Exp Brain Res* (2004) 154:109–12. doi:10.1007/s00221-003-1663-6
18. Ploner CJ, Gaymard BM, Rivaud-Pechoux S, Baulac M, Clemenceau S, Samson S, et al. Lesions affecting the parahippocampal cortex yield spatial memory deficits in humans. *Cereb Cortex* (2000) 10:1211–6. doi:10.1093/cercor/10.12.1211
19. Ploner CJ, Rivaud-Pechoux S, Gaymard BM, Agid Y, Pierrot-Deseilligny C. Errors of memory-guided saccades in humans with lesions of the frontal eye field and the dorsolateral prefrontal cortex. *J Neurophysiol* (1999) 82:1086–90.
20. Colnaghi S, Arbasino C, Beltrami G, Galimberti CA, Cosi V, Versino M. Memory guided saccades in mesial temporal lobe epilepsy with hippocampal sclerosis. *Clin Neurophysiol* (2006) 117:2392–8. doi:10.1016/j.clinph.2006.07.135
21. Raz N, Rodrigue KM. Differential aging of the brain: patterns, cognitive correlates and modifiers. *Neurosci Biobehav Rev* (2006) 30:730–48. doi:10.1016/j.neubiorev.2006.07.001
22. Robinson DA. A method of measuring eye movement using a scleral search coil in a magnetic field. *IEEE Trans Biomed Eng* (1963) 10:137–45.
23. Ploner CJ, Gaymard BM, Ehrle N, Rivaud-Pechoux S, Baulac M, Brandt SA, et al. Spatial memory deficits in patients with lesions affecting the medial temporal neocortex. *Ann Neurol* (1999) 45:312–9. doi:10.1002/1531-8249(199903)45:3<312::AID-ANA6>3.0.CO;2-J
24. Abrahams S, Pickering A, Polkey CE, Morris RG. Spatial memory deficits in patients with unilateral damage to the right hippocampal formation. *Neuropsychologia* (1997) 35:11–24. doi:10.1016/S0028-3932(96)00051-6
25. Owen AM, Morris RG, Sahakian BJ, Polkey CE, Robbins TW. Double dissociations of memory and executive functions in working memory tasks following frontal lobe excisions, temporal lobe excisions or amygdalo-hippocampectomy in man. *Brain* (1996) 119(Pt 5):1597–615. doi:10.1093/brain/119.5.1597
26. Owen AM, Sahakian BJ, Semple J, Polkey CE, Robbins TW. Visuo-spatial short-term recognition memory and learning after temporal lobe excisions, frontal lobe excisions or amygdalo-hippocampectomy in man. *Neuropsychologia* (1995) 33:1–24. doi:10.1016/0028-3932(94)00098-A
27. Rains GD, Milner B. Right-hippocampal contralateral-hand effect in the recall of spatial location in the tactual modality. *Neuropsychologia* (1994) 32:1233–42. doi:10.1016/0028-3932(94)90105-8
28. Smith ML, Milner B. The role of the right hippocampus in the recall of spatial location. *Neuropsychologia* (1981) 19:781–93. doi:10.1016/0028-3932(81)90090-7
29. Smith ML, Milner B. Right hippocampal impairment in the recall of spatial location: encoding deficit or rapid forgetting? *Neuropsychologia* (1989) 27:71–81. doi:10.1016/0028-3932(89)90091-2
30. Alhusaini S, Whelan CD, Doherty CP, Delanty N, Fitzsimons M, Cavalleri GL. Temporal cortex morphology in mesial temporal lobe epilepsy patients and their asymptomatic siblings. *Cereb Cortex* (2016) 26:1234–41. doi:10.1093/cercor/bhu315
31. Bernasconi N, Bernasconi A, Caramanos Z, Antel SB, Andermann F, Arnold DL. Mesial temporal damage in temporal lobe epilepsy: a volumetric MRI study of the hippocampus, amygdala and parahippocampal region. *Brain* (2003) 126:462–9. doi:10.1093/brain/awg034
32. Bernasconi N, Duchesne S, Janke A, Lerch J, Collins DL, Bernasconi A. Whole-brain voxel-based statistical analysis of gray matter and white matter in temporal lobe epilepsy. *Neuroimage* (2004) 23:717–23. doi:10.1016/j.neuroimage.2004.06.015
33. Bonilha L, Kobayashi E, Rorden C, Cendes F, Li LM. Medial temporal lobe atrophy in patients with refractory temporal lobe epilepsy. *J Neurol Neurosurg Psychiatry* (2003) 74:1627–30. doi:10.1136/jnnp.74.12.1627
34. Bonilha L, Rorden C, Castellano G, Pereira F, Rio PA, Cendes F, et al. Voxel-based morphometry reveals gray matter network atrophy in refractory medial temporal lobe epilepsy. *Arch Neurol* (2004) 61:1379–84. doi:10.1001/archneur.61.9.1379
35. Keller SS, Mackay CE, Barrick TR, Wieshmann UC, Howard MA, Roberts N. Voxel-based morphometric comparison of hippocampal and extrahippocampal abnormalities in patients with left and right hippocampal atrophy. *Neuroimage* (2002) 16:23–31. doi:10.1006/nimg.2001.1072
36. McDonald CR, Hagler DJ Jr, Ahmadi ME, Tecoma E, Iragui V, Gharapetian L, et al. Regional neocortical thinning in mesial temporal lobe epilepsy. *Epilepsia* (2008) 49:794–803. doi:10.1111/j.1528-1167.2008.01539.x
37. Hennessy MJ, Elwes RD, Honavar M, Rabe-Hesketh S, Binnie CD, Polkey CE. Predictors of outcome and pathological considerations in the surgical treatment of intractable epilepsy associated with temporal lobe lesions. *J Neurol Neurosurg Psychiatry* (2001) 70:450–8. doi:10.1136/jnnp.70.4.450
38. Wennberg R, Arruda F, Quesney LF, Olivier A. Preeminence of extrahippocampal structures in the generation of mesial temporal seizures: evidence from human depth electrode recordings. *Epilepsia* (2002) 43:716–26. doi:10.1046/j.1528-1157.2002.31101.x
39. Garcia M, Gaca LB, Sandim GB, Assuncao Leme IB, Carrete HJ, Centeno RS, et al. Morphometric MRI features are associated with surgical outcome in mesial temporal lobe epilepsy with hippocampal sclerosis. *Epilepsy Res* (2017) 132:78–83. doi:10.1016/j.eplepsyres.2017.02.022
40. Bonilha L, Rorden C, Appenzeller S, Coan AC, Cendes F, Li LM. Gray matter atrophy associated with duration of temporal lobe epilepsy. *Neuroimage* (2006) 32:1070–9. doi:10.1016/j.neuroimage.2006.05.038
41. Fuerst D, Shah J, Kupsky WJ, Johnson R, Shah A, Hayman-Abello B, et al. Volumetric MRI, pathological, and neuropsychological progression in hippocampal sclerosis. *Neurology* (2001) 57:184–8. doi:10.1212/WNL.57.2.184
42. Henshall DC, Simon RP. Epilepsy and apoptosis pathways. *J Cereb Blood Flow Metab* (2005) 25:1557–72. doi:10.1038/sj.jcbfm.9600149
43. Kalviainen R, Salmenpera T. Do recurrent seizures cause neuronal damage? A series of studies with MRI volumetry in adults with partial epilepsy. *Prog Brain Res* (2002) 135:279–95. doi:10.1016/S0079-6123(02)35026-X
44. Mathern GW, Adelson PD, Cahan LD, Leite JP. Hippocampal neuron damage in human epilepsy: Meyer's hypothesis revisited. *Prog Brain Res* (2002) 135:237–51. doi:10.1016/S0079-6123(02)35023-4
45. Bonilha L, Edwards JC, Kinsman SL, Morgan PS, Fridriksson J, Rorden C, et al. Extrahippocampal gray matter loss and hippocampal deafferentation in patients with temporal lobe epilepsy. *Epilepsia* (2010) 51:519–28. doi:10.1111/j.1528-1167.2009.02506.x

2

Characteristic Eye Movements in Ataxia-Telangiectasia-Like Disorder: An Explanatory Hypothesis

Pamela Federighi[1], Stefano Ramat[2], Francesca Rosini[1], Elena Pretegiani[3], Antonio Federico[4] and Alessandra Rufa[1]*

[1] *Eye Tracking and Visual Application Lab (EVA Lab), Department of Medicine, Surgery and Neuroscience, University of Siena, Siena, Italy,* [2] *Department of Electrical, Computer and Biomedical Engineering, University of Pavia, Pavia, Italy,* [3] *Laboratory of Sensorimotor Research, National Eye Institute, National Institutes of Health, Bethesda, MD, United States,* [4] *UOC Neurology and Neurometabolic Diseases, Department of Medicine, Surgery and Neuroscience, University of Siena, Siena, Italy*

Correspondence:
Pamela Federighi
federighi@unisi.it

Objective: To investigate cerebellar dysfunctions and quantitatively characterize specific oculomotor changes in ataxia-telangiectasia-like disorder (ATLD), a rare autosomal recessive disease caused by mutations in the *MRE11* gene. Additionally, to further elucidate the pathophysiology of cerebellar damage in the ataxia-telangiectasia (AT) spectrum disorders.

Methods: Saccade dynamics, metrics, and visual fixation deficits were investigated in two Italian adult siblings with genetically confirmed ATLD. Visually guided saccades were compared with those of 40 healthy subjects. Steady fixation was tested in primary and eccentric positions. Quantitative characterization of saccade parameters, saccadic intrusions (SI), and nystagmus was performed.

Results: Patients showed abnormally hypermetric and fast horizontal saccades to the left and greater inaccuracy than healthy subjects in all saccadic eye movements. Eye movement abnormalities included slow eye movements that preceded the initial saccade. Horizontal and vertical spontaneous jerk nystagmus, gaze-evoked, and rebound nystagmus were evident. Fixation was interrupted by large square-wave jerk SI and macrosaccadic oscillations.

Conclusion: Slow eye movements accompanying saccades, SI, and cerebellar nystagmus are frequently seen in AT patients, additionally our ATLD patients showed the presence of fast and hypermetric saccades suggesting damage of granule cell-parallel fiber-Purkinje cell synapses of the cerebellar vermis. A dual pathogenetic mechanism involving neurodevelopmental and neurodegenerative changes is hypothesized to explain the peculiar phenotype of this disease.

Keywords: ataxia-telangiectasia-like disorder, saccade hypermetria, granule cells, parallel fibers, Purkinje cells

INTRODUCTION

Autosomal recessive cerebellar ataxias with DNA-double strand break repair deficits are a group of severe neurodegenerative and systemic diseases featuring early-onset ataxia and radiosensitivity including ataxia-telangiectasia (AT), the most common disorder of this group, and ataxia-telangiectasia-like disorder (ATLD) (1). ATLD is a very rare autosomal recessive disease due to mutations in the *MRE11* gene (2). This gene encodes a protein (Mre11) with nuclease and DNA-binding activity;

together with Rad50 and Nbs1, it forms the MRN complex which is a target of ATM kinase and is involved in the signaling network of cellular response to DNA damage (3, 4). To date, reports document only 23 cases of ATLD belonging to two families from the United Kingdom (one native from Pakistan), one family from Italy, three families from Saudi Arabia, three families from Japan, and one family from Pakistan (2, 5–11). The clinical features of the majority of patients with ATLD resemble those of patients with AT including progressive cerebellar ataxia, oculomotor apraxia, and cellular hypersensitivity to ionizing radiations, with a generally mild presentation and slow progression (12). Like in AT, facial dyskinesia, choreoathetosis, and dystonia may also be present; whereas telangiectasia, immunodeficiency, and increased α-fetoprotein have not been reported (8, 13). Clinical descriptions of oculomotor changes in both AT and ATLD patients show inability to initiate voluntary saccades, saccade hypometria, delayed convergence and impaired smooth pursuit, vestibulo-ocular reflex (VOR), and optokinetic nystagmus (7, 10); fixation abnormalities such as saccadic intrusions (SI), drifts, spontaneous, gaze-evoked, and down-beat nystagmus (7).

Ataxia-telangiectasia-like disorder cases with a more severe phenotype have been observed: four subjects from two Saudi Arabian families showed microcephaly, as well as two unrelated patients from Japan who presented also a bird-headed facial appearance, mental retardation, no cerebellar ataxia or oculomotor apraxia (6, 11), and two Japanese siblings with minor dysmorphisms, cognitive delay, and lung adenocarcinoma (8). Overall these features recall Nijmegen breakage syndrome (NBS), due to mutations in Nbs1 of the MRN complex, which is characterized by microcephaly, growth retardation, immune dysfunction, and radiosensitivity with predisposition to cancer but no ataxia (3, 4). This suggests that some *MRE11* mutations could have a pivotal role during development giving rise to a wider clinical spectrum than that related solely to neurodegeneration.

The neural substrate of the network controlling eye movements is relatively well known. Therefore, the study of eye movement abnormalities, particularly in rare diseases with known genetic pathology, represents an ideal tool to investigate and model the function of discrete circuits of this network (14). The quantitative analysis of eye movement defects has not been reported in ATLD patients. Therefore, this study was principally designed to quantitatively characterize specific oculomotor changes in ATLD patients that may help to define diagnosis and contribute to better characterize cerebellar involvement in the control of eye movements. An additional purpose was to further elucidate the pathophysiology of cerebellar damage in ATLD. The main result of the study suggests that ATLD may damage granule cells (GCs) and their parallel fibers (PFs) in the cerebellar vermis. Finally, we propose a hypothetical scheme in which both neurodevelopmental and neurodegenerative components of cerebellar damage may account for the pathophysiology of the oculomotor changes observed in ATLD.

SUBJECTS

Two affected siblings, respectively, 45 (male, Patient 1) and 44 years old (female, Patient 2) were studied. Both wild-type for *ATM* and *NBS1*, but compound heterozygotes for *MRE11* gene mutations [1422C→A, T481K; 1714C→T, R571X]. The 1422C→A allele was inherited from the mother, whereas the paternally inherited 1714C→T allele was apparently null as a result of non-sense-mediated mRNA decay (5). Complete neurological, instrumental MRI, and cognitive investigations were obtained in these patients with a long clinical and MRI follow-up. The neuro-ophthalmological examination included visual acuity for distance and near, pupils and anterior segment evaluation, ocular alignment, nystagmus, conjugate eye movements, and ophthalmoscopy. Experimental protocols were approved by the Local Ethics Committee of the Azienda Ospedaliera Universitaria Senese and procedures performed in studies were in accordance with the 1964 Helsinki declaration and its later amendments or comparable ethical standards. Written informed consent was obtained from individual participants included in the study.

MATERIALS AND METHODS

Eye movements were measured using a video-based, remote, monocular recording, two-dimensional eye tracking technique (ASL 504, sample rate: 240 Hz) (15). The experiment was designed to study horizontal visually guided saccades (10°–18°) (16) and steady fixation in primary and eccentric positions (10°–18°), in order to study SI and nystagmus (17). Due to the head and neck dystonia which induced unbearable fatigue and poor compliance during the head constraint, patients performed a series of independent experiments on different sessions (in a period lasting 1 year). During this period, the disease remained clinically stable in both patients.

We performed a quantitative analysis of saccadic parameters of the first reflexive horizontal saccade executed in response to target presentation. We considered the following parameters: saccade duration (time interval between the start and the end of the saccade); saccade latency (time delay between target onset and saccade onset); saccade amplitude (change in eye position, in degrees of visual angle, between the start and end of the saccade); peak saccade velocity (maximum eye velocity, in degrees of visual angle/s); peak acceleration and peak deceleration (maximum eye acceleration and deceleration, in degrees of visual angle/s^2); and saccade accuracy, based on the absolute error (modulus of difference between target position and eye position at the end of the initial saccade, in degrees of visual angle). The main sequence relationships of peak velocity and duration versus amplitude were fitted using an exponential and a linear function, respectively. The saccade onset and offset times were based on a 10°/s velocity threshold. Recorded data were processed off-line using an interactive algorithm to identify each saccade, check automatic identification, and calculate saccadic parameters (18).

Saccadic intrusions were characterized by several types of inappropriate saccadic movements identified as square-wave SI and macrosaccadic oscillations (MSO). Square-wave SI were classified according to their waveform into two different types: monophasic or square-wave jerks (SWJs) and biphasic square-wave saccadic intrusions (BSWSI) (19, 20). SWJ were characterized by pairs of horizontal saccades: a first saccade was directed away from the target and a second saccade returned to it, generally after a period of time (intersaccadic interval) ranging 200–400 ms. BSWSI were characterized by three horizontal saccades: a saccade was directed away from the target, a following hypermetric saccade was directed in the opposite direction overshooting the target and, after an interval of time ranging 200–300 ms, a corrective saccade that returned back to the target. MSO were back to back hypermetric saccades, with an intersaccadic interval of about 200 ms; they oscillated around the target and spontaneously grew larger and then smaller (in amplitude). The quantitative characterization of SI included amplitude of saccades, their intersaccadic interval, and frequency of square-wave SI (17) or frequency of oscillations in MSO. Nystagmus was characterized by alternation of slow drift of the eye position (slow phase) followed by a rapid correction (quick phase). Nystagmus was described using slow phase velocity, amplitude, and frequency of fast phases. The rapid gaze shifts that intruded on visual fixation were identified automatically and their start and end were defined as the times when eye velocity exceeded or fell below 50°/s. All responses were tested by visual inspection of waveforms in eye position signals and the analysis was corrected interactively if necessary.

Forty age-matched healthy subjects (mean age: 35 years; range: 30–60) served as controls in saccade evaluation. Estimated descriptive parameters of SI were compared with the normal values previously reported (19). Differences in means of all saccadic parameters, which were calculated for each experiment of each patient, and differences of descriptive parameters of SI between patients and the healthy subjects were analyzed by the Mann-Whitney *U* test and Spearman correlation coefficients were estimated.

TABLE 1 | Demographics, clinical, and instrumental findings of patients with ataxia-telangiectasia-like disorder.

Clinical and instrumental findings	Patient 1	Patient 2
Sex/age at examination	M/45 years old	F/44 years old
Afferent visual functions	Normal	Normal
Ocular movements examination	Fast and inaccurate saccades, disrupted pursuit, abnormal VOR	Fast and inaccurate saccades, disrupted pursuit, abnormal VOR
Eye oscillations	Spontaneous GEN and rebound ny, SI	Spontaneous GEN and rebound ny, SI
Expressionless face	++	++
Head ataxia	++	++
Dysarthria	+++	+++
Hypotonia	++	++
Dysmetria/action tremor	+++	+++
Choreo-athetotic movements	++	+
Limbs dystonia	++	–
Joint laxity	++	++
Gait ataxia (with frequent falls)	+++	+++
EMG: axonal sensory neuropathy	+	+
MRI: cerebellar atrophy	+++	+++
ICARS subscores		
Posture and gait disturbances	26	26
Kinetic functions	31	31
Speech disorders	5	5
Oculomotor disorders	6	6
Global score	68	68

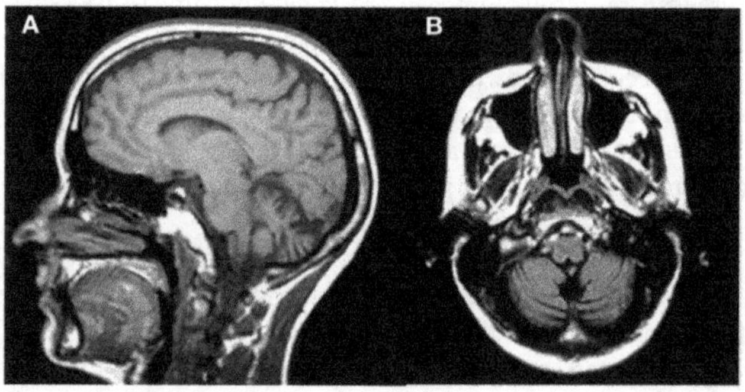

FIGURE 1 | Sagittal T1w **(A)** and coronal T2w-FLAIR **(B)** magnetic resonance images of Patient 2 show vermian and hemispheric cerebellar atrophy.

RESULTS

Clinical Neuro-Ophthalmological and MRI Profile

Table 1 summarizes a detailed report of clinical findings; neurological, MRI (see **Figure 1**), and cognitive follow-up of the two siblings have been recently updated and reported (20). Neurological examination showed a common clinical pattern in our two patients with a slow disease progression until age 14, followed by a long period of clinical, neurological, cognitive, and neuroimaging stability in adulthood with only dystonia of the arms and ataxic gait slightly deteriorating. No cancer was found.

Visual acuity, color vision, pupils, and ophthalmoscopy were not impaired and no conjunctival telangiectasias were evident. The evaluation of conjugate eye movements showed similar abnormalities in the two siblings (see **Table 1**).

Quantitative Characteristics of Saccade Abnormalities

Main eye movement abnormalities in both patients, pointed out by the analysis of saccade and fixation parameters, are shown in **Figure 2**.

Saccade amplitude was greater in ATLD patients than controls for both target jumps (10°: $P < 0.001$). The mean amplitude for the initial saccades was 13.8 ± 1.3° for 10° saccades and 19.0 ± 1.5° for 18° saccades (means for controls, 10°: 10.2 ± 0.5°; 18°: 18.1 ± 0.7°). Saccadic amplitude of each patient is summarized in **Table 2**. The mean amplitude for the initial leftward (LW) saccades was 15.8 ± 3.9° for 10° target jumps and 22.2 ± 5.7° for 18° target jumps (means for controls, 10°: 10.3 ± 1.1°; 18°: 18.1 ± 1.7°). The mean amplitude for 10° target jumps to the right was instead 11.1 ± 3.6° and 16.5 ± 4.0° for the 18° target jumps (means for controls, 10°: 10.1 ± 1.1°; 18°: 18.1 ± 1.6°). LW and rightward (RW) saccade amplitudes were significantly different (LW 10°: $P < 0.001$; 18°: $P < 0.001$; RW 10°: $P < 0.05$; 18°: $P < 0.001$) in our patients compared with controls. An example of very large LW hypermetric saccades, typically followed by corrective saccades to reach the target, is illustrated in **Figure 2A**.

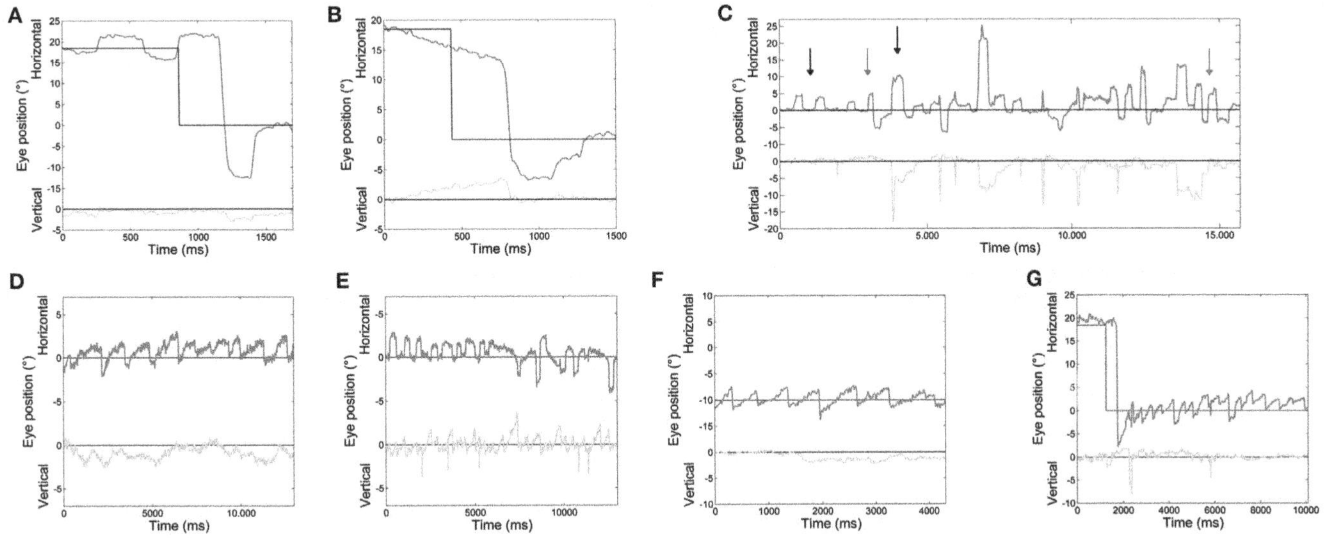

FIGURE 2 | An example of different oculomotor abnormalities found in both patients. **(A)** Very large hypermetric saccade, with higher than normal speed and followed by corrective saccades to reach the target. **(B)** Slow drifts preceding a centripetal saccade. **(C)** Large square-wave saccadic intrusions: square-wave jerk, macrosquare-wave jerks (black arrows), biphasic square-wave saccadic intrusions (blue arrow); and macrosaccadic oscillations (red arrow). **(D)** Spontaneous jerk nystagmus with mainly horizontal and, sometimes, **(E)** vertical component appearing as an oblique nystagmus. **(F)** Gaze-evoked nystagmus in eccentric gaze positions of 10°, and rebound nystagmus **(G)** after the eye was returned to central position. Horizontal and vertical eye positions are plotted in different shades of gray. The black line shows horizontal and vertical target position. Positive values correspond to rightward and upward.

TABLE 2 | Saccade metric parameters estimated for all saccades in each experiment.

Patients		Amplitude	Accuracy	Amplitude leftward saccades	Amplitude rightward saccades	Accuracy leftward saccades	Accuracy rightward saccades
Patient 1	10°	(14.6 ± 0.5)°	(5.9 ± 0.5)°	(17.8 ± 4.5)°	(10.7 ± 4.1)°	(8.0 ± 4.2)°	(3.2 ± 2.5)°
	18°	(19.3 ± 1.6)°	(5.8 ± 2.0)°	(25.4 ± 7.0)°	(15.4 ± 5.4)°	(8.4 ± 5.1)°	(5.1 ± 3.0)°
Patient 2	10°	(13.2 ± 1.5)°	(3.8 ± 1.4)°	(14.1 ± 2.3)°	(11.4 ± 3.2)°	(4.3 ± 2.1)°	(2.6 ± 2.5)°
	18°	(19.0 ± 1.7)°	(4.0 ± 1.9)°	(20.7 ± 4.4)°	(16.9 ± 3.0)°	(3.8 ± 3.0)°	(2.6 ± 2.1)°

Amplitude and accuracy (absolute error value is shown) for 10° and 18° saccades for Patient 1 and Patient 2. The first two columns show the mean of means and the SEM computed over each recording session for each patient. The rightmost four columns, instead, present the mean and the SD of the indicated parameters computed by pooling all appropriate saccades from all recordings.

Saccadic dysmetria, in which the eye overshoots or undershoots the target, was more accurately estimated using saccade accuracy. We found a higher absolute error of primary saccades (10°: $P < 0.001$; 18°: $P < 0.001$) in ATLD patients (mean, 10°: 4.7 ± 1.4°; 18°: 4.8 ± 2.0°) than in controls (mean, 10°: 0.8 ± 0.3°; 18°: 1.2 ± 0.5°). The mean absolute error was greater in Patient 1 than Patient 2. Saccadic absolute error of each patient is summarized in **Table 2**. The mean absolute error for the initial LW saccades was 5.9 ± 3.7° for 10° target jumps and 5.2 ± 4.3° for 18° target jumps (means for controls, 10°: 0.8 ± 0.8°; 18°: 1.2 ± 1.3°). The mean absolute error for RW saccades was 2.8 ± 2.5° for 10° target jumps and 3.5 ± 2.8° for the 18° target jumps (means for controls, 10°: 0.8 ± 0.7°; 18°: 1.2 ± 1.1°). LW and RW saccade absolute errors were significantly different (LW 10°: $P < 0.001$; 18°: $P < 0.001$; RW 10°: $P < 0.001$; 18°: $P < 0.001$) in our patients compared with controls.

Latency of saccades was prolonged, with a mean value of 296 ± 36 ms for 10° saccades and 292 ± 44 ms for 18° saccades (means for controls, 10°: 237 ± 88 ms; 18°: 241 ± 87 ms). The mean latency for the initial LW saccades was 284 ± 90 ms for 10° target jumps and 267 ± 54 ms for 18° target jumps (means for controls, 10°: 208 ± 85 ms; 18°: 220 ± 87 ms). The mean latency for 10° target jumps to the right was instead 294 ± 90 and 289 ± 97 ms for the 18° target jumps (means for controls, 10°: 215 ± 83 ms; 18°: 220 ± 76 ms). LW and RW saccade latencies were significantly different (LW 10°: $P < 0.001$; 18°: $P < 0.001$; RW 10°: $P < 0.001$; 18°: $P < 0.001$) in our patients compared with controls.

The duration of saccades to 10° target jumps was higher in patients than controls (10°: $P < 0.001$), the average values in patients were 65 ± 9 ms for 10° saccades and 72 ± 15 ms for 18° saccades (means for controls, 10°: 49 ± 5 ms; 18°: 65 ± 5 ms). The mean duration for the initial LW saccades was 69 ± 25 ms for 10° target jumps and 71 ± 24 ms for 18° target jumps (means for controls, 10°: 48 ± 9 ms; 18°: 65 ± 10 ms). The mean duration for 10° target jumps to the right was instead 58 ± 18 and 71 ± 20 ms for the 18° target jumps (means for controls, 10°: 48 ± 9 ms; 18°: 66 ± 12 ms). The duration of LW and RW saccades was significantly different in our patients compared with controls only for 10° target jumps (LW 10°: $P < 0.001$; 18°: $P > 0.05$; RW 10°: $P < 0.001$; 18°: $P > 0.05$).

Saccade peak velocity for saccades toward both eccentric targets (10°–18°) was higher in both patients than in controls, although the difference did not reach significance when we analyzed the saccade peak velocity without dealing separately with RW and LW saccades. The mean saccade peak velocity for the initial LW saccades was 467 ± 84°/s for 10° target jumps and 601 ± 116°/s for 18° target jumps (means for controls, 10°: 388 ± 65°/s; 18°: 497 ± 77°). The mean saccade peak velocity for 10° target jumps to the right was instead 356 ± 89° and 466 ± 96°/s for the 18° target jumps (means for controls, 10°: 378 ± 65°/s; 18°: 499 ± 94°). LW and RW saccade peak velocities were significantly different (LW 10°: $P < 0.001$; 18°: $P < 0.001$; RW 10°: $P = 0.002$; 18°: $P < 0.05$) in our patients with respect to controls.

Figure 3 shows the peak velocity versus amplitude main sequence relationship separately considering RW and LW saccades. The main sequence relationship was fitted using the classical exponential equation for healthy subjects and their 95% confidence interval is indicated. Larger saccades of both patients, especially Patient 2, were above the confidence interval bounds for controls. The relationship between peak velocity and amplitude in patients was better fitted by a linear model. To determine the accuracy of models on the entire dataset, model prediction was evaluated using percentage root mean square error, where large values of this parameter indicated poor fit. The slope of the linear equation was greater for LW than for RW saccades in both patients. Saccade acceleration ($P < 0.001$) and deceleration ($P < 0.001$) were significantly different in patients than controls. The amplitude-normalized average values of peak acceleration and deceleration normalized to amplitude in patients were 1,682 ± 635 and 1,661 ± 868 1/s^2, respectively, and 1,893 ± 744 and 1,866 ± 767 1/s^2 in controls.

Slow eye movements (**Figure 2B**) preceded 23% of initial saccades, 17% occurring in centripetal, and 6% in centrifugal saccades. Slow movements were centripetal when the subject attempted to hold the eyes in an eccentric position and centrifugal RW when attempting to hold the eyes in a central position. Slow movements were opposite with respect to the direction of upcoming saccades in 22% of cases. The mean amplitude of these slow eye movements was 2.9 ± 0.6°. Their velocity profile was relatively linear, with a mean velocity of 5.4 ± 1.6°/s. Their velocity also decreased with the reduction of eye position eccentricity, the mean velocity versus target eccentricity was: 3.9 ± 1.5°/s at 0°; 5.5 ± 0.8°/s at 10°; and 6.9 ± 1.5°/s at 18°.

Quantitative Characteristics of Fixation Abnormalities

Saccadic Intrusions

Square-wave SI and MSO were found in both patients (**Figure 2C**).

Square-wave jerk showed significantly larger amplitudes ($P = 0.002$) and abnormally higher frequencies than in healthy subjects. The average amplitude of SWJ was 3.6 ± 2.2° (normal amplitude in healthy subjects: 0.7 ± 0.5°) (19). Patient 2 showed SWJ, mainly macrosquare-wave jerks, with higher amplitude. The average intersaccadic interval was 212 ± 86 ms (normal interval in healthy subjects: 255 ± 147 ms) (19). **Figures 4A–D** show the distribution and a summary of amplitudes and intersaccadic intervals of SWJ in each patient. The frequency of SWJ was 5 intrusions/min in Patient 1 and 48 intrusions/min in Patient 2 (normal rate in healthy subjects: 12 ± 12 intrusions/min) (19). We found BSWSI only in Patient 2, which had larger amplitudes, greater intersaccadic intervals, and higher frequencies than healthy subjects. The average amplitude of BSWSI was (i) 7.6 ± 4.4°, (ii) 14.4 ± 7.1°, and (iii) 6.2 ± 3.3° for away, overshoot, and return saccades, respectively [normal amplitudes in healthy subjects: (i) 0.5 ± 0.2°, (ii) 1.1 ± 0.6°, and (iii) 0.7 ± 0.4°] (19). The average of first and second intersaccadic intervals was (i) 161 ± 74 ms and (ii) 160 ± 65 ms, respectively [normal intervals in healthy subjects: (i) 52 ± 24 ms and (ii) 124 ± 67 ms] (19). Finally, the frequency of BSWSI was 5 intrusions/min (normal rate in healthy subjects: 1 ± 3 intrusions/min) (19).

Macrosaccadic oscillations were especially prominent in Patient 2. Their amplitude ranged between 2.5° and 14.5° with an average value of 7.3 ± 3.3° and their mean intersaccadic interval was 188 ± 46 ms. The frequency of oscillation was 1.9 Hz.

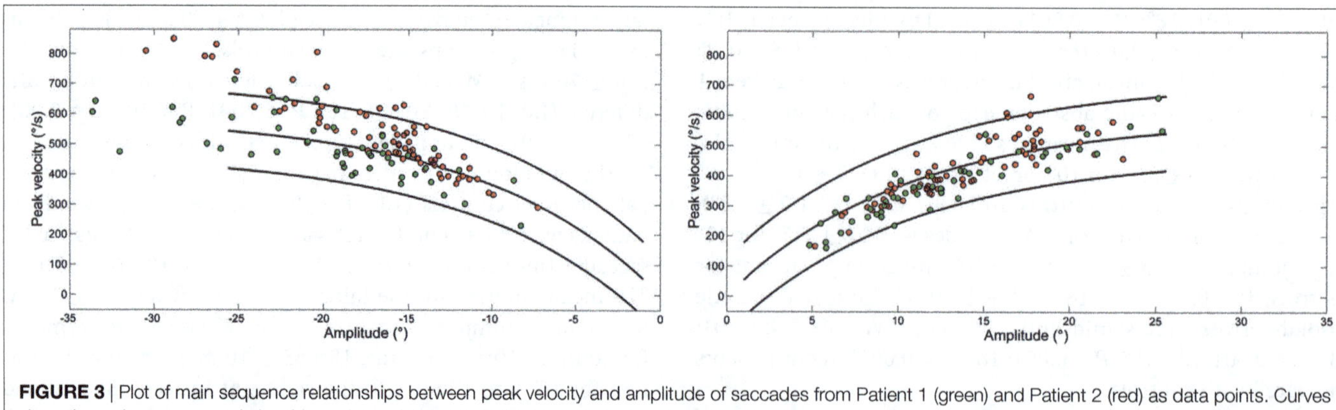

FIGURE 3 | Plot of main sequence relationships between peak velocity and amplitude of saccades from Patient 1 (green) and Patient 2 (red) as data points. Curves show the main sequence relationship and 5 and 95% prediction intervals for healthy subjects. Plot of peak velocity versus amplitude of leftward (LW) and rightward saccades from each ataxia-telangiectasia-like disorder patient. Larger LW saccades made by Patient 2 often exceeded the 95% confidence interval for healthy subjects.

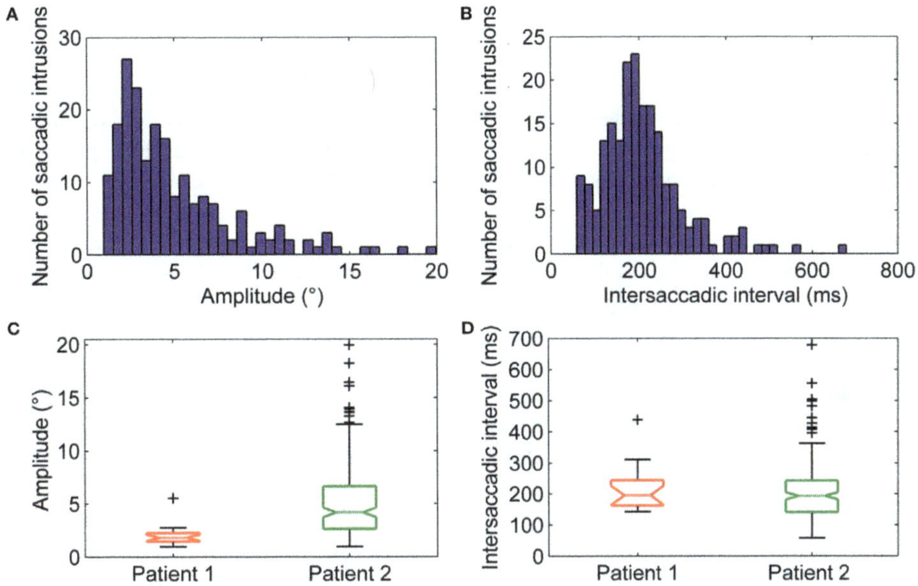

FIGURE 4 | **(A)** Amplitudes and **(B)** intersaccadic intervals distribution of square-wave jerks (SWJs). The *x*-axis in **(A,B)** represents bins of amplitudes and intersaccadic interval, respectively; the *y*-axis represents the number of the SWJs for the given bin. The box and whisker plots show summaries of the amplitudes **(C)** and intersaccadic intervals **(D)** of all SWJs in Patient 1 and Patient 2. The central horizontal bar in each box represents the median, lower, and upper borders are the lower and upper quartile values, whiskers indicate the 95% confidence interval around the median, and outliers (+) are shown individually.

Nystagmus

Spontaneous jerk nystagmus, gaze-evoked, and rebound nystamus were present in both patients (**Figures 2D–G**).

Spontaneous jerk nystagmus (**Figures 2D,E**) was mainly horizontal. Sometimes it presented a vertical component that, when it was in phase with the horizontal component, lead to an oblique nystagmus. Horizontal spontaneous nystagmus was left-beating in both patients, with a relatively constant slow phase velocity; the frequency was 1.0 Hz. **Figure 5A** summarizes the horizontal slow phase velocities. The amplitude was 1.8 ± 1.1° in Patient 1 and 3.1 ± 0.7° in Patient 2. Vertical spontaneous nystagmus was down-beating in both patients. Its slow phase eye velocity is summarized in **Figure 5B**. The amplitude was 1.1 ± 0.8° in Patient 1 and 1.0 ± 0.6° in Patient 2; the frequency was 0.8 Hz. The direction of the slow phase did not show a substantial change in any patient, although a little modulation in slow phase velocity appeared in Patient 1. Modulation showed a period of 40 s with an amplitude of 0.7° in horizontal nystagmus, and a period of 40 s with an amplitude of 0.4° in vertical nystagmus.

Gaze-evoked nystagmus was present in eccentric gaze positions of 10° and 18° (**Figure 2F**). The average velocity of the slow phases drift was 4.1 ± 1.9°/s with an amplitude of 2.2 ± 1.2°, and there was a gradual decay in velocity and amplitude during the 30 s of recording. Frequency of nystagmus beats was 1.4 Hz. After the eye returned to central position, a rebound nystagmus occurred in both siblings (**Figure 2G**). The rebound nystagmus showed a slow phase with an amplitude ranging 0.6°–4.2° and a velocity ranging 0.8°–8.2°/s. Frequency of the rebound nystagmus was 1.7 Hz. Both velocity and amplitude of slow phase drift showed a substantial reduction over 12 s.

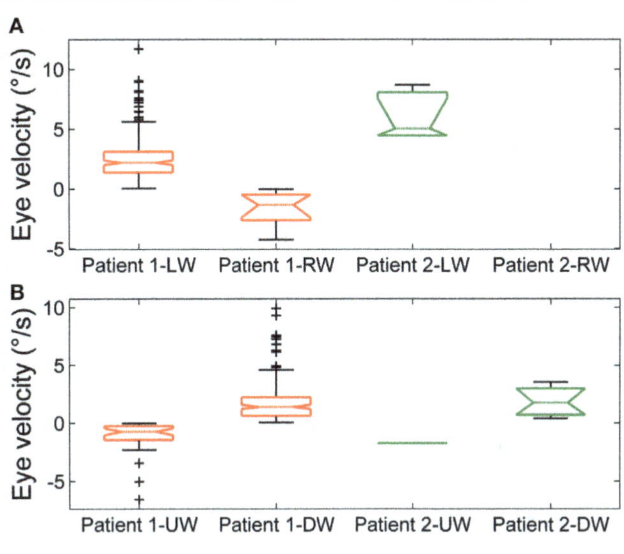

FIGURE 5 | Summary of slow phase eye velocity of **(A)** horizontal and **(B)** vertical spontaneous jerk nystagmus. The box and whisker plots show the slow phase eye velocity of spontaneous jerk nystagmus in Patient 1 and Patient 2. Rightward (RW) and leftward (LW) horizontal nystagmus and upward (UW) and downward (DW) vertical nystagmus are shown separately for each patient. Box plots as in **Figure 3**.

DISCUSSION

This study shows fast, hypermetric saccades sometimes preceded by slow eye movements, SI, MSO, and different types of nystagmus (spontaneous jerk type, gaze-evoked, and rebound nystagmus) in two siblings with ATLD.

Overall, these results confirm that oculomotor alterations are common to ATLD and AT including slow eye movements (drifts), especially following saccades in AT, SI, and different types of cerebellar nystagmus (21–23). Studies on AT patients have demonstrated a severe impairment of gaze fixation stability and VOR, providing elements in favor of a prominent role of Purkinje cells (PC) degeneration in the disinhibition of deep cerebellar nuclei, including the caudal fastigial oculomotor region (FOR), and vestibular nuclei (VN) (21). The loss of GABAergic inhibition on VN can cause nystagmus, including periodic alternating nystagmus (PAN), while disinhibition of FOR can result in instability of the feedback loop projecting to the saccadic burst neurons, leading to SI and oscillations, but also affect the saccade generating mechanisms (21). These abnormalities may explain the postural instability and the impaired gaze fixation due to nystagmus and ocular oscillations not only in AT but also in ATLD patients.

Slow drifts before or after saccades are characteristically seen in AT. Differently to AT patients who may exhibit pre- and post-saccadic drifts, our ATLD patients showed only pre-saccadic drifts. However, the dynamics of the drifts were comparable in AT and ATLD, both showing long duration and relatively linear velocity profiles (22). Slow drifts following saccades have been well characterized in AT, yet different but inconclusive explanations have been proposed to clarify the origin of these movements. They have been attributed to vestibular slow phases; abnormal VOR cancelation (head-free conditions); anticipatory pursuit; post-saccadic drift due to uncorrected pulse-step mismatch by a damaged flocculus, leaky neural integrator causing centripetal drifts, or aberrant suppression of burst cells by omipause neuron triggering slow saccades (22).

Eye movement defects, instead, have never been quantified in ATLD, although clinical qualitative inspections have documented ocular apraxia, SI, spontaneous nystagmus, gaze-evoked nystagmus, and down-beat nystagmus (7). Actually, the significant number of larger and faster LW saccades represents a distinctive oculomotor feature in our patients with ATLD (23, 24) suggesting a major damage of the cerebellar neural network controlling saccade amplitude in these subjects.

The neural substrate and mechanisms of saccadic motor control have been extensively clarified in recent years (25–27). It has been shown that the superior colliculus (SC), cerebellum, and brainstem participate in a network controlling saccade amplitude and accuracy. The displacement command for a saccade in a specific direction comes from the SC and goes to the pontine reticular formation where lies part of the cellular network responsible for generating the saccadic command. This network receives signals from dorsal cerebellar vermis lobule VII through the caudal fastigial nucleus (cFN). Through GC collaterals and PFs, signals for the control of saccade accuracy contact PC at the GC–PF–PC synapses (28), before reaching the cFN of the contralateral side (29, 30). Just before a horizontal saccade is triggered (14), neurons in the cFN of the contralateral side, with respect to the direction of the movement, discharge a burst of activity. Later, just before a saccade ends, neurons in the opposite cFN burst, in order to decelerate and stop the eyes exactly on target (31) (**Figure 6**). Support for this mechanism has been shown in monkeys with lesions of cFN that exhibited saccades overshooting the target ipsilaterally to the lesion (32).

We found that LW saccades of our ATLD patients were significantly hypermetric, while RW ones were hypometric at 18° and slightly but significantly hypermetric at 10° and saccades exhibited lower accuracy in both directions. They were faster to the left and their peak velocity was frequently above the upper limit of the interval of confidence of the main sequence for normal saccades.

It has been assumed from empirical models and experimental data (33, 34) that the slowing of PF conduction occurring in some degenerative cerebellar diseases may delay the cFN burst that chokes off saccades, making them hypermetric. Furthermore, damage to the GC–PF–PC synapses, possibly prevalent in the right cerebellar vermis (see **Figure 1**), would also reduce the inhibitory inputs to the right cFN causing abnormally fast LW saccades (33, 34), such as those observed in our patients (particularly in Patient 2).

The recent advances in the characterization of the molecular basis and pathologic changes underlying *MRE11* mutations (2) allow us to refine this model. Mre11 together with Rad50, Nbs1, and ATM kinase are key components of the signaling pathway participating in cellular response to DNA damage (35). Mutations in these three genes cause, respectively, ATLD, AT, and NBS, which share some common phenotypic features but also show some differences in clinical presentation and evolution, suggesting a diverse pathogenetic role of the three mutations. Unlike in AT and NBS, predisposition to cancer is uncommon in ATLD, while cerebellar involvement is atypical in NBS, which is mainly characterized by developmental anomalies. However, death from malignancy (8), and severe dysmorphisms (11) have been reported in few ATLD patients, widening the spectrum of possible implications of *MRE11* mutations in neurodegenerative as well as developmental changes. Postmortem studies of patients with ATLD (9) have demonstrated severe cerebellar atrophy, particularly in the vermis and medial part of the hemispheres, while other parts of the brain appeared normal. The number of GC and PF, Bergmann glial cells (BGC) and PC were dramatically reduced (reactive gliosis was very scarce), conversely neurons in the cerebellar cortex of the floccular and nodular lobe, deep cerebellar nuclei, brainstem, and olivary nuclei remained well represented as well as the cerebellar white matter. Moreover, intense immunoreactivity for DNA oxidative stress was evident in granule and BGC (9), suggesting an active neurodegenerative process. This pathologic substrate is slightly different with respect to that reported in AT consisting of a sharper loss of PC with abnormal residual PC often bigger and ectopic (36), but more preserved GC and volumetric density of PF varicosities, and limited qualitative and quantitative abnormalities in the granular layer (37). Changes in deep cerebellar nuclei, olivary nuclei, and cerebellar white matter have also been found in AT brains (38, 39).

According with this pathological substrate, our hypothesis supports the prevalent damage of the GC–PF–PC synapses and provides a possible explanation of the abnormal saccadic behavior observed in ATLD patients.

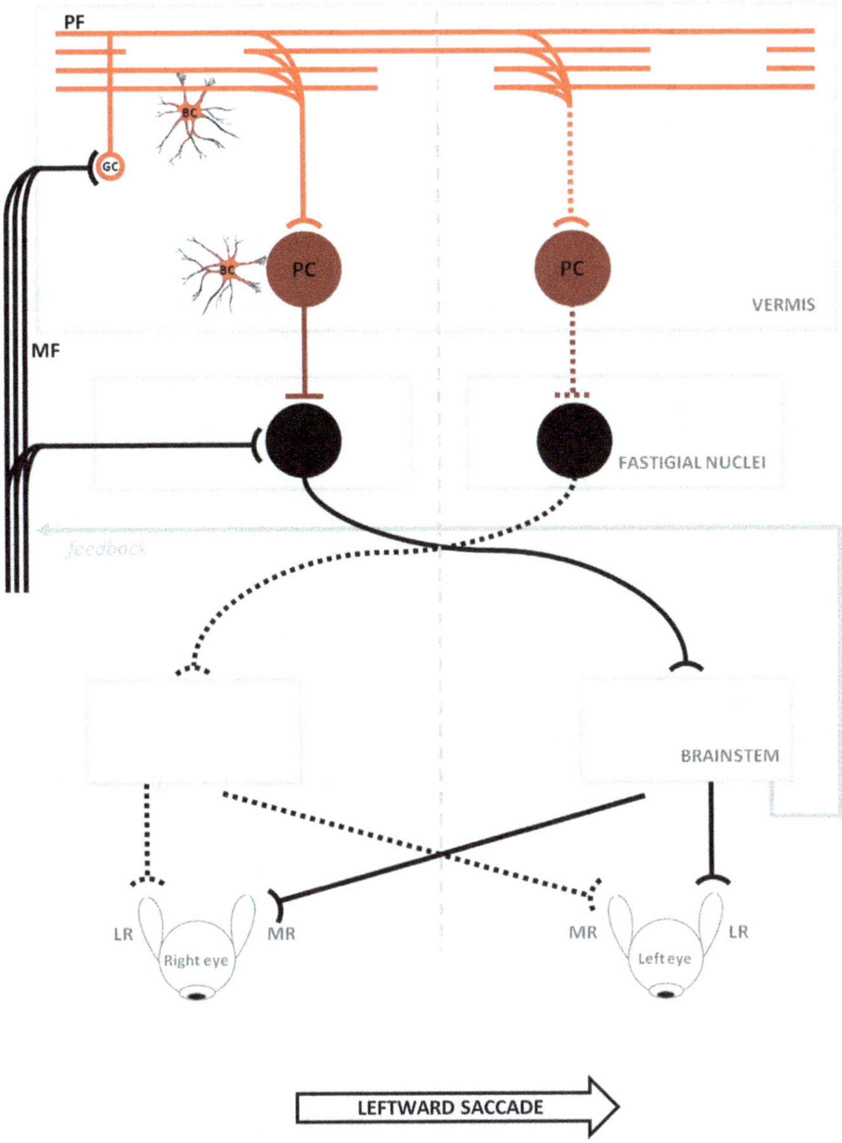

FIGURE 6 | Schematic circuitry for generating horizontal saccades (major active pathways are shown) is hypothesized to explain the disorder of our patients. Projections with curved endings are excitatory, while projections with flat endings are inhibitory. Bilateral input to the cerebellar cortical vermis goes from granule cells (GCs) to the caudal fastigial neurons through parallel fibers (PFs) and Purkinje cells (PC). The PC inhibit the fastigial neurons, canceling out the excitatory drive from the mossy fibers. Just before a horizontal saccade is triggered, neurons in the caudal fastigial nucleus (cFN) of the contralateral side with respect to the direction of the movement, discharge a burst of activity driving the excitatory burst neurons in the brainstem, which in turn drive the eyes in a contraversive saccade (continuous line circuit); later, just before a saccade is stopped, neurons in the opposite cFN burst, in order to decelerate and stop eyes exactly on target (broken line circuit). In ataxia-telangiectasia-like disorder, we consider a double pathogenetic effect that may explain its peculiar saccadic behavior: (1) a developmental anomaly principally affecting Bergmann cells associated with a reduction of the expansion of the GC–PF (light red circuit); (2) a neurodegenerative processes further affecting this circuit including PC synapses (dark red circuit). Slowing of parallel fibers conduction may delay the caudal fastigial neurons burst that blocks saccades, making them hypermetric. The damage of the GC–PF–PC synapses also reduces the inhibitory inputs to both caudal fastigial neurons causing abnormally fast contralateral saccades. The model is adapted from Optican and Quaia (31). ML, media recti; LR, lateral recti.

Here, the available MRI scan (**Figure 1**) shows extended atrophy of the hemispheres and of the cerebellar vermis, yet the technique does not allow elucidating further details such as, for instance, on the integrity of the cFN.

Hence, based on the results of previous postmortem studies (9) we will assume that the fastigial nuclei in our patients are spared. In this scenario, the findings of hypermetric LW saccades could be explained by hypothesizing that the reduced vermial inhibition is asymmetric, with the right fastigial nuclei being less inhibited by the greater extent of the damage on the right cerebellar vermis. The right fastigial nuclei would then be hyper active and this would cause the saccades to be programmed as excessively large toward the left (27, 34) as the pre-saccadic activity from the right cFN to the left EBN would be abnormally high.

The imbalance in cFN activity, or the slowing of PF conduction could also delay, or impair, the intervention of the ipsilateral cFN that would normally stop the saccade on target. During RW saccades, instead, the hyperactive right cFN, lacking proper cerebellar inhibition, would turn off the saccades too soon making them hypometric, although this reasoning would not explain why smaller RW saccades were not following a similar behavior.

Alternatively, a further hypothesis could be related to the role of the cerebellar vermis hypothesized in a recent work by Optican and Pretegiani (40), which considered that this structure, acting as a spatial integrator, determines when to stop a saccade by releasing the ipsiversive cFN from inhibition. The pause in the activity of the contraversive (right) vermis, identifying the target of the saccadic movement, should then spread to the ipsiversive (left) vermis to stop the saccade, and this mechanism, could have been damaged in our patients with ATLD by slowing the PF transmission within the cerebellar vermis, thus delaying the left cFN activation and making saccades hypermetric (33).

Clearly, if the hypothesis of spared FN was disproven, then the classical explanation of a more pronounced dysfunction of the left cFN, which would then cause hypermetric LW saccades, should be considered instead (32).

Moreover, the relative structural preservation of the nodulus-uvula region may justify the absence of PAN in these patients, wherein PAN has been reported in almost all patients with AT (20). The evidence of SWJ with higher amplitude, i.e., more than 7°, is also peculiar in our patients with respect to similar changes reported in AT and other cerebellar diseases. SWJ may seldom be correlated with quick phases of nystagmus in the orthogonal direction (i.e., down-beat nystagmus can have horizontal SWL), but we did not find any correlation.

The proposed hypothesis, based on the circuitry depicted in **Figure 6**, incorporates another cellular element, namely the BGC, which may be damaged early in ATLD. The BGC have a dual role in normal conditions: they provide a scaffold for the migration/differentiation of GCs in the developing cerebellum, and regulate PC functions in adulthood (41, 42). In this respect, the conditional inactivation of Mre11 determines early cerebellar atrophy and embryonic lethality in murine models (43). We suppose that an early dysfunction of BGC could be responsible for the abnormal development of GC and PF with primitive damage to the GC–PF–PC synapses, later the cerebellar damage may slowly progress due to the overlap of neurodegenerative processes leading to the reported changes (44).

In conclusion, we have reported two Italian adult patients with *MRE11* mutation as the only ATLD patients in whom the eye movements have been analyzed. Although slow eye movements accompanying saccades, various kinds of SI and cerebellar nystagmus are similar to those reported in AT patients, they show fast and overshooting LW saccades. The usually milder phenotype and slower neurological progression with respect to AT and these gaze detectable features may help to address the correct diagnosis in patients with familial neurodegenerative ataxias. A dual pathogenetic mechanism, which incorporates neurodevelopmental and neurodegenerative changes, could determine the phenotype observed in this disease.

AUTHOR CONTRIBUTIONS

PF and AR participated in the design of the work. AR and FR were responsible for patient's clinical data reporting. PF and FR participated in the acquisition of data. PF, FR, and SR participated in the analysis and interpretation of data. PF drafted the manuscript. PF, EP, and AR participated in editing the manuscript. PF, SR, and AR contributed to the manuscript preparation. AR, SR, and AF participated in the revising the manuscript critically. All authors read and approved the manuscript.

ACKNOWLEDGMENTS

We are grateful to Prof. Silvia Palmeri, recently retired, for her precious contribution in the study of patients with rare neurological disease; she diagnosed these two patients and followed their clinical evolution over 20 years. We also thank patients and their mother for the patience during experimental sessions. We wish to thank Dr. Lance M. Optican for his helpful critical comments, and Dr. A. Cerase for providing us with the MRI imaging of one patient.

FUNDING

This work was supported by the European Commission Framework Program for Research and Technological Development (EC-FP7), International Fellowships Research Executive Agency (REA), Marie Curie Actions People (grant: CERVISO 269263).

REFERENCES

1. Lavin MF. Ataxia-telangiectasia: from a rare disorder to a paradigm for cell signalling and cancer. *Nat Rev Mol Cell Biol* (2008) 9:759–69. doi:10.1038/nrm2598
2. Kulkarni A, Wilson DM III. The involvement of DNA-damage and -repair defects in neurological dysfunction. *Am J Hum Genet* (2008) 82:539–66. doi:10.1016/j.ajhg.2008.01.009
3. Stracker TH, Petrini JHJ. The MRE11 complex: starting from the ends. *Nat Rev Mol Cell Biol* (2011) 12:90–103. doi:10.1038/nrm3047
4. Stracker TH, Roig I, Knobel PA, Marjanović M. The ATM signaling network in development and disease. *Front Genet* (2013) 4:37. doi:10.3389/fgene.2013.00037
5. Delia D, Piane M, Buscemi G, Savio C, Palmeri S, Lulli P, et al. MRE11 mutations and impaired ATM-dependent responses in an Italian family with ataxia-telangiectasia-like disorder. *Hum Mol Genet* (2004) 13:2155–63. doi:10.1093/hmg/ddh221
6. Fernet M, Gribaa M, Salih MA, Seidahmed MZ, Hall J, Koenig M. Identification and functional consequences of a novel MRE11 mutation affecting 10 Saudi Arabian patients with the ataxia telangiectasia-like disorder. *Hum Mol Genet* (2005) 14:307–18. doi:10.1093/hmg/ddi027
7. Khan AO, Oystreck DT, Koenig M, Salih MA. Ophthalmic features of ataxia telangiectasia-like disorder. *J AAPOS* (2008) 12:186–9. doi:10.1016/j.jaapos.2007.09.016

8. Uchisaka N, Takahashi N, Sato M, Kikuchi A, Mochizuki S, Imai K, et al. Two brothers with ataxia-telangiectasia-like disorder with lung adenocarcinoma. *J Pediatr* (2009) 155:435–8. doi:10.1016/j.jpeds.2009.02.037
9. Oba D, Hayashi M, Minamitani M, Hamano S, Uchisaka N, Kikuchi A, et al. Autopsy study of cerebellar degeneration in siblings with ataxia-telangiectasia-like disorder. *Acta Neuropathol* (2010) 119:513–20. doi:10.1007/s00401-010-0639-4
10. Bohlega SA, Shinwari JM, Al Sharif LJ, Khalil DS, Alkhairallah TS, Al Tassan NA. Clinical and molecular characterization of ataxia with oculomotor apraxia patients in Saudi Arabia. *BMC Med Genet* (2011) 12:27. doi:10.1186/1471-2350-12-27
11. Matsumoto Y, Miyamoto T, Sakamoto H, Izumi H, Nakazawa Y, Ogi T, et al. Two unrelated patients with MRE11A mutations and Nijmegen breakage syndrome-like severe microcephaly. *DNA Repair* (2011) 10:314–21. doi:10.1016/j.dnarep.2010.12.002
12. Verhagen MM, Abdo WF, Willemsen MA, Hogervorst FB, Smeets DF, Hiel JA, et al. Clinical spectrum of ataxia-telangiectasia in adulthood. *Neurology* (2009) 73:430–7. doi:10.1212/WNL.0b013e3181af33bd
13. Taylor AM, Groom A, Byrd PJ. Ataxia-telangiectasia-like disorder (ATLD)—its clinical presentation and molecular basis. *DNA Repair* (2004) 3:1219–25. doi:10.1016/j.dnarep.2004.04.009
14. Optican LM. Sensorimotor transformation for visually guided saccades. *Ann N Y Acad Sci* (2005) 1039:132–48. doi:10.1196/annals.1325.013
15. Federighi P, Federico A, Rufa A. On the development of a data base for saccadic parameters and main sequence relationships—a quantitative study of video-base eye tracking. *Rom J Biophys* (2013) 23:125–38.
16. Rufa A, Federighi P. Fast versus slow: different saccadic behavior in cerebellar ataxias. *Ann N Y Acad Sci* (2011) 1233:148–54. doi:10.1111/j.1749-6632.2011.06126.x
17. Rosini F, Federighi P, Pretegiani E, Piu P, Leigh RJ, Serra A, et al. Ocular-motor profile and effects of memantine in a familial form of adult cerebellar ataxia with slow saccades and square wave saccadic intrusions. *PLoS One* (2013) 8(7):e69522. doi:10.1371/journal.pone.0069522
18. Federighi P, Cevenini G, Dotti MT, Rosini F, Pretegiani E, Federico A, et al. Differences in saccade dynamics between spinocerebellar ataxia 2 and late-onset cerebellar ataxias. *Brain* (2011) 134:879–91. doi:10.1093/brain/awr009
19. Abadi RV, Gowen E. Characteristics of saccadic intrusions. *Vision Res* (2004) 44:2675–90. doi:10.1016/j.visres.2004.05.009
20. Palmeri S, Rufa A, Pucci B, Santarnecchi E, Malandrini A, Stromillo ML, et al. Clinical course of two Italian siblings with ataxia-telangiectasia-like disorder. *Cerebellum* (2013) 12:596–9. doi:10.1007/s12311-013-0460-4
21. Shaikh AG, Marti S, Tarnutzer AA, Palla A, Crawford TO, Straumann D, et al. Gaze fixation deficits and their implication in ataxia telangiectasia. *J Neurol Neurosurg Psychiatry* (2009) 80:858–64. doi:10.1136/jnnp.2008.170522
22. Lewis RF, Crawford TO. Slow target-directed eye movements in ataxia-telangiectasia. *Invest Ophthalmol Vis Sci* (2002) 43:686–91.
23. Lewis RF, Lederman HM, Crawford TO. Ocular motor abnormalities in ataxia telangiectasia. *Ann Neurol* (1999) 46:287–95. doi:10.1002/1531-8249(199909)46:3<287::AID-ANA3>3.0.CO;2-0
24. Farr AK, Shalev B, Crawford TO, Lederman HM, Winkelstein JA, Repka MX. Ocular manifestations of ataxia-telangiectasia. *Am J Ophthalmol* (2002) 134: 891–6. doi:10.1016/S0002-9394(02)01796-8
25. Ramat S, Leigh RJ, Zee DS, Optican LM. What clinical disorders tell us about the neural control of saccadic eye movements. *Brain* (2007) 130:10–35. doi:10.1093/brain/awl309
26. Daye PM, Optican LM, Roze E, Gaymard B, Pouget P. Neuromimetic model of saccades for localizing deficits in an atypical eye-movement pathology. *J Transl Med* (2013) 11:125. doi:10.1186/1479-5876-11-125
27. Shaikh AG, Ramat S, Optican LM, Miura K, Leigh RJ, Zee DS. Saccadic burst cell membrane dysfunction is responsible for saccadic oscillations. *J Neuroophthalmol* (2008) 28(4):329–36. doi:10.1097/WNO.0b013e31818eb3a5
28. Hashimoto K, Yoshida T, Sakimura K, Mishina M, Watanabe M, Kano M. Influence of parallel fiber-Purkinje cell synapse formation on postnatal development of climbing fiber-Purkinje cell synapses in the cerebellum. *Neuroscience* (2009) 162:601–11. doi:10.1016/j.neuroscience.2008.12.037
29. Scudder CA, McGee DM. Adaptive modification of saccade size produces correlated changes in the discharge of fastigial nucleus neurons. *J Neurophysiol* (2003) 90:1011–26. doi:10.1152/jn.00193.2002
30. Noda H, Sugita S, Ikeda Y. Afferent and efferent connections of the oculomotor region of the fastigial nucleus in the macaque monkey. *J Comp Neurol* (1990) 302:330–48. doi:10.1002/cne.903020211
31. Optican LM, Quaia C. Distributed model of collicular and cerebellar function during saccades. *Ann N Y Acad Sci* (2002) 956:164–77. doi:10.1111/j.1749-6632.2002.tb02817.x
32. Robinson FR, Straube A, Fuchs AF. Role of the caudal fastigial nucleus in saccade generation. II. Effects of muscimol inactivation. *J Neurophysiol* (1993) 70:1741–58.
33. Swartz BE, Li S, Bespalova I, Burmeister M, Dulaney E, Robinson FR, et al. Pathogenesis of clinical signs in recessive ataxia with saccadic intrusions. *Ann Neurol* (2003) 54:824–8. doi:10.1002/ana.10758
34. Serra A, Liao K, Martinez-Conde S, Optican LM, Leigh RJ. Suppression of saccadic intrusions in hereditary ataxia by memantine. *Neurology* (2008) 70:810–2. doi:10.1212/01.wnl.0000286952.01476.eb
35. Gorodetsky E, Calkins S, Ahn J, Brooks PJ. ATM, the Mre11/Rad50/Nbs1 complex, and topoisomerase I are concentrated in the nucleus of Purkinje neurons in the juvenile human brain. *DNA Repair* (2007) 6:1698–707. doi:10.1016/j.dnarep.2007.06.011
36. Bottini AR, Gatti RA, Wirenfeldt M, Vinters HV. Heterotopic Purkinje cells in ataxia-telangiectasia. *Neuropathology* (2012) 32:23–9. doi:10.1111/j.1440-1789.2011.01210.x
37. Paula-Barbosa MM, Ruela C, Tavares MA, Pontes C, Saraiva A, Cruz C. Cerebellar cortex ultrastructure in ataxia-telangiectasia. *Ann Neurol* (1983) 13:297–302. doi:10.1002/ana.410130312
38. Crawford TO. Ataxia telangiectasia. *Semin Pediatr Neurol* (1998) 5:287–94. doi:10.1016/S1071-9091(98)80007-7
39. Kamiya M, Yamanouchi H, Yoshida T, Arai H, Yokoo H, Sasaki A, et al. Ataxia telangiectasia with vascular abnormalities in the brain parenchyma: report of an autopsy case and literature review. *Pathol Int* (2001) 51:271–6. doi:10.1046/j.1440-1827.2001.01199.x
40. Optican LM, Pretegiani E. What stops a saccade? *Philos Trans R Soc Lond B Biol Sci* (2017) 372(1718). doi:10.1098/rstb.2016.0194
41. Yamada K, Watanabe M. Cytodifferentiation of Bergmann glia and its relationship with Purkinje cells. *Anat Sci Int* (2002) 77:94–108. doi:10.1046/j.0022-7722.2002.00021.x
42. Xu H, Yang Y, Tang X, Zhao M, Liang F, Xu P, et al. Bergmann glia function in granule cell migration during cerebellum development. *Mol Neurobiol* (2013) 47:833–44. doi:10.1007/s12035-013-8405-y
43. Xiao Y, Weaver DT. Conditional gene targeted deletion by Cre recombinase demonstrates the requirement for the double-strand break repair Mre11 protein in murine embryonic stem cells. *Nucleic Acids Res* (1997) 25:2985–91. doi:10.1093/nar/25.15.2985
44. Millen KJ, Gleeson JG. Cerebellar development and disease. *Curr Opin Neurobiol* (2008) 18:12–9. doi:10.1016/j.conb.2008.05.010

3

Eyetracking Metrics in Young Onset Alzheimer's Disease: A Window into Cognitive Visual Functions

Ivanna M. Pavisic[1], Nicholas C. Firth[2], Samuel Parsons[3], David Martinez Rego[3], Timothy J. Shakespeare[1], Keir X. X. Yong[1], Catherine F. Slattery[1], Ross W. Paterson[1], Alexander J. M. Foulkes[1], Kirsty Macpherson[1], Amelia M. Carton[1], Daniel C. Alexander[2], John Shawe-Taylor[3], Nick C. Fox[1], Jonathan M. Schott[1], Sebastian J. Crutch[1] and Silvia Primativo[1]**

[1] Dementia Research Centre, Department of Neurodegenerative Diseases, Institute of Neurology, University College London, London, United Kingdom, [2] Centre for Medical Image Computing, Department of Computer Science, University College London, London, United Kingdom, [3] Centre for Computational Statistics and Machine Learning, Faculty of Engineering Science, Department of Computer Science, University College London, London, United Kingdom

Correspondence:
Ivanna M. Pavisic
ivanna.pavisic.15@ucl.ac.uk;
Silvia Primativo
s.primativo@ucl.ac.uk

Young onset Alzheimer's disease (YOAD) is defined as symptom onset before the age of 65 years and is particularly associated with phenotypic heterogeneity. Atypical presentations, such as the clinic-radiological visual syndrome posterior cortical atrophy (PCA), often lead to delays in accurate diagnosis. Eyetracking has been used to demonstrate basic oculomotor impairments in individuals with dementia. In the present study, we aim to explore the relationship between eyetracking metrics and standard tests of visual cognition in individuals with YOAD. Fifty-seven participants were included: 36 individuals with YOAD ($n = 26$ typical AD; $n = 10$ PCA) and 21 age-matched healthy controls. Participants completed three eyetracking experiments: fixation, pro-saccade, and smooth pursuit tasks. Summary metrics were used as outcome measures and their predictive value explored looking at correlations with visuoperceptual and visuospatial metrics. Significant correlations between eyetracking metrics and standard visual cognitive estimates are reported. A machine-learning approach using a classification method based on the smooth pursuit raw eyetracking data discriminates with approximately 95% accuracy patients and controls in cross-validation tests. Results suggest that the eyetracking paradigms of a relatively simple and specific nature provide measures not only reflecting basic oculomotor characteristics but also predicting higher order visuospatial and visuoperceptual impairments. Eyetracking measures can represent extremely useful markers during the diagnostic phase and may be exploited as potential outcome measures for clinical trials.

Keywords: young onset Alzheimer's disease, eye movements, eyetracking metrics, cognitive visual functions, machine learning, classification model

INTRODUCTION

Alzheimer's disease (AD) is the most common major neurodegenerative dementia type (1). While characterized by gradual and progressive episodic memory impairment, it is also associated with other cognitive impairments such as executive dysfunction, language, praxis, and complex visual processing deficits (2–5). Several phase three clinical trials have recently failed and there are no disease-modifying treatments available for AD (6, 7). Sensitive and sensible markers are needed to facilitate earlier diagnosis and to serve as outcome measures in clinical trials.

The focus of neuropsychological investigations in AD has previously been directed toward the study of anterograde episodic memory, and attentional and executive processes as primary consequences of AD and sources of functional impairment (8); by contrast, cognitive visual impairment has been widely overlooked (9). More recently, the presence of both low and high-level visual processing impairments has received more attention [for a review see Ref. (10)]. Deficits related to both the ventral and dorsal processing pathways have been described; impairments in object and facial recognition and color and pattern processing have been reported (11–13); abnormal performance has also been shown for tasks investigating visuospatial processing and motion perception (13–15). The presence of visual impairments has been associated with the severity of the disease (11, 13, 16, 17), leading to the possibility that visual testing could provide a method of screening and tracking AD. Studies suggest that cognitive visual deficits are more marked in young vs. late onset AD (18) and there may also be qualitative differences in the nature of the deficits. While some studies have highlighted the prominence of both ventral and dorsal stream deficits in late onset AD (13, 19), disproportionately impaired visuospatial ability has been described in young onset AD (18). Furthermore, the so called "visual variant" of AD—posterior cortical atrophy (PCA)—in which visual symptoms predominate (20–23) exhibits commonalities in cortical thinning with typical, amnestic AD particularly within temporoparietal regions (24), suggesting a continuum of visual impairment between typical AD (tAD) and PCA.

Posterior cortical atrophy is a progressive neurodegenerative syndrome mainly caused by AD pathology and characterized by progressive visuospatial and visuoperceptual dysfunction with relatively preserved memory, insight, and judgment (20). Individuals with PCA often manifest some or all of the features of Balint's syndrome such as simultanagnosia, oculomotor apraxia, optic ataxia, and environmental agnosia (21–23, 25–28). Not only differences but also similarities have been described between PCA and tAD in terms of visual processing deficits (29), emphasizing the need for further study on the cognitive visual deficits in AD.

Recently, eyetracking technology has become more widely available and the simplicity of the instruments needed to collect good quality eyetracking data has enabled the application of the methodology to clinical populations (29–32). The resulting literature has demonstrated the presence of oculomotor impairment in AD patients as compared to age-matched healthy controls: longer saccade latencies in pro-saccade tasks and lower accuracy than controls in anti-saccade tasks have been reported in AD (33–37), together with abnormalities in saccadic accuracy (38–41).

The study by Shakespeare et al. (29) represents, to our knowledge, the only direct comparison between the basic oculomotor characteristics of individuals with PCA, tAD, and healthy controls. PCA patients showed increased time to saccadic target fixation, increased first major saccade latency, and decreased saccadic amplitude as compared to both tAD and controls. The patients with PCA also showed more frequent large intrusive saccades and lower longest period of fixation in the fixation stability task and lower pursuit and more saccades per trial in the smooth pursuit task as compared to controls. The authors also described impaired performance in the fixation stability test in tAD patients, who produced a large proportion of square wave jerks as compared to controls and individuals with PCA. As in PCA, tAD patients also had shorter maximum fixation period than the healthy controls. In the smooth pursuit task, both PCA and tAD patients showed significantly lower gain than the control group (29).

In cognitive psychology, eyetracking metrics have frequently been used to study higher order cognitive functions (42, 43). However, few studies in the field of dementia have utilized this potential to date. Crutcher and colleagues (44) and Richmond and colleagues (45) used a visual paired-comparison task and showed that eye movement metrics, such as number of fixations and fixation duration, can be indicative of short-term memory difficulties in a group of patients with mild cognitive impairment (MCI) as compared to age-matched controls. Fernández et al. (46) have investigated the semantic, working, and retrieval memory deficits in individuals with young onset AD by looking at differences with controls when reading high- and low-predictability sentences.

Despite the above-reported evidence of visual cognitive processing impairments and oculomotor deficits in both AD and PCA, little has been done so far to exploit eyetracking metrics as a route to explore deficits in visual cognition.

There are multiple potential advantages of using eyetracking metrics for studying visual cognitive processing in dementia. In contrast to many traditional neuropsychological assessments, eye movement recording does not require additional behavioral responses, such as button presses or verbal responses to make inferences about psychological changes. Eyetracking is also non-invasive and does not have contraindications, making it particularly well suited for patient studies. Moreover, modern eyetracking systems have excellent recording frames of up to 1,000 Hz, enabling the building of very large datasets (time series of x and y coordinates) in a relatively short amount of time (e.g., a 1,000 Hz system generates 600,000 x–y data coordinates for a 10-min recording session). Such qualities represent incentives to fully explore the possible contribution of eyetracking metrics to an accurate and sensitive diagnosis and as outcome markers for clinical trials. An increasingly practical approach to take advantage of the volume of eyetracking datasets involves the application of machine-learning methods, in which automatically generated feature vectors of individual participants may be used to assign categories to each participant.

In the present study, we explored the relationship between eyetracking and standard visual cognitive tests in individuals with young onset AD (both tAD and PCA). We extracted standard eyetracking summary metrics and used them to test the hypothesis according to which such metrics well correlate with visuoperceptual and visuospatial metrics derived from standard cognitive tests. We then applied a machine-learning approach to a proportion of the data to explore the possibility of automatically discriminating patients and healthy individuals on the basis of raw eyetracking metrics only (i.e., time series of x and y coordinates). Therefore, our secondary hypothesis was that machine-learning classifiers would offer the discriminative power (47) for the diagnosis of young onset AD among healthy controls based on oculomotor profiles during a discrete task.

MATERIALS AND METHODS

Participants

The study was approved by the local Research Ethics Committee and all participants provided written informed consent according to guidelines established by the Declaration of Helsinki.

Data were collected from 36 individuals with young onset Alzheimer's disease (YOAD) (26 patients with tAD and 10 patients with PCA) and 21 age-matched healthy controls. Patients with PCA fulfilled standard criteria for PCA (21, 22). Patients with AD had a clinical diagnosis of probable AD and fulfilled the NIA (National Institute of Aging) clinical criteria (5). Healthy controls and patients with YOAD did not differ in terms of age at assessment (two sample t-test, $t = 0.09$, $p = 0.93$) or years of education (Wilcoxon Mann–Whitney U-test, $z = 1.57$, $p = 0.12$) (**Table 1**). Healthy controls and YOAD patients differed in terms of Mini-Mental State Examination (MMSE) scores (Wilcoxon Mann–Whitney U-test, $z = 6.21$, $p < 0.0001$). Within the YOAD patients, tAD and PCA were matched in terms of disease duration [tAD: 5.0 (2.8) years and PCA: 5.6 (3.4) years, Wilcoxon Mann–Whitney U-test, $z = -0.50$, $p = 0.62$] and MMSE scores [tAD: 20.1 (0.8) and PCA: 23.1 (1.5), Wilcoxon Mann–Whitney U-test, $z = -1.78$, $p = 0.07$].

All participants had a detailed neuropsychology assessment investigating memory, language, executive function, and vision. The battery included six standard visual tasks, which were the focus of the subsequent correlational analysis between eyetracking and traditional neuropsychological metrics. Early visual processing was examined using the shape detection subtest from the Visual and Object Space Perception battery (VOSP) (48) where individuals were presented with 20 patterns, 11 of which contained a faint cross. Participants were asked to express a judgment as to whether a faint cross was present or not with score ranging from 10 (chance) to 20. Visuoperceptual processing was assessed using the fragmented letters and object decision VOSP subtests (48). In the former, individuals were asked to identify 20-fragmented capital letters presented one at a time with score ranging from 0 to 20. In the latter, they were asked to identify, among four silhouettes, which one represented a real life object [score ranged from 5 (chance) to 20]. Visuospatial processing was assessed using the dot-counting VOSP subtest (48) and letter cancelation test (49). In the dot-counting test, individuals were presented with 10 pages containing from 5 to 9 dots in different positions and asked to identify the number of dots without using their fingers (score range: 0–10). In the "A" cancelation task, participants were presented with an A4 sheet and asked to mark all the letters "A" embedded among 69 distractors (other letters) within 90 s. Last, single word recognition was assessed using the National Adult Reading Test (NART) (50) where individuals were asked to read 50 words aloud (score ranged from 0 to 50).

Equipment

The experiment was run on a Dell 2120 desktop computer with a 23-inch screen at a viewing distance of 60 cm. Eye movements were recorded at 250 Hz using a head-mounted infrared video-based eye tracker (Eyelink II; SR Research). A chin rest was used to provide stability and maintain the viewing distance. The Eyelink system considered saccades using standard velocity and acceleration thresholds (30°/s and 8,000°/s^2) and automatically identified periods with no saccadic movement as fixations. A 9-point calibration and validation were performed prior to each experiment. All the data were obtained from recordings with an average Cartesian prediction error of <1° during the validation. A drift correction procedure was used before each individual trial.

Procedure

Three eyetracking experiments were performed:

Fixation stability: a red cross subtending at 0.5° of visual angle was presented in the center of the screen for 10 s. There was a practice trial followed by three test trials and participants were instructed to "look as closely as possible at the red cross without blinking for 10 s" (29, 51).

Pro-saccade: participants were initially presented with a black circle (subtending 0.4° of visual angle) having a white inner circle (0.1°) in the center of the screen lasting 500 ms. A blank screen was then displayed for 200 ms. After this, a target (black circle having a diameter of 0.75° and an inner white circle subtending 0.25°) was shown. The target remained on the screen until a fixation of minimum 250 ms duration was made within an area of 1.5° of visual angle from the center of the target (interest area) or after 5,000 ms from target onset. The participant's task was to look at the target as quickly and accurately as possible when it appeared. The target appeared in one of 10 possible locations: 5°, 10°, or 15° either on the left or on the right, 5° or 10° either up or down. There were four trials for each location, giving a total of 40 test trials. Trials were split into two blocks ($n = 20$ each) with target locations randomized and balanced within each block. Four practice trials were used. The target positions were pseudo-randomized but their order was kept constant for all participants.

Smooth pursuit: the target was a red circle subtending 0.5° of visual angle in diameter. Twelve trials of target sinusoidal movement followed (horizontal: $n = 6$; vertical: $n = 6$). Two target velocities were used (10° and 20° of visual angle/second). The frequency of the target oscillation was set at 0.25 Hz for a target speed of 10°/s and 0.5 Hz for a target speed of 20°/s. Each trial lasted 10 s. The task started with two practice trials. Participants were instructed to follow the target as closely as possible with their eyes.

Eyetracking Summary Metrics

All eyetracking recordings were visually inspected using Data Viewer and trials and/or participants were excluded if there was a significant signal loss that would have interfered with the data analysis and interpretation of results. Overall, 5.4% of the trials

TABLE 1 | Mean and SD demographic information and neuropsychology scores for the 36 patients with young onset Alzheimer's disease (YOAD) and 21 age-matched healthy controls.

	Max score	Controls (*N* = 21)	YOAD (*N* = 36)	*N* (%) below 5%[a]	Normative mean (SD)
Demographics					
Gender M:F		11:10	17:19	NA	NA
Age (years)		61.0 (5.3)	60.9 (5.2)	NA	NA
Education (years)		16.5 (3.2)	15.3 (2.7)	NA	NA
Disease duration (years)		NA	5.2 (2.9)	NA	NA
Background neuropsychology					
MMSE	30	29.5 (0.7)	20.9 (4.4)	NA	29.0 (1.3)
Visual acuity: Snellen[b]	6/9	NA	6/9	NA	NA
WASI vocabulary	80	69.0 (8.5)	53.4 (18.3)	1 (2.8%)	NA
WASI matrices	32	26.7 (2.7)	8.1 (7.1)	8 (22.2%)	NA
Digit span forward (max)	8	7.3 (1.2)	5.4 (1.5)	11 (30.6%)	NA
Digit span backward (max)	7	5.4 (0.9)	3.2 (1.5)	10 (27.8%)	NA
RMT for faces	25	24.7 (0.8)	19.5 (4.4)	11 (30.6%)	22.8 (1.9)
RMT for words	25	24.4 (1.4)	17.5 (3.2)	27 (75.0%)	23.7 (1.8)
GDA: oral	24	13.8 (6.6)	2.9 (4.7)	25 (69.4%)	11.95 (5.1)
Early visual processing					
Shape detection (VOSP)	20	19.5 (0.8)	18.0 (1.4)	NA	19.5 (0.7)
Visuoperceptual processing					
Object decision (VOSP)	20	18.2 (1.4)	14.7 (3.9)	12 (33.3%)	17.7 (1.9)
Fragmented letters (VOSP)	20	19.5 (0.7)	11.2 (7.2)	23 (63.9%)	18.8 (1.4)
Visuospatial processing					
Dot counting: *n* correct	10	9.9 (0.3)	7.6 (2.9)	16 (44.4%)	9.9 (0.2)
A cancelation time (s)	90	21.1 (6.0)	54.0 (22.8)	27 (75.0%)	20.5 (6.5)
Word recognition					
NART: number of errors	50	11.5 (8.0)	20.1 (11.0)	NA	NA

Mini-Mental State Examination (MMSE) (67); Cortical Vision Screening Test (CORVIST) (68); Wechsler Abbreviated Scale of Intelligence (WASI) (69); Wechsler Memory Scale Revised-digit span forwards and backwards (70); Matrices and Vocabulary subtest; Short Recognition Memory Test (RMT) for words and faces (71); oral Graded Difficulty Arithmetic (GDA) subtests addition and subtraction (72); Visual Object and Space Perception battery subtest object decision, shape detection, fragmented letters and dot counting (48); A cancelation (49); National Adult Reading Test (NART) (50). NA, not available.

[a]*Percentage of scores below 5% percentile are shown for the YOAD group (the performance of controls did not reach this level).*

[b]*Median value is reported.*

were excluded from the fixation stability task, 3.6% from the pro-saccade and 4% from the smooth pursuit tasks.

Blinks were identified and removed using Eyelink's automated blink detection and practice trials were discarded from the analysis. Vision was binocular but eye movements from the right eye were recorded. If a problem was detected (i.e., poor eyesight, watery, or dry eye) recordings were performed using the left eye.

Statistical analyses were carried out using Stata (v. 12.1).

Fixation Stability

All participants performed the fixation stability task but two controls were excluded from analysis because of failure in signal detection. The relevant eyetracking metrics for the fixation stability task were large intrusive saccades, square wave jerks, and maximum fixation duration (29).

Number of Large Intrusive Saccades

The number of saccades with an amplitude greater than 2° of visual angle were identified as large intrusive saccades (29, 35).

Number of Square Wave Jerks

Square wave jerks were identified as saccades smaller than 2° in amplitude which took the gaze away from the target position, were followed within 300 ms by another saccade with a similar amplitude (difference in amplitude <0.75°) and took the gaze back to the target position (29, 52).

Maximum Fixation Duration

The longest period of fixation on the target (length of time between saccades) was measured for each participant (29, 35).

Pro-Saccade

All participants performed the pro-saccade task but two individuals (a YOAD patient and a control) were excluded from the analysis due to a failure in signal detection. For this task, the following variables were taken into account: accuracy, time to fixate the target, and number of saccades necessary to fixate the target. For these metrics, fixations made within an area of 1.5° from the center of the target (interest area) were considered to have met the target.

Accuracy

This metric was defined as the ability of the participant to fixate the target (within 1.5° from its center) while it was presented on the screen.

Time to Fixate the Target

The time between the target onset and the first fixation reaching the target was calculated. Negative values due to anticipatory saccades were either corrected if another fixation reaching the interest area was detected (0.09%) or removed if no fixation reached the interest area after target onset (0.14%).

Number of Saccades Necessary to Fixate the Target

The minimum number of saccades necessary to fixate the target was calculated for each trial.

Smooth Pursuit Task

All but three patients performed the smooth pursuit task. A control and a patient were excluded from the analysis due to a signal failure. The following variables were extracted: pursuit gain and proportion of time pursuing the target.

Pursuit Gain

This was defined by the ratio between the eye and the target velocity (in the relevant direction). Saccades and blinks were excluded and only a ratio greater than 0.5 was considered as pursuit gain. This cut-off was applied to dismiss eye movements happening after anticipatory saccades and turnaround points in each trial.

Proportion of Time Pursuing the Target

The proportion of time the participant spent pursuing the target during the trial was reported. This was calculated taking into account the number of samples considered as pursuit gain and multiplying this value by four (recordings were made at 250 Hz).

Statistical Analysis

Differences in eyetracking metrics between the YOAD group and healthy controls were evaluated using linear regression models (clustered by participants) with robust SEs adjusted for repeated measures. Gender and age were considered as covariates for all metrics and stimulus distance and direction were considered as additional covariates for the pro-saccade task as well as target direction and velocity for the smooth pursuit task.

Normal distribution was assessed using the Shapiro–Wilk normality test. As the data were not normally distributed, a non-parametric measure of correlation (Spearman's correlations) was performed and the coefficients reported. Correlations were explored between all oculomotor metrics and six standard visual cognitive tests including measures of early visual processing (shape detection); visuoperceptual processing (fragmented letters and object decision); visuospatial processing (dot counting and "A" cancelation); and single word recognition tests (NART).

Machine Learning Classification Model

A machine-learning classification model is presented here as a proof of concept. As the statistical model aims to model movements in gaze location, the smooth pursuit experiment provided the most suitable data. The fixation stability and saccade experiments are designed to elicit 0 and one-gaze movements, respectively, and as such, their data did not provide enough information to discriminate between diagnostic classes on the basis of gaze movements. For this reason, the data from the smooth pursuit task were used in the pilot automatic classification procedure for the present study.

The automated classification procedure used the eyetracking data from the smooth pursuit task and modeled the movements in gaze location as the target moved. The gaze movements of each individual were used along with the statistical model to automatically generate feature vectors. These feature vectors were then used in a classification procedure that could predict the diagnoses of unseen individuals. The procedure, therefore, consisted of three components: (a) a fitted statistical model of each individual's data, (b) the generation of feature vectors for each individual *via* the fitted model, and (c) the classification of individuals *via* their feature vectors.

A hidden Markov model (HMM) (53) was the statistical model used. This considers movements in gaze location, and assumes that each gaze movement has an underlying "intended" movement direction. We have assumed that each gaze movement was a noisy application of one of the following possibilities: "no movement," "left," "right," "up," or "down." The HMM is slightly non-standard, in that fixed transformations of each gaze movement are applied before they are passed to the sub-model associated with each underlying intended movement direction. Furthermore, knowledge of where the gaze "should" be moving to was incorporated *via* the location of the target at each time. Intended movement directions that were more aligned to the target direction were given a higher likelihood. This implemented the natural assumption that individuals would follow the target as long as they were able to.

If $Y_{1:T}$ denotes the gaze movements for an individual over the course of one trial, $U_{1:T}$ denotes the direction of the target from the current gaze location at each time, and $X_{1:T}$ denotes the (unknown) underlying intended movement directions, then

$$\Pr(Y_{1:T}, U_{1:T} | X_{1:T}, \theta) = \prod_{t=1}^{T} N(Y_t^{(X_t)} | \mu_{X_t}, \Sigma_{X_t}) f(U_t | X_t)$$

$$Pr(X_{1:T} | \theta) = \pi_1(X_1) \prod_{t=2}^{T} P(X_t | X_{t-1}) \tag{1}$$

where $Y_t^{(X_t)}$ are the transformed data and $\theta = (\mu_{X_t}, \Sigma_{X_t}, \pi_1, P)$ are the parameters of the model. $N(|\mu, \Sigma)$ indicates the normal distribution with mean μ and covariance matrix Σ, and $f(U_t | X_t)$ are parameter-free logarithmic distributions that go to 0 as the target direction diverges from the intended direction X_t.

The model could be fit to the data using the EM algorithm (54). For every trial in the experiment, we fit the model to the data for one control. The individual that could follow the dot most accurately was subjectively chosen.

Once a model for each trial in the smooth pursuit experiment had been fitted, this could be used to generate feature vectors for each individual. The feature vectors are composites, made as the sum of "Fisher" feature vectors from the fitted models for each trial. Fisher feature vectors were computed as the gradient vectors of the data log-likelihood, evaluated at the fitted parameter settings. If $Z^{(j)}$ is the Fisher feature vector for an individual in trial j, $Y_{1:T}$ are the gaze movement data for that trial, and $\hat{\theta}$ is the fitted parameter vector, then

$$Z^{(j)} = \nabla_\theta \log Pr(Y_{1:T} | \theta)|_{\theta=\hat{\theta}} \tag{2}$$

which is a vector with as many dimensions as the model has parameters. The sum over trials gave the un-normalized feature vectors for each individual:

$$\hat{Z} = \sum_j Z^{(j)} \tag{3}$$

Once all un-normalized feature vectors for an experiment had been computed, they were normalized element-wise by their SDs (over individuals):

$$Z_i = \frac{\hat{Z}_i}{std\{\hat{Z}_i\}} \tag{4}$$

where Z_i and $\tilde{Z}_i$ are the ith elements of the normalized and un-normalized feature vectors, respectively.

These feature vectors can be used in many classification algorithms. We chose to use logistic regression to classify individuals. As there are approximately as many individuals in the dataset as there are dimensions to the feature vectors, the logistic regression classifier required some regularization. We used the Bayesian methodology to regularize the classifier, placing a sparsity prior on the weights in the classifier. If $d(Z)$ is the diagnosis of the patient associated with feature vector Z (with 0 meaning control and 1 meaning either tAD or PCA), and w are the weights of the model, then

$$\begin{aligned} Pr(d(Z)=1\,|\,w) &= \sigma(Zw) \\ Pr(w\,|\,\alpha) &= \prod_i N(w_i\,|\,0,\alpha_i^{-1}) \end{aligned} \tag{5}$$

where $\sigma()$ is the sigmoid function, and α are the Bayesian hyper-parameters of the model.

The performance of the classifier was assessed through cross-validation tests. Leave-one-out, leave-two-out, and leave-half-out tests were performed. In each of these tests, the data was partitioned multiple times into training and test sets. The classifier was trained on the training sets, and its predictions for the test sets were compared to the true diagnoses. If the proportion of correct predictions for each group class was high, then the classifier had high predictive power on the data within the dataset.

RESULTS

Eyetracking Summary Metrics

Mean and SD performance metrics for fixation stability, pro-saccade and smooth pursuit tasks are shown in **Table 2**.

Fixation Stability

Results from the fixation stability task are represented in **Figure 1** and in **Table 2**.

Number of Large Intrusive Saccades

Young onset Alzheimer's disease patients made a statistically significant higher number of large intrusive saccades compared to healthy controls [YOAD: 2.5 (4.3), healthy controls: 0.7 (1.7), $t = 2.5$, $p = 0.02$].

TABLE 2 | Mean and SD of fixation stability, pro-saccade, and smooth pursuit metrics for young onset Alzheimer's disease (YOAD) patients and age-matched healthy controls.

		YOAD	Controls
		Mean (SD)	**Mean (SD)**
Fixation stability			
Number of large intrusive saccades		2.5 (4.3)*	0.7 (1.7)*
Number of square wave jerks		0.9 (1.6)	0.9 (1.6)
Maximum fixation duration (ms)		1,950.7 (1,352.8)*	2,908.5 (2,062.1)*
Pro-saccade			
Accuracy	Overall	0.85 (0.35)*	0.94 (0.24)*
	5°	0.90 (0.31)	0.96 (0.19)
	10°	0.84 (0.37)*	0.92 (0.27)*
	15°	0.81 (0.39)*	0.93 (0.26)*
	Up	0.86 (0.35)	0.90 (0.30)
	Down	0.86 (0.32)*	0.93 (0.22)*
	Right	0.83 (0.38)*	0.97 (0.18)*
	Left	0.86 (0.35)	0.93 (0.25)
Time taken to reach the target (ms)	Overall	538.7 (682.3)*	328.7 (329.8)*
	5°	437.1 (583.0)*	306.1 (366.6)*
	10°	613.8 (777.3)*	337.4 (333.4)*
	15°	609.0 (650.4)*	358.8 (222.9)*
	Up	537.8 (648.5)*	365.6 (468.4)*
	Down	518.5 (571.2)*	329.2 (163.4)*
	Right	591.0 (827.1)*	300.6 (180.7)*
	Left	501.9 (613.8)*	333.6 (413.8)*
Saccades made to reach the target	Overall	3.1 (2.3)*	2.1 (1.2)*
	5°	2.7 (1.9)*	2.0 (1.2)*
	10°	3.4 (2.7)*	2.1 (1.1)*
	15°	3.4 (2.4)*	2.2 (1.2)*
	Up	3.3 (2.4)*	2.3 (1.3)*
	Down	3.1 (2.5)*	2.1 (1.1)*
	Right	3.0 (2.1)*	2.1 (1.2)*
	Left	3.0 (2.2)*	2.0 (1.1)*
Smooth pursuit			
Pursuit gain	Overall	1.4 (0.4)	1.4 (0.4)
	10°/s	1.4 (0.3)	1.4 (0.4)
	20°/s	1.3 (0.4)	1.4 (0.4)
	Horizontal	1.3 (0.3)	1.3 (0.3)
	Vertical	1.5 (0.4)	1.4 (0.4)
Prop. of time pursuing the target	Overall	0.4 (0.2)*	0.6 (0.2)*
	10°/s	0.5 (0.2)*	0.6 (0.1)*
	20°/s	0.3 (0.2)*	0.5 (0.2)*
	Horizontal	0.5 (0.2)*	0.7 (0.1)*
	Vertical	0.3 (0.1)*	0.5 (0.1)*

Statistically significant differences are highlighted in blue and marked with an asterisk (*) (for specific p values see text).

Number of Square Wave Jerks

Healthy controls and YOAD patients did not show a statistically significant difference in terms of the average number of square wave jerks [YOAD: 0.9 (1.6); healthy controls 0.9 (1.6); $t = 0.4$, $p = 0.60$].

Maximum Fixation Duration

The longest period of fixation was significantly shorter for YOAD patients as compared to healthy controls [YOAD: 1,950.7 (1,352.8) ms; healthy controls: 2,908.5 (2,062.1) ms; $t = -2.3$, $p = 0.02$].

Pro-Saccade

Results from the pro-saccade task are represented in **Figure 2** and in **Table 2**.

Accuracy

Young onset Alzheimer's disease patients had an overall significantly lower accuracy compared to healthy controls ($z = -2.1$, $p = 0.04$). The effect of stimulus distance was statistically significant: the greater the distance from the center, the lower the accuracy ($z = -3.5$, $p < 0.001$). When looking at the accuracy for specific stimulus distances YOAD patients showed a trend toward lower accuracy than controls at 10° and 15° ($z = -1.81$, $p = 0.07$) but not at 5° ($z = -1.64$, $p = 0.10$). The effect of stimulus direction was not statistically significant when comparing the accuracy of YOAD patients and healthy controls ($z = 0.79$, $p = 0.40$).

Time Taken to Fixate the Target

Young onset Alzheimer's disease patients took significantly longer to fixate the target compared to healthy controls ($t = 3.7$, $p = 0.001$). The effect of the stimulus distance was significant on the time taken to fixate the target: the time increased with stimulus distance ($t = 4.2$, $p < 0.001$). A statistical trend was observed for the effect of stimulus direction ($t = -1.9$, $p = 0.06$). YOAD patients took more time to reach the target at all stimulus distances (all $p < 0.01$) as well as all stimulus directions (all $p < 0.01$) compared to controls.

Number of Saccades Necessary to Fixate the Target

Young onset Alzheimer's disease patients made a statistically higher number of saccades in order to fixate the target ($t = 3.65$, $p = 0.001$). The effect of the stimulus distance ($t = -3.7$, $p < 0.001$) and the stimulus direction ($t = 4.9$, $p < 0.001$) both had a significant effect on the number of saccades necessary to reach the target. The number of saccades increased with stimulus distance and the greatest number of saccades for both groups was made when the stimulus moved upwards. YOAD patients made a greater number of saccades to reach the target for all stimulus distances (all $p < 0.001$) and stimulus directions (all $p < 0.001$) compared to controls.

Smooth Pursuit

Results from the smooth pursuit task are represented in **Figure 3** and are reported in **Table 2**.

Pursuit Gain

Young onset Alzheimer's disease patients and healthy controls did not differ in terms of pursuit gain ($t = 0.52$, $p = 0.60$). Stimulus velocity did not have a statistically significant effect ($t = -0.95$, $p = 0.30$) but stimulus direction did ($t = 4.06$, $p < 0.001$). Pursuit gain was closer to one (one: eye velocity = target velocity, eyes moving at the exact target's velocity) when the target moved horizontally (as opposed to vertically) for both groups.

Proportion of Time Pursuing the Target

Young onset Alzheimer's disease patients spent significantly less time pursing the target compared to controls ($t = -5.5$, $p < 0.001$). Stimulus direction ($t = -10.31$, $p < 0.001$) and velocity ($t = -10.84$, $p < 0.001$) were both statistically significant: the proportion of time pursuing the target was greater when the target moved at 10°/s (as opposed to 20°/s) and horizontally (compared to vertically). YOAD patients spent less time pursuing the target when it was presented either horizontally ($t = -4.29$, $p < 0.001$) or vertically ($t = -5.79$, $p < 0.001$) as well as at both stimulus

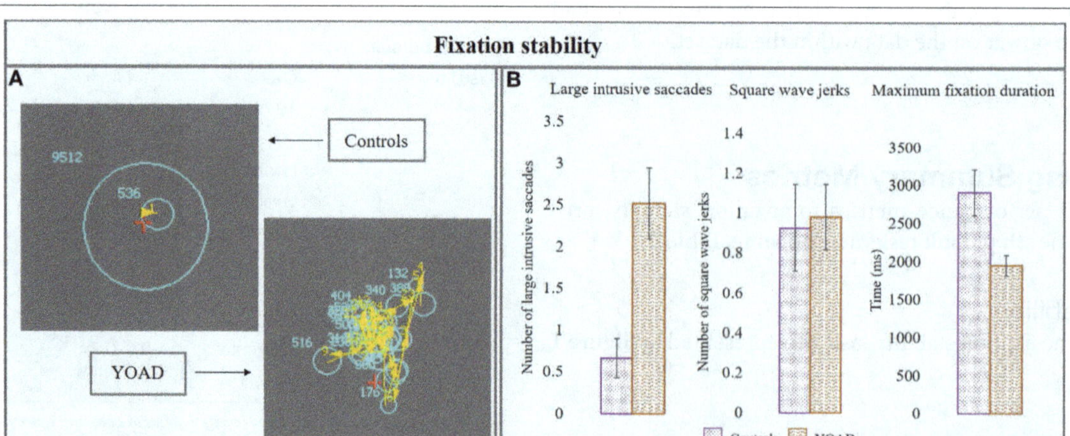

FIGURE 1 | (A) Performance of a control and a young onset Alzheimer's disease (YOAD) patient in the fixation stability task: light blue circles show fixations, yellow arrows indicate saccades, and red crosses represent target position. **(B)** Group means for controls and YOAD patients for the different task metrics. Error bars represent SE.

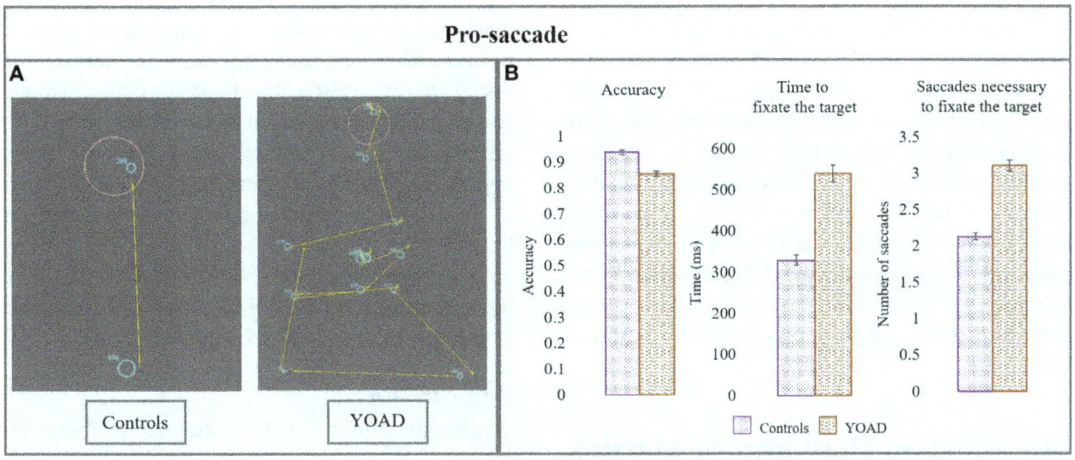

FIGURE 2 | (A) Performance of a control and a patient with young onset Alzheimer's disease (YOAD) in the pro-saccade task: light blue circles show fixations, yellow arrows indicate saccades, red crosses represent target position and orange circles outline the interest area (1.5° from the center of the target). **(B)** Group means for controls and YOAD patients for the different task metrics. Error bars represent standard error.

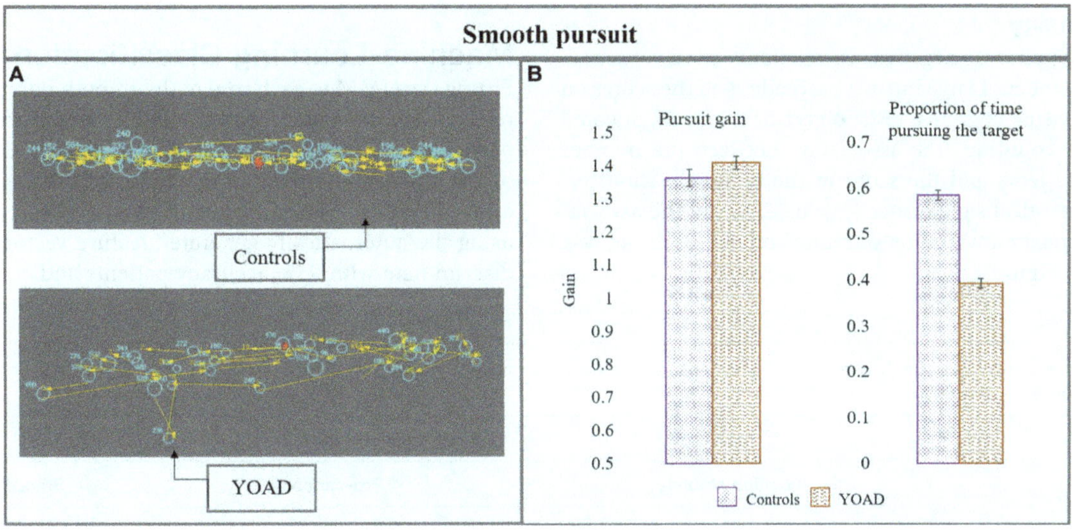

FIGURE 3 | (A) Performance of a control and a young onset Alzheimer's disease (YOAD) patient in the smooth pursuit task: light blue circles show fixations, yellow arrows indicate saccades, and red crosses represent target position. **(B)** Group means for controls and YOAD patients for the different task metrics. Error bars represent SE.

velocities (10°/s: $t = -5.02, p < 0.001$, 20°/s: $t = -5.59, p < 0.001$) when compared to controls.

Comparisons between Eyetracking Metrics in tAD and PCA Patients

Given the aims of the present study, all the described analyses were conducted by examining individuals with tAD and PCA as part of the same group of individuals with YOAD. There were statistically significant differences between the two groups of patients in only three out of the eight eyetracking metrics all of which showed a poorer performance of PCA compared to tAD: maximum fixation duration (controls: 2,908.5 ms, tAD: 2,183.6 ms, PCA: 1,342.4 ms, $t = 2.85, p = 0.006$); time to fixate the target (controls: 328.7 ms, tAD: 428.4 ms, PCA: 924.4 ms, $t = 5.13, p < 0.001$) and number of saccades necessary to reach the target (controls = 2.13, tAD:2.59, PCA: 4.86, $t = 5.13$, $p < 0.001$). PCA and tAD individual group performance was worse than that of healthy controls on all metrics for the three tasks (all $p < 0.001$).

No statistically significant differences were observed between tAD and PCA in the remaining five-eyetracking metrics. There was no difference in the number of square wave jerks (controls: 0.93, tAD: 1.04, PCA: 0.82, $t = 0.11, p = 0.91$) or pursuit gain (controls: 1.36, tAD: 1.35, PCA: 1.62, $t = 1.50, p = 0.14$) between tAD and PCA nor was there an effect of the phenotype in general ($t = 0.36$, $p = 0.72$ and $t = 1.50$, $p = 0.14$, respectively). No differences were observed between tAD and PCA in the number large intrusive saccades (controls: 0.67, tAD: 1.81, PCA: 4.39, $t = -1.56$, $p = 0.12$) and accuracy in the pro-saccade task (controls: 0.94, tAD: 0.89, PCA: 0.75, $z = 1.55$, $p = 0.12$). For these two metrics patients performed worse than controls but only PCA were statistically worse ($t = 2.38$, $p = 0.02$ and $z = -2.62$, $p = 0.01$, respectively). No difference was observed between the two groups of patients in the proportion of time pursuing the target (controls: 0.58, tAD: 0.40, PCA: 0.34, $t = 1.11$, $p = 0.27$) and the two performed statistically worse compared to controls (both $p < 0.001$).

Relationship between Oculomotor Metrics and Standard Visual Cognitive Tests

In **Table 3** coefficients and p values of correlations between estimates of visual cognitive processing and eyetracking metrics for the fixation stability, pro-saccade and smooth pursuit tasks are reported.

Fixation Stability

Statistically significant negative correlations were observed between the number of large intrusive saccades and the scores on the following visual cognitive tests: object decision, fragmented letter, and dot counting. The association between the number of square wave jerks and the score in the object decision test approached statistical significance ($p = 0.06$) as did the association between maximum fixation duration and dot-counting task ($p = 0.07$) (see **Figure 4**).

Pro-Saccade

Statistically significant negative correlations were reported between the time taken to fixate the target and the following visual cognitive tests: object decision, fragmented letters, and dot counting. The association between the time taken to fixate the target and the scores corresponding to the "A" cancelation task approached statistical significance ($p = 0.07$).

Statistically significant negative correlations were found between the number of saccades necessary to fixate the target and the shape detection, object decision, fragmented letters, and dot-counting tests as well as a positive correlation with the "A" cancelation test scores (see **Figure 5**).

Smooth Pursuit

Statistically significant correlations were observed between visual cognitive scores and both the pursuit gain and the proportion of time spent pursuing the target during the trial. In particular, the pursuit gain scores for YOAD patients negatively correlated with the object decision and dot-counting tests. The proportion of time spent pursuing the target positively correlated with the fragmented letters, dot counting and negatively with the "A" cancelation test scores (see **Figure 6**).

Machine-Learning Classification Model

Fitting the HMM to each trial of the smooth pursuit experiment resulted in fitted parameters that conformed to expectations. In particular, the fitted model placed significantly more likelihood on the movement directions that followed the target than on any other direction. The results of the logistic regression classifier using the automatically generated feature vectors were able to discriminate with 95% accuracy patients and controls. Feature

TABLE 3 | Spearman's rank coefficient (Spearman's rho) and p values for correlations between visual cognitive tests and eyetracking metrics for the fixation stability, pro-saccade and smooth pursuit tasks.

	Eyetracking metrics							
	Fixation stability			Pro-saccade			Smooth pursuit	
Visual Cognitive Test	No. of large intrusive saccades	No. of square wave jerks	Max. fixation duration (ms)	Accuracy	Time to reach the target (ms)	Saccades made to fixate the target	Pursuit gain	Prop. of time pursuing the target
VOSP shape detection	$r = -0.16$	$r = 0.04$	$r = 0.19$	$r = -0.26$	$r = -0.19$	$r = -0.38$	$r = -0.09$	$r = 0.04$
	$p = 0.38$	$p = 0.81$	$p = 0.28$	$p = 0.14$	$p = 0.71$	$p = 0.03$*	$p = 0.61$	$p = 0.81$
VOSP object decision	$r = -0.49$	$r = -0.32$	$r = 0.26$	$r = 0.09$	$r = -0.44$	$r = -0.64$	$r = -0.39$	$r = 0.29$
	$p = 0.003$*	$p = 0.06$	$p = 0.13$	$p = 0.61$	$p = 0.009$*	$p < 0.001$*	$p = 0.03$*	$p = 0.11$
VOSP fragmented letters	$r = -0.41$	$r = -0.16$	$r = 0.26$	$r = 0.14$	$r = -0.40$	$r = -0.61$	$r = -0.23$	$r = 0.41$
	$p = 0.02$*	$p = 0.36$	$p = 0.14$	$p = 0.44$	$p = 0.02$*	$p < 0.001$*	$p = 0.22$	$p = 0.02$*
VOSP dot counting	$r = -0.48$	$r = 0.07$	$r = 0.32$	$r = 0.18$	$r = -0.60$	$r = -0.54$	$r = -0.46$	$r = 0.66$
	$p = 0.005$*	$p = 0.70$	$p = 0.07$	$p = 0.32$	$p = 0.002$*	$p < 0.001$*	$p = 0.01$*	$p < 0.001$*
A cancelation time	$r = 0.29$	$r = -0.15$	$r = -0.10$	$r = -0.04$	$r = 0.32$	$r = 0.45$	$r = 0.25$	$r = -0.49$
	$p = 0.10$	$p = 0.42$	$p = 0.57$	$p = 0.79$	$p = 0.07$	$p = 0.009$*	$p = 0.19$	$p = 0.006$*
National adult reading test	$r = -0.23$	$r = -0.06$	$r = 0.14$	$r = 0.08$	$r = 0.18$	$r = -0.08$	$r = -0.14$	$r = 0.03$
	$p = 0.18$	$p = 0.72$	$p = 0.44$	$p = 0.64$	$p = 0.32$	$p = 0.66$	$p = 0.48$	$p = 0.88$

Statistically significant correlations are highlighted in blue and their p values marked with an asterisk (*).

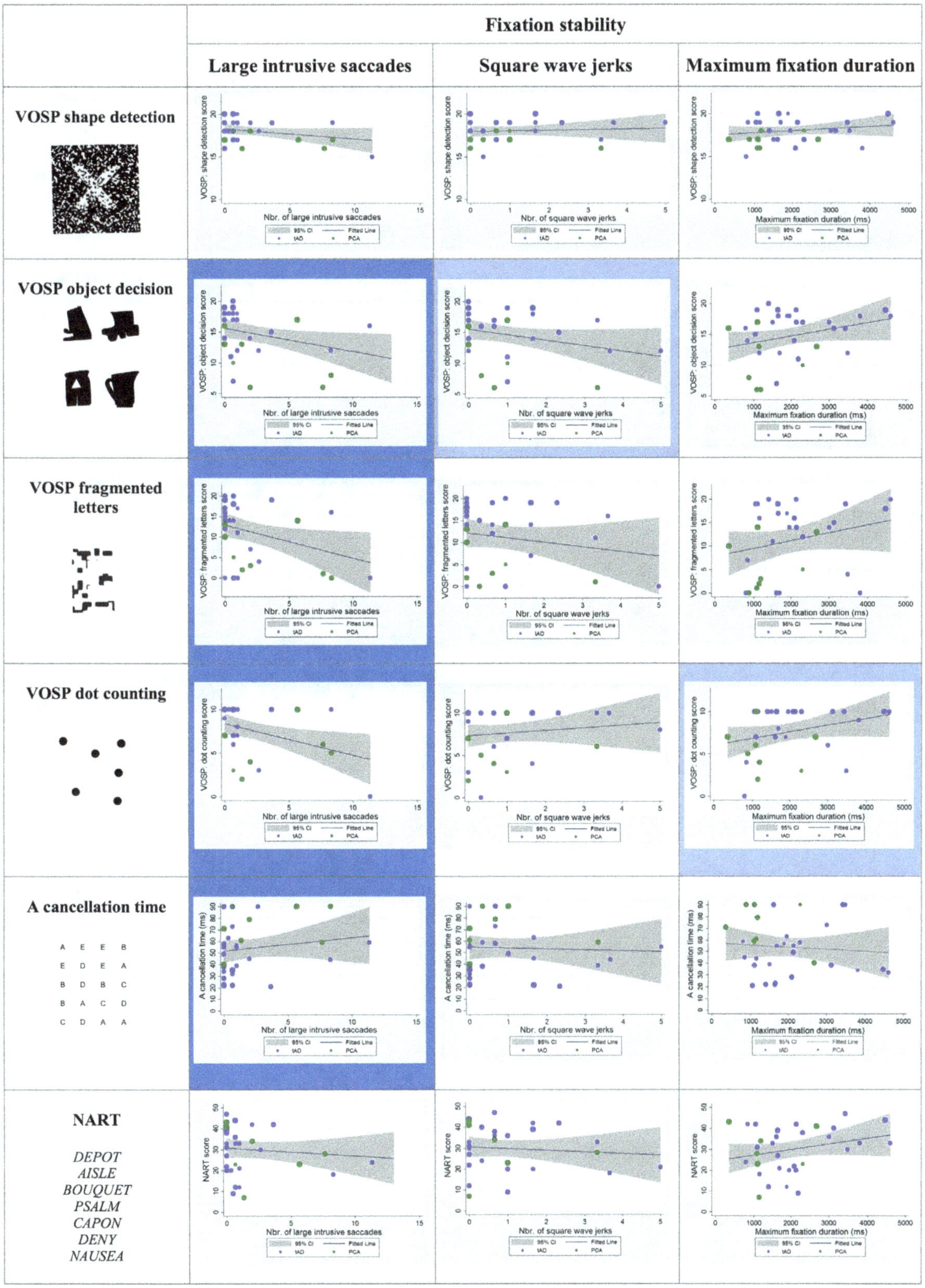

FIGURE 4 | Scatter plots showing correlations between fixation stability metrics and visual cognitive scores for young onset Alzheimer's disease patients. Statistically significant correlations are marked with a blue background and statistical trends ($p > 0.05$ and $p < 0.10$) in a lighter blue. Best fit line and 95% CI are shown. Each data point corresponds to a participant and its size is proportionate to the Mini-Mental State Examination score (indication of disease severity). typical AD (tAD) patients are shown in blue and posterior cortical atrophy (PCA) in green.

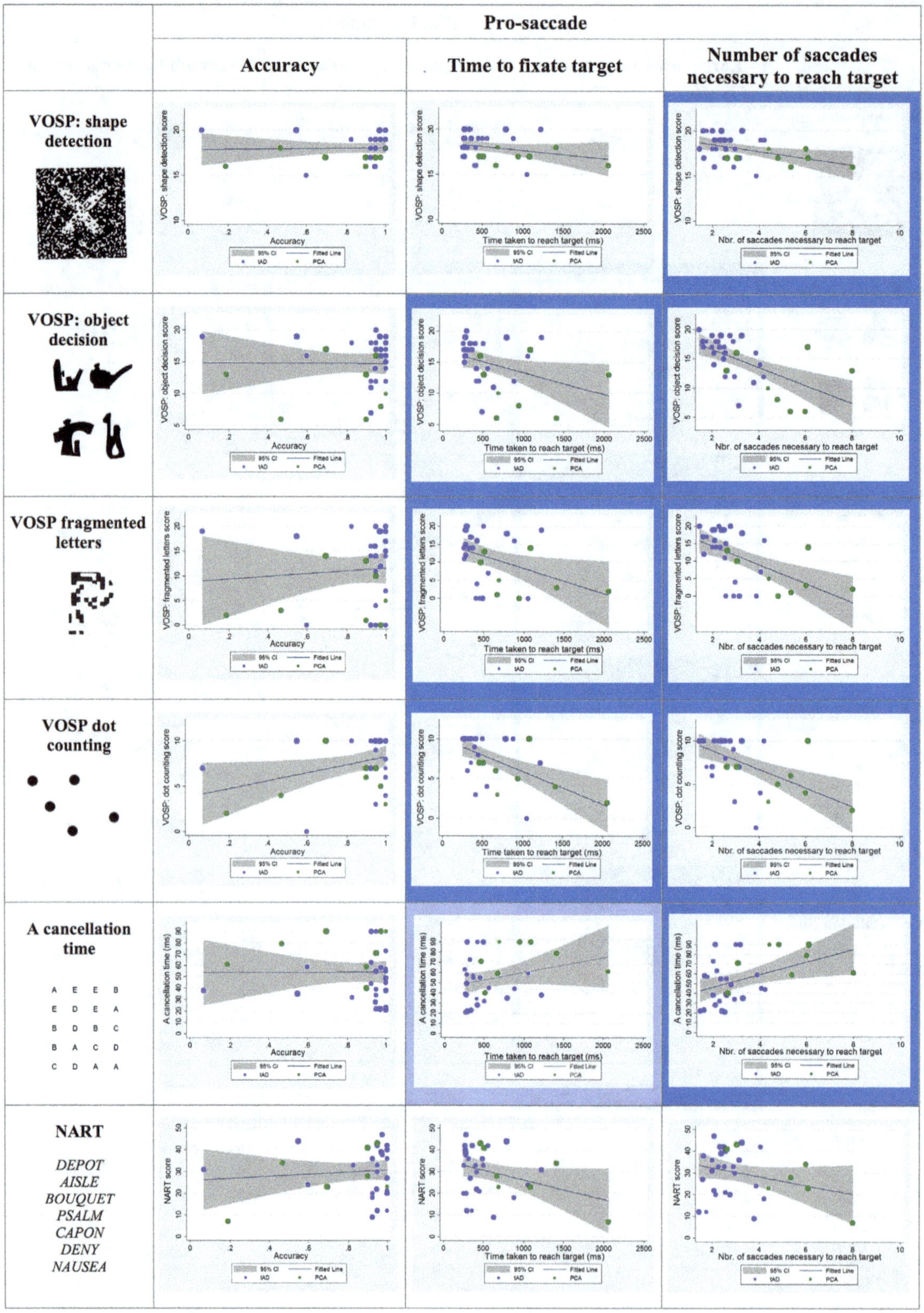

FIGURE 5 | Scatter plots showing correlations between pro-saccade metrics and visual cognitive scores for young onset Alzheimer's disease patients. Statistically significant correlations are marked with a blue background and statistical trends ($p > 0.05$ and $p < 0.10$) in a lighter blue. Best fit line and 95% CI are shown. Each data point corresponds to a participant and its size is proportionate to the Mini-Mental State Examination score (disease severity). typical AD (tAD) individuals are shown in blue and posterior cortical atrophy (PCA) in green.

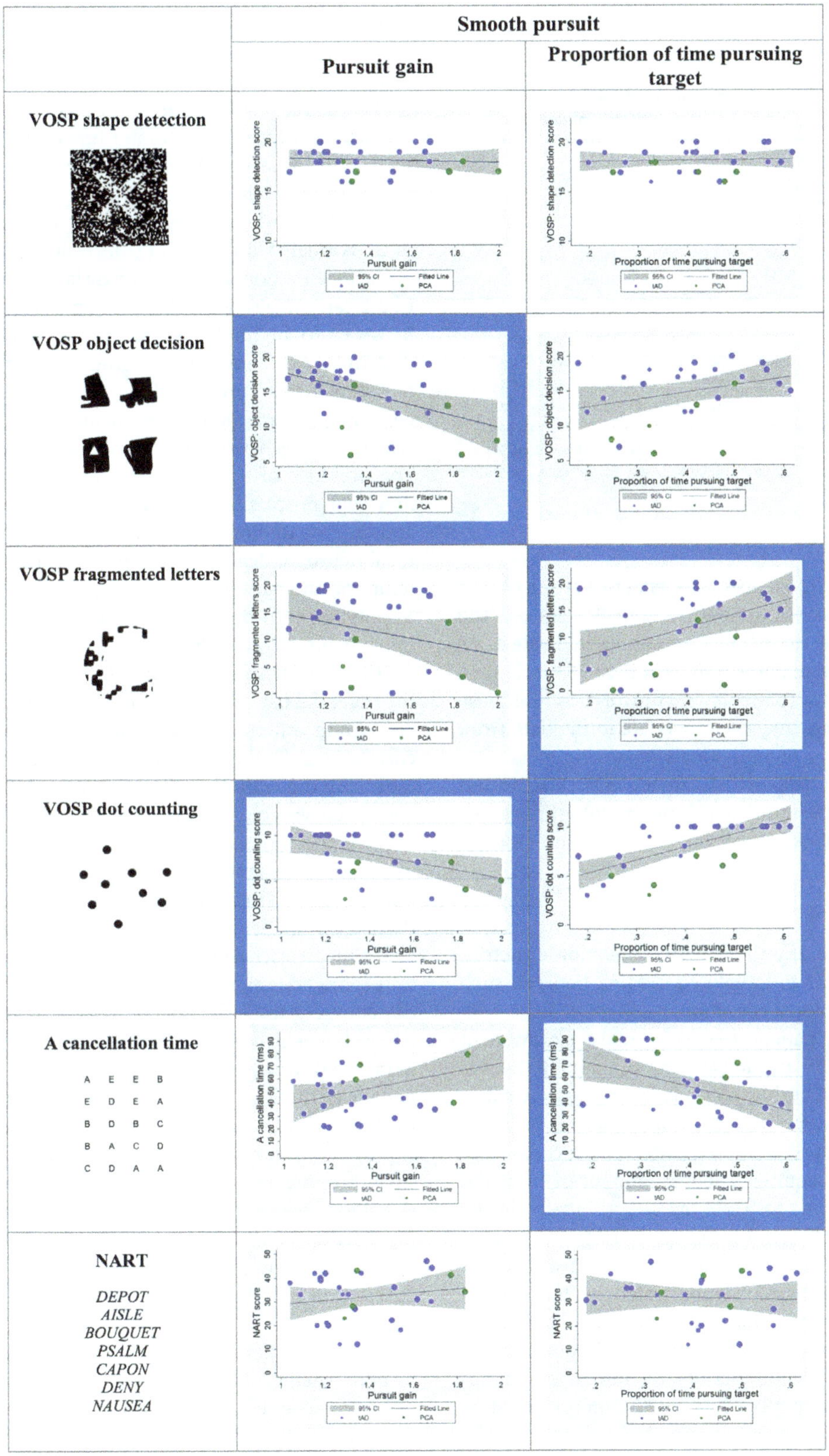

FIGURE 6 | Scatter plots showing correlations between smooth pursuit metrics and visual cognitive scores for young onset Alzheimer's disease patients. Statistically significant correlations are marked with a blue background and statistical trends ($p > 0.05$ and $p < 0.10$) in a lighter blue. Best fit line and 95% CI are shown. Each data point corresponds to a participant and its size is proportionate to the Mini-Mental State Examination score (disease severity). typical AD (tAD) individuals are shown in blue and posterior cortical atrophy (PCA) in green.

TABLE 4 | Table showing the results of cross-validation tests for the predictive power of the Bayesian logistic regression classifier.

Test	Actual diagnosis	Predicted diagnosis	
		Control	Young onset Alzheimer's disease (YOAD) patient
L-1-O	Control	0.95	0.05
	YOAD patient	0.03	0.97
L-2-O	Control	0.95	0.05
	YOAD patient	0.03	0.97
L-H-O	Control	0.94	0.06
	YOAD patient	0.04	0.96

Leave-one-out (L-1-O) tests take each individual in turn and train the classifier on all other individuals' feature vectors. The diagnostic status of that individual is predicted by the classifier and compared to the actual diagnosis (YOAD patient vs. control). Leave-two-out (L-2-O) tests take each possible pair of one control individual and one patient, train on all other individuals, and then predict the diagnosis of the original pair. The leave-half-out (L-H-O) test takes 500 random partitions of the data, with half of each diagnostic class in each partition, trains on one partition and predicts the diagnoses of the other. The columns of the table represent predicted diagnostic classes, and the rows represent actual diagnoses.

vectors generated as described above are effective at separating the patients in the dataset into their diagnostic classes. The results of each test for the experiment are shown in **Table 4**. As can be seen, the predicted diagnoses show at least 95% accuracy for both diagnostic classes (patients vs. controls). While these results are very promising, they do only relate to the data from a relatively small number of individuals on a single test. An expanded experimental set-up, with a larger sample size, would be able to further verify the utility of this methodology for accurately predicting the diagnoses of previously unseen individuals.

DISCUSSION

In the present study, we examined basic oculomotor metrics in individuals with YOAD and explored the link between such metrics and measures of visual cognition.

Results confirmed that patients have abnormal eye movement patterns in fixation stability, saccade and smooth pursuit tasks as compared to age-matched healthy controls. In the fixation stability task, YOAD patients showed a larger number of large intrusive saccades and shorter fixation duration. In the pro-saccade task, they were less accurate, required a longer amount of time and greater saccadic movements to fixate the target. Finally, in the smooth pursuit task, YOAD patients spent a shorter amount of time pursuing the target and made more interruptive saccades compared to controls. Results also demonstrated that these established basic control and movement metrics were significantly associated with measures of higher order visual cognition. In the fixation stability task the number of large intrusive saccades negatively correlated with performance in the object decision, fragmented letters and dot-counting tests. Pro-saccade metrics such as the time taken to reach the target and the number of saccades made in the process negatively correlated with object decision, fragmented letters, and dot-counting test scores. Additionally the "number of saccades necessary to reach the target" also correlated with shape detection scores and as the time taken to complete the "A" cancelation task. The eyetracking metrics extracted from the smooth pursuit task correlated with object decision, fragmented letters, dot counting and time to complete the "A" cancelation tests.

To our knowledge, this is the first time that the systematic impairment of basic oculomotor functions is reported in patients with young onset dementia as a single group and that the relationship between such impairment and visual cognition is explored.

Our data underline the extent of visual cognitive impairments in individuals with YOAD (18). Awareness of dementia-related visual dysfunction in tAD is increasing (11, 12, 55) but, especially in the early stages of the disease, sensitive measures are required in order to highlight subtle changes that can potentially be discriminated from normal aging. For example, a recent study has shown that an eyetracking behavioral task can predict the conversion from cognitively normal to MCI and from MCI to AD up to three years prior to a change in clinical diagnosis (56). The presence of both eye movement deficits and impairments in visual processing is in accordance with the neuroimaging and neuropathological literature showing that in AD multifocal neuronal degeneration affects visual areas in the occipital, temporal and parietal lobes (57–59) and subcortical regions such as pulvinar (60) that process visual information and orient eye movements accordingly (61, 62).

The present study provides preliminary evidence suggesting the potential use of eyetracking metrics as markers of high-level vision and other cognitive domains. Examining the pattern of correlations, it should be noted that some eyetracking metrics, especially the "number of saccades needed to fixate the target," correlated with most of the visual cognitive tests, possibly reflecting non-specific associations with disease severity or the ubiquity of pro-saccade generation deficits in YOAD patients. However, not all eyetracking metrics had such widespread associations. Particularly evident were the impact of "large intrusive saccades" and "time to reach a pro-saccade target" upon the visuoperceptual tests (object decision and fragmented letters) and the visuospatial dot-counting test. All three of these tests require scanning over relatively small visual areas and across multiple discrete perceptual items, all of which are relevant to the task demands. By contrast, neither of these eyetracking metrics was correlated significantly with the "A" cancelation test, in which visual attention must be deployed over a much wider visual area and across items, only a small proportion of which constitute task-relevant targets. Also possibly noteworthy are the significant correlations between the "proportion of time pursuing target" metric from the smooth pursuit task and the fragmented letter, dot counting and "A" cancelation tests. Unlike the other tests with which these correlations were not observed, these three tests all require participants to trace a specific continuous visual route through separated stimuli, whether that route pertains to the shape of a large letter (fragmented letter), the path through a group of dots that permits them to be counted (and not accidentally re-counted) in an efficient manner (dot counting), or the line-by-line orderly searching for target "A"s among other distractor letters (A cancelation).

Of equal note is the relative absence of correlations between eyetracking metrics and either shape detection or reading. In the case of shape detection, which was only correlated with the number of saccades required to reach the pro-saccade target, this may relate in part to the limited dynamic range of the test (all patient scores between 15 and 20 out of 20). However, for single word reading, with which there were no significant correlations and which with small print can be achieved in a single fixation, disordered eye movements such as large saccadic intrusions appear to have relatively little impact on accuracy (though note that reading latencies, if recorded, may have elicited a different result).

Naturally, such a qualitative examination of patterns of association has inherent limitations in determining causal relations between cognitive functions and observed behaviors. However, the current data arguably provide a useful starting point for generating testable hypotheses regarding the ability of certain eye movement patterns and paradigms to index specific cognitive abilities and deficits among dementia patients and other clinical populations.

Eyetracking-based measures of cognition may offer certain advantages over traditional pen and paper-based cognitive tests in some dementia contexts. Eyetracking data by definition do not suffer from ceiling and floor effects, which are instead common problems when exploring cognitive performance in patients (floor effect) and comparing it with performance in age-matched healthy controls (ceiling effect). Tasks such a fixation stability, saccade generation and smooth pursuit require minimal verbal instructions. Eye movement metrics derived from appropriate test designs may also be less vulnerable to the practice effects normally observed in standard cognitive testing, allowing for re-testing in the context of longitudinal assessments or before/after a trial phase.

One further potential advantage of eyetracking-based measures of visual cognition and other cognitive capacities is the type and scale of data generated. The large datasets that can be extracted in terms of time series of *x* and *y* coordinates open up new avenues of statistical analysis on individual trials. This may contribute to the design of shorter, less stressful cognitive assessments for patients. In the current study, we have provided proof of principle evidence for the feasibility of using an eyetracking dataset as the input for a machine-learning classification model to discriminate YOAD patients and controls on the basis of eye movements alone. While eyetracking in isolation is unlikely to ever be a primary determinant of clinical decision making, the application of a machine-learning approach to such examinations may add value in detecting change in at risk and presymptomatic individuals, monitoring progression over time (especially in the context of clinical trials), improving the discrimination and characterization disease and syndromic phenotypes.

The study had a number of potential limitations. First, the sample size was relatively small, and thus we have not been able to clarify whether the eye movement impairment is more widely a consequence of the disease severity rather than being a direct indication of visual cognition. Nonetheless, previous studies exploring eyetracking metrics in individuals affected by different types of dementia but matched for disease severity have shown that eye movement deficits can be disease-specific (33, 63). Second, the study did not include markers of focal and sustained attention, deficits in which may have contributed to both eyetracking metrics and visual cognition estimates. Third, we only found limited evidence of differences between PCA and tAD in terms of eyetracking metrics. This result can have several explanations. The PCA group size was very small and the individual variability within each group was very large, as is frequently described within this literature (28, 64, 65). This might reflect the biological reality of YOAD where a greater prevalence of visual deficits across the population has already been suggested (18) and/or the phenotypic continuum of visual impairment across the tAD-PCA spectrum (64, 66). To address further the issue of individual phenotypic differences, rather than a binary PCA/tAD diagnostic category, future studies involving a larger sample size should take into account the possibility of using a quantitative continuous metric of visual cognitive impairment, such as a ratio of memory to perceptual and/or spatial scores.

In conclusion, we have demonstrated that basic oculomotor metrics can provide information about not only the oculomotor system and its functionality *per se*, but also about high-level visual cognition. We have also shown that such metrics can be used in a machine-learning approach to discriminate between YOAD patients and healthy controls. Visual deficits represent a common feature in AD and eyetracking metrics may have potential as sensitive markers, particularly as outcome measures for clinical trials.

AUTHOR CONTRIBUTIONS

IP and SPrimativo: conception of the work, analysis and interpretation of data, drafting, final approval of the manuscript, and agreement to be accountable for all aspects of the work in ensuring that questions related to the accuracy or integrity of any part of the work are investigated and resolved. SParsons and DR: analysis of the data, drafting, final approval of the manuscript, and agreement to be accountable for all aspects of the work in ensuring that questions related to the accuracy or integrity of any part of the work are investigated and resolved. TS, CS, RP, KM, AC, KY, NFirth, AF, DA, JT, NFox, and JS: contribution to the conception and design of the study, collection of the data, revising it, final approval of the manuscript, and agreement to be accountable for all aspects of the work in ensuring that questions related to the accuracy or integrity of any part of the work are investigated and resolved. SC: conception of the work, interpretation of data, contributed to the drafting of the manuscript, final approval, and agreement to be accountable for all aspects of the work in ensuring that questions related to the accuracy or integrity of the work are investigated and resolved.

ACKNOWLEDGMENTS

This work was supported by Alzheimer's Research UK (ARUK 2012-6-ICE) and was undertaken at UCLH/UCL, which received a proportion of funding from the Department of Health's NIHR Biomedical Research funding scheme. The Dementia Research Centre is supported by Alzheimer's Research UK, Brain Research Trust, and The Wolfson Foundation. This work was supported by the NIHR Queen Square Dementia Biomedical Research Unit and by an Alzheimer's Research UK Senior Research Fellowship (ART-SRF2010-3) and ESRC/NIHR (ES/L001810/1) and EPSRC (EP/M006093/1) grants to SC. TS was supported by Alzheimer's Research UK Fellowship (ARUK-RF2013-5). The authors would also like to thank patients and controls for taking part in the study and Sam Hutton for his helpful suggestions in terms of data analysis.

REFERENCES

1. Alzheimer's Association. 2015 Alzheimer's disease facts and figures. *Alzheimers Dement* (2015) 11(3):332. doi:10.1016/j.jalz.2015.02.003
2. Dubois B, Feldman HH, Jacova C, Dekosky ST, Barberger-Gateau P, Cummings J, et al. Research criteria for the diagnosis of Alzheimer's disease: revising the NINCDS-ADRDA criteria. *Lancet Neurol* (2007) 6(8):734–46. doi:10.1016/S1474-4422(07)70178-3
3. Dubois B, Feldman HH, Jacova C, Cummings JL, Dekosky ST, Barberger-Gateau P, et al. Revising the definition of Alzheimer's disease: a new lexicon. *Lancet Neurol* (2010) 9(11):1118–27. doi:10.1016/S1474-4422(10)70223-4
4. Dubois B, Feldman HH, Jacova C, Hampel H, Molinuevo JL, Blennow K, et al. Advancing research diagnostic criteria for Alzheimer's disease: the IWG-2 criteria. *Lancet Neurol* (2014) 13(6):614–29. doi:10.1016/S1474-4422(14)70090-0
5. McKhann GM, Knopman DS, Chertkow H, Hyman BT, Jack CR, Kawas CH, et al. The diagnosis of dementia due to Alzheimer's disease: recommendations from the national institute on aging-Alzheimer's association workgroups on diagnostic guidelines for Alzheimer's disease. *Alzheimers Dement* (2011) 7(3):263–9. doi:10.1016/j.jalz.2011.03.005
6. Doody RS, Thomas RG, Farlow M, Iwatsubo T, Vellas B, Joffe S, et al. Phase 3 trials of solanezumab for mild-to-moderate Alzheimer's disease. *N Engl J Med* (2014) 370(4):311–21. doi:10.1056/NEJMoa1312889
7. Gauthier S, Feldman HH, Schneider LS, Wilcock GK, Frisoni GB, Hardlund JH, et al. Efficacy and safety of tau-aggregation inhibitor therapy in patients with mild or moderate Alzheimer's disease: a randomised, controlled, double-blind, parallel-arm, phase 3 trial. *Lancet* (2016) 388(10062):2873–84. doi:10.1016/S0140-6736(16)31275-2
8. Weintraub S, Wicklund AH, Salmon DP. The neuropsychological profile of Alzheimer disease. *Cold Spring Harb Perspect Med* (2012) 2(4):a006171. doi:10.1101/cshperspect.a006171
9. Hodges JR. Alzheimer's centennial legacy: origins, landmarks and the current status of knowledge concerning cognitive aspects. *Brain* (2006) 129(11):2811–22. doi:10.1093/brain/awl275
10. Kirby E, Bandelow S, Hogervorst E. Visual impairment in Alzheimer's disease: a critical review. *J Alzheimers Dis* (2010) 21(1):15–34. doi:10.3233/JAD-2010-080785
11. Cronin-Golomb A, Corkin S, Rizzo JF, Cohen J, Growdon JH, Banks KS. Visual dysfunction in Alzheimer's disease: relation to normal aging. *Ann Neurol* (1991) 29(1):41–52. doi:10.1002/ana.410290110
12. Mendola JD, Cronin-Golomb A, Corkin S, Growdon JH. Prevalence of visual deficits in Alzheimer's disease. *Optom Vis Sci* (1995) 72(3):155–67. doi:10.1097/00006324-199503000-00003
13. Rizzo M, Anderson SW, Dawson J, Nawrot M. Vision and cognition in Alzheimer's disease. *Neuropsychologia* (2000) 38(8):1157–69. doi:10.1016/S0028-3932(00)00023-3
14. Kurylo DD, Corkin S, Rizzo JF, Growdon JH. Greater relative impairment of object recognition than of visuospatial abilities in Alzheimer's disease. *Neuropsychology* (1996) 10:74–81. doi:10.1037/0894-4105.10.1.74
15. Rizzo M, Nawrot M. Perception of movement and shape in Alzheimer's disease. *Brain* (1998) 121(12):2259–70. doi:10.1093/brain/121.12.2259
16. Uhlmann RF, Larson EB, Koepsell TD, Rees TS, Duckert LG. Visual impairment and cognitive dysfunction in Alzheimer's disease. *J Gen Intern Med* (1991) 6(2):126–32. doi:10.1007/BF02598307
17. Cronin-Golomb A, Gilmore GC, Neargarder S, Morrison SR, Laudate TM. Enhanced stimulus strength improves visual cognition in aging and Alzheimer's disease. *Cortex* (2007) 43(7):952–66. doi:10.1016/S0010-9452(08)70693-2
18. Fujimori M, Imamura T, Yamashita H, Hirono N, Ikejiri Y, Shimomura T, et al. Age at onset and visuocognitive disturbances in Alzheimer disease. *Alzheimer Dis Assoc Disord* (1998) 12(3):163–6. doi:10.1097/00002093-199809000-00007
19. Cronin-Golomb A, Sugiura R, Corkin S, Growdon JH. Incomplete achromatopsia in Alzheimer's disease. *Neurobiol Aging* (1993) 14(5):471–7. doi:10.1016/0197-4580(93)90105-K
20. Benson D, Davis R, Snyder BD. Posterior cortical atrophy. *Arch Neurol* (1988) 45(7):789–93. doi:10.1001/archneur.1988.00520310107024
21. Mendez MF, Ghajarania M, Perryman KM. Posterior cortical atrophy: clinical characteristics and differences compared to Alzheimer's disease. *Dement Geriatr Cogn Disord* (2002) 14(1):33–40. doi:10.1159/000058331
22. Tang-Wai DF, Graff-Radford NR, Boeve BF, Dickson DW, Parisi JE, Crook R, et al. Clinical, genetic, and neuropathologic characteristics of posterior cortical atrophy. *Neurology* (2004) 63(7):1168–74. doi:10.1212/01.WNL.0000140289.18472.15
23. Crutch SJ, Schott JM, Rabinovici GD, Murray M, Snowden JS, van der Flier WM, et al. Consensus classification of posterior cortical atrophy. *Alzheimers Dement* (2017). doi:10.1016/j.jalz.2017.01.014
24. Ridgway GR, Lehmann M, Barnes J, Rohrer JD, Warren JD, Crutch SJ, et al. Early-onset Alzheimer disease clinical variants. *Neurology* (2012) 79(1):80–4. doi:10.1212/WNL.0b013e31825dce28
25. Renner JA, Burns JM, Hou CE, McKeel DW, Storandt M, Morris JC. Progressive posterior cortical dysfunction: a clinicopathologic series. *Neurology* (2004) 63(7):1175–80. doi:10.1212/01.WNL.0000140290.80962.BF
26. Charles RF, Hillis AE. Posterior cortical atrophy: clinical presentation and cognitive deficits compared to Alzheimer's disease. *Behav Neurol* (2005) 16(1):15–23. doi:10.1155/2005/762569
27. McMonagle P, Deering F, Berliner Y, Kertesz A. The cognitive profile of posterior cortical atrophy. *Neurology* (2006) 66(3):331–8. doi:10.1212/01.wnl.0000196477.78548.db
28. Lehmann M, Barnes J, Ridgway GR, Wattam-Bell J, Warrington EK, Fox NC, et al. Basic visual function and cortical thickness patterns in posterior cortical atrophy. *Cereb Cortex* (2011) 21(9):2122–32. doi:10.1093/cercor/bhq287
29. Shakespeare TJ, Kaski D, Yong KX, Paterson RW, Slattery CF, Ryan NS, et al. Abnormalities of fixation, saccade and pursuit in posterior cortical atrophy. *Brain* (2015) 138(7):1976–91. doi:10.1093/brain/awv103
30. Michaelis JR, McConnell DS, Smither JA. Attention deficit/hyperactivity disorder's effects on individuals' scan paths during a simulated drive. *Work* (2012) 41(Suppl 1):5833–5. doi:10.3233/WOR-2012-0967-5833
31. Sasson NJ, Elison JT. Eye tracking young children with autism. *J Vis Exp* (2012) 61:3675. doi:10.3791/3675
32. Molitor RJ, Ko PC, Ally BA. Eye movements in Alzheimer's disease. *J Alzheimers Dis* (2015) 44(1):1–12. doi:10.3233/JAD-141173
33. Boxer AL, Garbutt S, Seeley WW, Jafari A, Heuer HW, Mirsky J, et al. Saccade abnormalities in autopsy-confirmed frontotemporal lobar degeneration and Alzheimer disease. *Arch Neurol* (2012) 69(4):509–17. doi:10.1001/archneurol.2011.1021
34. Fletcher WA, Sharpe JA. Saccadic eye movement dysfunction in Alzheimer's disease. *Ann Neurol* (1986) 20(4):464–71. doi:10.1002/ana.410200405
35. Bylsma FW, Rasmusson DX, Rebok GW, Keyl PM, Tune L, Brandt J. Changes in visual fixation and saccadic eye movements in Alzheimer's disease. *Int J Psychophysiol* (1995) 19(1):33–40. doi:10.1016/0167-8760(94)00060-R
36. Yang Q, Wang T, Su N, Liu Y, Xiao S, Kapoula Z. Long latency and high variability in accuracy-speed of prosaccades in Alzheimer's disease at mild to moderate stage. *Dement Geriatr Cogn Dis Extra* (2011) 1(1):318–29. doi:10.1159/000333080
37. Yang Q, Wang T, Su N, Xiao S, Kapoula Z. Specific saccade deficits in patients with Alzheimer's disease at mild to moderate stage and in patients with amnestic mild cognitive impairment. *Age (Dordr)* (2013) 35(4):1287–98. doi:10.1007/s11357-012-9420-z
38. Garbutt S, Matlin A, Hellmuth J, Schenk AK, Johnson JK, Rosen H, et al. Oculomotor function in frontotemporal lobar degeneration, related disorders

and Alzheimer's disease. *Brain* (2007) 131(5):1268–81. doi:10.1093/brain/awn047

39. Abel LA, Bowman EA, Velakoulis D, Fahey MC, Desmond P, Macfarlane MD, et al. Saccadic eye movement characteristics in adult Niemann-pick type C disease: relationships with disease severity and brain structural measures. *PLoS One* (2012) 7(11):e50947. doi:10.1371/journal.pone.0050947
40. Crawford TJ, Higham S, Renvoize T, Patel J, Dale M, Suriya A, et al. Inhibitory control of saccadic eye movements and cognitive impairment in Alzheimer's disease. *Biol Psychiatry* (2005) 57(9):1052–60. doi:10.1016/j.biopsych.2005.01.017
41. Shafiq-Antonacci R, Maruff P, Masters C, Currie J. Spectrum of saccade system function in Alzheimer disease. *Arch Neurol* (2003) 60(9):1272–8. doi:10.1001/archneur.60.9.1272
42. Pereira MLF, Camargo MV, Aprahamian I, Forlenza OV. Eye movement analysis and cognitive processing: detecting indicators of conversion to Alzheimer's disease. *Neuropsychiatr Dis Treat* (2014) 10:1273–85. doi:10.2147/NDT.S55371
43. Forssman L, Ashorn P, Ashorn U, Maleta K, Matchado A, Kortekangas E, et al. Eye-tracking-based assessment of cognitive function in low-resource settings. *Arch Dis Child* (2016) 102(4):301–2. doi:10.1136/archdischild-2016-310525
44. Crutcher MD, Calhoun-Haney R, Manzanares CM, Lah JJ, Levey AI, Zola SM. Eye tracking during a visual paired comparison task as a predictor of early dementia. *Am J Alzheimers Dis Other Demen* (2009) 24(3):258–66. doi:10.1177/1533317509332093
45. Richmond J, Sowerby P, Colombo M, Hayne H. The effect of familiarization time, retention interval, and context change on adults' performance in the visual paired-comparison task. *Dev Psychobiol* (2004) 44(2):146–55. doi:10.1002/dev.10161
46. Fernández G, Manes F, Rotstein NP, Colombo O, Mandolesi P, Politi LE, et al. Lack of contextual-word predictability during reading in patients with mild Alzheimer disease. *Neuropsychologia* (2014) 62:143–51. doi:10.1016/j.neuropsychologia.2014.07.023
47. Costa L, Gago MF, Yelshyna D, Ferreira J, David Silva H, Rocha L, et al. Application of machine learning in postural control kinematics for the diagnosis of Alzheimer's disease. *Comput Intell Neurosci* (2016) 2016:15. doi:10.1155/2016/3891253
48. Warrington EK, James M. *Visual Object and Space Perception Battery (VOSP).* Pearson Assessment (2017). Available from: http://www.pearson-clinical.co.uk/Psychology/AdultCognitionNeuropsychologyandLanguage/AdultPerceptionandVisuomotorAbilities/VisualObjectandSpacePerception-Battery(VOSP)/VisualObjectandSpacePerceptionBattery(VOSP).aspx
49. Willison JR, Warrington EK. Cognitive retardation in a patient with preservation of psychomotor speed. *Behav Neurol* (1992) 5(2):113–6. doi:10.3233/BEN-1992-5207
50. Nelson HE. *National Adult Reading Test.* Windsor: NFER-Nelson (1982).
51. Crossland MD, Rubin GS. The use of an infrared eyetracker to measure fixation stability. *Optom Vis Sci* (2002) 79(11):735–9. doi:10.1097/00006324-200211000-00011
52. Zee DS, Leigh RJ. *The Neurology of Eye Movements.* Oxford: Oxford University Press (2006).
53. Baum LE, Petrie T. Statistical inference for probabilistic functions of finite state Markov chains. *Ann Math Stat* (1966) 37(6):1554–63. doi:10.1214/aoms/1177699147
54. Dempster AP, Laird NM, Rubin DB. Maximum likelihood from incomplete data via the EM algorithm. *J R Stat Soc Ser B Methodol* (1977) 39:1–38.
55. Cronin-Golomb A, Corkin S, Growdon JH. Visual dysfunction predicts cognitive deficits in Alzheimer's disease. *Optom Vis Sci* (1995) 72(3):168–76. doi:10.1097/00006324-199503000-00004
56. Zola SM, Manzanares CM, Clopton P, Lah JJ, Levey AI. A behavioral task predicts conversion to mild cognitive impairment and Alzheimer's disease. *Am J Alzheimers Dis Other Demen* (2013) 28(2):179–84. doi:10.1177/1533317512470484
57. Beach TG, McGeer EG. Cholinergic fiber loss occurs in the absence of synaptophysin depletion in Alzheimer's disease primary visual cortex. *Neurosci Lett* (1992) 142(2):253–6. doi:10.1016/0304-3940(92)90385-K
58. Buck BH, Black SE, Behrmann M, Caldwell C, Bronskill MJ. Spatial- and object-based attentional deficits in Alzheimer's disease. Relationship to HMPAO-SPECT measures of parietal perfusion. *Brain* (1997) 120(7):1229–44. doi:10.1093/brain/120.7.1229
59. Mielke R, Kessler J, Fink G, Herholz K, Heiss W-D. Dysfunction of visual cortex contributes to disturbed processing of visual information in Alzheimer's disease. *Int J Neurosci* (1995) 82(1–2):1–9. doi:10.3109/00207459508994285
60. Kuljis RO. Lesions in the pulvinar in patients with Alzheimer's disease. *J Neuropathol Exp Neurol* (1994) 53(2):202–11. doi:10.1097/00005072-199403000-00012
61. Ogren MP, Mateer CA, Wyler AR. Alterations in visually related eye movements following left pulvinar damage in man. *Neuropsychologia* (1984) 22(2):187–96. doi:10.1016/0028-3932(84)90061-7
62. Robinson DL, Petersen SE. Responses of pulvinar neurons to real and self-induced stimulus movement. *Brain Res* (1985) 338(2):392–4. doi:10.1016/0006-8993(85)90176-3
63. Boxer AL, Garbutt S, Rankin KP, Hellmuth J, Neuhaus J, Miller BL, et al. Medial versus lateral frontal lobe contributions to voluntary saccade control as revealed by the study of patients with frontal lobe degeneration. *J Neurosci* (2006) 26(23):6354–63. doi:10.1523/JNEUROSCI.0549-06.2006
64. Crutch SJ, Lehmann M, Schott JM, Rabinovici GD, Rossor MN, Fox NC. Posterior cortical atrophy. *Lancet Neurol* (2012) 11(2):170–8. doi:10.1016/S1474-4422(11)70289-7
65. Primativo S, Yong KX, Shakespeare TJ, Crutch SJ. The oral spelling profile of posterior cortical atrophy and the nature of the graphemic representation. *Neuropsychologia* (2017) 94:61–74. doi:10.1016/j.neuropsychologia.2016.11.021
66. Migliaccio R, Agosta F, Rascovsky K, Karydas A, Bonasera S, Rabinovici GD, et al. Clinical syndromes associated with posterior atrophy early age at onset AD spectrum. *Neurology* (2009) 73(19):1571–8. doi:10.1212/WNL.0b013e3181c0d427
67. Folstein MF, Folstein SE, McHugh PR. "Mini-mental state". A practical method for grading the cognitive state of patients for the clinician. *J Psychiatr Res* (1975) 12(3):189–98.
68. Warrington E, James M, Plant GT. *CORVIST: Cortical Vision Screening Test: Manual & Test Materials.* Thames Valley Test Company. (2001).
69. Wechsler D. *Wechsler Abbreviated Scale of Intelligence (WASI) Manual.* The Psychological Corporation (1999).
70. Wechsler D. A standardized memory scale for clinical use. *J Psychol* (1945) 19(1):87–95.
71. Warrington EK. *The Camden Memory Tests.* Psychology Press (1996). 140 p.
72. Jackson M, Warrington EK. Arithmetic skills in patients with unilateral cerebral lesions. *Cortex* (1986) 22(4):611–20.

4

Spontaneous Nystagmus in the Dark in an Infantile Nystagmus Patient may Represent Negative Optokinetic Afternystagmus

*Ting-Feng Lin[1,2], Christina Gerth-Kahlert[3], James V. M. Hanson[3,4], Dominik Straumann[1,2] and Melody Ying-Yu Huang[1,2]**

[1] Department of Neurology, University Hospital Zurich, University of Zurich, Zurich, Switzerland, [2] Neuroscience Center Zurich (ZNZ), University of Zurich and ETH Zurich, Zurich, Switzerland, [3] Department of Ophthalmology, University Hospital Zurich, Zurich, Switzerland, [4] Neuroimmunology and Multiple Sclerosis Research, Clinic for Neurology, University Hospital Zurich, University of Zurich, Zurich, Switzerland

Correspondence:
Melody Ying-Yu Huang
melody.yingyu.huang@gmail.com

Abnormal projection of the optic nerves to the wrong cerebral hemisphere transforms the optokinetic system from its usual negative feedback loop to a positive feedback loop with characteristic ocular motor instabilities including directional reversal of the optokinetic nystagmus (OKN) and spontaneous nystagmus, which are common features of infantile nystagmus syndrome (INS). Visual input plays a critical role in INS linked to an underlying optic nerve misprojection such as that often seen in albinism. However, spontaneous nystagmus often continues in darkness, making the visual, sensory-driven etiology questionable. We propose that sensorimotor adaptation during the constant nystagmus of patients in the light could account for continuing nystagmus in the dark. The OKN is a stereotyped reflexive eye movement in response to motion in the surround and serves to stabilize the visual image on the retina, allowing high resolution vision. Robust negative optokinetic afternystagmus (negative OKAN), referring to the continuous nystagmus in the dark with opposite beating direction of the preceding OKN, has been identified in various non-foveated animals. In humans, a robust afternystagmus in the same direction as previous smooth-pursuit movements (the eye's continuous tracking and foveation of a moving target) induced by visual stimuli has been known to commonly mask negative OKAN. Some INS patients are often associated with ocular hypopigmentation, foveal hypoplasia, and compromised smooth pursuit. We identified an INS case with negative OKAN in the dark, in contrast to the positive afternystagmus in healthy subjects. We hypothesize that spontaneous nystagmus in the dark in INS patients may be attributable to sensory adaptation in the optokinetic system after a sustained period of spontaneous nystagmus with directional visual input in light.

Keywords: infantile nystagmus syndrome, optokinetic response, optokinetic afternystagmus, smooth pursuit, smooth pursuit afternystagmus, albinism

INTRODUCTION

Infantile nystagmus syndrome (INS), also known as congenital nystagmus, is an ocular motor disorder which is commonly identified in infants less than 2–3 months old (1). INS patients usually exhibit involuntary horizontal eye movements (1). Genetic sequences have suggested that a variety of gene mutations lead to the disruption of neurophysiological functions in afferent visual pathways, ocular motor system, and the mechanisms involved with extraocular muscle innervations (2). Different disease mechanisms and models have been proposed for INS: Yonehara et al. reported that the FRMD7 gene mutation caused a significantly reduced asymmetric inhibition of starburst amacrine cells to direction-selective ganglion cells in the retina (3). Huang and colleagues suggested that a positive feedback optokinetic controlling system underlying optic nerve fiber misrouting can lead to INS-like ocular motor behaviors in animal models and in humans (4–7). Earlier, Optican and Zee also proposed a positive feedback loop model which results in an unstable neural integrator (8). Jacobs and Dell'Osso developed a model based on an underdamped smooth-pursuit system (9, 10). Further, Brodsky and Dell'Osso proposed that malfunction of the smooth-pursuit system would cause an uncontrolled optokinetic system (11). Harris and Berry suggested that abnormal eye oscillations may develop due to a poor, high spatial frequency, contrast sensitivity (12, 13). Akman et al. used a nonlinear dynamics model based on an abnormal saccadic system to predict nystagmus (14). Berg et al. reported changes to extraocular muscle properties in INS patients, which suggested an adaptation mechanism at the effector level due to deficient motor innervations (15). Even though all of these models were proposed to help explain the pathological mechanism underlying INS, to date no consensus exists as to which is most credible (2).

Among the known genetic mutations, there is a group of patients who share a common pathological phenotype, ocular hypopigmentation, which is caused by the reduction of melanogenesis. Oculocutaneous albinism (OCA) is an autosomal-recessive disorder in which pigmentation of the hair, skin, and eyes is reduced (16). Ocular albinism (OA) is an X-linked disorder, which shows hypopigmentation only in the eyes (17, 18). All types of OCA and OA patients have been reported to exhibit INS (17–25). Huang et al. demonstrated that the zebrafish mutant *belladonna* (*bel*), which exhibit abnormal retinal ganglion cell (RGC) projections (a defect also commonly found in albino patients), exhibited reversed optokinetic nystagmus (OKN) and spontaneous nystagmus, both of which are often seen in INS patients (4, 5). In a subsequent publication, the same authors demonstrated that the nystagmic eye movements found in *bel* qualitatively resemble those seen in INS patients (26). It was proposed that the reversed OKN and spontaneous nystagmus were caused by the underlying abnormal RGC projection causing a transformation of the optokinetic system from a negative feedback loop to a positive feedback loop (4, 6). With normal negative feedback control, the retinal slip velocity is used as the error signal, which drives the eyes to move with the moving surround in order to reduce the retinal slip; in contrast, the motor output (i.e., eye movement) of a positive feedback loop would further increase the error signal (i.e., retinal slip velocity). However, while data from INS models (4–7) supporting the abnormal pathway hypothesis of INS can be taken as evidence for the causal role of afferent visual deficits, one remaining challenge is elucidating how the primary sensory input contributes to the pathological mechanism of INS without visual input, since patients also show nystagmus in the dark (27). Shawkat reported the spontaneous reversal of nystagmus beating direction in the dark in manifest latent nystagmus (MLN) and INS patients (28). While the author proposed the non-seeing eye in these patients as the potentially dominant eye and adapted the MLN mechanism to explain the nystagmus in the dark, the evident reversal of nystagmus beating directions from light to dark could actually be attributed to a visual sensory adaptation during the nystagmus in the light.

Both smooth-pursuit and optokinetic ocular motor subsystems have been suggested to contribute to the pathological eye movements in INS (2, 11). Smooth pursuit (or foveal pursuit) refers to the voluntary tracking of moving objects *via* cortical pursuit pathways (11, 27). During the foveal smooth pursuit, it is necessary for the visual target to be located in the visual field of the fovea or, in the case of perifoveal smooth pursuit, perifovea so that the eyes can lock onto the target (27); in other words, a functional fovea is essential in order to perform smooth pursuit. Continued smooth-pursuit behavior was reported to induce an afternystagmus in darkness in the same beating direction for at least 3 min (29). Afoveation is commonly found in INS patients, of whom many are affected with albinism (2). Thus, it is conceivable that smooth-pursuit function may be compromised in INS due to afoveation as well as the nystagmic eye movements. The subcortical optokinetic pathways are responsible for the OKN, which is an involuntary tracking of a moving surround or a large field of motion in the surround (11, 30). Positive optokinetic afternystagmus (OKAN) describes a short-lived (<1 min) persisting eye movement in darkness after the cessation of optokinetic stimulation (31–33). Besides positive OKAN, a reversed afternystagmus (i.e., associated with beating in the opposite direction) of longer duration has been reported in different species including human adults (32), infants (34), monkeys (35, 36), rabbits (37–39), cats (40, 41), and rats (42). This condition is also known as negative OKAN or, in some cases, secondary OKAN or reversed post-optokinetic nystagmus. However, the underlying mechanisms relating to this phenomenon remain unknown and existing studies show wide variability. In general, the presence of negative OKAN depends on the duration of the optokinetic stimulation. Animal studies have shown that a longer period of stimulation leads to a shorter positive OKAN followed by a longer negative OKAN (36, 39).

Abnormal binocular vision (i.e., monocular occlusion or strabismus) has been reported to result in impaired smooth-pursuit function, which may further lead to lack of the normal cortical suppression of the optokinetic pathways by the smooth-pursuit system (11, 28, 43, 44). Based on clinical observations of the spontaneous reversal of nystagmus beating direction in darkness in MLN patients with single healthy eyes or an INS patient with convergent strabismus (28), and the robust negative OKAN observed in animals lacking evident smooth-pursuit functions (37, 38, 42), we propose a new hypothesis of the pathological mechanism underlying INS in darkness. The nystagmus in darkness can develop *via* an adaptive process in the optokinetic system during a sustained period of spontaneous nystagmus in the light. In our present study, we recorded a clear negative OKAN in an INS patient with iris transillumination and foveal hypoplasia. In a healthy subject examined using the same experimental paradigm, we observed an aftereffect of eye movements predominantly in the same direction of the preceding stimulus, which we believed

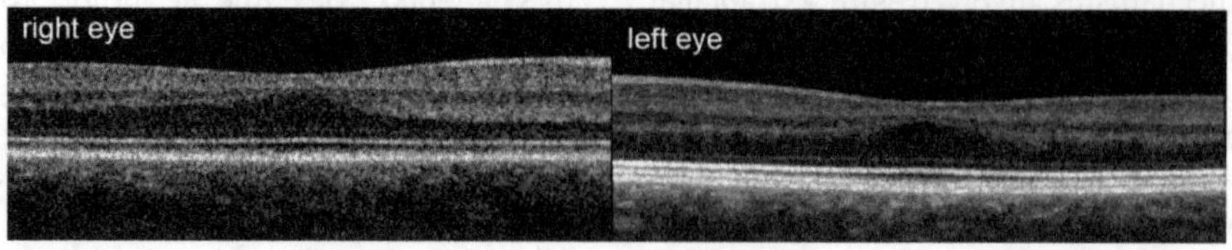

FIGURE 1 | Optical coherence tomography scan showed the foveal hypoplasia.

to be afternystagmus following smooth pursuit. Until now, there has been no plausible explanation for the occurrence of the spontaneous nystagmus in darkness following the visual input-related nystagmus in the light, which brings into question the role of aberrant visual sensory processing in INS etiology (4, 6). Based on the outcome of our current study, we hypothesize that nystagmus in the dark in INS patients may be a result of sensorimotor adaptation in the optokinetic system, *via* a similar adaptive process to that observed commonly in afoveated animals and manifested as negative OKAN.

MATERIALS AND METHODS

Medical Information of the Participants

This was an observational study on a 19-year-old female INS patient with mild OCA. The diagnosis was based on the results of the clinical examination; no genetic analysis was performed. There was no family history of OCA or OA. Visual acuity with her myopic astigmatism corrected was 20/50 and 20/40 in the right and left eye, respectively. Ophthalmological examination revealed iris transillumination, chorioretinal hypopigmentation, and macular hypoplasia, but no optic nerve hypoplasia. Foveal hypoplasia was defined as grade 2 to 3 in both eyes (45) by optical coherence tomography (OCT) (**Figure 1**). Analysis of multi-channel pattern-appearance visual evoked potentials (VEP) revealed asymmetric response localization over the two cerebral hemispheres consistent with previously described findings in albinism (**Figure 2**) (46).

The healthy subject was a 29-year-old male, who had no ocular or ocular motor abnormalities. Both subjects described herein gave their informed consent for inclusion in this report.

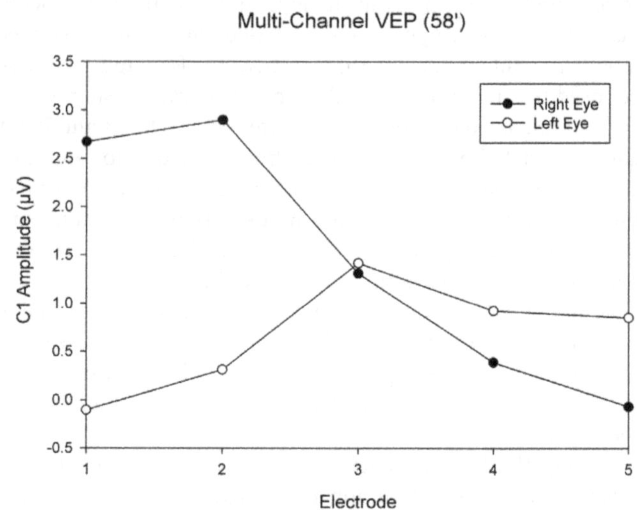

FIGURE 2 | Visual evoked potential (VEP) topography revealed asymmetric response localization over the two cerebral hemispheres in the left and right eye pattern onset responses.

Experimental Apparatus

Subjects sat upright on a fixed chair surrounded by a custom-built optokinetic drum, which was constructed by a horizontally rotatable cylinder (radius: 74 cm) painted with black and white vertical stripes of width: 9.69 cm (spatial frequency 0.067 cycles/degree). The rotation of the optokinetic drum was driven by a servo-controlled motor-driven axes turntable system (Acutrol® ACT2000, Acutronic, Switzerland Ltd.). A remotely controlled light source was mounted on the ceiling of the cylinder. During the recording, the subject was restrained by safety belts around the feet and trunk with the head being stabilized by a headrest.

Recording of Eye Movements

Horizontal eye movements were recorded using a head-mounted monocular video-oculography (VOG) device (EyeSeeCam), running at 220 Hz (47, 48), employing an infrared light source and an infrared sensitive camera. Pupil positions were detected by the camera and analyzed by the VOG system online. Eye positions were calibrated before each recording and the data were analyzed offline by custom-built software written in MATLAB (Mathworks, Natick, MA, USA), version (R2014a).

Experimental Procedure

Before the experiment, the INS patient was first tested for directional bias of eye beating in each eye. The patient sat inside the optokinetic drum and was instructed to look at the stationary vertical stripes for 5 min. During the monocular testing, only the viewing eye was recorded. After both eyes were tested, the left eye was chosen for the subsequent optokinetic test as it showed less directional bias during its spontaneous nystagmus. The control subject showed no clear eye dominance and, therefore, the left eye was also chosen for the test.

During the experiment, the left eye position was recorded while the right eye was covered by soft tissues. The subject was recorded in complete darkness for 1 min followed by a 10-min optokinetic stimulation with a constant stimulus velocity of 30°/s in the clockwise direction. Subsequently, the light was switched off for another minute before the stimulus changed to the counterclockwise direction for another 10-min period. The experiment was concluded with another 1-min recording in total darkness. During the optokinetic stimulation, subjects were instructed to follow the horizontally moving vertical stripes. Left eye movements were recorded throughout the entire experimental procedure.

RESULTS

During the optokinetic stimulation with a constant stimulus velocity of 30°/s in both clockwise and counterclockwise directions, the INS patient showed a reversed optokinetic eye reflex (**Figures 3A,C**); by contrast, the healthy subject displayed a typical optokinetic eye reflex with the slow tracking eye movement in the same direction of the drum rotation (**Figures 4A,C**). After the clockwise optokinetic stimulation, the eye movements of the healthy subject continued in the same direction, with reduced velocity, in the subsequent complete darkness (**Figure 4B**); in contrast to this, eye movements of the INS patient reversed, with the eye beating in the opposite direction (**Figure 3B**). In the complete darkness following counterclockwise optokinetic stimulation, the eye movements of the healthy subject continued with reduced velocity mainly in the same direction, but with occasional isolated reversed beatings (**Figure 4D**). In the case of the INS patient, interestingly, eye movements continued in the same beating direction in complete darkness during the first 50 s and then reversed to the opposite direction (**Figure 3D**). However, under binocular viewing conditions, both the forward afternystagmus in the healthy and the reversed afternystagmus in the INS patient were much more pronounced (data not shown).

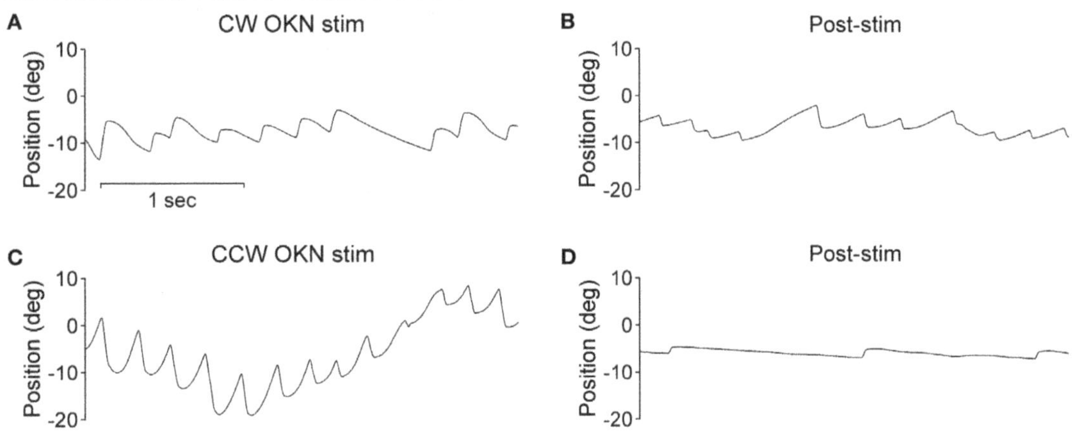

FIGURE 3 | Optokinetic nystagmus (OKN) and afternystagmus of the infantile nystagmus syndrome patient. Plots on the left demonstrate eye position traces during optokinetic stimulation in **(A)** CW (clockwise) and **(C)** CCW (counterclockwise) directions. Plots on the right demonstrate eye position traces in darkness subsequent to the 10-min optokinetic stimulations in **(B)** CW (clockwise) and **(D)** CCW (counterclockwise) directions. OKN stim, optokinetic stimulation phase; post-stim, post-stimulation phase.

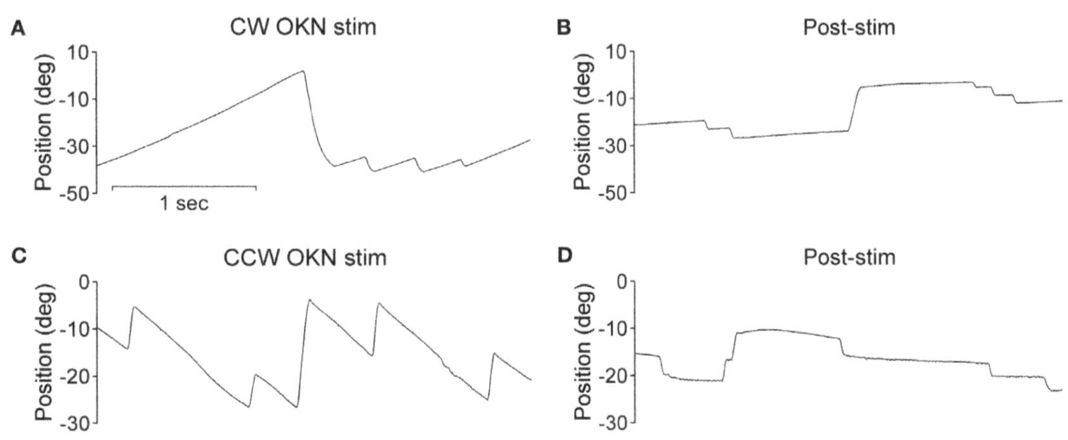

FIGURE 4 | Optokinetic nystagmus (OKN) and afternystagmus of the healthy subject. Plots on the left demonstrate eye position traces during optokinetic stimulation in **(A)** CW (clockwise) and **(C)** CCW (counterclockwise) directions. Plots on the right demonstrate eye position traces in darkness subsequent to the 10-min optokinetic stimulations in **(B)** CW (clockwise) and **(D)** CCW (counterclockwise) directions. OKN stim, optokinetic stimulation phase; post-stim, post-stimulation phase.

To better visualize the directional relationship of the eye velocities over time under different visual conditions, we computed the velocity distribution of the eye movements in each viewing condition within time windows of 20 s. Data numbers were plotted versus velocity ranks (every 1°/s) and we compared the three 20-s time windows of the pre-stimulation dark phase (eye movements in darkness before the stimulation), the final 20 s of the optokinetic stimulation phases, and the three 20-s time windows of the post-stimulation dark phases (eye movements in darkness after optokinetic stimulation) (**Figure 5**). The healthy subject's eye velocity distribution peaks fell tightly around 0°/s for all three 20-s periods of the pre-stimulation dark phase (**Figures 5A,B**); in comparison, the INS patient showed a broader velocity distribution, as well as a directional bias toward the positive velocity (i.e., clockwise direction) during the pre-stimulation dark phase (**Figures 5C,D**). However, during this 1-min dark period the eye velocity markedly reduced over time with the distribution peak shifting toward 0°/s (**Figures 5C,D**).

During the final 20 s of the optokinetic stimulation phases in both directions, the healthy subject showed clear velocity distributions consistent with the stimulus directions (**Figures 5A,B**); however, the INS patient showed a broad velocity distribution with more data falling over velocities in the opposite direction of the stimulus (**Figures 5C,D**). After the clockwise optokinetic stimulation, the healthy subject showed a clear data distribution over velocities in the same direction as during the stimulation phase (**Figure 5A**); for the post counterclockwise optokinetic stimulation phase, the healthy subject again showed a data distribution over velocities in the same direction as during the stimulation phase (**Figure 5B**). Moreover, the velocity distributions of both post-stimulation dark phases were broader than in the pre-stimulation dark phase (**Figures 5A,B**). After the clockwise optokinetic stimulation, the INS patient showed a data distribution over velocities in the opposite direction compared to the stimulation phase (**Figure 5C**). However, after the counterclockwise optokinetic stimulation, the patient showed a data distribution first over velocities in the same direction as during the stimulation phase, but then eye velocities markedly reduced over time (**Figure 5D**).

DISCUSSION

Comparison of Nystagmus in Darkness After Prolonged Smooth Pursuit and Optokinetic Tracking

Previous studies have reported that background movements of the whole visual field while the eyes remained fixed on a stationary central target led to afternystagmus in darkness with slow phase eye movements in the opposite direction of the preceding background movement (49, 50). This suggested that, without eye movement, a large field of motion in the visual background is sufficient to induce an afternystagmus similar to negative OKAN. In contrast, eye tracking of a single moving target with a dark background led to afternystagmus of smooth pursuit in the subsequent dark condition, in which the eyes moved in the same

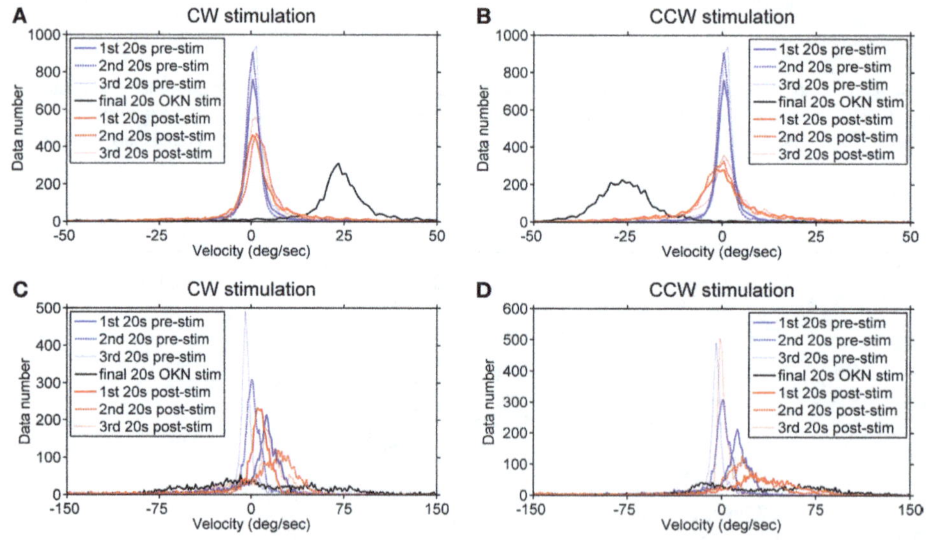

FIGURE 5 | Velocity distribution before, during, and after the optokinetic stimulation. The data numbers within each time window of 20 s were plotted against velocity ranks (every 1°/s). Plots on the top demonstrate the velocity distribution of the healthy subject **(A,B)** and, at the bottom, of the infantile nystagmus syndrome (INS) patient **(C,D)**. The velocity distributions during the pre-stimulation phase are shown in **(A,B)** of the healthy subject and **(C,D)** of the INS patient. Plots on the left demonstrate the velocity distribution during and after the clockwise (positive) stimulation while the plots on the right demonstrate the velocity distribution during and after the counterclockwise (negative) stimulation. The velocity distributions during the pre-stimulation phase are shown as blue line (first 20 s), blue dashed line (second 20 s), and blue dotted line (third 20 s); during the final 20-s stimulation phase as black line; during the post-stimulation phases as red line (first 20 s), red dashed line (second 20 s), and red dotted line (third 20 s). 1st 20 s pre-stim = first 20 s of the pre-stimulation phase; 2nd 20 s pre-stim = second 20 s of the pre-stimulation phase; 3rd 20 s pre-stim = third 20 s of the pre-stimulation phase; final 20 s optokinetic nystagmus (OKN) stim = final 20 s of the optokinetic stimulation phase; 1st 20 s post-stim = first 20 s of the post-stimulation phase; 2nd 20 s post-stim = second 20 s of the post-stimulation phase; 3rd 20 s post-stim = third 20 s of the post-stimulation phase.

direction as the previous moving target (29, 51). This behavior depends mainly upon eye movements, and not retinal slip, as the high gain of the smooth-pursuit tracking of a small moving target minimizes the retinal slip. We propose that this negative OKAN in darkness is an outcome of a sensory adaptation triggered by the retinal slip of a large moving field during a sustained period of optokinetic stimulation. Conversely, continued eye tracking by the smooth-pursuit system leads to a motor adaptation that yields an aftereffect of continuing eye movements in the same direction in darkness.

Negative OKAN has been previously documented in both animal and human subjects, albeit with evident variability in study designs and methods. However, with binocular viewing conditions we did not observe any negative OKAN in our healthy subject tested up to and after a 15-min optokinetic stimulation period with our experimental apparatus, instead, we observed a long-lasting positive afternystagmus (data not shown). We deduce that whilst sitting inside the optokinetic drum, our healthy subject tended to fixate sharp borders of the vertical stripes with the fovea, thus, the smooth pursuit overshadowed the optokinetic behavior during the drum rotation. In this situation, afternystagmus of smooth pursuit most likely masked the negative OKAN. Under monocular viewing conditions while tracking the stripes of the optokinetic drum, a representative healthy subject displayed afternystagmus with markedly reduced velocity in the same direction (**Figures 4B,D**). In contrast to the healthy subject, the INS patient exhibited afternystagmus in the opposite direction (**Figures 3B,D**).

Previous studies have reported that background movements of the whole visual field whilst the eyes remained fixed on a stationary central target led to afternystagmus in darkness with slow phase eye movements in the opposite direction of the preceding background movement (49, 50). This suggested that, without eye movement, a large field of motion in the visual background is sufficient to induce an afternystagmus similar to negative OKAN. In contrast, eye tracking of a single moving target with a dark background led to afternystagmus of smooth pursuit in the subsequent dark condition, in which the eyes moved in the same direction as the previous moving target (29, 51). This behavior depends mainly upon eye movements, and not retinal slip, as the high gain of the smooth-pursuit tracking of a small moving target minimizes the retinal slip. We propose that this negative OKAN in darkness is an outcome of a sensory adaptation triggered by the retinal slip of a large moving field during a sustained period of optokinetic stimulation. Conversely, continued eye tracking by the smooth-pursuit system leads to a motor adaptation that yields an aftereffect of continuing eye movements in the same direction in darkness.

In our pilot study with zebrafish larvae that do not possess a fovea, we recorded only a robust negative OKAN (without observing positive OKAN) in darkness after cessation of continuous optokinetic visual stimulation (unpublished data). Rats, also afoveal, exhibited both positive and negative OKAN in darkness if the preceding OKN reached a steady-state velocity (42). We interpreted the data as indicating that without foveal tracking by a smooth-pursuit system, the optokinetic system might undergo an adaptive process, most likely *via* a sensory adaptation related to the input of a continuous retinal slip signal, resulting in subsequent afternystagmus in the dark. Rabbits (37–39) and cats (40, 41), which have visual streaks, as well as monkeys (35, 36) and humans (32), who have foveas, were all reported to show afternystagmus in darkness in both directions after optokinetic stimulations. However, two components are known to contribute to the afternystagmus moving in the same direction of the preceding visual stimuli: positive OKAN and the afternystagmus of smooth pursuit. It is difficult to differentiate these two mechanisms, particularly in foveated animals. In a previous study, rabbits were reported to exhibit afternystagmus for 50 min in darkness in the same direction as the previous 15-h visual stimulation (39). However, such long-lasting afternystagmus does not match our current knowledge of positive OKAN, the duration of which is typically up to 1 min. Rather, these data suggested that the visual streak could be trained to perform smooth-pursuit tracking, an observation which was reported in a study in cats (52).

In addition to the maladaptive eye movements, INS is often linked to OA with foveal hypoplasia, a condition in which smooth-pursuit function was found to be impaired (53, 54). In contrast, in healthy humans the smooth-pursuit system dominates the optokinetic system with a much higher gain of tracking. Without a healthy smooth-pursuit system, INS patients generally present lower or even reversed (53–55) optokinetic gains during motion tracking and hence maintain considerably higher retinal slip velocities compared to healthy subjects who can rely on the smooth-pursuit system for almost perfect tracking. Following a sustained period of visual motion stimulation, the mechanisms underlying afternystagmus of smooth pursuit and negative OKAN may mask or cancel each other, depending on which of the two and/or how much of each tracking system has been activated during the visual motion stimulation.

In our present study, the INS patient showed a clear reversal of the beating direction during and after the visual stimulation, which we never recorded in our healthy subject. Since the INS patient lacks a normal smooth-pursuit function, the afternystagmus in darkness with an opposite beating direction most likely was an unmasked negative OKAN. In the healthy control, in contrast, the negative OKAN was probably masked by the afternystagmus of smooth pursuit, as the smooth-pursuit system dominated the optokinetic system during the visual stimulation. In other words, with the same experimental paradigm we would expect to record more pronounced negative OKAN in patient populations affected with nystagmus and/or foveal defects such as macular hypoplasia and age-related macular degeneration.

Set-Point Adaptation and Ocular Motor Behavior

Negative OKAN is usually recorded in the laboratory under specific experimental conditions and not in the natural environment. However, this does not mean that the neural circuits underlying this behavior are superfluous. On the contrary, these circuits could provide an important environmental advantage. We propose that the negative OKAN is a demonstration of retinal slip velocity set-point adaptation, similar to the recently discovered vestibular set-point adaptation elicited by magneto-hydrodynamic stimulation using a MRI machine (56, 57). This adaptation is hypothesized to work as a calibration between the eye movement velocity and the retinal slip velocity, similar to earlier proposals by Leigh et al. (58). Environmental changes and nervous system development/ injuries, as well as inherent variability, all affect the accuracy of velocity detection and/or eye movements. The fundamental function of this set-point adaptation in the natural environment is to provide how fast "0" is as a reference value for the retinal slip. Under experimental conditions, a sustained retinal slip input during long visual stimulation shifts the set-point to an extreme value; therefore, the eyes continue to move in the dark since the ocular motor system has an incorrect "0" setting.

Sensory/motor adaptation is essential for animals to exhibit sensory–motor coordination during various actions, as well as for sensorimotor learning. However, erroneous sensory input might also be memorized and lead to problems in behaviors. The constant moving images on the retina during pathological nystagmus would be an erroneous visual input which would exacerbate the instability of the ocular motor system.

In rabbits, negative OKAN can last for 70 h following a 48-h period of visual stimulation. Furthermore, long-term optokinetic stimulation is known to regulate transcriptions and translations in rabbit's cerebellum (59–61). The molecular and biochemical events in these neurons are commonly linked to long-term memory formation (62). We, therefore, hypothesize that constant negative OKAN could possibly lead to a long-term ocular motor instability. In other words, the new condition can be memorized and lead to a change in ocular motor behaviors over a certain period if the stimulation is of sufficiently long duration. In INS patients, spontaneous nystagmus and the lack of normal smooth pursuit can lead to continuous retinal slip input signal and a constant high gain in the ocular motor system. We propose that at an early disease stage, nystagmus in the dark may develop due to the negative OKAN. However, after a longer period of impaired motor learning, eye movements may develop in a complex and unpredictable manner, depending upon genetic, environmental, and other factors.

Instead of the retinal slip, asymmetric optokinetic signal input may also adjust the set-point. Children with MLN or INS with a latent component exhibited reversed nystagmus in the dark (28), similar to previous reports by Dell'Osso et al. (63). Latent nystagmus is commonly associated with the nasotemporal asymmetry of the optokinetic pathways (11, 64, 65). This inherent asymmetry is normally compensated for by the top-down control of the smooth-pursuit system (66, 67). The smooth-pursuit system is mal-developed in patients with amblyopia or strabismus from an early age because of the unequal visual input from the two eyes (68, 69). Without a functional pursuit system, the nasotemporal asymmetric input from the single healthy eye can lead to latent nystagmus (66, 70). In the case of MLN, it has been proposed that the nystagmus beating direction depends on the side of the healthy eye in light and changed to the direction based on its inherent/preprogrammed dominant eye in darkness (28). Another possible explanation is that the asymmetric signal not only drives the eyes to move to the contralateral side of the healthy eye, but also adjusts the set-point of the optokinetic system.

Set-point adaptation presents in a variety of different behaviors. Similar to the optokinetic system, the vestibular system shows set-point adaptation of velocity during a sustained magnetic field stimulation (56). Moreover, in a manner which is different from velocity, set-point adaptation of position can be demonstrated as gaze-evoked nystagmus decays and rebound nystagmus (57).

In conclusion, we propose a new hypothesis that the spontaneous nystagmus in the dark can be a negative OKAN in some of the INS patients whose nystagmus symptoms in light can be linked to aberrant visual inputs and erroneous visual processing. We further suggest that patients with foveal defects may display more pronounced negative OKAN than healthy subjects due to compromised smooth-pursuit tracking. However, our hypothesis should not infer common pathological mechanisms underlying various types of nystagmus presented in all of these patient groups. In order to identify different mechanisms, understanding the correlation between genotypes and phenotypes is important. Following our hypothesis, a longitudinal study of INS from infanthood to old age would help to understand how impaired sensorimotor learning leads to new behavioral features through brain adaptations.

AUTHOR CONTRIBUTIONS

MH, T-FL, and DS conceived the study. T-FL, MH, CG-K, and JH performed the experiments and analyzed the data. T-FL and MH drafted the article. All authors approved the final version of the article.

ACKNOWLEDGMENTS

The authors thank Monika Molnar for providing essential help and input to the experiments and eye measurements, Nicoletta Caramia for the fruitful discussions and help with pilot experiments, Fausto Romano for the assist with experimentation and data analysis, and Marco Penner for the technical support.

FUNDING

This work was supported by the Betty and David Koetser Foundation for Brain Research (T-FL and MH), the Oxford McGill ZNZ Partnership in the Neurosciences Pilot Project Funding (MH), and the Dr. Dabbous Foundation (DS). JH is partially funded by the Clinical Research Priority Programme of the University of Zurich.

REFERENCES

1. Maybodi M. Infantile-onset nystagmus. *Curr Opin Ophthalmol* (2003) 14(5):276–85. doi:10.1097/00055735-200310000-00008
2. Gottlob I, Proudlock FA. Aetiology of infantile nystagmus. *Curr Opin Neurol* (2014) 27(1):83–91. doi:10.1097/WCO.0000000000000058
3. Yonehara K, Fiscella M, Drinnenberg A, Esposti F, Trenholm S, Krol J, et al. Congenital nystagmus gene FRMD7 is necessary for establishing a neuronal circuit asymmetry for direction selectivity. *Neuron* (2016) 89(1):177–93. doi:10.1016/j.neuron.2015.11.032
4. Huang YY, Rinner O, Hedinger P, Liu SC, Neuhauss SCF. Oculomotor instabilities in zebrafish mutant belladonna: a behavioral model for congenital nystagmus caused by axonal misrouting. *J Neurosci* (2006) 26(39):9873–80. doi:10.1523/jneurosci.2886-06.2006
5. Huber-Reggi SP, Chen CC, Grimm L, Straumann D, Neuhauss SCF, Huang MYY. Severity of infantile nystagmus syndrome-like ocular motor phenotype is linked to the extent of the underlying optic nerve projection defect in zebrafish belladonna mutant. *J Neurosci* (2012) 32(50):18079–86. doi:10.1523/jneurosci.4378-12.2012
6. Chen CC, Bockisch CJ, Olasagasti I, Weber KP, Straumann D, Huang MY. Positive or negative feedback of optokinetic signals: degree of the misrouted optic flow determines system dynamics of human ocular motor behavior. *Invest Ophthalmol Vis Sci* (2014) 55(4):2297–306. doi:10.1167/iovs.13-12750
7. Traber GL, Chen CC, Huang YY, Spoor M, Roos J, Frens MA, et al. Albino mice as an animal model for infantile nystagmus syndrome. *Invest Ophthalmol Vis Sci* (2012) 53(9):5737–47. doi:10.1167/iovs.12-10137
8. Optican LM, Zee DS. A hypothetical explanation of congenital nystagmus. *Biol Cybern* (1984) 50(2):119–34. doi:10.1007/BF00337159
9. Jacobs JB, Dell'Osso LF. Congenital nystagmus: hypotheses for its genesis and complex waveforms within a behavioral ocular motor system model. *J Vis* (2004) 4(7):604–25. doi:10.1167/4.7.7
10. Wang ZI, Dell'Osso LF. A unifying model-based hypothesis for the diverse aveforms of infantile nystagmus syndrome. *J Eye Mov Res* (2011) 4(1):11–8. doi:10.16910/jemr.4.1.1
11. Brodsky MC, Dell'Osso LF. A unifying neurologic mechanism for infantile nystagmus. *JAMA Ophthalmol* (2014) 132(6):761–8. doi:10.1001/jamaophthalmol.2013.5833
12. Harris C, Berry D. A developmental model of infantile nystagmus. *Semin Ophthalmol* (2006) 21(2):63–9. doi:10.1080/08820530600613746
13. Harris CM, Berry DL. A distal model of congenital nystagmus as nonlinear adaptive oscillations. *Nonlinear Dyn* (2006) 44(1–4):367–80. doi:10.1007/s11071-006-2021-6
14. Akman OE, Broomhead DS, Abadi RV, Clement RA. Eye movement instabilities and nystagmus can be predicted by a nonlinear dynamics model of the saccadic system. *J Math Biol* (2005) 51(6):661–94. doi:10.1007/s00285-005-0336-4
15. Berg KT, Hunter DG, Bothun ED, Antunes-Foschini R, McLoon LK. Extraocular muscles in patients with infantile nystagmus: adaptations at the effector level. *Arch Ophthalmol* (2012) 130(3):343–9. doi:10.1001/archophthalmol.2011.381
16. Montoliu L, Gronskov K, Wei AH, Martinez-Garcia M, Fernandez A, Arveiler B, et al. Increasing the complexity: new genes and new types of albinism. *Pigment Cell Melanoma Res* (2014) 27(1):11–8. doi:10.1111/pcmr.12167
17. Lewis RA. *Ocular Albinism, X-Linked. GeneReviews(R)*. Seattle, WA: University of Washington, Seattle (1993).
18. Rosenberg T, Schwartz M, Simonsen SE. Aland eye disease (Forsius-Eriksson-Miyake syndrome) with probability established in a Danish family. *Acta Ophthalmol (Copenh)* (1990) 68(3):281–91. doi:10.1111/j.1755-3768.1990.tb01923.x
19. Bertolotti A, Lasseaux E, Plaisant C, Trimouille A, Morice-Picard F, Rooryck C, et al. Identification of a homozygous mutation of SLC24A5 (OCA6) in two patients with oculocutaneous albinism from French Guiana. *Pigment Cell Melanoma Res* (2016) 29(1):104–6. doi:10.1111/pcmr.12425
20. Gronskov K, Dooley CM, Ostergaard E, Kelsh RN, Hansen L, Levesque MP, et al. Mutations in c10orf11, a melanocyte-differentiation gene, cause autosomal-recessive albinism. *Am J Hum Genet* (2013) 92(3):415–21. doi:10.1016/j.ajhg.2013.01.006
21. Kausar T, Bhatti MA, Ali M, Shaikh RS, Ahmed ZM. OCA5, a novel locus for non-syndromic oculocutaneous albinism, maps to chromosome 4q24. *Clin Genet* (2013) 84(1):91–3. doi:10.1111/cge.12019
22. Lewis RA. *Oculocutaneous Albinism Type 1. GeneReviews(R)*. Seattle, WA: University of Washington, Seattle (1993).
23. Lewis RA. *Oculocutaneous Albinism Type 2. GeneReviews(R)*. Seattle, WA: University of Washington, Seattle (1993).
24. Suzuki T, Hayashi M. *Oculocutaneous Albinism Type 4. GeneReviews(R)*. Seattle, WA: University of Washington, Seattle (1993).
25. Zhang KH, Li Z, Lei J, Pang T, Xu B, Jiang WY, et al. Oculocutaneous albinism type 3 (OCA3): analysis of two novel mutations in TYRP1 gene in two Chinese patients. *Cell Biochem Biophys* (2011) 61(3):523–9. doi:10.1007/s12013-011-9234-0
26. Huang MY, Chen CC, Huber-Reggi SP, Neuhauss SC, Straumann D. Comparison of infantile nystagmus syndrome in achiasmatic zebrafish and humans. *Ann N Y Acad Sci* (2011) 1233:285–91. doi:10.1111/j.1749-6632.2011.06150.x
27. Leigh RJ, Zee DS. *The Neurology of Eye Movements*. New York: Oxford University Press (2006).
28. Shawkat FS. Spontaneous reversal of nystagmus in the dark. *Br J Ophthalmol* (2001) 85(4):428–31. doi:10.1136/bjo.85.4.428
29. Marti S, Bockisch CJ, Straumann D. Prolonged asymmetric smooth-pursuit stimulation leads to downbeat nystagmus in healthy human subjects. *Invest Ophthalmol Vis Sci* (2005) 46(1):143–9. doi:10.1167/iovs.04-0235
30. Huang YY, Neuhauss SC. The optokinetic response in zebrafish and its applications. *Front Biosci* (2008) 13:1899–916. doi:10.2741/2810
31. Laurens J, Angelaki DE. The functional significance of velocity storage and its dependence on gravity. *Exp Brain Res* (2011) 210(3–4):407–22. doi:10.1007/s00221-011-2568-4
32. Brandt T, Dichgans J, Buchle W. Motion habituation: inverted self-motion perception and optokinetic after-nystagmus. *Exp Brain Res* (1974) 21(4):337–52. doi:10.1007/BF00237897
33. Cohen B, Henn V, Raphan T, Dennett D. Velocity storage, nystagmus, and visual-vestibular interactions in humans. *Ann N Y Acad Sci* (1981) 374:421–33. doi:10.1111/j.1749-6632.1981.tb30888.x
34. Schor CM, Narayan V, Westall C. Postnatal development of optokinetic after nystagmus in human infants. *Vision Res* (1983) 23(12):1643–7. doi:10.1016/0042-6989(83)90178-5
35. Waespe W, Henn V. Reciprocal changes in primary and secondary optokinetic after-nystagmus (OKAN) produced by repetitive optokinetic stimulation in the monkey. *Archiv Psychiatr Nervenkr* (1978) 225(1):23–30. doi:10.1007/bf00367349
36. Buttner U, Waespe W, Henn V. Duration and direction of optokinetic after-nystagmus as a function of stimulus exposure time in the monkey. *Arch Psychiatr Nervenkr* (1976) 222(4):281–91. doi:10.1007/BF00343237
37. Bures J, Neverov VP. Reversed postoptokinetic nystagmus: a model of plasticity in the vestibuloocular system. *Acta Neurobiol Exp (Wars)* (1979) 39(6):477–90.
38. Neverov VP, Burešová O, Bureš J. Effect of ECS on the neural traces underlying the reversive postoptokinetic nystagmus in the rabbit. *Physiol Behav* (1977) 18(1):7–11. doi:10.1016/0031-9384(77)90085-3
39. Barmack NH, Nelson BJ. Influence of long-term optokinetic stimulation on eye movements of the rabbit. *Brain Res* (1987) 437(1):111–20. doi:10.1016/0006-8993(87)91532-0
40. Maioli C, Precht W. The horizontal optokinetic nystagmus in the cat. *Exp Brain Res* (1984) 55(3):494–506. doi:10.1007/BF00235280
41. Maioli C. Optokinetic nystagmus: modeling the velocity storage mechanism. *J Neurosci* (1988) 8(3):821–32.
42. Hess BJM, Precht W, Reber A, Cazin L. Horizontal optokinetic ocular nystagmus in the pigmented rat. *Neuroscience* (1985) 15(1):97–107. doi:10.1016/0306-4522(85)90126-5
43. Tychsen L, Hurtig RR, Scott WE. Pursuit is impaired but the vestibulo-ocular reflex is normal in infantile strabismus. *Arch Ophthalmol* (1985) 103(4):536–9. doi:10.1001/archopht.1985.01050040078022
44. Kiorpes L, Walton PJ, O'Keefe LP, Movshon JA, Lisberger SG. Effects of early-onset artificial strabismus on pursuit eye movements and on neuronal responses in area MT of macaque monkeys. *J Neurosci* (1996) 16(20):6537–53.

45. Thomas MG, Kumar A, Mohammad S, Proudlock FA, Engle EC, Andrews C, et al. Structural grading of foveal hypoplasia using spectral-domain optical coherence tomography. *Ophthalmology* (2011) 118(8):1653–60. doi:10.1016/j.ophtha.2011.01.028
46. Apkarian P, Shallo-Hoffmann J. VEP projections in congenital nystagmus; VEP asymmetry in albinism: a comparison study. *Invest Ophthalmol Vis Sci* (1991) 32(9):2653–61.
47. Schneider E, Dera T, Bartl K, Boening G, Bardins S, Brandt T. Eye movement driven head-mounted camera: it looks where the eyes look. *IEEE Xplore* (2005) 3:2437–42. doi:10.1109/icsmc.2005.1571514
48. Ko CH, Hung YP. Real time large motion feature tracking by matching characteristic curves via dynamic programming. *IEEE Xplore* (2006):5185–90. doi:10.1109/ICSMC.2006.385131
49. Chen CC, Huang MYY, Weber KP, Straumann D, Bockisch CJ. Afternystagmus in darkness after suppression of optokinetic nystagmus: an interaction of motion aftereffect and retinal afterimages. *Exp Brain Res* (2014) 232(9): 2891–8. doi:10.1007/s00221-014-3971-4
50. Ventre-Dominey J, Luyat M. Asymmetry of visuo-vestibular mechanisms contributes to reversal of optokinetic after-nystagmus. *Exp Brain Res* (2009) 193(1):55–67. doi:10.1007/s00221-008-1595-2
51. Muratore R, Zee DS. Pursuit after-nystagmus. *Vision Res* (1979) 19(9):1057–9. doi:10.1016/0042-6989(79)90233-5
52. Evinger C, Fuchs AF. Saccadic, smooth pursuit, and optokinetic eye movements of the trained cat. *J Physiol* (1978) 285:209–29. doi:10.1113/jphysiol.1978.sp012568
53. Collewijn H, Apkarian P, Spekreijse H. The oculomotor behaviour of human albinos. *Brain* (1985) 108(1):1–28. doi:10.1093/brain/108.1.1
54. John RS, Fisk JD, Timney B, Goodale MA. Eye movements of human albinos. *Optom Vis Sci* (1984) 61(6):377–85. doi:10.1097/00006324-198406000-00007
55. Self JE, Shawkat F, Malpas CT, Thomas NS, Harris CM, Hodgkins PR, et al. Allelic variation of the FRMD7 gene in congenital idiopathic nystagmus. *Arch Ophthalmol* (2007) 125(9):1255–63. doi:10.1001/archopht.125.9.1255
56. Jareonsettasin P, Otero-Millan J, Ward BK, Roberts DC, Schubert MC, Zee DS. Multiple time courses of vestibular set-point adaptation revealed by sustained magnetic field stimulation of the labyrinth. *Curr Biol* (2016) 26(10):1359–66. doi:10.1016/j.cub.2016.03.066
57. Zee DS, Jareonsettasin P, Leigh RJ. Ocular stability and set-point adaptation. *Philos Trans R Soc Lond B Biol Sci* (2017) 372(1718):20160199. doi:10.1098/rstb.2016.0199
58. Leigh RJ, Robinson DA, Zee DS. A hypothetical explanation for periodic alternating nystagmus: instability in the optokinetic-vestibular system. *Ann N Y Acad Sci* (1981) 374:619–35. doi:10.1111/j.1749-6632.1981.tb30906.x
59. Barmack NH, Qian Z, Yakhnitsa V. Long-term climbing fibre activity induces transcription of microRNAs in cerebellar Purkinje cells. *Philos Trans R Soc Lond B Biol Sci* (2014) 369(1652):20130508. doi:10.1098/rstb.2013.0508
60. Barmack NH, Qian Z, Yakhnitsa V. Climbing fibers induce microRNA transcription in cerebellar Purkinje cells. *Neuroscience* (2010) 171(3):655–65. doi:10.1016/j.neuroscience.2010.09.039
61. Barmack NH, Qian Z. Activity-dependent expression of calbindin in rabbit floccular Purkinje cells modulated by optokinetic stimulation. *Neuroscience* (2002) 113(1):235–50. doi:10.1016/S0306-4522(02)00008-8
62. Malenka RC, Nicoll RA. Long-term potentiation – a decade of progress? *Science* (1999) 285(5435):1870–4. doi:10.1126/science.285.5435.1870
63. Dell'Osso LF, Abel LA, Daroff RB. Latent/manifest latent nystagmus reversal using an ocular prosthesis. Implications for vision and ocular dominance. *Invest Ophthalmol Vis Sci* (1987) 28(11):1873–6.
64. Brodsky MC, Tusa RJ. Latent nystagmus: vestibular nystagmus with a twist. *Arch Ophthalmol* (2004) 122(2):202–9. doi:10.1001/archopht.122.2.202
65. Braddick O. Where is the naso-temporal asymmetry? Motion processing. *Curr Biol* (1996) 6(3):250–3. doi:10.1016/S0960-9822(02)00470-0
66. Schor CM. Subcortical binocular suppression affects the development of latent and optokinetic nystagmus. *Am J Optom Physiol Opt* (1983) 60(6): 481–502. doi:10.1097/00006324-198306000-00009
67. Atkinson J. Development of optokinetic nystagmus in the human infant and monkey infant: an analogue to development in kittens. In: Freeman RD. *Developmental Neurobiology of Vision*. Boston, MA: Springer US (1979). p. 277–87.
68. Mustari MJ, Tusa RJ, Burrows AF, Fuchs AF, Livingston CA. Gaze-stabilizing deficits and latent nystagmus in monkeys with early-onset visual deprivation: role of the pretectal not. *J Neurophysiol* (2001) 86(2):662–75. doi:10.1152/jn.2001.86.2.662
69. Tusa RJ, Mustari MJ, Burrows AF, Fuchs AF. Gaze-stabilizing deficits and latent nystagmus in monkeys with brief, early-onset visual deprivation: eye movement recordings. *J Neurophysiol* (2001) 86(2):651–61. doi:10.1152/jn.2001.86.2.651
70. Tusa RJ, Mustari MJ, Das VE, Boothe RG. Animal models for visual deprivation-induced strabismus and nystagmus. *Ann N Y Acad Sci* (2002) 956:346–60. doi:10.1111/j.1749-6632.2002.tb02833.x

5

The Intersection between Ocular and Manual Motor Control: Eye–Hand Coordination in Acquired Brain Injury

John-Ross Rizzo[1,2], Maryam Hosseini[1], Eric A. Wong[1], Wayne E. Mackey[3], James K. Fung[1], Edmond Ahdoot[1], Janet C. Rucker[2,4], Preeti Raghavan[1], Michael S. Landy[3] and Todd E. Hudson[1,2]*

[1] Department of Rehabilitation Medicine, New York University Langone Medical Center, New York, NY, United States, [2] Department of Neurology, New York University Langone Medical Center, New York, NY, United States, [3] Department of Psychology and Center for Neural Science, New York University, New York, NY, United States, [4] Department of Ophthalmology, New York University Langone Medical Center, New York, NY, United States

***Correspondence:**
John-Ross Rizzo
johnross.rizzo@nyumc.org

Acute and chronic disease processes that lead to cerebral injury can often be clinically challenging diagnostically, prognostically, and therapeutically. Neurodegenerative processes are one such elusive diagnostic group, given their often diffuse and indolent nature, creating difficulties in pinpointing specific structural abnormalities that relate to functional limitations. A number of studies in recent years have focused on eye–hand coordination (EHC) in the setting of acquired brain injury (ABI), highlighting the important set of interconnected functions of the eye and hand and their relevance in neurological conditions. These experiments, which have concentrated on focal lesion-based models, have significantly improved our understanding of neurophysiology and underscored the sensitivity of biomarkers in acute and chronic neurological disease processes, especially when such biomarkers are combined synergistically. To better understand EHC and its connection with ABI, there is a need to clarify its definition and to delineate its neuroanatomical and computational underpinnings. Successful EHC relies on the complex feedback- and prediction-mediated relationship between the visual, ocular motor, and manual motor systems and takes advantage of finely orchestrated synergies between these systems in both the spatial and temporal domains. Interactions of this type are representative of functional sensorimotor control, and their disruption constitutes one of the most frequent deficits secondary to brain injury. The present review describes the visually mediated planning and control of eye movements, hand movements, and their coordination, with a particular focus on deficits that occur following neurovascular, neurotraumatic, and neurodegenerative conditions. Following this review, we also discuss potential future research directions, highlighting objective EHC as a sensitive biomarker complement within acute and chronic neurological disease processes.

Keywords: coordination, eye, hand, stroke, brain injuries

INTRODUCTION

Acute and chronic disease processes that lead to cerebral injury can often be clinically challenging diagnostically, prognostically, and therapeutically. Neurodegenerative processes are one such elusive diagnostic group, given their often diffuse and indolent nature, creating difficulties in pinpointing specific structural abnormalities that relate to functional limitations. Historically, experiments have concentrated on cerebral lesion-based approaches, significantly improving our understanding of the neurophysiology and underscoring the sensitivity of behavioral biomarkers to detect as well as predict the outcomes of cerebral injury. These focal lesion-based models and associated biomarkers can be combined synergistically and have significant potential in shedding light on acute and chronic neurological disease processes.

Eye–hand coordination (EHC) can be defined as the complex relationship between our visual system and our manual motor system. Visually guided reaching, grasping, and object manipulation depend on the ability to visually decipher environmental details and finely coordinate motor responses of the eye and hand to produce controlled, rapid and accurate movements. Independent deficits of either ocular or manual motor control have been studied extensively after acquired brain injury (ABI). More recently, the coordination between eye and hand movements in patients with central nervous system injury, as related to neurovascular, neurotraumatic, and neurodegenerative conditions, has been highlighted as a critical concept in understanding brain-behavior relationships.

Over the course of the past two decades, a number of studies have demonstrated that EHC deficits (i.e., eye–hand incoordination or dyssynergia) resulting from ABI are important thematic concepts within the field of rehabilitation following neurological injury (1–3). In response, a focused review was performed on the PubMed database using a series of key words that included the following phrases and/or words: eye–hand coordination, acquired brain injury, stroke, cerebrovascular accident (CVA), traumatic brain injury, and brain injury (including acute, subacute, and chronic time scales). The research included articles published over the past two decades. A total of 74 articles were surveyed, which varied significantly in scope and merit.

The aim of this narrative review on EHC was to clarify its conceptual importance in the setting of ABI, to improve understanding neuroanatomically, and to address implications therapeutically. The articles reviewed were focused on EHC or the integration of visual input secondary to ocular motor control and manual motor output and related pathology, including neurovascular, neurotraumatic, and neurodegenerative conditions. The overarching goal of this review is to engender dialogue between clinicians and scientists in a framework that will provide clarity, improve comprehension and precipitate translational, clinical research.

LITERATURE SEARCH STRATEGY

Our literature review was performed by J.R. and E.W. on publications available in the National Center for Biotechnology Information's PubMed database using key words containing the phrase "eye hand coordination" and key words relevant to ABI (specific key words are listed in **Table 1**). The search of the literature included seminal and contemporary peer-reviewed articles on EHC in the setting of ABI, including injuries that were either secondary to trauma or CVAs. The research articles spanned publication dates between 1998 and 2015. The quality and the relevance of the resultant literature varied significantly in caliber and applicability. Articles were utilized based on their pertinence to ABI and its associated effects on EHC. Pertinence was determined by consensus between two authors based on whether there was a thematic focus on EHC, and also discussion of at least one of the patient populations of interest. A total of 74 articles were originally reviewed (surveyed); this compilation was ultimately distilled to 8 pertinent (utilized) references (see **Figure 1** and **Table 2**).

TABLE 1 | Literature search strategy details.

Key words	Articles surveyed	Articles utilized
Eye hand coordination acute brain injury	3	2
Eye hand coordination chronic brain injury	2	2
Eye hand coordination subacute brain injury	0	0
Eye hand coordination ABI	1	1
Eye hand coordination stroke	14	5
Eye hand coordination acute stroke	14	5
Eye hand coordination chronic stroke	0	0
Eye hand coordination CVA	14	5
Eye hand coordination cerebrovascular accident	14	5
Eye hand coordination traumatic brain injury	5	3
Eye hand coordination TBI	1	1
Eye hand coordination traumatic injury	6	3
Total listed items	74	32
Total articles (duplicate articles removed)	20	8

EHC DEFINITION

Eye–hand coordination is the complex relationship between the visual and manual motor systems, at the intersection between vision and dexterity. EHC depends on vision to aid in directing goal-oriented hand movements, including pointing, reaching, grasping, object manipulation, and tool use, and encompasses many functionally relevant motor activities (4, 5). Optimal coordination relies on precise ocular motor control for high acuity visual perception and sound manual motor control, yielding robust effector coaction (6, 7). This visuomotor integration requires complex motor programs and near continuous, multimodal sensory feedback, and predictions thereof, to produce controlled and rapid task-specific movements (8).

EHC NEUROPHYSIOLOGY AND NEUROANATOMY

The Visual System (Eye)

Primary visual cortex (V1), also known as striate cortex, is the first cortical region that processes visual input. V1 is located in the posterior pole of the occipital lobe. It mainly serves to process primitive visual features, such as bars of a specific orientation or edges and contours of solid objects within a specific portion of the retina's visual field. From V1, visual processing continues through a sequence of adjacent cortical regions known as extrastriate cortex. A fundamental organizing principle of these visual areas is a topographic representation of the contralateral visual field. The spatial layout of a scene is represented in an orderly manner across a population of neurons that reflect input from

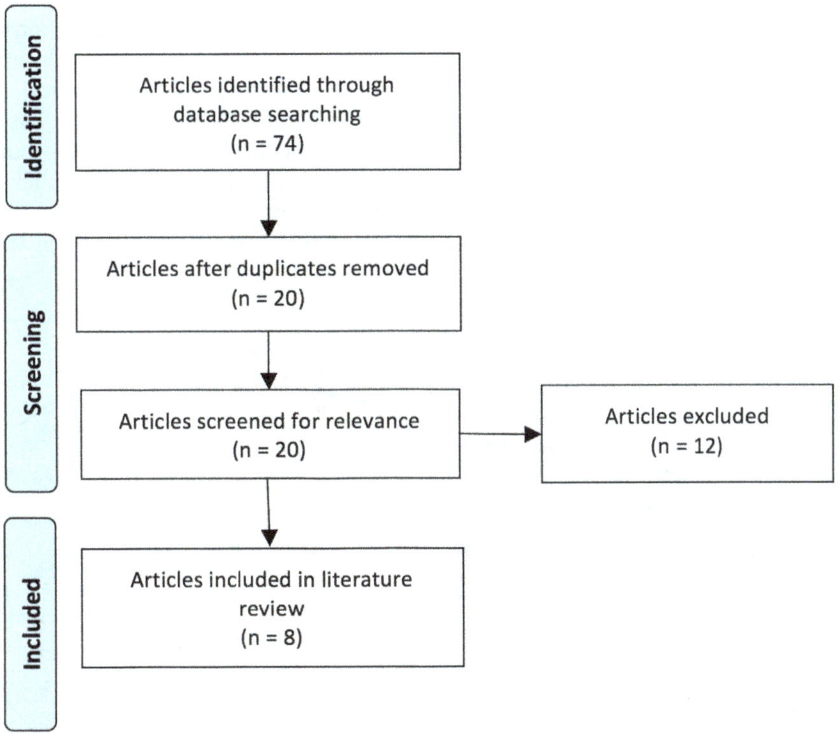

FIGURE 1 | **Flow diagram of literature search.**

TABLE 2 | Key comparisons of the articles utilized in the review following the literature search and selection process.

Author	Year	Journal	Cohort	Obj. eye[a]	Obj. hand[b]
Caeyenberghs et al. (1)	2009	*J Head Trauma Rehabil*	ABI	[–]	(+)/2D
Caeyenberghs et al. (210)	2010	*Neuropsychologia*	TBI	[–]	(+)/2D
Brown et al. (215)	2015	*BMC Sports Sci Med Rehabil*	TBI	[–]	(+)/2D
Gao et al. (2)	2010	*J Rehabil Med*	CVA	[–]	(+)/2D
Ghika et al. (3)	1998	*Clin Neurol Neurosurg*	CVA	[–]	(–)
Tsang et al. (142)	2013	*Am J Phys Med Rehabil*	CVA	[–]	(+)/2D
Procacci et al. (106)	2009	*Neurocase*	CVA	[+]	(+)/2D
Vesia et al. (74)	2012	*Exp Brain Res*	Review	[n/a]	(n/a)

[a]Obj. eye = objective eye recording was performed [+] or not performed [–].
[b]Obj. hand = objective hand recording was performed (+) or not performed (–) and, if performed, were the recordings in 1D, 2D, or 3D.
ABI = acquired brain injury; TBI = traumatic brain injury; CVA = cerebrovascular stroke.

the retina. This population of neurons constitutes a visual field map whereby adjacent neurons represent adjacent points in space (9), preserving the spatial layout of the retinal image in each of these cortical areas. This systematic organization is computationally and metabolically efficient as it shortens connection lengths between similarly tuned neurons. Interestingly, topographic organization extends beyond retinotopic coordinate space. Relevant for EHC, other areas represent space in head-centered coordinates (10–12), or a combination of coordinate systems (13, 14). The interactions between these areas likely facilitate sensorimotor transformations fundamental to EHC. Extrastriate regions (such as V2/V3), which emanate rostrally from V1, are believed to be responsible for processing features of progressively increasing complexity (15–17). This processing stream bifurcates into a ventral "what" pathway, processing object identity and visual features, and a dorsal "where" pathway, processing spatial attention and movement (15, 18). The dorsal pathway has also been implicated in processing visual input for predictive and anticipatory movements, including those coordinated between the eye and hand (17, 19, 20). The dorsal and ventral streams are thought to aid EHC (21, 22).

The Ocular Motor System

In order to examine our environment, we alternate between fixating a point of interest and making fast, darting eye movements (saccades) from one point of interest to another. For well over a century, scientists have measured saccades to investigate the link between brain and behavior (23, 24). Broadly, along with the subcortical superior colliculus (SC), four cortical areas contribute to the control of saccades: the frontal eye field (FEF), the supplementary eye field (SEF), the parietal eye field (PEF), and the cingulate eye field (CEF). Each region appears to play a distinct role in controlling eye movements. The FEF, SEF, and PEF directly project to the SC, while the CEF influences ocular motor control more indirectly through connections with the FEF, SEF, and PEF (25–29). Additionally, the FEF connects directly to the brainstem ocular motor nuclei, which house the ocular motor neurons that innervate the extraocular muscles (**Figure 2**).

Frontal Eye Field

The FEF is crucial for the preparation and execution of voluntary saccades to either external (visually guided saccades) or internal targets (memory-guided saccades) (30–34). The majority of research characterizing the FEF has been with respect to the monkey ocular motor system, ever since Ferrier discovered that electrical stimulation of the FEF elicited eye movements (23). In the monkey, FEF is located in the anterior bank of the arcuate sulcus, just posterior to the principal sulcus (31). The FEF both

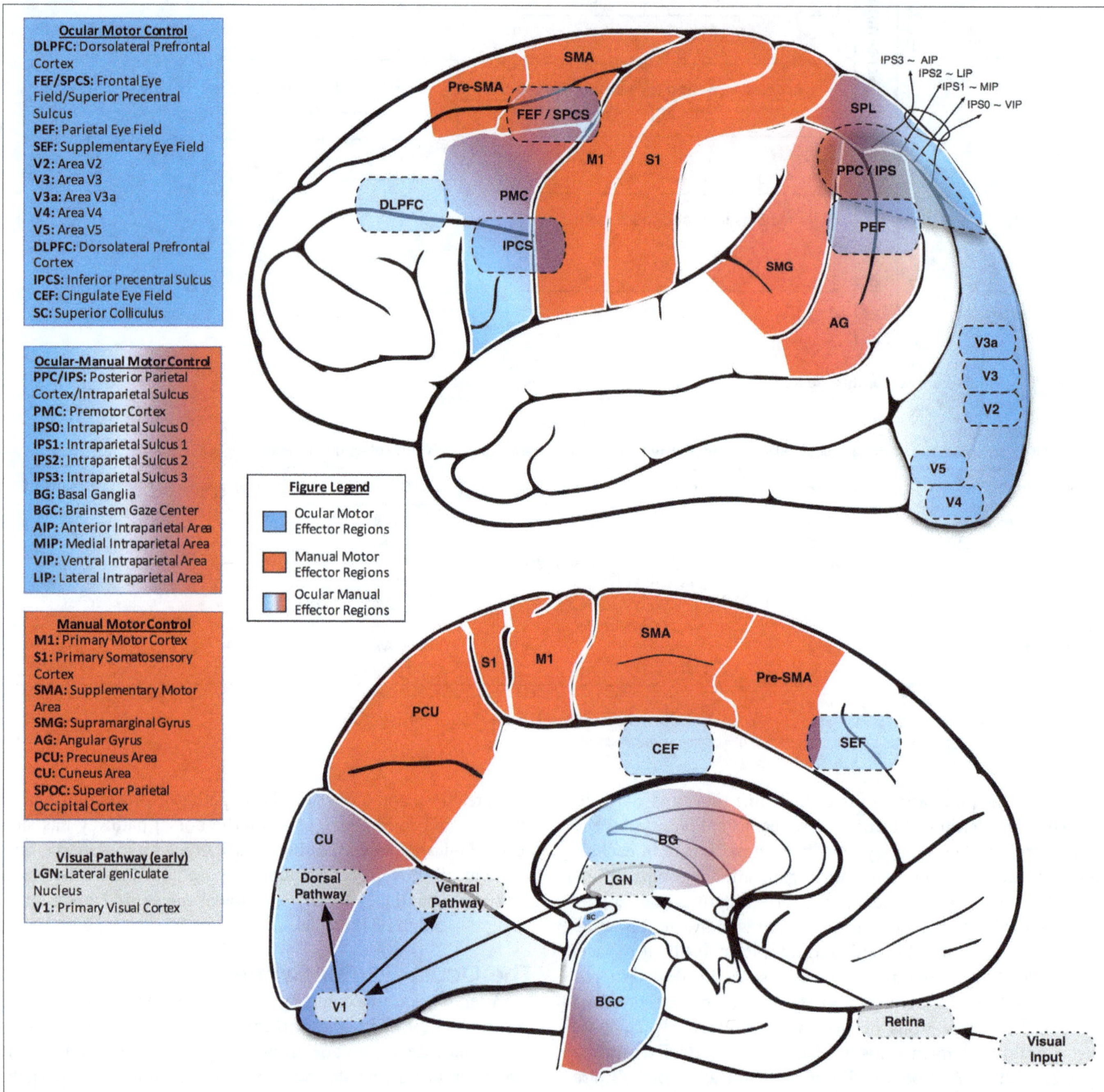

FIGURE 2 | Lateral (upper) and midsaggital (lower) views of the human brain, labeled with neuroanatomical regions of interest related to eye–hand coordination. In both views, ocular motor areas are colored blue, manual motor areas red, and combined ocular-manual motor areas a blend of red and blue.

projects to and receives connections from numerous cortical and subcortical brain regions (35, 36). It is retinotopically organized and primarily comprised of neurons that contribute to the holding or shifting of gaze (fixation neurons and saccade neurons, respectively) or neurons that generally respond to stimuli within their receptive field (visual neurons) (37, 38). Neurons within the FEF also have a preference for the contralateral visual field (31). In monkeys, there is also a rough topographic organization with regards to saccade amplitude. The superior portion of the FEF is responsible for generating larger amplitude saccades and shares connections with the dorsal visual stream, while the inferior portion of the FEF is responsible for generating smaller amplitude saccades and shares connections with the ventral visual stream (39). Interestingly, this topography and connectivity organized by dorsal and ventral streams has yet to be demonstrated in the human FEF. Instead, the putative human homolog of FEF, located in the superior precentral sulcus (SPCS), is organized into distinct visual field map clusters similar to early visual cortex (40).

Supplementary Eye Field

The SEF is involved in more indirect aspects of saccade control, such as monitoring the consequences or context of eye movements (41) and coordinating sequences of successive saccades (42, 43). Although believed to typically be found in the posteromedial part of the human superior frontal gyrus, there exists a great amount of variability between individuals in the exact location of the SEF, thus rendering it difficult to define by anatomy alone (44). The activity of neurons in the SEF is modulated by target position in multiple reference frames, aiding in maintaining eye position despite changes in body and head position (14, 45). This region receives both sensory and motor inputs and supplies outgoing connections to both the FEF and PEF (46). Although electrical stimulation of an FEF neuron elicits an eye movement of a fixed magnitude and direction, SEF stimulation elicits an eye movement to a fixed region of the visual field relative to the position of the head, irrespective of the starting position of the eye (47). Although much less is known about topographic organization in SEF, a recent human neuroimaging study suggests it also contains an orderly map of continuous space similar to other visual areas (48).

Parietal Eye Field

Visual input is received by the PEF and aids in triggering reflexive saccades toward visual stimuli found within the peripheral field of vision, as well as managing alterations in attention (49) and performing memory-guided saccades (40, 50). The PEF is located in the lateral intraparietal (LIP) area in monkeys and the intraparietal sulcus (IPS) in humans, and contains strong and reciprocal connections with the FEF. Similar to early visual areas, the IPS contains multiple visual field maps of contralateral space that have led to further parcelation (34, 51). These subregions are labeled numerically (IPS0, IPS1, IPS2, IPS3, etc.), starting from the most posterior area, IPS0, which borders V3A/V3B. Each of these subdivisions are activated during human neuroimaging studies involving eye movements (52). Therefore, which of these individual maps, if any, directly correspond to subdivisions of the monkey IPS (LIP, AIP, VIP, MIP) is still up for debate (52–55). It is also possible that some of the retinotopic IPS subdivisions are unique to humans.

Cingulate Eye Field

The CEF is involved in intentional but not reflexive saccade control (56), and projects to both the FEF and SEF (57). In non-human primates, the CEF is located on the medial wall in each hemisphere, ventral and partly anterior to the SEF. In humans, however, the CEF is located more posterior and ventral to the SEF (57). In humans, lesions of the CEF impair many types of saccades, including sequences of visually-guided saccades, memory-guided saccades, and antisaccades (56). Compared to the other ocular motor regions listed here, the CEF is the least studied and least understood.

Superior Colliculus

The SC plays a crucial role in saccade execution, as it projects directly to the brainstem ocular motor nuclei. It receives projections from a multitude of areas including FEF, SEF, and PEF. Like FEF, electrical stimulation of SC elicits saccades of a particular magnitude and direction. SC is also organized similarly to FEF, except in a rostral-caudal, rather than an inferior–superior, gradient of increasing saccade amplitude. Recent human neuroimaging studies have demonstrated that human SC contains a retinotopic map of the entire contralateral visual field (58, 59). In non-human primates, lesions of the SC alone impair but do not abolish eye movements, but lesions of SC and FEF together have catastrophic consequences for eye movements that do not recover with time (60).

Other Areas

The aforementioned areas are clearly not an exhaustive list of brain regions associated with ocular motor control, although they are the most studied. For example, dorsomedial frontal cortex, sometimes referred to as the presupplementary motor area, is critical for inhibition of reflexive saccades in humans (61). It has also been implicated in selecting among competing movements during action selection (62). Additionally, V1 also plays a role in ocular motor control and has projections directly to the SC. In the rhesus monkey, electrical stimulation of V1 can elicit saccades, but the required level of stimulation is much higher than what is necessary to elicit saccades via FEF or SC stimulation (63).

The role of human dorsolateral prefrontal cortex (dlPFC) in ocular motor control is still unclear. Electrophysiological and lesion studies in non-human primates show that the dlPFC contains spatially selective neurons that are critical for memory-guided saccades (64, 65). However, lesions to human dlPFC do not impair memory-guided saccades (34), and do not show spatial selectivity (34, 66). A handful of studies have examined the effects of transcranial magnetic stimulation (TMS) on dlPFC during a memory-guided saccade task (67–69). These results seem to parallel the results from non-human primate lesion studies, finding effects of TMS on memory-guided saccade performance. However, it is likely that the stimulation site in these studies overlapped with the FEF. All three papers used the identical method to localize and define dlPFC, first finding the motor hand area and then moving anteriorly a few centimeters; this method has also been described as an effective way to localize the human FEF (70). A more recent study using TMS to disrupt activity in human dlPFC found no impairment on memory-guided saccades (48).

The Manual Motor System (Hand)

Within EHC, the end goal is to place the hand/finger(s) or the manual effector in the position required for motor program execution or, in a dynamic sense, to work seamlessly and reciprocally with the eye to build and actualize complex motor programs. The neuroanatomical reach network most directly responsible for voluntary movements of the arm and hand includes motor cortical regions such as primary motor cortex (M1) and the supplementary and premotor cortices. The primary motor cortex begins on the anterior wall of the central sulcus and continues rostrally to comprise what is the anterior paracentral lobule. It is the cortical region responsible for the collective generation of action potentials that relay neural information to the descending corticospinal tract to produce hand movements (71). The premotor cortex (PMC) is located anterior to the primary motor cortex (M1) and in a lateral position from midline; this region is in close spatial proximity to the inferior precentral sulcus (70). PMC is the planning region for anticipatory movements, provides spatial guidance during hand movements, and processes the sensory input used to aid the guidance of hand movements. The supplementary motor cortex is closer to the midline and anterior to the primary motor cortex, and is used to plan sequential manual movements. These motor areas supply the bulk of the neurons whose axons compose the corticospinal tract (in conjunction with smaller inputs from somatosensory, posterior parietal, and cingulate cortex), which travels through the internal capsule and pons, decussates at the level of the medulla, and ultimately activates the alpha motorneurons in the spinal cord (primarily the lower cervical and first thoracic levels) either directly or via spinal interneurons.

This cortical reach network is supplemented by a larger network of cortical and subcortical regions, including the posterior parietal cortex (PPC), somatosensory cortex, basal ganglia, and cerebellum. The PPC is an associative region that translates visual information and input from the somatosensory cortex into motor commands (72, 73). Based on functional neuroimaging, TMS studies, and human case series with parietal injuries, a functional topography for reach, as it relates to the planning and control of visuomotor action, has been described within the human PPC (74). More specifically, midposterior intraparietal sulcus (mIPS), superior parietal occipital cortex (SPOC), and angular gyrus (AG) are reach-specific areas (**Figure 2**). Three main aspects in reach-dominant areas include effector specificity, hemispheric laterality and computational specificity. The area posteromedial to IPS contributes to the planning of reaching, while the area anterolateral to the IPS has a role in grasp-related information integration. Cortex anterior to the intraparietal area (AIP) is involved in object-directed hand grasping and hand preshaping. In hemispheric lateralization, bilateral activation due to reaching with more emphasis on contralateral movements has been identified (75).

The anterior portion of IPS monitors the compatibility of a planned reach/grasp with outgoing movement commands and incoming sensory inputs (74, 76). Eye movements frequently take place before a hand movement and may be spatially fixated on the object of interest until the end of reaching to improve accuracy (77–79). Decoupling of eye and hand movements requires reach and saccade goal separation (80–83). SPOC is more active in reaches toward peripheral (non-foveal) targets independent of gaze signals, while mIPS is more active in reach toward foveated targets with spatial congruence between gaze and reach goal (74).

In cortical reach-dominant regions, the anterior precuneus (aPCu) area, expanding into the medial IPS, is equally active in visual and non-visual reaching. Medial, anterior intraparietal and superior parietal cortices are also activated in both visual and non-visual reaching; areas located in the anterior distribution are more active during hand movements in comparison to those in the posterior distribution, which are more active during combined eye and hand movements. Another area, at the superior end of the parieto-occipital sulcus (sPOS), is more active during visual reaching. Taken together, aPCu may be a sensorimotor area with a prominent proprioceptive sensory input and sPOS, a visuomotor area that receives visual feedback during reaching (84).

In addition to these cortical contributions, the cerebellum plays a critical role in the timing and control aspects of manual dexterity, particularly multijoint movements, through both reciprocal connections with frontal motor areas, and through connections to the descending motor pathway through the red nucleus (85). The cerebellum receives inputs from a cortical network composed of motor, somatosensory, and posterior parietal areas via the pons. These inputs allow the cerebellum to compare the desired consequences of a movement (e.g., touching an elevator button), with the future progression of the hand through space as predicted from current motor commands. The cerebellum is often said to act as a "forward modeler" of the arm/hand for this reason (it can predict the consequences of the descending motor commands sent to the arm) (86, 87). The cerebellum is then able to modulate the ongoing stream of motor commands to correct anticipated errors, either through connections to SMA, or via a more direct modulation of the descending motor pathway via the red nucleus (86). Cerebellar damage results in motor incoordination, and a loss of the typical smoothness of manual motor trajectories through space (85, 88).

This highly interconnected reach network is further complicated by additional interconnections with the basal ganglia, the set of subcortical structures including the striatum (caudate nucleus and putamen), globus pallidus, subthalamic nucleus, and substantia nigra. Inputs to this functional grouping of nuclei from reach-related cortical areas are received by the striatum and processed by the remaining basal ganglia before being returned to the cortex (SMA) via the thalamus. The basal ganglia have a complex modulatory role in the reach motor network that appears to involve the choice of which movement to make, from among the possible alternatives, as well as the related function of assigning values to different possible movements (e.g., based on which are expected to be most rewarding) (89, 90).

SENSORIMOTOR CONTROL: OCULAR (EYE) AND MANUAL (HAND)

Overview

In humans, sensorimotor control strategies are essential for skilled somatic behavior; object manipulation performance aids in characterizing the interactions between the body and the article of interest (91). Before initiating a manual motor movement, the eyes very often fixate on the preferred object (92); however, a more invariant feature is that the eyes will spatially direct gaze on the target prior to the arrival of the hand (93), typically near the peak acceleration of the reach (94–96). The ocular motor system enables the needed visual information to direct the hand and successfully accomplish the task requirements; this is performed so fixations are "just in time," providing information at the moment the additional foveal-based fine detail would be required for the task at hand (97). Change blindness and short-term memory limitations, features of normal visual function, support the notion that information acquired during prior fixations factors minimally into computation (98–100). The information that is integrated across the fixations when a visual scene, for example, is largely semantic in nature, i.e., the memory of an object's identity but not specific features or the memory of a global scene but not particular details (101, 102). Therefore, eye movements are closely coupled to motor action in both time and space (103).

Sensorimotor coupling involves the fusion of visual perception and somatic motor control for action planning and behavioral execution; in fact, vision may best be understood through the "lens" of action production (104, 105). The line of sight is often directed at items of interest in an environment, upon which manual interactions may subsequently be focused. Based on the final goal of an intended manual interaction, grasping choices will be affected; this not only has relevance for motor control and planning requisite to finger position but also for eye fixation position, as gaze is paramount to precise manual action before execution (71). Eye fixations suggest a multitiered manual motor planning hierarchy. At the first level, it is determined where to grasp the object of interest, given the current descriptive content and the orientation of the object. If needed, at the second level the grasp is altered based on the type of secondary task to be accomplished with the grasped object, e.g., tool movement from location A to B. If needed, at the third level the movement plan incorporates a joint action component reflecting, e.g., the final resting place for the tool, handing it to a second person or placing it in a convenient location. Changes in the second and third levels of motor planning alter eye movement patterns and suggest a bidirectional sensorimotor coupling of eye to hand in coordinated activities (71).

The brain putatively plans visually guided action in the PPC, as suggested by neurophysiological studies in non-human primates, in imaging studies in healthy humans, and in human patients with cerebral injuries (74, 106–108). In non-human primate studies, electrophysiological results have revealed effector-specific regions in the PPC, with the parietal reach region relating to arm movements and the LIP area relating to saccadic activity. Given the relationship to effector preference but not dominance in these PPC subregions, functional imaging studies have sought to determine similar degrees of effector selectivity in human PPC, including area V7 and IPS areas 1 and 2 (IPS1 and IPS2) (109). Results indicate a limited degree of effector selectivity in the cortex and that transitions from the specificity surrounding one effector to another are gradual through the cerebral hierarchy in association with the frontal, parietal, and occipital cortices (109). In the visual cortex, there is a general preference noted for saccades, the PPC subregion, V7, has been specifically noted to activate relative to these fast eye movements. In the parietal cortex, IPS1 reflects a balance of saccade and reach activity, while IPS2 appears to be biased somewhat toward representing reach planning. In the frontal cortex, while regions near the central sulcus are more active for reach, FEF displays no effector preference (109), which may indirectly indicate a form of balance between eye and hand (**Figure 2**).

The PPC is of central importance given its strong feedforward connections to premotor and primary motor cortex (110). It has been suggested that the cytoarchitecture of networks between frontal and parietal cortices and their associative connections is ideal for integrating visual and somatic information (111). In fact, connections between the parietal and the dorsolateral (e.g., PMC) and medial (e.g., SMA) frontal motor areas may link vital neural information that assists in determining the visually deciphered target location and the somatic hand configuration required for execution (112). Expanding the integration network, the parieto-occipital junction shows activation when hand-motor goals are directed by a combination of gaze-oriented and proprioceptive body cues, suggesting some level of segregation within the reach-related regions of the PPC, while purely gaze-centered motor goals demonstrate activation in the anterior cuneus (113).

In visually guided reaching, studies in the macaque have shown that the ventral aspect of the parieto-occipital sulcus may act as a potential early node of the distributed eye–hand network, serving as a possible source of visual- and eye-position signals to parietal and frontal areas; this process has been described as re-entrant signaling, reciprocal associative connections leading to the interaction of eye and hand motor commands (110, 114). The ventral bank of the parieto-occipital sulcus, areas V6 and V6A, operates as an integrator of visual and somatic spatial information (115). There might be overlap between these two areas and the "parieto-occipital area" (PO) (116), but recent studies comparing the connections emphasize that V6Av (the ventral subregion of area V6A) is cytoarchitectonically and functionally distinct from the adjoining areas (V6 and V6Ad, the dorsal subregion) (117). More specifically, V6Av may serve as an integrator of visual and somatic/motor inputs (118). PPC is not only considered the sensorimotor interface for the planning and control of visually guided movements, but also conveys initial sensory-to-motor signals and online updates for the integration of sensory information from prior and current manual motor movement (119). The spatial position of the target is compared to the current spatial position of the hand which is thought to be represented in an eye-centered reference frame, mapping directly into motor error signals in a hand-centered reference frame; the superior parietal lobule (SPL) in the PPC is the primary location where these transformations are thought to occur with activation patterns mapped along a ventral–dorsal axis (119).

Coordinate Mapping Based on Visual Cues

Visual cues that translate into retinotopically coded information must be converted into meaningful output for effector-specific, goal-directed activity. The PPC may direct and plan movement by establishing a head/body-centered coordinate system, through both visual input and motor/proprioceptive cues, or, in contrast, utilize an eye-centered coordinate system (120, 121). An eye-centered frame of reference proves useful when considering the optimal dual-effector coordination, as eye movements are coded in eye-centered coordinates: extending this into PPC would ostensibly be strategic (122). In addition, the eye-centered reference frame used in PPC would help in accounting for online obstacles during visuomotor action and during error correction (123, 124). Evidence from macaque supports the concept of PPC operating under a common reference frame, where sensory targets are computationally processed for transformation from head-, body-, eye-, and limb-based coordinates into one eye-centered representation; this simplifies inter-effector motor planning (122).

The brain maintains a dynamic map of memory-based, geometric space in a gaze-centered coordinate system (125). On a cellular level, in the primate parietal cortex, the receptive fields of neurons have been shown to shift transiently in anticipation of an eye movement, predicting the sensory consequences of the intended eye movement (126). Given natural delays in sensory feedback and the anticipatory nature of this physiologic phenomenon, the mechanism is likely a forward model similar to what has been described for arm movements (87, 127, 128), which would combine sensory feedback with the predicted consequences of motor commands to facilitate online feedback control; additionally, this may impact the process by which the brain monitors and stores memories of previous movement execution and performance (125, 129, 130).

IMPAIRMENT OF THE VISUOMOTOR SYSTEM

Pathology and Clinical Disease

Pathology and clinical disease provides neuroanatomical and neurophysiological "knockouts" that can be diagnosed and characterized behaviorally, shedding light on cerebral function. Connecting empirical data on clinical deficits with neuroimaging and anatomical correlates yields greater understanding behind the nature of specific visuomotor pathologies and more significantly on relevant connections, associations, pathways, and networks. Optic ataxia (OA), as a clinical entity, is an archetype; patients demonstrate difficulty in executing visually guided reaching without additional sensory cues, accompanied by deficits in prehension and hand orientation. As opposed to Balint's syndrome or OA plus ocular apraxia and simultagnosia, an isolated optic ataxia often manifests with intact ocular motor function, full visual fields, normal depth perception, complete motor ability, and cerebellar function and no known cause of reaching ataxia. These clinical signs and disease patterns are attributed to lesions in the PPC or, more specifically, neurovascular injuries in the superior and inferior parietal lobule (SPL and IPL, respectively), around the IPS (131–134).

Optic ataxia, again defined as the inability to properly reach or grasp objects under visual control, particularly under peripheral vision, is associated neuroanatomically with dysfunction at the border of the SPL, near the IPS, but superior to the IPL, and behaviorally with poor motor performance when faced with moving targets that pose immediate motor programming challenges (135, 136). More precisely, the SPL receives afferent signals from the extrastriate areas of the occipital lobe and has reciprocal connections to and from the premotor and primary motor cortices of the frontal lobe, serving as a multisensory integration hub planning motor commands (137, 138). Optic ataxia has been interpreted as a combinatorial dysfunction in the ability of parietal neurons to integrate retinal, eye, and hand signals utilized for EHC (134). The neural mechanisms of hand movement corrections given rapid target changes shed light on the functional abilities of the eye and hand to maintain coupling and assist in further understanding the pathology of optic ataxia, highlighting clinical deficits that manifest as an inability to quickly adjust in-flight hand movement trajectories aimed at moving objects (132).

Sensorimotor Impairment

Cerebrovascular accident leads to sensorimotor impairments that result in a myriad of deficits in visually guided reaching and pointing movements, impairments that are noted in both the contralateral and ipsilateral hands (2, 139–145). The focus post-injury has been to examine the hand objectively during visually guided action without objective eye movement assessment, leaving one to question the abnormalities that may exist between effectors. In fact, the ocular motor system, when objectively assessed, has been shown to be a powerful tool in clinical neuroscience, serving as a marker of cerebral function (146–148). Recently, eye movements have been shown in stroke investigations to be a sensitive biomarker for cognitive and motor recovery (149, 150). Additionally, poststroke patients display unique pathophysiologic phenotypes that may include tactile deficits (151–153), proprioceptive losses (154, 155), hemiparesis and related motor synergies (156–158), and spasticity (159–161), which would suggest that these new sensory and motor "states" postinjury create new relationships between receptor and effector, requiring the need for re-integration (162–164).

In fact, poor visuomotor performance (EHC) has been associated with poorer accuracy and longer movement times in visually guided action poststroke, and these deficits have correlated significantly with impairments at the sensory and motor level; more specifically, poor chronometric and spatial performance in the more affected limbs of stroke subjects have correlated with tactile insensitivity, handgrip strength deficits and more severe motor impairment scores, as assessed by the Fugl-Meyer (2). It is well known that reaching depends on inputs from both vision and proprioception; tactile sensation is a component of proprioception, particularly when proprioceptive inputs may be impaired (165, 166). Evidence of this sensori-motor coupling in control physiology during multi-joint action tasks is well documented (167,168). Optimality in functionally oriented somatic movements of the upper extremity is demonstrated through hand paths that are straight, smooth, and with bell-shaped velocity profiles that scale with distance, implying advance planning (169, 170). These control markers set comparative baselines for investigations into impairment and not surprisingly suggest impairments in motor control programming at the planning level and at the sensorimotor interface level (162, 171, 172).

Following stroke, sensorimotor uncoupling is a byproduct of new relationships between impaired sensory input and poor motor output (163). As these new relationships are learned, the execution of limb movements is altered, above and beyond what would be expected from the individual deficits themselves: take for example a velocity curve that has an earlier peak and a prolonged deceleration phase, allowing greater opportunity for feedback mechanisms to improve endpoint accuracy (141, 163, 173). An intriguing experimental paradigm is the double-step saccade task (174), in that goal-directed action can be tested while a spatial target is displaced between two locations during the primary saccade, a period in which there is no visual perception. This paradigm can be deployed as a part of a visually guided reach to point task and will decrease the performance of the arm movement without mechanical perturbation or cognitive understanding of the manipulation. It has been suggested that during visually guided rapid arm-movement control, in which saccadic double-stepped targets are implemented, that spatial corrections of the hand are driven by ocular motor corrections following spatial target shifting (175).

Vision is essential to the sensori-motor integration required for visuomotor action. Gaze position is a consequence of ocular motor control and supports hand movement planning. These spatial locations or fixations often mark key positions for fingertip placement and are a byproduct of the functional requirements of the task at hand (91, 176). Furthermore, vision-based hand feedback is vital to motor adjustments during online control, as saccadic behavior updates spatial understanding and improves goal localization (177); in fact, it has been suggested that there is parallel processing between effectors (77, 178). This could be particularly problematic in patients with ABI with eye movement deficits (179–185), in addition to somatic motor deficits (e.g., hemiparesis). While manual motor deficits are typically evident on clinical examination, ocular motor deficits frequently require objective recording techniques (186–194) for identification and prognostication (181, 183, 195). Nevertheless, even if eye movements are found to be sound post-ABI, clinically and subclinically, following objective recordings, an impaired limb with poor functional performance may lead to maladaptive ocular motor behavior to compensate for lost task ability.

An eye-hand dyssynergia, or a lack of coordination between effectors, may operate in suboptimal modes to re-establish premorbid skill level, impeding recovery. This sensorimotor impairment may by multifactorial and compromised secondary to not only ocular motor deficits but also visuospatial and visuoperceptual abnormalities (196–200), in addition to balance deficits; in fact, decreases in balance have been noted during EHC tasks with stroke patients (142). This may all be of significant interest given the increased sensitivity during poststroke periods to sensory reweighting (201).

Deficits of Predictive Control

Our visual world is ever changing and prediction is a necessary part of object manipulation and consequently an important aspect of eye–hand control. Catching a ball or grasping a pen being handed to you requires anticipating the motion and direction of the object, and planning a motor response that will intersect successfully with the predicted trajectory. If the afferent end of visual processing or perception was simply used to generate spatial cues for EHC, our hand would consistently miss the spatial target; rather, an integrated construct replete with anticipation and prediction is pivotal to successful outcomes, which translate into functional performance (202). Superior skill in sports demonstrates finely tuned ocular motor control that drives complex somatic motor control (203–207). For example, soccer goalkeepers at the expert level demonstrate more accurate soccer ball prediction during anticipation tasks, as compared to novice level players; differences also include efficient and more effective strategies during visual search, which consist in part of longer fixations that are less frequent and directed at disparate regions of interest (208, 209).

In ABI, including injuries secondary to neurovascular and neurotraumatic insults significant predictive control deficits have been demonstrated during dynamic EHC tasks in the absence of deficits during static visuomotor tasks, highlighting difficulties in rapidly processing sensory information rather than motor execution errors. Delaying or inefficiently managing sensory information may not only lead to problems with target anticipation during dynamic tasks (feedforward impairment), but also the use of sensory feedback for error correction (1, 210). In fact, studies have demonstrated ocular motor deficits in predictive control within ABI for moving targets with and without intermittent stimulus blanking, and these impairments have been correlated with cognitive performance (211–213). Moreover, increasing cognitive load during predictive ocular motor tasks degrades performance in ABI and may suggest an "overload" to the impaired neural network (214).

This opens several broader questions, as patients with ABI who suffer from impaired eye movements, or even decreases in exploratory eye movements, may have perceptual limitations that hampers the understanding of scenes and spatial relationships between objects. This, in combination with loss of sensory feedback systems typically in place during action production, may increase the cognitive complexity of the task at hand (3). This may be more problematic in tasks for which EHC needs to flexibly convert from coupled function to uncoupled or decoupled function. For example, consider reaching for your cell phone while reading a newspaper, thus executing a somatic motor movement toward one spatial target while simultaneously executing saccades during the reading task elsewhere (74). Even asymptomatic post-ABI patients have shown difficulty in visually guided action when there is a level of dissociation between the visual information used to guide the required motoric action, decoupling the eye and the hand and perhaps increasing the task complexity. Similarly, multidomain tasks that encompass cognitive and motoric skill are effective at "pushing" the brain during functionally relevant performance; these constructs must be viewed on a spectrum. A cognitive "load" in such dual tasks can be experimentally manipulated and made more or less challenging for more effective screening; at the mild end, this may be accomplished by increasing the cognitive difficulty (e.g., visually guided pointing coupled with a serial sevens countdown), or decreased for those on the severe end by decreasing the cognitive difficulty (e.g., adding an easily predictable element to a spatial sequence of visually guided pointing) (215).

These predictive control deficits are provocative when framed in neurovascular and neurotraumatic conditions, particularly when visually guided action is uncoupled and spatial targets are dynamic. However, in the setting of neurodegeneration, whether one considers vascular dementia following repeated multistepped strokes or chronic traumatic encephalopathy following repeated traumatic brain injuries, these constructs are even more compelling, given the cognitive impairments that may be superimposed on ocular motor and/or visual deficits (216–219).

Disorders in Visuomotor Planning

Predictive control is a central element of visuomotor planning; this is particularly relevant during dynamic motor tasks with spatial targets that are in motion and that require anticipation for successful interaction (202). However, at a more basic level, if one considers motor programming or feedforward control during tasks without dynamically moving targets, the planning of hand movements during reach is impaired after stroke or post-ABI (171, 172, 220, 221). Impaired planning results in an inability to program sequences of motor action in space and time (139, 222–225). As the environment undergoes incessant change, our body must adapt, a fundamental element to spatially accurate motoric action. During adaptation, previously observed errors in one's own performance inform the correction of future motor plans. It has been suggested that sensory prediction errors are a primary input for motor programming revisions, during which planning is adjusted following a comparison between motor output and the predicted sensory outcomes of the original plan (226).

While planning is contingent on sensory information, e.g., vision and proprioception, laterality may also play a significant role. It has been even suggested that hemispheric specialization is paramount, producing dissociable differences in poststroke motor control. The left hemisphere is theorized to be motor-planning dominant for feedforward control while the right hemisphere is theorized to be feedback dominant for error correction during position control. Following this construct, a limb stabilized on a visual target may leverage right hemisphere resources, while a limb attempting to catch a moving ball may leverage left. In concert, optimizing ongoing action is undoubtedly the integration of feedforward and feedback control, and ABI has revealed deficits in initial trajectory profiles in left-brain injury and deficits in spatial accuracy in right-brain damage (227–230). Thorough assessment and targeted treatment of planning deficits may lead to improved motor relearning and functional recovery in ABI (221).

Clinical Implications and Outcome Measures

Acute and chronic disease processes that lead to cerebral injury are often challenging from a diagnostic and therapeutic standpoint; this is particularly true with neurodegenerative disorders secondary to their often diffuse and indolent nature, constraining our ability to isolate specific structural abnormalities with associations to functional limitations (231). To improve our understanding of neurophysiology and enhance our understanding of the clinical implications, experiments have historically concentrated on focal lesion-based approaches. These lesion-based models and associated biomarkers can be combined synergistically with the goal of detecting and characterizing the preclinical evolution of the neurobiological events that precede the cognitive impairments associated with neurodegeneration (232–235).

Objective eye movement recordings, when approached with methodological rigor, have already proven valuable as a research tool within ABI (236–238). In fact, ocular motor recordings have been used for their screening utility in a diagnostic capacity (211–214). As a response, rapid, vision-based performance measures that depend on time taken and errors made during visually presented number reading or object naming have been developed and extensively studied in the setting of ABI (239–244). More broadly, eye movements and visuomotor skill of the upper limb have been sensitive markers of cerebral injury (245). Taken further, eye and arm function following acute ABI has demonstrated good predictive capacity for outcomes in the subacute and chronic stages following injury with superior performance when compared to health status on self-report or based on neuropsychologic assessment (1, 246, 247). These prognostic capabilities have also enabled the identification of individuals who are poor responders or those who may require more aggressive intervention (248, 249). Ocular motor performance has even been demonstrated to be a biomarker of cognitive recovery beyond the times at which apparent full recovery had been deemed, as assessed by conventional metrics (150). While the literature is more extensive for neurovascular and neurotraumatic etiologies, the evidence base does extend into neurodegeneration (250, 251).

Given this framework, it is not difficult to see that there are extensive opportunities for translational ocular motor investigations that extend beyond the research setting and into the clinic. These opportunities are multiplied when ocular motor investigations are juxtaposed with manual motor investigations in ABI. While the clinical implications are significant, the literature has yet to see objective ocular motor and somatic motor control recordings enter the setting of ABI for unconstrained, coordinated eye and hand movements and frequently the motor output that is quantified during visually guided action is simply somatic in nature (**Table 2**). Though examples certainly exist where these two effectors have been objectively recorded, the movements have been constrained to one or two spatial dimensions, limiting the ecological validity; such constrained movements may require altered programmatic control between effectors, as a limb restricted to execute somatic motor output in an unnatural mode may have problematic effects on the ocular motor output, restricting comparisons. In the present narrative review, there was only one study that simultaneously recorded ocular and manual motor activity; the remaining manuscripts quantified movements of a single effector system (**Table 2**).

In fact, objective EHC tasks have already been designed for neurodegenerative disease processes, incorporating simultaneous ocular and manual motor recordings (252, 253). These investigations focused on integrated eye and hand assessments have yielded promising results and used simple tasks during which subjects are merely asked to perform a "look and reach," revealing quantifiable deficits in visually guided action (254). Additionally, and perhaps more promising, are tasks that have combined more cognitively demanding elements, e.g., antisaccades and antitapping, as part of an effort to increase the diagnostic power of the measures (252, 253, 255). While it has been suggested that objectified visuomotor tasks and related deficits may assist in diagnosing prodromal neurodegenerative disease entities and monitoring their progression, similar tasks that further increase complexity with distractors and/or feedback perturbations may assist in preclinical detection.

Currently, a central focus of rehabilitative interventions for cerebral injury is to restore motor ability and increase function. However, the return of motor ability often does not ensure ecologically valid, meaningful gains in function (222, 256). A clearer characterization of ocular motor control and its relationship to manual motor control will improve our understanding of EHC in a functional context. The quantitative relationships and motor outputs from both effectors are likely to yield metrics that can be correlated and compared to existing assessments and outcome measures utilized in current care models. Positive relationships will yield significant opportunities on the diagnostic, prognostic and therapeutic fronts, driving toward the development of algorithmic approaches with tailored, patient-specific management plans.

CONCLUSION

During goal-directed movement, first-rate function often requires that visual perception, under precise ocular motor control, be translated optimally into somatic action. Leveraging focal lesion-based models and associated eye–hand biomarkers is a robust approach toward significantly improving our understanding of acute and chronic neurological disease processes. In recent years, a number of studies have focused on EHC in ABI. The present review describes a series of studies that directly or indirectly highlight EHC in ABI and the neuroanatomic, computational, and broader clinical implications. While there is ample evidence to suggest that coupling is essential to EHC and that it is a sensitive biomarker for cerebral injury, visually guided action in the experimental setting has typically been limited to quantifying one effector or two effectors in a limited or constrained fashion. As such, it is recommended that future studies addressing related behavior should concurrently objectify ocular and manual motor control in unconstrained and natural modes. These studies, while technically more challenging, are likely to further characterize coupling and potentially yield high-impact results along the care spectrum from diagnosis to neurorehabilitative treatment in the setting of neurovascular, neurotraumatic, and neurodegenerative pathology.

AUTHOR CONTRIBUTIONS

Conception and design of the review: J-RR and EW. Substantial manuscript drafting: J-RR, MH, JF, WM, EA, PR, JR, ML, and TH.

ACKNOWLEDGMENTS

We would like to thank Dr. David S. Zee and Dr. Tamara Bushnik for their thoughts, suggestions, and contributions.

FUNDING

This research was supported in part by National Institutes of Health Grants EY08266 (to MSL), HD071978 (to PR), TR000038 (to J-RR), R03 AG042379 (to J-RR, ML, and PR), and 5K12 HD001097 (to J-RR, ML, and PR).

REFERENCES

1. Caeyenberghs K, van Roon D, van Aken K, De Cock P, Linden CV, Swinnen SP, et al. Static and dynamic visuomotor task performance in children with acquired brain injury: predictive control deficits under increased temporal pressure. *J Head Trauma Rehabil* (2009) 24:363–73. doi:10.1097/HTR.0b013e3181af0810
2. Gao KL, Ng SS, Kwok JW, Chow RT, Tsang WW. Eye-hand coordination and its relationship with sensori-motor impairments in stroke survivors. *J Rehabil Med* (2010) 42:368–73. doi:10.2340/16501977-0520
3. Ghika J, Ghika-Schmid F, Bogousslasvky J. Parietal motor syndrome: a clinical description in 32 patients in the acute phase of pure parietal strokes studied prospectively. *Clin Neurol Neurosurg* (1998) 100:271–82. doi:10.1016/S0303-8467(98)00054-7
4. Bard C, Fleury M, Hay L. *Development of Eye Hand Coordination across the Lifespan*. Columbia, SC: University of South Carolina Press (1990).
5. Crawford JD, Medendorp WP, Marotta JJ. Spatial transformations for eye-hand coordination. *J Neurophysiol* (2004) 92:10–9. doi:10.1152/jn.00117.2004
6. Farber SD. *Assessing Neuromotor Performance Enablers*. Thorofare, NJ: Slack (1991).
7. Zoltan B, Pedretti LW. *Evaluation of Muscle Tone and Coordination*. St. Louis: Mosby (1990).
8. Desrosiers J, Hebert R, Bravo G, Dutil E. Upper-extremity motor co-ordination of healthy elderly people. *Age Ageing* (1995) 24:108–12. doi:10.1093/ageing/24.2.108
9. Mountcastle VB. Modality and topographic properties of single neurons of cat's somatic sensory cortex. *J Neurophysiol* (1957) 20:408–34.
10. Sereno MI, Huang RS. A human parietal face area contains aligned head-centered visual and tactile maps. *Nat Neurosci* (2006) 9:1337–43. doi:10.1038/nn1777
11. McKyton A, Zohary E. Beyond retinotopic mapping: the spatial representation of objects in the human lateral occipital complex. *Cereb Cortex* (2007) 17:1164–72. doi:10.1093/cercor/bhl027
12. Goossens HH, van Opstal AJ. Influence of head position on the spatial representation of acoustic targets. *J Neurophysiol* (1999) 81:2720–36.
13. Andersen RA, Zipser D. The role of the posterior parietal cortex in coordinate transformations for visual-motor integration. *Can J Physiol Pharmacol* (1988) 66:488–501. doi:10.1139/y88-078
14. Mushiake H, Fujii N, Tanji J. Visually guided saccade versus eye-hand reach: contrasting neuronal activity in the cortical supplementary and frontal eye fields. *J Neurophysiol* (1996) 75:2187–91.
15. Mishkin M, Ungerleider LG, Macko KA. Object vision and spatial vision: two cortical pathways. *Trends Neurosci* (1983) 6:414–7. doi:10.1016/0166-2236(83)90190-X

16. Goodale MA, Milner AD. Separate visual pathways for perception and action. *Trends Neurosci* (1992) 15:20–5. doi:10.1016/0166-2236(92)90344-8
17. Milner AD, Goodale MA. Two visual systems re-viewed. *Neuropsychologia* (2008) 46:774–85. doi:10.1016/j.neuropsychologia.2007.10.005
18. Ungerleider LG, Mishkin M. Two cortical visual systems. In: Goodale MA, Mansfield RJW, Ingle DJ, editors. *Analysis of Visual Behavior*. Cambridge, MA: MIT Press (1982). p. 549–86.
19. Sheth BR, Young R. Two visual pathways in primates based on sampling of space: exploitation and exploration of visual information. *Front Integr Neurosci* (2016) 10:37. doi:10.3389/fnint.2016.00037
20. Goodale MA, Westwood DA. An evolving view of duplex vision: separate but interacting cortical pathways for perception and action. *Curr Opin Neurobiol* (2004) 14:203–11. doi:10.1016/j.conb.2004.03.002
21. Sereno AB, Sereno ME, Lehky SR. Recovering stimulus locations using populations of eye-position modulated neurons in dorsal and ventral visual streams of non-human primates. *Front Integr Neurosci* (2014) 8:28. doi:10.3389/fnint.2014.00028
22. van Polanen V, Davare M. Interactions between dorsal and ventral streams for controlling skilled grasp. *Neuropsychologia* (2015) 79:186–91. doi:10.1016/j.neuropsychologia.2015.07.010
23. Ferrier D. The croonian lecture: experiments on the brain of monkeys (second series). *Philos Trans R Soc Lond* (1875) 165:433–88. doi:10.1098/rstl.1875.0016
24. Huey EB. *The Psychology and Pedagogy of Reading: With a Review of the History of Reading and Writing and of Methods, Texts, and Hygiene in Reading*. New York, NY: Macmillan Company (1908).
25. Parthasarathy HB, Schall JD, Graybiel AM. Distributed but convergent ordering of corticostriatal projections: analysis of the frontal eye field and the supplementary eye field in the macaque monkey. *J Neurosci* (1992) 12:4468–88.
26. Huerta MF, Kaas JH. Supplementary eye field as defined by intracortical microstimulation: connections in macaques. *J Comp Neurol* (1990) 293: 299–330. doi:10.1002/cne.902930211
27. Luppino G, Rozzi S, Calzavara R, Matelli M. Prefrontal and agranular cingulate projections to the dorsal premotor areas F2 and F7 in the macaque monkey. *Eur J Neurosci* (2003) 17:559–78. doi:10.1046/j.1460-9568.2003.02476.x
28. Small DM, Gitelman DR, Gregory MD, Nobre AC, Parrish TB, Mesulam MM. The posterior cingulate and medial prefrontal cortex mediate the anticipatory allocation of spatial attention. *Neuroimage* (2003) 18:633–41. doi:10.1016/S1053-8119(02)00012-5
29. Wang SY, Wollin J. Falls among older people: identifying those at risk. *Nurs Older People* (2004) 15:14–6. doi:10.7748/nop2004.02.15.10.14.c2242
30. Keating EG. Frontal eye field lesions impair predictive and visually-guided pursuit eye movements. *Exp Brain Res* (1991) 86:311–23. doi:10.1007/BF00228954
31. Bruce CJ, Goldberg ME. Primate frontal eye fields. I. Single neurons discharging before saccades. *J Neurophysiol* (1985) 53:603–35.
32. Rivaud S, Muri RM, Gaymard B, Vermersch AI, Pierrot-Deseilligny C. Eye movement disorders after frontal eye field lesions in humans. *Exp Brain Res* (1994) 102:110–20. doi:10.1007/BF00232443
33. Dias EC, Segraves MA. Muscimol-induced inactivation of monkey frontal eye field: effects on visually and memory-guided saccades. *J Neurophysiol* (1999) 81:2191–214.
34. Mackey WE, Devinsky O, Doyle WK, Meager MR, Curtis CE. Human dorsolateral prefrontal cortex is not necessary for spatial working memory. *J Neurosci* (2016) 36:2847–56. doi:10.1523/jneurosci.3618-15.2016
35. Huerta MF, Krubitzer LA, Kaas JH. Frontal eye field as defined by intracortical microstimulation in squirrel monkeys, owl monkeys, and macaque monkeys. II. Cortical connections. *J Comp Neurol* (1987) 265:332–61. doi:10.1002/cne.902650304
36. Stanton GB, Bruce CJ, Goldberg ME. Topography of projections to posterior cortical areas from the macaque frontal eye fields. *J Comp Neurol* (1995) 353:291–305. doi:10.1002/cne.903530210
37. Bruce C, Friedman H, Kraus M, Stanton G. The primate frontal eye field. In: Chalupa LM, Werner JS, editors. *The Visual Neurosciences* (Vol. 1). Cambridge, MA: MIT Press (2004). p. 1428–48.
38. Schall JD, Stuphorn V, Brown JW. Monitoring and control of action by the frontal lobes. *Neuron* (2002) 36:309–22. doi:10.1016/S0896-6273(02)00964-9
39. Schall JD, Morel A, King DJ, Bullier J. Topography of visual-cortex connections with frontal eye field in macaque – convergence and segregation of processing streams. *J Neurosci* (1995) 15:4464–87.
40. Mackey WE, Devinsky O, Doyle WK, Golfinos JG, Curtis CE. Human parietal cortex lesions impact the precision of spatial working memory. *J Neurophysiol* (2016) 116:1049–54. doi:10.1152/jn.00380.2016
41. Stuphorn V, Bauswein E, Hoffmann KP. Neurons in the primate superior colliculus coding for arm movements in gaze-related coordinates. *J Neurophysiol* (2000) 83:1283–99.
42. Gaymard B, Pierrot-Deseilligny C, Rivaud S. Impairment of sequences of memory-guided saccades after supplementary motor area lesions. *Ann Neurol* (1990) 28:622–6. doi:10.1002/ana.410280504
43. Isoda M, Tanji J. Cellular activity in the supplementary eye field during sequential performance of multiple saccades. *J Neurophysiol* (2002) 88:3541–5. doi:10.1152/jn.00299.2002
44. Tehovnik EJ. The dorsomedial frontal cortex: eye and forelimb fields. *Behav Brain Res* (1995) 67:147–63. doi:10.1016/0166-4328(94)00151-5
45. Tehovnik EJ, Slocum WM, Tolias AS, Schiller PH. Saccades induced electrically from the dorsomedial frontal cortex: evidence for a head-centered representation. *Brain Res* (1998) 795:287–91. doi:10.1016/S0006-8993(98)00302-3
46. Pierrot-Deseilligny C, Muri RM, Nyffeler T, Milea D. The role of the human dorsolateral prefrontal cortex in ocular motor behavior. *Ann N Y Acad Sci* (2005) 1039:239–51. doi:10.1196/annals.1325.023
47. Tehovnik EJ, Lee K. The dorsomedial frontal cortex of the rhesus monkey: topographic representation of saccades evoked by electrical stimulation. *Exp Brain Res* (1993) 96:430–42. doi:10.1007/BF00234111
48. Mackey WE, Curtis CE. Distinct contributions by frontal and parietal cortices support working memory. *bioRxiv* (2017) (in press).
49. Pierrot-Deseilligny C, Milea D, Muri RM. Eye movement control by the cerebral cortex. *Curr Opin Neurol* (2004) 17:17–25. doi:10.1097/00019052-200402000-00005
50. Li CS, Mazzoni P, Andersen RA. Effect of reversible inactivation of macaque lateral intraparietal area on visual and memory saccades. *J Neurophysiol* (1999) 81:1827–38.
51. Silver MA, Ress D, Heeger DJ. Topographic maps of visual spatial attention in human parietal cortex. *J Neurophysiol* (2005) 94:1358–71. doi:10.1152/jn.01316.2004
52. Silver MA, Kastner S. Topographic maps in human frontal and parietal cortex. *Trends Cogn Sci* (2009) 13:488–95. doi:10.1016/j.tics.2009.08.005
53. Grefkes C, Fink GR. The functional organization of the intraparietal sulcus in humans and monkeys. *J Anat* (2005) 207:3–17. doi:10.1111/j.1469-7580.2005.00426.x
54. Shikata E, McNamara A, Sprenger A, Hamzei F, Glauche V, Buchel C, et al. Localization of human intraparietal areas AIP, CIP, and LIP using surface orientation and saccadic eye movement tasks. *Hum Brain Mapp* (2008) 29:411–21. doi:10.1002/hbm.20396
55. Bosley TM, Dann R, Silver FL, Alavi A, Kushner M, Chawluk JB, et al. Recovery of vision after ischemic lesions: positron emission tomography. *Ann Neurol* (1987) 21:444–50. doi:10.1002/ana.410210505
56. Gaymard B, Rivaud S, Cassarini JF, Dubard T, Rancurel G, Agid Y, et al. Effects of anterior cingulate cortex lesions on ocular saccades in humans. *Exp Brain Res* (1998) 120:173–83. doi:10.1007/s002210050391
57. Amiez C, Petrides M. Anatomical organization of the eye fields in the human and non-human primate frontal cortex. *Prog Neurobiol* (2009) 89:220–30. doi:10.1016/j.pneurobio.2009.07.010
58. Katyal S, Zughni S, Greene C, Ress D. Topography of covert visual attention in human superior colliculus. *J Neurophysiol* (2010) 104:3074–83. doi:10.1152/jn.00283.2010
59. DeSimone K, Viviano JD, Schneider KA. Population receptive field estimation reveals new retinotopic maps in human subcortex. *J Neurosci* (2015) 35:9836–47. doi:10.1523/jneurosci.3840-14.2015
60. Schiller PH, True SD, Conway JL. Deficits in eye movements following frontal eye-field and superior colliculus ablations. *J Neurophysiol* (1980) 44:1175–89.
61. Ploner CJ, Gaymard BM, Rivaud-Pechoux S, Pierrot-Deseilligny C. The prefrontal substrate of reflexive saccade inhibition in humans. *Biol Psychiatry* (2005) 57:1159–65. doi:10.1016/j.biopsych.2005.02.017

62. Nachev P, Wydell H, O'Neill K, Husain M, Kennard C. The role of the pre-supplementary motor area in the control of action. *Neuroimage* (2007) 36:T155–63. doi:10.1016/j.neuroimage.2007.03.034
63. Tehovnik EJ, Slocum WM, Schiller PH. Saccadic eye movements evoked by microstimulation of striate cortex. *Eur J Neurosci* (2003) 17:870–8. doi:10.1046/j.1460-9568.2003.02489.x
64. Funahashi S, Bruce CJ, Goldman-Rakic PS. Mnemonic coding of visual space in the monkey's dorsolateral prefrontal cortex. *J Neurophysiol* (1989) 61:331–49.
65. Funahashi S, Bruce CJ, Goldman-Rakic PS. Dorsolateral prefrontal lesions and oculomotor delayed-response performance: evidence for mnemonic "scotomas". *J Neurosci* (1993) 13:1479–97.
66. Kastner S, DeSimone K, Konen CS, Szczepanski SM, Weiner KS, Schneider KA. Topographic maps in human frontal cortex revealed in memory-guided saccade and spatial working-memory tasks. *J Neurophysiol* (2007) 97:3494–507. doi:10.1152/jn.00010.2007
67. Muri RM, Vermersch AI, Rivaud S, Gaymard B, Pierrot-Deseilligny C. Effects of single-pulse transcranial magnetic stimulation over the prefrontal and posterior parietal cortices during memory-guided saccades in humans. *J Neurophysiol* (1996) 76:2102–6.
68. Nyffeler T, Pierrot-Deseilligny C, Felblinger J, Mosimann UP, Hess CW, Muri RM. Time-dependent hierarchical organization of spatial working memory: a transcranial magnetic stimulation study. *Eur J Neurosci* (2002) 16:1823–7. doi:10.1046/j.1460-9568.2002.02252.x
69. Nyffeler T, Pierrot-Deseilligny C, Pflugshaupt T, von Wartburg R, Hess CW, Muri RM. Information processing in long delay memory-guided saccades: further insights from TMS. *Exp Brain Res* (2004) 154:109–12. doi:10.1007/s00221-003-1663-6
70. Ro T, Farne A, Chang E. Locating the human frontal eye fields with transcranial magnetic stimulation. *J Clin Exp Neuropsychol* (2002) 24:930–40. doi:10.1076/jcen.24.7.930.8385
71. Belardinelli A, Stepper MY, Butz MV. It's in the eyes: planning precise manual actions before execution. *J Vis* (2016) 16:18. doi:10.1167/16.1.18
72. Guyton AC, Hall JE. *Textbook of Medical Physiology*. Philadelphia: Saunders (2005).
73. Rathelot JA, Strick PL. Muscle representation in the macaque motor cortex: an anatomical perspective. *Proc Natl Acad Sci U S A* (2006) 103:8257–62. doi:10.1073/pnas.0602933103
74. Vesia M, Crawford JD. Specialization of reach function in human posterior parietal cortex. *Exp Brain Res* (2012) 221:1–18. doi:10.1007/s00221-012-3158-9
75. Blangero A, Menz MM, McNamara A, Binkofski F. Parietal modules for reaching. *Neuropsychologia* (2009) 47:1500–7. doi:10.1016/j.neuropsychologia.2008.11.030
76. Tunik E, Frey SH, Grafton ST. Virtual lesions of the anterior intraparietal area disrupt goal-dependent on-line adjustments of grasp. *Nat Neurosci* (2005) 8:505–11. doi:10.1038/nn1430
77. Prablanc C, Echallier JF, Komilis E, Jeannerod M. Optimal response of eye and hand motor systems in pointing at a visual target. I. Spatio-temporal characteristics of eye and hand movements and their relationships when varying the amount of visual information. *Biol Cybern* (1979) 35:113–24. doi:10.1007/BF00337063
78. Vercher JL, Magenes G, Prablanc C, Gauthier GM. Eye-head-hand coordination in pointing at visual targets: spatial and temporal analysis. *Exp Brain Res* (1994) 99:507–23. doi:10.1007/BF00228987
79. Henriques DY, Klier EM, Smith MA, Lowy D, Crawford JD. Gaze-centered remapping of remembered visual space in an open-loop pointing task. *J Neurosci* (1998) 18:1583–94.
80. Grol MJ, Majdandzic J, Stephan KE, Verhagen L, Dijkerman HC, Bekkering H, et al. Parieto-frontal connectivity during visually guided grasping. *J Neurosci* (2007) 27:11877–87. doi:10.1523/jneurosci.3923-07.2007
81. Cavina-Pratesi C, Monaco S, Fattori P, Galletti C, McAdam TD, Quinlan DJ, et al. Functional magnetic resonance imaging reveals the neural substrates of arm transport and grip formation in reach-to-grasp actions in humans. *J Neurosci* (2010) 30:10306–23. doi:10.1523/jneurosci.2023-10.2010
82. Gorbet DJ, Staines WR, Sergio LE. Brain mechanisms for preparing increasingly complex sensory to motor transformations. *Neuroimage* (2004) 23:1100–11. doi:10.1016/j.neuroimage.2004.07.043
83. Prado J, Clavagnier S, Otzenberger H, Scheiber C, Kennedy H, Perenin MT. Two cortical systems for reaching in central and peripheral vision. *Neuron* (2005) 48:849–58. doi:10.1016/j.neuron.2005.10.010
84. Filimon F, Nelson JD, Huang RS, Sereno MI. Multiple parietal reach regions in humans: cortical representations for visual and proprioceptive feedback during on-line reaching. *J Neurosci* (2009) 29:2961–71. doi:10.1523/jneurosci.3211-08.2009
85. Gibbon J, Malapani C, Dale CL, Gallistel C. Toward a neurobiology of temporal cognition: advances and challenges. *Curr Opin Neurobiol* (1997) 7:170–84. doi:10.1016/S0959-4388(97)80005-0
86. Desmurget M, Grafton S. Forward modeling allows feedback control for fast reaching movements. *Trends Cogn Sci* (2000) 4:423–31. doi:10.1016/S1364-6613(00)01537-0
87. Miall RC, Weir DJ, Wolpert DM, Stein JF. Is the cerebellum a smith predictor? *J Mot Behav* (1993) 25:203–16. doi:10.1080/00222895.1993.9942050
88. Bienkiewicz MM, Craig CM. Parkinson's is time on your side? Evidence for difficulties with sensorimotor synchronization. *Front Neurol* (2015) 6:249. doi:10.3389/fneur.2015.00249
89. Piray P, Toni I, Cools R. Human choice strategy varies with anatomical projections from ventromedial prefrontal cortex to medial striatum. *J Neurosci* (2016) 36:2857–67. doi:10.1523/jneurosci.2033-15.2016
90. Jocham G, Brodersen KH, Constantinescu AO, Kahn MC, Ianni AM, Walton ME, et al. Reward-guided learning with and without causal attribution. *Neuron* (2016) 90:177–90. doi:10.1016/j.neuron.2016.02.018
91. Flanagan JR, Bowman MC, Johansson RS. Control strategies in object manipulation tasks. *Curr Opin Neurobiol* (2006) 16:650–9. doi:10.1016/j.conb.2006.10.005
92. Carlton LG. Visual information: the control of aiming movements. *Q J Exp Psychol* (1981) 33:87–93. doi:10.1080/14640748108400771
93. Binsted G, Elliott D. Ocular perturbations and retinal/extraretinal information: the coordination of saccadic and manual movements. *Exp Brain Res* (1999) 127:193–206. doi:10.1007/s002210050789
94. Helsen WF, Elliott D, Starkes JL, Ricker KL. Temporal and spatial coupling of point of gaze and hand movements in aiming. *J Mot Behav* (1998) 30:249–59. doi:10.1080/00222899809601340
95. Helsen WF, Elliott D, Starkes JL, Ricker KL. Coupling of eye, finger, elbow, and shoulder movements during manual aiming. *J Mot Behav* (2000) 32:241–8. doi:10.1080/00222890009601375
96. Starkes J, Helsen W, Elliott D. A menage a trois: the eye, the hand and on-line processing. *J Sports Sci* (2002) 20:217–24. doi:10.1080/026404102317284772
97. Hayhoe MM, Shrivastava A, Mruczek R, Pelz JB. Visual memory and motor planning in a natural task. *J Vis* (2003) 3:49–63. doi:10.1167/3.1.6
98. Irwin DE. Information integration across saccadic eye movements. *Cogn Psychol* (1991) 23:420–56. doi:10.1016/0010-0285(91)90015-G
99. Irwin DE, Zacks JL, Brown JS. Visual memory and the perception of a stable visual environment. *Percept Psychophys* (1990) 47:35–46. doi:10.3758/BF03208162
100. Ballard DH, Hayhoe MM, Pelz JB. Memory representations in natural tasks. *J Cogn Neurosci* (1995) 7:66–80. doi:10.1162/jocn.1995.7.1.66
101. Irwin DE. Integrating information across saccadic eye movements. *Curr Dir Psychol Sci* (1996) 5:94–100. doi:10.1111/1467-8721.ep10772833
102. O'Regan JK. Solving the "real" mysteries of visual perception: the world as an outside memory. *Can J Psychol* (1992) 46:461–88. doi:10.1037/h0084327
103. Land M, Mennie N, Rusted J. The roles of vision and eye movements in the control of activities of daily living. *Perception* (1999) 28:1311–28. doi:10.1068/p2935
104. Ballard DH. Animate vision. *Artif Intell* (1991) 48:57–86. doi:10.1016/0004-3702(91)90080-4
105. Cilo M, Politzer T, Ripley DL, Weintraub A. Vision examination of TBI patients in an acute rehabilitation hospital. *NeuroRehabilitation* (2010) 27:237–42. doi:10.3233/NRE-2010-0603
106. Procacci NM, Stanford TR, Wittenberg GF. The relationship between visual orienting and interlimb synchrony in a patient with a superior parietal infarction: a case study. *Neurocase* (2009) 15:73–88. doi:10.1080/13554790802620558
107. Jeannerod M, Arbib MA, Rizzolatti G, Sakata H. Grasping objects: the cortical mechanisms of visuomotor transformation. *Trends Neurosci* (1995) 18:314–20. doi:10.1016/0166-2236(95)93921-J
108. Snyder LH, Batista AP, Andersen RA. Coding of intention in the posterior parietal cortex. *Nature* (1997) 386:167–70. doi:10.1038/386167a0

109. Levy I, Schluppeck D, Heeger DJ, Glimcher PW. Specificity of human cortical areas for reaches and saccades. *J Neurosci* (2007) 27:4687–96. doi:10.1523/jneurosci.0459-07.2007
110. Caminiti R, Genovesio A, Marconi B, Mayer AB, Onorati P, Ferraina S, et al. Early coding of reaching: frontal and parietal association connections of parieto-occipital cortex. *Eur J Neurosci* (1999) 11:3339–45. doi:10.1046/j.1460-9568.1999.00801.x
111. Johnson PB, Ferraina S, Bianchi L, Caminiti R. Cortical networks for visual reaching: physiological and anatomical organization of frontal and parietal lobe arm regions. *Cereb Cortex* (1996) 6:102–19. doi:10.1093/cercor/6.2.102
112. Johnson PB, Ferraina S. Cortical networks for visual reaching: intrinsic frontal lobe connectivity. *Eur J Neurosci* (1996) 8:1358–62. doi:10.1111/j.1460-9568.1996.tb01598.x
113. Bernier PM, Grafton ST. Human posterior parietal cortex flexibly determines reference frames for reaching based on sensory context. *Neuron* (2010) 68:776–88. doi:10.1016/j.neuron.2010.11.002
114. Tanne J, Boussaoud D, Boyer-Zeller N, Rouiller EM. Direct visual pathways for reaching movements in the macaque monkey. *Neuroreport* (1995) 7:267–72. doi:10.1097/00001756-199512000-00064
115. Galletti C, Fattori P, Battaglini PP, Shipp S, Zeki S. Functional demarcation of a border between areas V6 and V6A in the superior parietal gyrus of the macaque monkey. *Eur J Neurosci* (1996) 8:30–52. doi:10.1111/j.1460-9568.1996.tb01165.x
116. Colby CL, Gattass R, Olson CR, Gross CG. Topographical organization of cortical afferents to extrastriate visual area PO in the macaque: a dual tracer study. *J Comp Neurol* (1988) 269:392–413. doi:10.1002/cne.902690307
117. Galletti C, Gamberini M, Kutz DF, Baldinotti I, Fattori P. The relationship between V6 and PO in macaque extrastriate cortex. *Eur J Neurosci* (2005) 21:959–70. doi:10.1111/j.1460-9568.2005.03911.x
118. Passarelli L, Rosa MG, Gamberini M, Bakola S, Burman KJ, Fattori P, et al. Cortical connections of area V6Av in the macaque: a visual-input node to the eye/hand coordination system. *J Neurosci* (2011) 31:1790–801. doi:10.1523/jneurosci.4784-10.2011
119. Buneo CA, Andersen RA. The posterior parietal cortex: sensorimotor interface for the planning and online control of visually guided movements. *Neuropsychologia* (2006) 44:2594–606. doi:10.1016/j.neuropsychologia.2005.10.011
120. Connolly JD, Vuong QC, Thiele A. Gaze-dependent topography in human posterior parietal cortex. *Cereb Cortex* (2015) 25:1519–26. doi:10.1093/cercor/bht344
121. Soechting JF, Flanders M. Moving in three-dimensional space: frames of reference, vectors, and coordinate systems. *Annu Rev Neurosci* (1992) 15:167–91. doi:10.1146/annurev.ne.15.030192.001123
122. Cohen YE, Andersen RA. A common reference frame for movement plans in the posterior parietal cortex. *Nat Rev Neurosci* (2002) 3:553–62. doi:10.1038/nrn873
123. Batista AP, Buneo CA, Snyder LH, Andersen RA. Reach plans in eye-centered coordinates. *Science* (1999) 285:257–60. doi:10.1126/science.285.5425.257
124. McGuire LM, Sabes PN. Sensory transformations and the use of multiple reference frames for reach planning. *Nat Neurosci* (2009) 12:1056–61. doi:10.1038/nn.2357
125. Medendorp WP, Beurze SM, Van Pelt S, Van Der Werf J. Behavioral and cortical mechanisms for spatial coding and action planning. *Cortex* (2008) 44:587–97. doi:10.1016/j.cortex.2007.06.001
126. Duhamel JR, Colby CL, Goldberg ME. The updating of the representation of visual space in parietal cortex by intended eye movements. *Science* (1992) 255:90–2. doi:10.1126/science.1553535
127. Sommer MA, Wurtz RH. A pathway in primate brain for internal monitoring of movements. *Science* (2002) 296:1480–2. doi:10.1126/science.1069590
128. Sommer MA, Wurtz RH. Brain circuits for the internal monitoring of movements. *Annu Rev Neurosci* (2008) 31:317–38. doi:10.1146/annurev.neuro.31.060407.125627
129. Vaziri S, Diedrichsen J, Shadmehr R. Why does the brain predict sensory consequences of oculomotor commands? Optimal integration of the predicted and the actual sensory feedback. *J Neurosci* (2006) 26:4188–97. doi:10.1523/jneurosci.4747-05.2006
130. Wolpert DM, Kawato M. Multiple paired forward and inverse models for motor control. *Neural Netw* (1998) 11:1317–29. doi:10.1016/S0893-6080(98)00066-5
131. Andersen RA, Andersen KN, Hwang EJ, Hauschild M. Optic ataxia: from Balint's syndrome to the parietal reach region. *Neuron* (2014) 81:967–83. doi:10.1016/j.neuron.2014.02.025
132. Battaglia-Mayer A, Archambault PS, Caminiti R. The cortical network for eye-hand coordination and its relevance to understanding motor disorders of parietal patients. *Neuropsychologia* (2006) 44:2607–20. doi:10.1016/j.neuropsychologia.2005.11.021
133. Perenin MT, Vighetto A. Optic ataxia: a specific disruption in visuomotor mechanisms. I. Different aspects of the deficit in reaching for objects. *Brain* (1988) 111(Pt 3):643–74. doi:10.1093/brain/111.3.643
134. Battaglia-Mayer A, Caminiti R. Optic ataxia as a result of the breakdown of the global tuning fields of parietal neurones. *Brain* (2002) 125:225–37. doi:10.1093/brain/awf034
135. Rossetti Y, Pisella L, Vighetto A. Optic ataxia revisited: visually guided action versus immediate visuomotor control. *Exp Brain Res* (2003) 153:171–9. doi:10.1007/s00221-003-1590-6
136. Milner AD, Paulignan Y, Dijkerman HC, Michel F, Jeannerod M. A paradoxical improvement of misreaching in optic ataxia: new evidence for two separate neural systems for visual localization. *Proc Biol Sci* (1999) 266:2225–9. doi:10.1098/rspb.1999.0912
137. Andersen RA, Buneo CA. Intentional maps in posterior parietal cortex. *Annu Rev Neurosci* (2002) 25:189–220. doi:10.1146/annurev.neuro.25.112701.142922
138. Battaglia-Mayer A, Caminiti R, Lacquaniti F, Zago M. Multiple levels of representation of reaching in the parieto-frontal network. *Cereb Cortex* (2003) 13:1009–22. doi:10.1093/cercor/13.10.1009
139. Beer RF, Dewald JP, Rymer WZ. Deficits in the coordination of multijoint arm movements in patients with hemiparesis: evidence for disturbed control of limb dynamics. *Exp Brain Res* (2000) 131:305–19. doi:10.1007/s002219900275
140. Fisher BE, Winstein CJ, Velicki MR. Deficits in compensatory trajectory adjustments after unilateral sensorimotor stroke. *Exp Brain Res* (2000) 132:328–44. doi:10.1007/s002210000391
141. McCrea PH, Eng JJ. Consequences of increased neuromotor noise for reaching movements in persons with stroke. *Exp Brain Res* (2005) 162:70–7. doi:10.1007/s00221-004-2106-8
142. Tsang WW, Ng SS, Lee MW, Tse SP, Yip EW, Yuen JK. Does postural stability affect the performance of eye-hand coordination in stroke survivors? *Am J Phys Med Rehabil* (2013) 92:781–8. doi:10.1097/PHM.0b013e3182876adb
143. Velicki MR, Winstein CJ, Pohl PS. Impaired direction and extent specification of aimed arm movements in humans with stroke-related brain damage. *Exp Brain Res* (2000) 130:362–74. doi:10.1007/s002219900262
144. Wenzelburger R, Kopper F, Frenzel A, Stolze H, Klebe S, Brossmann A, et al. Hand coordination following capsular stroke. *Brain* (2005) 128:64–74. doi:10.1093/brain/awh317
145. Zackowski KM, Dromerick AW, Sahrmann SA, Thach WT, Bastian AJ. How do strength, sensation, spasticity and joint individuation relate to the reaching deficits of people with chronic hemiparesis? *Brain* (2004) 127:1035–46. doi:10.1093/brain/awh116
146. Leigh RJ, Kennard C. Using saccades as a research tool in the clinical neurosciences. *Brain* (2004) 127:460–77. doi:10.1093/brain/awh035
147. White OB, Fielding J. Cognition and eye movements: assessment of cerebral dysfunction. *J Neuroophthalmol* (2012) 32:266–73. doi:10.1097/WNO.0b013e3182688230
148. Ramat S, Leigh RJ, Zee DS, Optican LM. What clinical disorders tell us about the neural control of saccadic eye movements. *Brain* (2007) 130:10–35. doi:10.1093/brain/awl309
149. Anderson T. Could saccadic function be a useful marker of stroke recovery? *J Neurol Neurosurg Psychiatry* (2013) 84:242. doi:10.1136/jnnp-2012-304481
150. Dong W, Yan B, Johnson BP, Millist L, Davis S, Fielding J, et al. Ischaemic stroke: the ocular motor system as a sensitive marker for motor and cognitive recovery. *J Neurol Neurosurg Psychiatry* (2013) 84:337–41. doi:10.1136/jnnp-2012-303926
151. Lima NM, Menegatti KC, Yu E, Sacomoto NY, Scalha TB, Lima IN, et al. Sensory deficits in ipsilesional upper-extremity in chronic stroke patients. *Arq Neuropsiquiatr* (2015) 73:834–9. doi:10.1590/0004-282X20150128
152. Meyer S, Karttunen AH, Thijs V, Feys H, Verheyden G. How do somatosensory deficits in the arm and hand relate to upper limb impairment, activity,

and participation problems after stroke? A systematic review. *Phys Ther* (2014) 94:1220–31. doi:10.2522/ptj.20130271
153. Scalha TB, Miyasaki E, Lima NM, Borges G. Correlations between motor and sensory functions in upper limb chronic hemiparetics after stroke. *Arq Neuropsiquiatr* (2011) 69:624–9. doi:10.1590/S0004-282X2011000500010
154. Findlater SE, Dukelow SP. Upper extremity proprioception after stroke: bridging the gap between neuroscience and rehabilitation. *J Mot Behav* (2017) 49:27–34. doi:10.1080/00222895.2016.1219303
155. Hughes CM, Tommasino P, Budhota A, Campolo D. Upper extremity proprioception in healthy aging and stroke populations, and the effects of therapist- and robot-based rehabilitation therapies on proprioceptive function. *Front Hum Neurosci* (2015) 9:120. doi:10.3389/fnhum.2015.00120
156. Ekstrand E, Lexell J, Brogardh C. Grip strength is a representative measure of muscle weakness in the upper extremity after stroke. *Top Stroke Rehabil* (2016) 23:400–5. doi:10.1080/10749357.2016.1168591
157. McCrea PH, Eng JJ, Hodgson AJ. Saturated muscle activation contributes to compensatory reaching strategies after stroke. *J Neurophysiol* (2005) 94:2999–3008. doi:10.1152/jn.00732.2004
158. Rohafza M, Fluet GG, Qiu Q, Adamovich S. Correlation of reaching and grasping kinematics and clinical measures of upper extremity function in persons with stroke related hemiplegia. *Conf Proc IEEE Eng Med Biol Soc* (2014) 2014:3610–3. doi:10.1109/EMBC.2014.6944404
159. Kong KH, Lee J, Chua KS. Occurrence and temporal evolution of upper limb spasticity in stroke patients admitted to a rehabilitation unit. *Arch Phys Med Rehabil* (2012) 93:143–8. doi:10.1016/j.apmr.2011.06.027
160. Opheim A, Danielsson A, Alt Murphy M, Persson HC, Sunnerhagen KS. Upper-limb spasticity during the first year after stroke: stroke arm longitudinal study at the University of Gothenburg. *Am J Phys Med Rehabil* (2014) 93:884–96. doi:10.1097/PHM.0000000000000157
161. Opheim A, Danielsson A, Alt Murphy M, Persson HC, Sunnerhagen KS. Early prediction of long-term upper limb spasticity after stroke: part of the SALGOT study. *Neurology* (2015) 85:873–80. doi:10.1212/WNL.0000000000001908
162. Levin MF. Interjoint coordination during pointing movements is disrupted in spastic hemiparesis. *Brain* (1996) 119(Pt 1):281–93. doi:10.1093/brain/119.1.281
163. Trombly CA. Deficits of reaching in subjects with left hemiparesis: a pilot study. *Am J Occup Ther* (1992) 46:887–97. doi:10.5014/ajot.46.10.887
164. Raghavan P. Upper limb motor impairment after stroke. *Phys Med Rehabil Clin N Am* (2015) 26:599–610. doi:10.1016/j.pmr.2015.06.008
165. Rao AK, Gordon AM. Contribution of tactile information to accuracy in pointing movements. *Exp Brain Res* (2001) 138:438–45. doi:10.1007/s002210100717
166. Van Beers RJ, Sittig AC, Denier Van Der Gon JJ. Localization of a seen finger is based exclusively on proprioception and on vision of the finger. *Exp Brain Res* (1999) 125:43–9. doi:10.1007/s002210050656
167. Flanagan JR, Ostry DJ, Feldman AG. Control of trajectory modifications in target-directed reaching. *J Mot Behav* (1993) 25:140–52. doi:10.1080/00222895.1993.9942045
168. Ghafouri M, Feldman AG. The timing of control signals underlying fast point-to-point arm movements. *Exp Brain Res* (2001) 137:411–23. doi:10.1007/s002210000643
169. Hogan N, Flash T. Moving gracefully: quantitative theories of motor coordination. *Trends Neurosci* (1987) 10:170–4. doi:10.1016/0166-2236(87)90043-9
170. Gordon J, Ghilardi MF, Ghez C. Accuracy of planar reaching movements. I. Independence of direction and extent variability. *Exp Brain Res* (1994) 99:97–111. doi:10.1007/BF00241415
171. Raghavan P, Krakauer JW, Gordon AM. Impaired anticipatory control of fingertip forces in patients with a pure motor or sensorimotor lacunar syndrome. *Brain* (2006) 129:1415–25. doi:10.1093/brain/awl070
172. Raghavan P, Santello M, Gordon AM, Krakauer JW. Compensatory motor control after stroke: an alternative joint strategy for object-dependent shaping of hand posture. *J Neurophysiol* (2010) 103:3034–43. doi:10.1152/jn.00936.2009
173. Nagasaki H. Asymmetric velocity and acceleration profiles of human arm movements. *Exp Brain Res* (1989) 74:319–26. doi:10.1007/BF00248865
174. Becker W, Jurgens R. An analysis of the saccadic system by means of double step stimuli. *Vision Res* (1979) 19:967–83. doi:10.1016/0042-6989(79)90222-0
175. Blouin J, Teasdale N, Bard C, Fleury M. Control of rapid arm movements when target position is altered during saccadic suppression. *J Mot Behav* (1995) 27:114–22. doi:10.1080/00222895.1995.9941704
176. Johansson RS, Westling G, Backstrom A, Flanagan JR. Eye-hand coordination in object manipulation. *J Neurosci* (2001) 21:6917–32.
177. Gaveau V, Pisella L, Priot AE, Fukui T, Rossetti Y, Pelisson D, et al. Automatic online control of motor adjustments in reaching and grasping. *Neuropsychologia* (2014) 55:25–40. doi:10.1016/j.neuropsychologia.2013.12.005
178. Prablanc C, Echallier JE, Jeannerod M, Komilis E. Optimal response of eye and hand motor systems in pointing at a visual target. II. Static and dynamic visual cues in the control of hand movement. *Biol Cybern* (1979) 35:183–7. doi:10.1007/BF00337436
179. Bogousslavsky J. Impairment of visually evoked eye movements with a unilateral parieto-occipital lesion. *J Neurol* (1987) 234:160–2. doi:10.1007/BF00314136
180. Bogousslavsky J, Meienberg O. Eye-movement disorders in brain-stem and cerebellar stroke. *Arch Neurol* (1987) 44:141–8. doi:10.1001/archneur.1987.00520140013011
181. Catz A, Ron S, Solzi P, Korczyn AD. Saccade characteristics in patients with hemispheric stroke. *J Neurol Rehabil* (1997) 11:175–80.
182. Colombo A, Gibertoni M, Sorgato P. [Clinical study of disorders of eye movements (voluntary and following) after acute vascular accidents involving the cerebral hemispheres (author's transl)]. *Riv Patol Nerv Ment* (1981) 102:38–46.
183. Lekwuwa GU, Barnes GR. Cerebral control of eye movements. II. Timing of anticipatory eye movements, predictive pursuit and phase errors in focal cerebral lesions. *Brain* (1996) 119(Pt 2):491–505. doi:10.1093/brain/119.2.491
184. Pierrot-Deseilligny C, Ploner CJ, Muri RM, Gaymard B, Rivaud-Pechoux S. Effects of cortical lesions on saccadic: eye movements in humans. *Ann N Y Acad Sci* (2002) 956:216–29. doi:10.1111/j.1749-6632.2002.tb02821.x
185. Waespe W, Baumgartner R. Enduring dysmetria and impaired gain adaptivity of saccadic eye movements in Wallenberg's lateral medullary syndrome. *Brain* (1992) 115(Pt 4):1123–46. doi:10.1093/brain/115.4.1125
186. Agrawal Y, Schubert MC, Migliaccio AA, Zee DS, Schneider E, Lehnen N, et al. Evaluation of quantitative head impulse testing using search coils versus video-oculography in older individuals. *Otol Neurotol* (2014) 35:283–8. doi:10.1097/MAO.0b013e3182995227
187. Eggert T. Eye movement recordings: methods. *Dev Ophthalmol* (2007) 40:15–34. doi:10.1159/000100347
188. Houben MM, Goumans J, van der Steen J. Recording three-dimensional eye movements: scleral search coils versus video oculography. *Invest Ophthalmol Vis Sci* (2006) 47:179–87. doi:10.1167/iovs.05-0234
189. Imai T, Sekine K, Hattori K, Takeda N, Koizuka I, Nakamae K, et al. Comparing the accuracy of video-oculography and the scleral search coil system in human eye movement analysis. *Auris Nasus Larynx* (2005) 32:3–9. doi:10.1016/j.anl.2004.11.009
190. Kimmel DL, Mammo D, Newsome WT. Tracking the eye non-invasively: simultaneous comparison of the scleral search coil and optical tracking techniques in the macaque monkey. *Front Behav Neurosci* (2012) 6:49. doi:10.3389/fnbeh.2012.00049
191. McCamy MB, Otero-Millan J, Leigh RJ, King SA, Schneider RM, Macknik SL, et al. Simultaneous recordings of human microsaccades and drifts with a contemporary video eye tracker and the search coil technique. *PLoS One* (2015) 10:e0128428. doi:10.1371/journal.pone.0128428
192. Stahl JS, van Alphen AM, De Zeeuw CI. A comparison of video and magnetic search coil recordings of mouse eye movements. *J Neurosci Methods* (2000) 99:101–10. doi:10.1016/S0165-0270(00)00218-1
193. van der Geest JN, Frens MA. Recording eye movements with video-oculography and scleral search coils: a direct comparison of two methods. *J Neurosci Methods* (2002) 114:185–95. doi:10.1016/S0165-0270(01)00527-1
194. Yee RD, Schiller VL, Lim V, Baloh FG, Baloh RW, Honrubia V. Velocities of vertical saccades with different eye movement recording methods. *Invest Ophthalmol Vis Sci* (1985) 26:938–44.
195. Machado L, Rafal RD. Control of fixation and saccades in humans with chronic lesions of oculomotor cortex. *Neuropsychology* (2004) 18:115–23. doi:10.1037/0894-4105.18.1.115
196. Kaplan J, Hier DB. Visuospatial deficits after right hemisphere stroke. *Am J Occup Ther* (1982) 36:314–21. doi:10.5014/ajot.36.5.314

197. Machner B, Sprenger A, Kompf D, Sander T, Heide W, Kimmig H, et al. Visual search disorders beyond pure sensory failure in patients with acute homonymous visual field defects. *Neuropsychologia* (2009) 47:2704–11. doi:10.1016/j.neuropsychologia.2009.05.016
198. Malhotra P, Coulthard E, Husain M. Hemispatial neglect, balance and eye-movement control. *Curr Opin Neurol* (2006) 19:14–20. doi:10.1097/01.wco.0000198101.87670.7e
199. Mennem TA, Warren M, Yuen HK. Preliminary validation of a vision-dependent activities of daily living instrument on adults with homonymous hemianopia. *Am J Occup Ther* (2012) 66:478–82. doi:10.5014/ajot.2012.004762
200. Rowe F. Visual perceptual consequences of stroke. *Strabismus* (2009) 17:24–8. doi:10.1080/09273970802678537
201. Bonan IV, Gaillard F, Ponche ST, Marquer A, Vidal PP, Yelnik AP. Early post-stroke period: a privileged time for sensory re-weighting? *J Rehabil Med* (2015) 47:516–22. doi:10.2340/16501977-1968
202. Hudson TE, Maloney LT, Landy MS. Movement planning with probabilistic target information. *J Neurophysiol* (2007) 98:3034–46. doi:10.1152/jn.00858.2007
203. Mann DT, Williams AM, Ward P, Janelle CM. Perceptual-cognitive expertise in sport: a meta-analysis. *J Sport Exerc Psychol* (2007) 29:457–78. doi:10.1123/jsep.29.4.457
204. McRobert AP, Williams AM, Ward P, Eccles DW. Tracing the process of expertise in a simulated anticipation task. *Ergonomics* (2009) 52:474–83. doi:10.1080/00140130802707824
205. Piras A, Lobietti R, Squatrito S. A study of saccadic eye movement dynamics in volleyball: comparison between athletes and non-athletes. *J Sports Med Phys Fitness* (2010) 50:99–108.
206. Willams AM, Hodges NJ, North JS, Barton G. Perceiving patterns of play in dynamic sport tasks: investigating the essential information underlying skilled performance. *Perception* (2006) 35:317–32. doi:10.1068/p5310
207. Williams AM. Perceptual skill in soccer: implications for talent identification and development. *J Sports Sci* (2000) 18:737–50. doi:10.1080/02640410050120113
208. Savelsbergh GJ, Williams AM, Van der Kamp J, Ward P. Visual search, anticipation and expertise in soccer goalkeepers. *J Sports Sci* (2002) 20:279–87. doi:10.1080/026404102317284826
209. Savelsbergh GJ, Van der Kamp J, Williams AM, Ward P. Anticipation and visual search behaviour in expert soccer goalkeepers. *Ergonomics* (2005) 48:1686–97. doi:10.1080/00140130500101346
210. Caeyenberghs K, Leemans A, Geurts M, Taymans T, Vander Linden C, Smits-Engelsman BC, et al. Brain-behavior relationships in young traumatic brain injury patients: fractional anisotropy measures are highly correlated with dynamic visuomotor tracking performance. *Neuropsychologia* (2010) 48:1472–82. doi:10.1016/j.neuropsychologia.2010.01.017
211. Suh M, Basu S, Kolster R, Sarkar R, McCandliss B, Ghajar J, et al. Increased oculomotor deficits during target blanking as an indicator of mild traumatic brain injury. *Neurosci Lett* (2006) 410:203–7. doi:10.1016/j.neulet.2006.10.001
212. Suh M, Kolster R, Sarkar R, McCandliss B, Ghajar J; Cognitive and Neurobiological Research Consortium. Deficits in predictive smooth pursuit after mild traumatic brain injury. *Neurosci Lett* (2006) 401:108–13. doi:10.1016/j.neulet.2006.02.074
213. Maruta J, Suh M, Niogi SN, Mukherjee P, Ghajar J. Visual tracking synchronization as a metric for concussion screening. *J Head Trauma Rehabil* (2010) 25:293–305. doi:10.1097/HTR.0b013e3181e67936
214. Contreras R, Ghajar J, Bahar S, Suh M. Effect of cognitive load on eye-target synchronization during smooth pursuit eye movement. *Brain Res* (2011) 1398:55–63. doi:10.1016/j.brainres.2011.05.004
215. Brown JA, Dalecki M, Hughes C, Macpherson AK, Sergio LE. Cognitive-motor integration deficits in young adult athletes following concussion. *BMC Sports Sci Med Rehabil* (2015) 7:25. doi:10.1186/s13102-015-0019-4
216. Armstrong R, Kergoat H. Oculo-visual changes and clinical considerations affecting older patients with dementia. *Ophthalmic Physiol Opt* (2015) 35:352–76. doi:10.1111/opo.12220
217. Rosler A, Billino J, Muller NG, Weidauer S, Steinmetz H, Kleinschmidt A. Visual search in patients with subcortical vascular dementia: short fixations but long reaction times. *Dement Geriatr Cogn Disord* (2005) 20:375–80. doi:10.1159/000089104
218. Schewe HJ, Uebelhack R, Vohs K. Abnormality in saccadic eye movement in dementia. *Eur Psychiatry* (1999) 14:52–3. doi:10.1016/S0924-9338(99)80716-0
219. Ling H, Kara E, Revesz T, Lees AJ, Plant GT, Martino D, et al. Concomitant progressive supranuclear palsy and chronic traumatic encephalopathy in a boxer. *Acta Neuropathol Commun* (2014) 2:24. doi:10.1186/2051-5960-2-24
220. Beer R, Dewald J, Rymer Z. Disturbances of voluntary movement coordination in stroke: problems of planning or execution? *Prog Brain Res* (1999) 123:455–60. doi:10.1016/S0079-6123(08)62881-2
221. Rizzo JR, Hudson TE, Abdou A, Rashbaum IG, George AE, Raghavan P, et al. Motor planning poststroke: impairment in vector-coded reach plans. *Physiol Rep* (2015) 3:e12650. doi:10.14814/phy2.12650
222. Cirstea MC, Levin MF. Compensatory strategies for reaching in stroke. *Brain* (2000) 123(Pt 5):940–53. doi:10.1093/brain/123.5.940
223. Ketcham CJ, Rodriguez TM, Zihlman KA. Targeted aiming movements are compromised in nonaffected limb of persons with stroke. *Neurorehabil Neural Repair* (2007) 21:388–97. doi:10.1177/1545968306297872
224. Kusoffsky A, Apel I, Hirschfeld H. Reaching-lifting-placing task during standing after stroke: coordination among ground forces, ankle muscle activity, and hand movement. *Arch Phys Med Rehabil* (2001) 82:650–60. doi:10.1053/apmr.2001.22611
225. Takahashi CD, Reinkensmeyer DJ. Hemiparetic stroke impairs anticipatory control of arm movement. *Exp Brain Res* (2003) 149:131–40. doi:10.1007/s00221-002-1340-1
226. Tseng YW, Diedrichsen J, Krakauer JW, Shadmehr R, Bastian AJ. Sensory prediction errors drive cerebellum-dependent adaptation of reaching. *J Neurophysiol* (2007) 98:54–62. doi:10.1152/jn.00266.2007
227. Sarlegna FR, Sainburg RL. The roles of vision and proprioception in the planning of reaching movements. *Adv Exp Med Biol* (2009) 629:317–35. doi:10.1007/978-0-387-77064-2_16
228. Schaefer SY, Mutha PK, Haaland KY, Sainburg RL. Hemispheric specialization for movement control produces dissociable differences in online corrections after stroke. *Cereb Cortex* (2012) 22:1407–19. doi:10.1093/cercor/bhr237
229. Schaefer SY, Haaland KY, Sainburg RL. Ipsilesional motor deficits following stroke reflect hemispheric specializations for movement control. *Brain* (2007) 130:2146–58. doi:10.1093/brain/awm145
230. Shabbott BA, Sainburg RL. Differentiating between two models of motor lateralization. *J Neurophysiol* (2008) 100:565–75. doi:10.1152/jn.90349.2008
231. Roy OW, Cohen NR, Nicoll JA. Pathophysiology of dementias and implications for therapy. *Indian J Pathol Microbiol* (2005) 48:289–99.
232. Masdeu JC. Future directions in imaging neurodegeneration. *Curr Neurol Neurosci Rep* (2017) 17:9. doi:10.1007/s11910-017-0718-1
233. Sperling RA, Aisen PS, Beckett LA, Bennett DA, Craft S, Fagan AM, et al. Toward defining the preclinical stages of Alzheimer's disease: recommendations from the National Institute on aging-Alzheimer's Association workgroups on diagnostic guidelines for Alzheimer's disease. *Alzheimers Dement* (2011) 7:280–92. doi:10.1016/j.jalz.2011.03.003
234. Velazquez-Perez L, Rodriguez-Labrada R, Laffita-Mesa JM. Prodromal spinocerebellar ataxia type 2: prospects for early interventions and ethical challenges. *Mov Disord* (2017) 32:708–18. doi:10.1002/mds.26969
235. Meissner WG. When does Parkinson's disease begin? From prodromal disease to motor signs. *Rev Neurol (Paris)* (2012) 168:809–14. doi:10.1016/j.neurol.2012.07.004
236. Rizzo JR, Hudson TE, Dai W, Birkemeier J, Pasculli RM, Selesnick I, et al. Rapid number naming in chronic concussion: eye movements in the King–Devick test. *Ann Clin Transl Neurol* (2016) 3:801–11. doi:10.1002/acn3.345
237. Rizzo JR, Hudson TE, Dai W, Desai N, Yousefi A, Palsana D, et al. Objectifying eye movements during rapid number naming: methodology for assessment of normative data for the King–Devick test. *J Neurol Sci* (2016) 362:232–9. doi:10.1016/j.jns.2016.01.045
238. Hutton SB. Cognitive control of saccadic eye movements. *Brain Cogn* (2008) 68:327–40. doi:10.1016/j.bandc.2008.08.021
239. Cobbs L, Hasanaj L, Amorapanth P, Rizzo JR, Nolan R, Serrano L, et al. Mobile universal lexicon evaluation system (MULES) test: a new measure of rapid picture naming for concussion. *J Neurol Sci* (2017) 372:393–8. doi:10.1016/j.jns.2016.10.044
240. Galetta KM, Barrett J, Allen M, Madda F, Delicata D, Tennant AT, et al. The King–Devick test as a determinant of head trauma and concussion

in boxers and MMA fighters. *Neurology* (2011) 76:1456–62. doi:10.1212/WNL.0b013e31821184c9

241. Galetta KM, Brandes LE, Maki K, Dziemianowicz MS, Laudano E, Allen M, et al. The King–Devick test and sports-related concussion: study of a rapid visual screening tool in a collegiate cohort. *J Neurol Sci* (2011) 309:34–9. doi:10.1016/j.jns.2011.07.039
242. Galetta KM, Liu M, Leong DF, Ventura RE, Galetta SL, Balcer LJ. The King–Devick test of rapid number naming for concussion detection: meta analysis and systematic review of the literature. *Concussion* (2015) 15:1–15.
243. Leong DF, Balcer LJ, Galetta SL, Evans G, Gimre M, Watt D. The King–Devick test for sideline concussion screening in collegiate football. *J Optom* (2015) 8:131–9. doi:10.1016/j.optom.2014.12.005
244. Ventura RE, Balcer LJ, Galetta SL, Rucker JC. Ocular motor assessment in concussion: current status and future directions. *J Neurol Sci* (2016) 361:79–86. doi:10.1016/j.jns.2015.12.010
245. Heitger MH, Anderson TJ, Jones RD, Dalrymple-Alford JC, Frampton CM, Ardagh MW. Eye movement and visuomotor arm movement deficits following mild closed head injury. *Brain* (2004) 127:575–90. doi:10.1093/brain/awh066
246. Heitger MH, Jones RD, Dalrymple-Alford JC, Frampton CM, Ardagh MW, Anderson TJ. Mild head injury – a close relationship between motor function at 1 week post-injury and overall recovery at 3 and 6 months. *J Neurol Sci* (2007) 253:34–47. doi:10.1016/j.jns.2006.11.007
247. Heitger MH, Jones RD, Dalrymple-Alford JC, Frampton CM, Ardagh MW, Anderson TJ. Motor deficits and recovery during the first year following mild closed head injury. *Brain Inj* (2006) 20:807–24. doi:10.1080/02699050600676354
248. Heitger MH, Jones RD, Anderson TJ. A new approach to predicting post-concussion syndrome after mild traumatic brain injury based upon eye movement function. *Conf Proc IEEE Eng Med Biol Soc* (2008) 2008:3570–3. doi:10.1109/IEMBS.2008.4649977
249. Heitger MH, Jones RD, Macleod AD, Snell DL, Frampton CM, Anderson TJ. Impaired eye movements in post-concussion syndrome indicate suboptimal brain function beyond the influence of depression, malingering or intellectual ability. *Brain* (2009) 132:2850–70. doi:10.1093/brain/awp181
250. Galetta KM, Chapman KR, Essis MD, Alosco ML, Gillard D, Steinberg E, et al. Screening utility of the King–Devick test in mild cognitive impairment and Alzheimer disease dementia. *Alzheimer Dis Assoc Disord* (2016) 31:152–8. doi:10.1097/WAD.0000000000000157
251. van Stockum S, MacAskill M, Anderson T, Dalrymple-Alford J. Don't look now or look away: two sources of saccadic disinhibition in Parkinson's disease? *Neuropsychologia* (2008) 46:3108–15. doi:10.1016/j.neuropsychologia.2008.07.002
252. de Boer C, Pel JJ, van den Dorpel JJ, Boon AJ, van der Steen J. Behavioral inhibition errors in Parkinson's disease tested using an antisaccade and antitapping task. *J Parkinsons Dis* (2014) 4:599–608. doi:10.3233/JPD-140401
253. Muilwijk D, Verheij S, Pel JJ, Boon AJ, van der Steen J. Changes in timing and kinematics of goal directed eye-hand movements in early-stage Parkinson's disease. *Transl Neurodegener* (2013) 2:1. doi:10.1186/2047-9158-2-1
254. Verheij S, Muilwijk D, Pel JJ, van der Cammen TJ, Mattace-Raso FU, van der Steen J. Visuomotor impairment in early-stage Alzheimer's disease: changes in relative timing of eye and hand movements. *J Alzheimers Dis* (2012) 30:131–43. doi:10.3233/JAD-2012-111883
255. Tippett WJ, Krajewski A, Sergio LE. Visuomotor integration is compromised in Alzheimer's disease patients reaching for remembered targets. *Eur Neurol* (2007) 58:1–11. doi:10.1159/000102160
256. O'Dell MW, Lin CC, Harrison V. Stroke rehabilitation: strategies to enhance motor recovery. *Annu Rev Med* (2009) 60:55–68. doi:10.1146/annurev.med.60.042707.104248

6

Microsaccade Characteristics in Neurological and Ophthalmic Disease

Robert G. Alexander, Stephen L. Macknik and Susana Martinez-Conde*

State University of New York (SUNY) Downstate Medical Center, Brooklyn, NY, United States

Correspondence:
Susana Martinez-Conde
smart@neuralcorrelate.com

Microsaccade research has recently reached a critical mass of studies that allows, for the first time, a comprehensive review of how microsaccadic dynamics change in neurological and ophthalmic disease. We discuss the various pathological conditions that affect microsaccades, their impact on microsaccadic and other fixational eye movement dynamics, and the incipient studies that point to microsaccadic features as potential indicators of differential and early diagnoses of multiple clinical conditions, from movement disorders to attention-deficit hyperactivity disorder to amblyopia. We propose that the objective assessment of fixational eye movement parameters may help refine differential diagnostics in neurological disease and assist in the evaluation of ongoing therapy regimes. In addition, determining the effects of ophthalmic disease on fixational eye movement features may help evaluate visual impairment in an objective manner, particularly in young patients or those experiencing communication difficulties.

Keywords: microsaccades, fixational eye movements, square-wave jerks, Parkinson's disease, progressive supranuclear palsy, amblyopia, strabismus, fixational saccades

INTRODUCTION

When we attempt to fixate our gaze on a target, our eyes are never still, but produce small "fixational eye movements," which include tremor, drift, and microsaccades. Microsaccades (also called fixational saccades) occur at a typical rate of 1–2 Hz. Converging research points to a saccadic generation continuum, which extends from the smallest fixational microsaccades to the largest exploratory saccades (1–5). Drift is a slow (typically less than 2°/s) motion that occurs between microsaccades and saccades, and travels in an erratic pattern that has been modeled as a random walk (6). Tremor (or ocular microtremor) occurs simultaneously with drift, during intersaccadic intervals. This is the smallest fixational eye movement, with amplitudes that approximate the width of a single photoreceptor and dominant frequencies between 70 and 103 Hz (averaging 84 Hz) (7, 8). Tremor studies are much scarcer than those centered on microsaccades and/or drift, due to the technical difficulties inherent to measuring this tiny motion (8, 9). Thus, we do not address tremor in this review.

Because we spend approximately 80% of our waking hours fixating our gaze [not only in a sustained way but also in transient fashion, between large saccades (10)], understanding fixational dynamics is critical to advance current knowledge of oculomotor and visual function. Fixational eye movement assessments may also help further our understanding of central and peripheral pathologies that result in impaired fixation.

Various neurological and ophthalmic disorders produce abnormal fixational eye movement patterns, with distinctive characteristics. Thus, establishing how neurological and ophthalmic disease affects fixational dynamics holds the potential to help in the early and differential diagnosis of such disorders, clarify their pathophysiology, and quantify their progression and response to treatment. Recent research efforts have set out to characterize fixational dynamics in a growing record of neurological and ophthalmological conditions, which we discuss in this review.

A classification of abnormal eye movements in different disorders of fixation was previously published [see Table 1 of Martinez-Conde (10)]. The intervening decade has seen an upsurge in fixational eye movement research, with an emphasis on microsaccade studies. In addition, cross-fertilization between fundamental and translational approaches to fixational dynamics has facilitated the identification of previously unknown links between (micro)saccadic eye movements and saccadic intrusions (the latter formerly relegated to the clinical literature).

Such recent developments have resulted in a critical mass of studies that allows us, for the first time, to offer a comprehensive review of how microsaccadic dynamics change in neurological and ophthalmic pathologies, from movement disorders to attention-deficit hyperactivity disorder (ADHD) to amblyopia.

MICROSACCADES IN NEUROLOGICAL DISEASE

The balance that fixational eye movement system must achieve in healthy oculomotor function is quite delicate: whereas insufficient eye motion can result in visual losses due to neural adaptation and visual fading, excessive eye motion leads to blurred and unstable vision. This fine calibration is disrupted in patients of various neurological and neurodegenerative disorders who display increased gaze instability during the attempt to fixate (11). Recent research efforts aimed to characterize such fixation instability—with an emphasis on the dynamic of microsaccades and drift—in neurological disease seek not only to improve early and differential diagnosis and help evaluate the efficacy of concurrent treatments but also to gain a deeper understanding of the pathophysiology and pathogenesis of such disorders.

Microsaccades, Saccades, and Saccadic Intrusions in the Healthy Brain and in Neurological Disease

Converging evidence from physiological and behavioral studies conducted over the last decade has led to the current consensus that microsaccades and saccades—though previously considered as two different eye movement types—share a common oculomotor generator [(3); for review see Ref. (12)]. More recently, the proposal of a microsaccade-to-saccade continuum has been expanded to saccadic intrusions (3, 13, 14), defined as involuntary saccades that interrupt, or intrude on, precise fixation. Sacccadic intrusions are prevalent in certain neurodegenerative disorders, although healthy individuals also produce them. The most common saccadic intrusion is the square-wave jerk (SWJ), which consists of a small, horizontal saccade moving away from the fixation target, quickly followed by a corrective return saccade of equivalent amplitude and opposite direction. Though microsaccades and SWJs have most often been studied as two separate types of eye movements, recent work has put forward the notion that they, too, may be fundamentally the same kind of eye movement with different names (4, 5, 13, 14).

Progressive Supranuclear Palsy (PSP) and Other Movement Disorders

Pinnock and colleagues found larger and more frequent saccadic intrusions (including small intrusions due to microsaccades) in patients with Parkinson's disease, multiple system atrophy, and PSP, than in healthy age-matched controls (15). Otero-Millan et al. subsequently set out to study the characteristics of microsaccades and SWJs in patients with PSP—a parkinsonian disorder that affects the basal ganglia, mesencephalon, and frontal lobe—in which SWJs are a distinctive clinical feature (14) (**Figure 1**).

Though normal microsaccades were found to be rare in PSP, microsaccade magnitude was linked to SWJ coupling in both PSP patients and in healthy participants, with large microsaccades being more likely to trigger return saccades (forming SWJs) than small microsaccades (**Figure 2**). In addition, microsaccades and SWJs were slower in PSP patients than in controls, and they

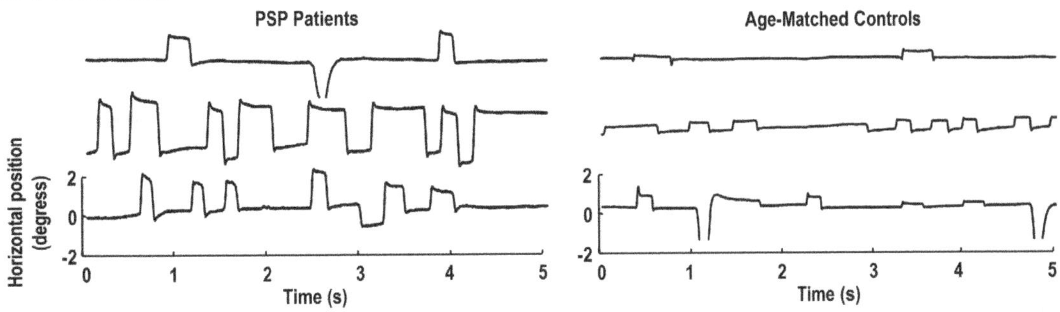

FIGURE 1 | Square-wave jerks (SWJs) from three progressive supranuclear palsy (PSP) patients (left) and three age-matched controls (right). In both populations, (micro)saccades with amplitudes equal to or larger than half a degree of visual angle are paired as SWJs. Only the horizontal eye positions are shown. Modified from Otero-Millan et al. (14).

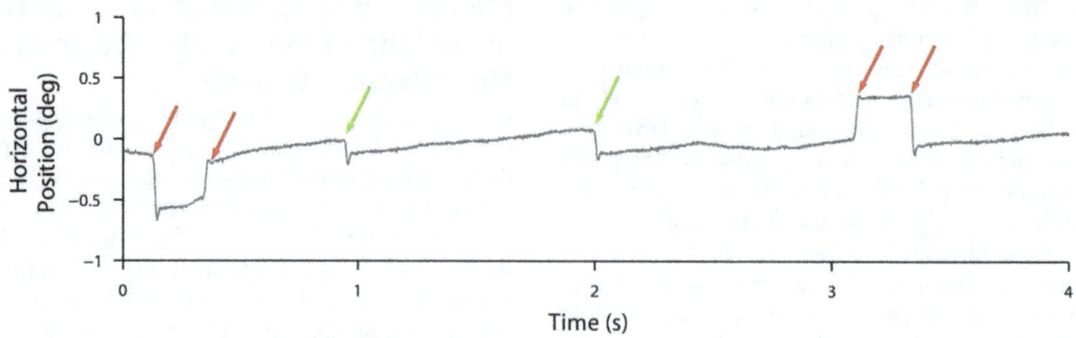

FIGURE 2 | Square-wave coupling takes place for large but not small (micro)saccades. In this eye position trace from a healthy participant, red arrows point to pairs of larger microsaccades forming square-wave jerks; green arrows point to smaller unpaired microsaccades. From Otero-Millan et al. (14).

had a diminished vertical component, consistent with the vertical saccadic palsy that sets apart PSP from other parkinsonian patients. The results supported the hypothesis that a common mechanism may account for microsaccade and SWJ generation (13, 14) and explained how the position error from a large first saccade could serve as the trigger for the return saccade in SWJs produced by both PSP patients and healthy participants (16). The study concluded that the apparent distinction between microsaccades and SWJs could be due to two complementary mechanisms, underlying: (1) microsaccade production and (2) correction of gaze fixation errors due to oversized microsaccades (14). These two factors, combined, could explain square-wave coupling, both for microsaccade pairs in healthy subjects and for saccadic intrusions in neurological patients suffering from PSP, Parkinson's disease, and other movement disorders, including multiple system atrophy, corticobasal syndrome, and spinocerebellar ataxia (5, 14).

Mild Cognitive Impairment and Alzheimer's Disease

Kapoula and colleagues recorded the eye movements of Alzheimer's disease patients, patients with mild cognitive impairment, and healthy age-matched participants during the attempt to fixate. Whereas most microsaccadic features, including magnitude, velocity, duration, and intersaccadic intervals were equivalent across the three groups, oblique microsaccade directions were more prevalent in mild cognitive impairment and Alzheimer's disease patients than in healthy participants (17). Layfield and colleagues wondered about potential links (positive or negative) between microsaccade dynamics and the amelioration of cognitive deficits in aging adults—following from targeted interventions known as "Speed Processing Training"—but found no relationship (18).

Attention-Deficit Hyperactivity Disorder (ADHD)

The neural system that controls attention and the system that generates (micro) saccadic eye movements overlap extensively. Thus, multiple research studies have examined the connection between microsaccades, attention, and distractors [for review see Ref. (3)]. The superior colliculus, which plays a central role in (micro)saccade triggering, has moreover attracted recent interest as a potential site of dysfunction in ADHD (19, 20). A handful of studies have examined the connection between ADHD and gaze instability during fixation (21–23). Most recently, two studies have focused on the characteristics of microsaccades in individuals with ADHD (24) and ADHD traits (20). Fried et al. found a higher microsaccade rate in adult individuals with ADHD who were off medication than in control participants. Methylphenidate medication served to normalize microsaccade rates in the ADHD group. Panagiotidi and colleagues similarly found differing microsaccade rates in non-clinical participants with high and low levels of ADHD-like traits (20), assessed with the Adult ADHD Self-Report Scale (25). These combined results suggested that abnormal fixation behavior is a core deficit in ADHD, which could aid in the development of a biomarker for the disorder (20). Another recent study set out to investigate the impairment of temporal expectations in ADHD, by examining the inhibition of microsaccades prior to the onset of predicted stimuli. The data indicated decreased microsaccade inhibition in participants with ADHD than in controls, suggesting that microsaccade characterization may help enhance current understanding of the range of cognitive deficits that affect ADHD individuals (26).

Autism Spectrum Disorder (ASD)

Recent research has found increased drift in autistic individuals (27). Microsaccade sizes and rates during fixation of a small target were comparable in ASD and neurotypical participants (27, 28), but those with ASD presented greater fixation instability, more microsaccades, and larger microsaccades when asked to maintain fixation on a blank screen with no target (28).

Tourette Syndrome

A recent study found patients with Tourette syndrome to have reduced microsaccade amplitudes and increased intersaccadic intervals, along with increased fixation instability and drift velocities (29).

Schizophrenia

Egaña and colleagues (30) found that previously reported decreased oculomotor function—in terms of decreased saccade and fixation rate—in schizophrenic patients (31) no longer differed from that of control participants once they included microsaccades in the analyses. In other words, schizophrenic patients made similar numbers of overall eye movements as healthy individuals, but produced fewer large, exploratory saccades to scan wide regions of the visual field. This study shows that fixational eye movement analyses in neurological and psychiatric disorders can be valuable not only to differentiate across populations but also to reveal previously unknown similarities between groups.

Cerebral Palsy

Kozeis and colleagues proposed that microsaccadic impairment might complicate the acquisition of reading skills in children with cerebral palsy (32), but no studies to date have directly characterized fixational eye movements in this disorder.

Hemianopia and Cortical Blindness

Hemianopia, or blindness in one-half of the visual field, can result from any lesion impairing post-chiasmatic central visual pathways. Reinhard and colleagues found microsaccadic distributions in hemianopic patients to be asymmetrical, with microsaccade directions biased toward the blind hemifield (33).

Gao and Sabel (34) subsequently investigated the characteristics of microsaccades in hemianopic stroke patients, to determine their potential relationship with visual performance and to assess how microsaccadic direction might be related to visual defect topography. They found that hemianopia resulted in enlarged microsaccades with impaired binocular conjugacy. Alterations of microsaccade dynamics worsened over time, being most prominent for older lesions. The data also revealed a microsaccade bias toward the seeing field, which was associated with faster reaction times to super-threshold visual stimuli in areas of residual vision, and suggested greater allocation of attention. Visual acuity was highest in patients with more binocular microsaccades and lower microsaccade velocities. The authors proposed that microsaccades may help compensate visual impairment in hemianopia and provide a basis for vision restoration and plasticity.

Blindsight is a rare phenomenon in which patients who have cortical blindness (due to lesions to the primary visual cortex) produce appropriate behavioral responses to visual stimuli they do not consciously see. Though no studies to date have systematically characterized microsaccadic properties in blindsighted patients, researchers in a recent case report studied microsaccadic inhibition (i.e., the transient suppression of microsaccade production after the presentation of a peripheral stimulus) in a patient who suffered from blindsight due to traumatic brain injury. The investigators observed that the patient's microsaccade rates dropped briefly after the presentation of high- and low-contrast peripheral stimuli, in both the left (blind) and the right visual fields. In the case of low-contrast stimuli, the release from microsaccadic inhibition was slower in the blind field than in the sighted field, however (35).

Short-Term Hypoxia

Di Stasi and colleagues found that saccadic velocity decreased and intersaccadic drift velocity increased, in connection with short-term hypobaric hypoxia in aviators. The finding that acute hypoxia diminishes eye stability, the authors proposed, may help to better understand the relationship between hypoxia episodes and central nervous system impairments (36).

MICROSACCADES IN OPHTHALMIC DISEASE

Vision and eye movements are intrinsically linked. Whereas it may seem intuitive to consider vision primarily in terms of its spatial characteristics, the process of seeing is a spatiotemporal one, where many timing features and constraints that impact our visual experience derive from the timing of eye movement production and targeting. Eye movements shape what we see, and our visual perception, in turn, affects the way we move our eyes. Ophthalmic disease, due to its deleterious effects on visual quality, tends to result in measurable abnormalities in eye movement properties, which extend to the fixational domain.

Because human beings are typically unaware of their fixational eye movements, studying their characteristics in ophthalmic disease may help evaluate the extent of a patient's visual impairment in an objective manner—particularly in very young patients or those experiencing communication difficulties.

Amblyopia and Strabismus

Most studies of fixational eye movements in ophthalmic disease to date have centered on amblyopia and strabismus. Amblyopia is defined as underdeveloped vision of one eye due to any condition that interferes with focusing during early childhood, including strabismus (in which the two eyes do not align correctly during fixation) and uncorrected refractive error (with anisometropia, or unequal refractive power in the two eyes).

Starting in the late 1970s, Ciuffreda and his colleagues conducted a series of pioneering studies on how amblyopia and strabismus affected fixation behavior (37–39). They found that, whereas amblyopic patients produced normal fixational eye movements during binocular fixation (and during monocular fixation with the fellow eye), monocular fixation with the amblyopic eye resulted in increased drift (whether or not strabismus was also present) (11, 37–40). If the amblyopia was due to strabismus, or in cases of alternating strabismus, this increase in drift was accompanied by sizable and frequent saccadic intrusions (37–39). By contrast, amblyopic fixation in dark-adaptation conditions was found to be normal or close to normal (41, 42).

More recently, Shi and colleagues found less frequent but larger microsaccades during monocular fixation with the amblyopic eye than with the fellow eye (43) and proposed that the objective evaluation of oculomotor function in amblyopia includes a microsaccade assessment. Otero-Millan et al. (44) noted that microsaccades produced during normal binocular fixation of large targets have similar features to those reported by Shi et al. during monocular fixation with the amblyopic eye, which might indicate a common lack of fixation precision in both scenarios. This possibility is consistent with work finding reduced fixation stability in the amblyopic eye, as compared to the fellow eye and to binocular viewing (45) (**Figure 3**).

Ghasia et al. found that fixational saccades and ocular drift were more disconjugate for patients with strabismus than for control participants. This disconjugacy was greater for patients with large-angle strabismus and impaired stereopsis (as a result of the misalignment of their eyes) than for patients with small-angle strabismus and preserved stereopsis (**Figure 4**). This study also found that drift was faster in patients with strabismus than in control subjects (46).

Fixation stability, usually measured as the eye position dispersion [i.e., bivariate contour elliptical area (BCEA)] during the attempt to fixate, combines the effects of microsaccades and drifts, without making a distinction between the two types of eye motion (44). Subramanian et al. (47) found that the BCEA was larger in the amblyopic eye than in the fellow eye, especially along the horizontal axis, and that patients with larger BCEAs tend to have lower visual acuities.

Increased drift and decreased microsaccade production in severe amblyopia may lead to perceptual fading of large portions of the visual field, including the "small fixation spot, small and large acuity targets, and even portions of the laboratory" during monocular fixation with the amblyopic eye (37, 48–50). One patient reportedly "made saccades to revive the faded or blanked-out portions" of the image in such situations (37), suggesting that visual fading in amblyopia might be related to ordinary Troxler fading [i.e., the kind of visual fading that normally sighted individuals can experience during fixation in the absence of microsaccades (10, 51)].

Increased drift in amblyopia could also produce lower visual acuity—and increased variability in visual acuity measurements—by shifting retinal images to more eccentric positions (39, 52). Such links exemplify the tight bond between the motor and sensory aspects of fixational eye movements (44).

Aiming to increase fixation stability for the amblyopic eye (and thus produce bifoveal fixation), Raveendran et al. (53) decreased the contrast of the image viewed by the fellow eye until it was equivalent to the contrast perceived by the amblyopic eye. Fixation stability in the amblyopic eye improved as a result, but bifoveal fixation was nevertheless temporary (due to the amblyopic eye drifting away from foveal alignment).

Loudon and colleagues used a binocularity score to assess how well subjects fixated a target with both eyes and proposed that the presence of fixation instability can help detect amblyopia at an early age (when it otherwise goes undetected up to a third of the time) (54).

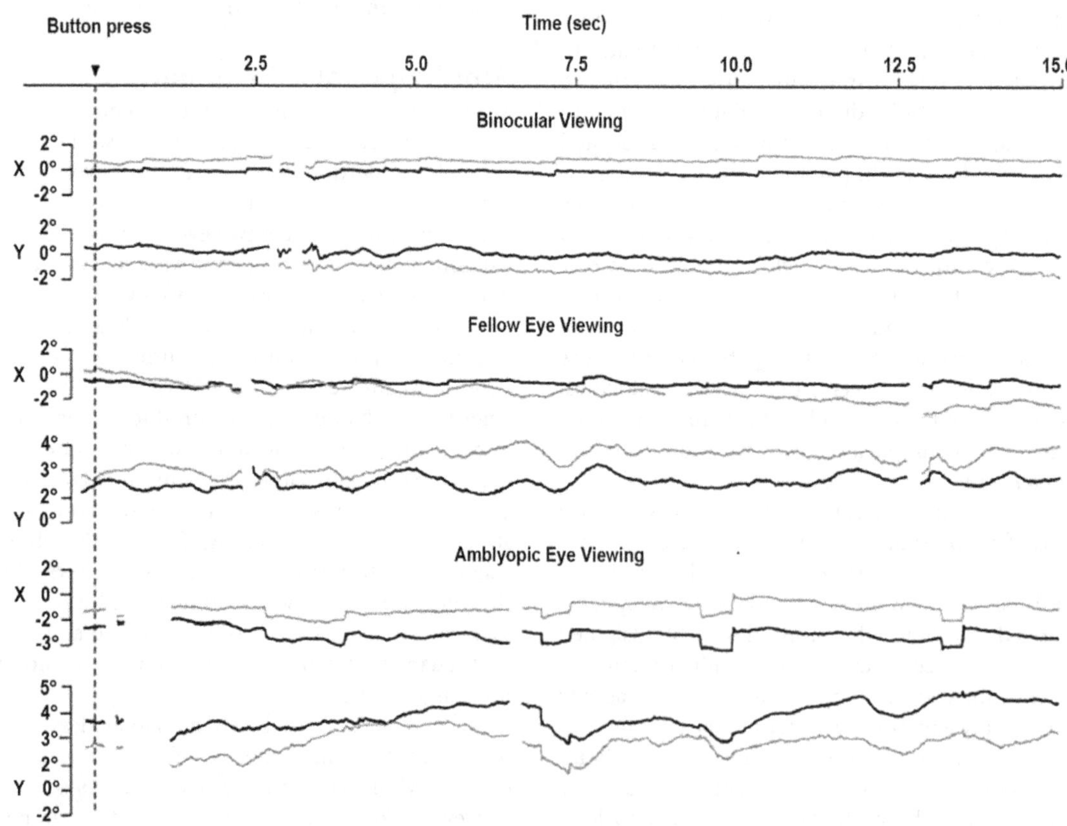

FIGURE 3 | Eye movements of a patient with strabismic amblyopia. Horizontal (X) and vertical (Y) positions are plotted for the left eye (gray, amblyopic eye) and the right eye (black, fellow eye). Amblyopic eye viewing results in larger microsaccades in both eyes. Monocular viewing with the fellow eye is tied to increased instability in the amblyopic eye. Monocular viewing with the amblyopic eye produces increased instability in the two eyes. From González et al. (45).

Successful orthoptics therapy tends to normalize fixational eye movements in amblyopia [though not all oculomotor and visual functions may improve concurrently (52, 55)]. Thus, Ciuffreda and colleagues have proposed that amblyopic therapies should not be interrupted when patients achieve normal visual acuity and centralized fixation, but should continue until they produced normal or stabilized fixational eye movements. Because critical periods for some aspects of oculomotor plasticity may extend into adulthood, lack of fixational eye movement normalization in amblyopic patients could be a factor in their reverting to the pre-treatment condition once therapy is discontinued (52). Thus, fixational eye movement assessments may help establish the optimal duration of treatments.

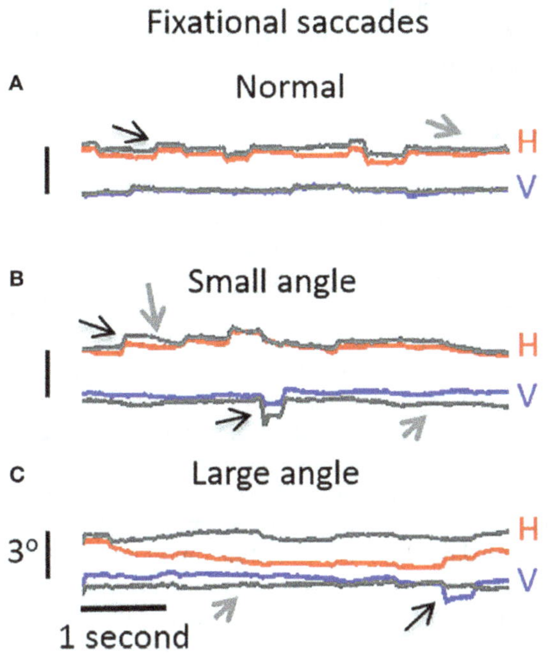

FIGURE 4 | Visual fixation of a target for 5 s, under monocular viewing conditions. **(A)** Participant with normal vision: both microsaccades and intersaccadic drift are conjugate. **(B)** Participant with small-angle strabismus and stereopsis present: disconjugancy across the two eyes is mild for both microsaccades and drift. **(C)** Participant with large-angle strabismus and absent stereopsis: disconjugancy is pronounced for both microsaccades and drift. **(A–C)** Horizontal (red: right eye, gray: left eye) and vertical (blue: right eye, gray: left eye) eye positions are presented. Black arrows indicate microsaccades, and gray arrows represent intersaccadic drift. From Ghasia et al. (46).

Central Scotoma due to Macular Disease or Dysfunction

Macular scotomas, and other pathologies producing prolonged monocular visual deprivation, have also been connected to increased drift, with comparable characteristics to drift in amblyopes (11, 56). A recent study by Kumar and Chung (57) found that patients with macular disease presented not only increased drift amplitudes but also larger microsaccadic amplitudes (**Figure 5**) than healthy subjects, without a corresponding change in microsaccade rate. The authors concluded that an increase in drift and microsaccade amplitudes—as opposed to changes in velocity or rate—is the strongest predictor of overall fixation instability in macular disease. Moller et al. previously found, in a group of diabetic maculopathy patients, that microsaccade magnitude increased as visual acuity decreased (58). A more recent study set out to determine if saccades in an eye affected by diabetic maculopathy were influenced by the other eye during binocular fixation. The results revealed that microsaccades during monocular fixation with the eye most affected by macular edema were larger, more frequent, and involved a larger retinal area than those produced during binocular fixation. A significant negative correlation was found between area of fixation and visual acuity during monocular, but not binocular, fixation. The authors concluded that binocular fixation can reduce the fixation area and microsaccade amplitude in the "worst eye" of diabetic maculopathy patients and advised that microsaccades in diabetic maculopathy are studied during monocular fixation (59).

Myopia

Recent work found increased microsaccade amplitude—without a corresponding change in microsaccade velocity or microsaccade

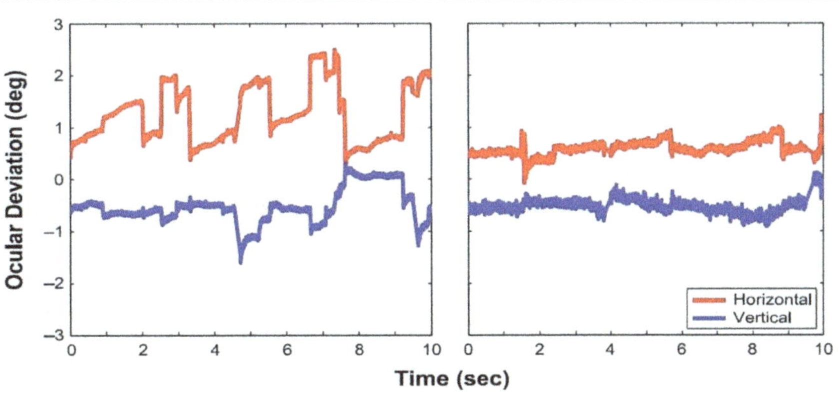

FIGURE 5 | Eye positions during fixation in a patient with macular disease (left) and a healthy control subject (right). From Kumar and Chung (57).

rate—in myopic individuals (60). As the severity of uncorrected refractive error increased, so did the sizes of microsaccades. This suggested that the control of microsaccade amplitude relies on the precision of visual information on the fovea, with blurred information leading to fixational instability.

Retinal Implants

Here, we discuss current efforts to characterize fixational eye movements, including microsaccades, in patients with subretinal implants. Because subretinal implants are placed below the retina (unlike epiretinal implants such as the Argus II, where an external camera is used to capture an image), the eye movements of implanted patients have the potential to affect—and be affected by—their visual perception.

In recent research, patients with a subretinal Alpha IMS scanned their visual field to locate a fixation target that appeared at random locations. Upon target fixation, the patients produced fixational eye movements—including microsaccades (with and without square-wave coupling) and drifts—that were analogous to those produced by control participants (61). A previous study by the same group made similar observations (62). The properties of (micro)saccades moreover depended on the shape of the stimulus being viewed. For instance, both patients and control participants made more horizontal eye movements when viewing a rectangle than when viewing a square (61). These data suggest that (micro) saccadic dynamics might help provide an objective measure of the success of an implant, especially in situations where subjective reports are questionable or inviable: if eye movements characteristics change in response to changes in the stimulus, it would indicate that visual inputs have been processed appropriately (61).

One limitation of subretinal implants such as the Alpha IMS is that visible stimuli typically fade from perception within seconds (61–63). Understanding the relationship between fixational eye movement dynamics and image fading in prosthetic vision may prove key to improving future subretinal implants. Microsaccades have been shown to counteract, and to help prevent, perceptual fading in natural vision (51, 64–68). Similarly, microsaccade occurrence has been connected to fading prevention in patients with subretinal implants (61). It has also been proposed that the characterization of microsaccade patterns in patients could help fine-tune the frequency of stimulation that results in optimal visibility in specific individuals. That is, depending on a particular observer's fixational eye movement patterns, he/she may need higher or lower stimulation frequencies to maintain visibility (69). Future research may investigate the translational value of this potential relationship.

It remains currently unknown why visual fading is more severe in patients with prosthetic implants than in healthy observers. One possibility is that fixational eye movements counteract and prevent perceptual fading less effectively in implanted patients than in natural vision (70). Recent modeling work has suggested that increased fading in prosthetic vision might be due to a lack of OFF responses and to lower contrast sensitivity than in natural vision (71); thus, the quality of the visual input may be too low for eye movements to refresh retinal images effectively. Fading may also be more or less prevalent depending on the size of electrodes used: stimulation from a single electrode may affect such a large visual region that even when microsaccades shift the stimulus to adjacent electrodes, they may not significantly change the activated neurons (70, 72).

CONCLUSION

We have reviewed the characteristics of fixational eye movements in neurological and ophthalmic disease, with an emphasis on microsaccades. Though studies addressing microsaccadic impairments in patient populations remain relatively scarce, this has recently become an area of active inquiry, with valuable implications for both clinical and basic research (3). Converging studies have made significant headway vis-à-vis the potential of microsaccade and other fixational eye movement dysfunctions as indicators of ongoing pathologies beyond the oculomotor realm. Thus, the objective assessment of fixational eye movement parameters may help refine differential diagnostics and assist in the evaluation of ongoing therapy regimes (i.e., successful treatments should result in the normalization of previously impaired fixational eye movements). These measures will also help refine current understanding of the pathogenesis of neural disease, as well as place constraints on—and guide the development of—future saccadic generation models, especially with regards to the relationship of (micro)saccades to saccadic intrusions in neurological disease.

AUTHOR CONTRIBUTIONS

SM-C, RGA, and SLM wrote and edited the manuscript. SM-C and RGA conducted the literature review.

ACKNOWLEDGMENTS

The authors thank Rosario Malpica and Daniel Cortes-Rastrollo for administrative and technical assistance.

FUNDING

This work was supported by the Empire Innovation Program (Awards to SM-C and SLM) and the National Science Foundation (Award 1523614 to SLM and Award 1734887 to SLM and SM-C).

REFERENCES

1. Otero-Millan J, Troncoso XG, Macknik SL, Serrano-Pedraza I, Martinez-Conde S. Saccades and microsaccades during visual fixation, exploration, and search: foundations for a common saccadic generator. *J Vis* (2008) 8(14):21–21. doi:10.1167/8.14.21
2. Rolfs M, Kliegl R, Engbert R. Toward a model of microsaccade generation: the case of microsaccadic inhibition. *J Vis* (2008) 8(11):5.1–23. doi:10.1167/8.11.5
3. Martinez-Conde S, Otero-Millan J, Macknik SL. The impact of microsaccades on vision: towards a unified theory of saccadic function. *Nat Rev Neurosci* (2013) 14(2):83–96. doi:10.1038/nrn3405

4. Otero-Millan J, Macknik SL, Langston RE, Martinez-Conde S. An oculomotor continuum from exploration to fixation. *Proc Natl Acad Sci U S A* (2013) 110(15):6175–80. doi:10.1073/pnas.1222715110
5. Otero-Millan J, Schneider R, Leigh RJ, Macknik SL, Martinez-Conde S. Saccades during attempted fixation in parkinsonian disorders and recessive ataxia: from microsaccades to square-wave jerks. *PLoS One* (2013) 8(3): e58535. doi:10.1371/journal.pone.0058535
6. Engbert R, Kliegl R. Microsaccades keep the eyes' balance during fixation. *Psychol Sci* (2004) 15(6):431–6. doi:10.1111/j.0956-7976.2004.00697.x
7. Bolger C, Bojanic S, Sheahan NF, Coakley D, Malone JF. Dominant frequency content of ocular microtremor from normal subjects. *Vision Res* (1999) 39(11):1911–5. doi:10.1016/S0042-6989(98)00322-8
8. Martinez-Conde S, Macknik SL, Hubel DH. The role of fixational eye movements in visual perception. *Nat Rev Neurosci* (2004) 5(3):229–40. doi:10.1038/nrn1348
9. Alexander RG, Martinez-Conde S. Fixational eye movements. In: Reuter M, Montag C, Klein C, Ettinger U, editors. *Studies in Neuroscience, Psychology and Behavioral Economics: An Introduction to the Scientific Foundations of Eye Movement Research and Its Applications*. New York: Springer (Forthcoming).
10. Martinez-Conde S. Fixational eye movements in normal and pathological vision. *Prog Brain Res* (2006) 154:151–76. doi:10.1016/s0079-6123(06)54008-7
11. Ciuffreda KJ, Tannen B. *Eye Movement Basics for the Clinician*. St. Louis: Mosby-Year Book, Inc. (1995).
12. Rolfs M. Microsaccades: small steps on a long way. *Vision Res* (2009) 49(20):2415–41. doi:10.1016/j.visres.2009.08.010
13. Gowen E, Abadi RV, Poliakoff E, Hansen PC, Miall RC. Modulation of saccadic intrusions by exogenous and endogenous attention. *Brain Res* (2007) 1141:154–67. doi:10.1016/j.brainres.2007.01.047
14. Otero-Millan J, Serra A, Leigh RJ, Troncoso XG, Macknik SL, Martinez-Conde S. Distinctive features of saccadic intrusions and microsaccades in progressive supranuclear palsy. *J Neurosci* (2011) 31(12):4379–87. doi:10.1523/JNEUROSCI.2600-10.2011
15. Pinnock RA, McGivern RC, Forbes R, Gibson JM. An exploration of ocular fixation in Parkinson's disease, multiple system atrophy and progressive supranuclear palsy. *J Neurol* (2010) 257(4):533–9. doi:10.1007/s00415-009-5356-3
16. Otero-Millan J, Macknik SL, Serra A, Leigh RJ, Martinez-Conde S. Triggering mechanisms in microsaccade and saccade generation: a novel proposal. *Ann N Y Acad Sci* (2011) 1233:107–16. doi:10.1111/j.1749-6632.2011.06177.x
17. Kapoula Z, Yang Q, Otero-Millan J, Xiao S, Macknik SL, Lang A, et al. Distinctive features of microsaccades in Alzheimer's disease and in mild cognitive impairment. *Age* (2014) 36(2):535–43. doi:10.1007/s11357-013-9582-3
18. Layfield S, Burge W, Mitchell W, Ross L, Denning C, Amthor F, et al. The effect of speed of processing training on microsaccade amplitude. *PLoS One* (2014) 9(9):e107808. doi:10.1371/journal.pone.0107808
19. Clements K, Devonshire I, Reynolds J, Overton P. Enhanced visual responses in the superior colliculus in an animal model of attention-deficit hyperactivity disorder and their suppression by D-amphetamine. *Neuroscience* (2014) 274:289–98. doi:10.1016/j.neuroscience.2014.05.054
20. Panagiotidi M, Overton P, Stafford T. Increased microsaccade rate in individuals with ADHD traits. *J Eye Mov Res* (2017) 10(1):1–9. doi:10.16910/jemr.10.1.6
21. Gould TD, Bastain TM, Israel ME, Hommer DW, Castellanos FX. Altered performance on an ocular fixation task in attention-deficit/hyperactivity disorder. *Biol Psychiatry* (2001) 50(8):633–5. doi:10.1016/S0006-3223(01)01095-2
22. Armstrong I, Munoz D. Attentional blink in adults with attention-deficit hyperactivity disorder. *Exp Brain Res* (2003) 152(2):243–50. doi:10.1007/s00221-003-1535-0
23. Munoz DP, Armstrong IT, Hampton KA, Moore KD. Altered control of visual fixation and saccadic eye movements in attention-deficit hyperactivity disorder. *J Neurophysiol* (2003) 90(1):503–14. doi:10.1152/jn.00192.2003
24. Fried M, Tsitsiashvili E, Bonneh YS, Sterkin A, Wygnanski-Jaffe T, Epstein T, et al. ADHD subjects fail to suppress eye blinks and microsaccades while anticipating visual stimuli but recover with medication. *Vision Res* (2014) 101:62–72. doi:10.1016/j.visres.2014.05.004
25. Kessler RC, Adler L, Ames M, Demler O, Faraone S, Hiripi E, et al. The World Health Organization Adult ADHD Self-Report Scale (ASRS): a short screening scale for use in the general population. *Psychol Med* (2005) 35(2):245–56. doi:10.1017/S0033291704002892
26. Dankner Y, Shalev-Mevorach L, Carrasco M, Yuval-Greenberg S. Pre-stimulus inhibition of microsaccades in adults with and without ADHD as an index for temporal expectations. *J Vis* (2016) 16(12):598–598. doi:10.1167/16.12.598
27. Frey HP, Molholm S, Lalor EC, Russo NN, Foxe JJ. Atypical cortical representation of peripheral visual space in children with an autism spectrum disorder. *Eur J Neurosci* (2013) 38(1):2125–38. doi:10.1111/ejn.12243
28. Shirama A, Kanai C, Kato N, Kashino M. Ocular fixation abnormality in patients with autism spectrum disorder. *J Autism Dev Disord* (2016) 46(5): 1613–22. doi:10.1007/s10803-015-2688-y
29. Shaikh AG, Finkelstein SR, Schuchard R, Ross G, Juncos JL. Fixational eye movements in Tourette syndrome. *Neurol Sci* (2017) 38(11):1977–84. doi:10.1007/s10072-017-3069-4
30. Egaña JI, Devia C, Mayol RV, Parrini J, Orellana G, Ruiz A, et al. Small saccades and image complexity during free viewing of natural images in schizophrenia. *Front Psychiatry* (2013) 4:37. doi:10.3389/fpsyt.2013.00037
31. Beedie SA, Clair DMS, Benson PJ. Atypical scanpaths in schizophrenia: evidence of a trait-or state-dependent phenomenon? *J Psychiatry Neurosci* (2011) 36(3):150. doi:10.1503/jpn.090169
32. Kozeis N, Anogeianaki A, Mitova DT, Anogianakis G, Mitov T, Felekidis A, et al. Visual function and execution of microsaccades related to reading skills, in cerebral palsied children. *Int J Neurosci* (2006) 116(11):1347–58. doi:10.1080/00207450500514011
33. Reinhard JI, Damm I, Ivanov IV, Trauzettel-Klosinski S. Eye movements during saccadic and fixation tasks in patients with homonymous hemianopia. *J Neuroophthalmol* (2014) 34(4):354–61. doi:10.1097/wno.0000000000000146
34. Gao Y, Sabel BA. Microsaccade dysfunction and adaptation in hemianopia after stroke. *Restor Neurol Neurosci* (2017) 35(4):365–76. doi:10.3233/RNN-170749
35. Sacher Y, Bonneh Y, Doron R, Fried M, Kadosh O, Lev M, et al. Unilateral blindsight following traumatic brain injury: a case report. *Presented at: Rehab Science and Technology Update*. Tel Aviv (2016).
36. Di Stasi LL, Cabestrero R, McCamy MB, Ríos F, Catena A, Quirós P, et al. Intersaccadic drift velocity is sensitive to short-term hypobaric hypoxia. *Eur J Neurosci* (2014) 39(8):1384–90. doi:10.1111/ejn.12482
37. Ciuffreda KJ, Kenyon RV, Stark L. Fixational eye movements in amblyopia and strabismus. *J Am Optom Assoc* (1979) 50(11):1251–8.
38. Ciuffreda KJ, Kenyon RV, Stark L. Suppression of fixational saccades in strabismic and anisometropic amblyopia. *Ophthalmic Res* (1979) 11(1):31–9. doi:10.1159/000264983
39. Ciuffreda KJ, Kenyon RV, Stark L. Increased drift in amblyopic eyes. *Br J Ophthalmol* (1980) 64(1):7–14. doi:10.1136/bjo.64.1.7
40. Srebro R. Fixation of normal and amblyopic eyes. *Arch Ophthalmol* (1983) 101(2):214–7. doi:10.1001/archopht.1983.01040010216006
41. Wald G, Burian HM. The dissociation of form and light perception in strabismus amblyopia. *Am J Ophthalmol* (1944) 27:950–63. doi:10.1016/S0002-9394(44)92327-5
42. von Noorden GK, Burian HM. An electro-oculographic study of the behavior of the fixation in amblyopic eyes in light- and dark-adapted state: a preliminary report. *Am J Ophthalmol* (1958) 46:68. doi:10.1016/0002-9394(58)90037-0
43. Shi XF, Xu LM, Li Y, Wang T, Zhao KX, Sabel BA. Fixational saccadic eye movements are altered in anisometropic amblyopia. *Restor Neurol Neurosci* (2012) 30(6):445–62. doi:10.3233/RNN-2012-129000
44. Otero-Millan J, Macknik SL, Martinez-Conde S. Fixational eye movements and binocular vision. *Front Integr Neurosci* (2014) 8:52. doi:10.3389/fnint.2014.00052
45. González EG, Wong AMF, Niechwiej-Szwedo E, Tarita-Nistor L, Steinbach MJ. Eye position stability in amblyopia and in normal binocular vision. *Invest Ophthalmol Vis Sci* (2012) 53(9):5386–94. doi:10.1167/iovs.12-9941
46. Ghasia FF, Otero-Millan J, Shaikh AG. Abnormal fixational eye movements in strabismus. *Br J Ophthalmol* (2018) 102:253–9. doi:10.1136/bjophthalmol-2017-310346
47. Subramanian V, Jost RM, Birch EE. A quantitative study of fixation stability in amblyopiafixation stability in amblyopia. *Invest Ophthalmol Vis Sci* (2013) 54(3):1998–2003. doi:10.1167/iovs.12-11054
48. Lawwill T. Local adaptation in functional amblyopia. *Am J Ophthalmol* (1968) 65(6):903–6. doi:10.1016/0002-9394(68)92219-8

49. Hess RF, Campbell FW, Greenhalgh T. On the nature of the neural abnormality in human amblyopia; neural aberrations and neural sensitivity loss. *Pflugers Arch* (1978) 377(3):201–7. doi:10.1007/BF00584273
50. Ciuffreda KJ, Kenyon RV, Stark L. Saccadic intrusions in strabismus. *Arch Ophthalmol* (1979) 97(9):1673–9. doi:10.1001/archopht.1979.01020020241012
51. Martinez-Conde S, Macknik SL, Troncoso XG, Dyar TA. Microsaccades counteract visual fading during fixation. *Neuron* (2006) 49(2):297–305. doi:10.1016/j.neuron.2005.11.033
52. Ciuffreda KJ, Kenyon RV, Stark L. Different rates of functional recovery of eye movements during orthoptics treatment in an adult amblyope. *Invest Ophthalmol Vis Sci* (1979) 18(2):213–9.
53. Raveendran RN, Babu RJ, Hess RF, Bobier WR. Transient improvements in fixational stability in strabismic amblyopes following bifoveal fixation and reduced interocular suppression. *Ophthalmic Physiol Opt* (2014) 34(2): 214–25. doi:10.1111/opo.12119
54. Loudon SE, Rook CA, Nassif DS, Piskun NV, Hunter DG. Rapid, high-accuracy detection of strabismus and amblyopia using the pediatric vision scanner. *Invest Ophthalmol Vis Sci* (2011) 52(8):5043–8. doi:10.1167/iovs.11-7503
55. Selenow A, Ciuffreda KJ. Vision function recovery during orthoptic therapy in an exotropic amblyope with high unilateral myopia. *Am J Optom Physiol Opt* (1983) 60(8):659–66. doi:10.1097/00006324-198308000-00003
56. Leigh RJ, Thurston SE, Tomsak RL, Grossman GE, Lanska DJ. Effect of monocular visual loss upon stability of gaze. *Invest Ophthalmol Vis Sci* (1989) 30(2):288–92.
57. Kumar G, Chung ST. Characteristics of fixational eye movements in people with macular disease. *Invest Ophthalmol Vis Sci* (2014) 55(8):5125–33. doi:10.1167/iovs.14-14608
58. Moller F, Laursen ML, Sjolie AK. Binocular fixation topography in patients with diabetic macular oedema: possible implications for photocoagulation therapy (3rd revision). *Graefes Arch Clin Exp Ophthalmol* (2005) 243(9): 903–10. doi:10.1007/s00417-004-1120-7
59. Jakobsen NS, Larsen DA, Bek T. Binocular fixation reduces fixational eye movements in the worst eye of patients with center-involving diabetic macular edema. *Ophthalmic Res* (2017) 58(3):142–9. doi:10.1159/000476038
60. Ghasia FF, Shaikh AG. Uncorrected myopic refractive error increases microsaccade amplitude. *Invest Ophthalmol Vis Sci* (2015) 56(4):2531–5. doi:10.1167/iovs.14-15882
61. Hafed ZM, Stingl K, Bartz-Schmidt K-U, Gekeler F, Zrenner E. Oculomotor behavior of blind patients seeing with a subretinal visual implant. *Vision Res* (2016) 118:119–31. doi:10.1016/j.visres.2015.04.006
62. Stingl K, Bartz-Schmidt KU, Besch D, Chee CK, Cottriall CL, Gekeler F, et al. Subretinal visual implant Alpha IMS – clinical trial interim report. *Vis Res* (2015) 111:149–60. doi:10.1016/j.visres.2015.03.001
63. Zrenner E, Bartz-Schmidt KU, Benav H, Besch D, Bruckmann A, Gabel V-P, et al. Subretinal electronic chips allow blind patients to read letters and combine them to words. *Proc R Soc Lond B Biol Sci* (2011) 278(1711):1489–97. doi:10.1098/rspb.2010.1747
64. Troncoso XG, Macknik SL, Martinez-Conde S. Microsaccades counteract perceptual filling-in. *J Vis* (2008) 8(14):15.1–9. doi:10.1167/8.14.15
65. McCamy MB, Otero-Millan J, Macknik SL, Yang Y, Troncoso XG, Baer SM, et al. Microsaccadic efficacy and contribution to foveal and peripheral vision. *J Neurosci* (2012) 32(27):9194–204. doi:10.1523/JNEUROSCI.0515-12.2012
66. Costela FM, McCamy MB, Macknik SL, Otero-Millan J, Martinez-Conde S. Microsaccades restore the visibility of minute foveal targets. *PeerJ* (2013) 1:e119. doi:10.7717/peerj.119
67. McCamy MB, Macknik SL, Martinez-Conde S. Different fixational eye movements mediate the prevention and the reversal of visual fading. *J Physiol* (2014) 592(19):4381–94. doi:10.1113/jphysiol.2014.279059
68. Costela FM, McCamy MB, Coffelt M, Otero-Millan J, Macknik S, Martinez-Conde S. Changes in visibility as a function of spatial frequency and microsaccade occurrence. *Eur J Neurosci* (2017) 45:433–9. doi:10.1111/ejn.13487
69. Stingl K, Bartz-Schmidt KU, Besch D, Braun A, Bruckmann A, Gekeler F, et al. Artificial vision with wirelessly powered subretinal electronic implant Alpha-IMS. *Proc R Soc Lond B Biol Sci* (2013) 280(1757):20130077. doi:10.1098/rspb.2013.0077
70. Weiland JD, Walston ST, Humayun MS. Electrical stimulation of the retina to produce artificial vision. *Annu Rev Vis Sci* (2016) 2:273–94. doi:10.1146/annurev-vision-111815-114425
71. Goetz G, Palanker D. Electronic approaches to restoration of sight. *Rep Prog Phys* (2016) 79(9):096701. doi:10.1088/0034-4885/79/9/096701
72. Behrend MR, Ahuja AK, Humayun MS, Chow RH, Weiland JD. Resolution of the epiretinal prosthesis is not limited by electrode size. *IEEE Trans Neural Syst Rehabil Eng* (2011) 19(4):436–42. doi:10.1109/TNSRE.2011.2140132

7

Disrupted Saccade Control in Chronic Cerebral Injury: Upper Motor Neuron-Like Disinhibition in the Ocular Motor System

John-Ross Rizzo[1,2], Todd E. Hudson[1,2], Andrew Abdou[3], Yvonne W. Lui[4], Janet C. Rucker[2], Preeti Raghavan[1] and Michael S. Landy[5]*

[1] Department of Rehabilitation Medicine, New York University Langone Medical Center, New York, NY, USA, [2] Department of Neurology, New York University Langone Medical Center, New York, NY, USA, [3] Rutgers School of Biomedical and Health Sciences, New Brunswick, NJ, USA, [4] Department of Radiology, New York University Langone Medical Center, New York, NY, USA, [5] Department of Psychology and Center for Neural Science, New York University, New York, NY, USA

***Correspondence:**
John-Ross Rizzo
johnross.rizzo@nyumc.org

Saccades rapidly direct the line of sight to targets of interest to make use of the high acuity foveal region of the retina. These fast eye movements are instrumental for scanning visual scenes, foveating targets, and, ultimately, serve to guide manual motor control, including eye–hand coordination. Cerebral injury has long been known to impair ocular motor control. Recently, it has been suggested that alterations in control may be useful as a marker for recovery. We measured eye movement control in a saccade task in subjects with chronic middle cerebral artery stroke with both cortical and substantial basal ganglia involvement and in healthy controls. Saccade latency distributions were bimodal, with an early peak at 60 ms (anticipatory saccades) and a later peak at 250 ms (regular saccades). Although the latencies corresponding to these peaks were the same in the two groups, there were clear differences in the size of the peaks. Classifying saccade latencies relative to the saccade "go signal" into anticipatory (latencies up to 80 ms), "early" (latencies between 80 and 160 ms), and "regular" types (latencies longer than 160 ms), stroke subjects displayed a disproportionate number of anticipatory saccades, whereas control subjects produced the majority of their saccades in the regular range. We suggest that this increase in the number of anticipatory saccade events may result from a disinhibition phenomenon that manifests as an impairment in the endogenous control of ocular motor events (saccades) and interleaved fixations. These preliminary findings may help shed light on the ocular motor deficits of neurodegenerative conditions, results that may be subclinical to an examiner, but clinically significant secondary to their functional implications.

Keywords: cortex, saccades, stroke, latency, disinhibition

INTRODUCTION

Interventions that drive neurorehabilitation are centered on strategies to restore motor ability and improve function. However, restoration of motor ability does not ensure gains in function (1, 2). We propose that a barrier to functional progress post-injury may be the lack of understanding and characterization of subtle eye movement deficits that have been found in individuals with unilateral cerebral damage (3, 4). Impaired eye movements can impede visually guided movements, such as eye–hand coordination (5–8), which can impact function. In this study, we assess eye-movement control in a paradigm used previously to study upper limb control in chronic stroke as an initial step toward advancing knowledge of poststroke eye–hand coordination (9, 10). This may provide further insight into characterizing the ocular motor control of chronic cerebral injury in neurodegeneration.

A central element of eye–hand coordination is the timing and accuracy of eye movements that enable the acquisition of visual information (11, 12). Studies have shown that highly skilled athletes, in whom excellent eye–hand coordination is critical, utilize more efficient eye movement strategies relative to novices (8, 13–15). For example, an elite volleyball player, as compared to a novice, performs fewer fixations, of longer duration, to extract more task-relevant information, suggesting that visual strategy may coincide with skill (15). In fact, comparisons between different players in various positions engaged in the same sport reveal disparate strategies or patterns of eye control, serving their particular role on the team. For example, a defensive player uses different visual search behavior when compared with an offensive player on a soccer team (16). These results underscore the crucial role of eye movements in a dynamic environment that integrates coordinated eye and limb motion (17).

Visual dysfunction following cerebral injury can be divided into sensory (including visual acuity and visual field), motor (including extraocular muscle control), and perceptual (including neglect) disorders (18). Given this framework, previous work has verified that hemispheric stroke can significantly alter ocular motor control, including control of fast eye movements (saccades). These deficits often go undetected without objective recording techniques (3, 4, 19–22). Recent work has described the ocular motor system as a sensitive marker in ischemic stroke for motor and cognitive recovery (23, 24). The neuroanatomic underpinnings for human eye movement control, now better understood through work involving transcranial magnetic stimulation and functional imaging (19, 20), emphasize the importance of a large interconnected network of cortical and subcortical structures. The frontal eye field (FEF) and the parietal eye field (PEF) are critical control centers for intentional and reflexive saccades (25, 26). In addition, the PEF has been considered necessary for perceptual (27, 28) and value-based decision-making (29). The supplementary eye field (SEF) is considered a monitoring area to evaluate the context and consequence of eye movements, regulating saccade production during performance and for anticipated task requirements (30, 31). The pre-SEF contributes to learning motor programs while the dorsolateral prefrontal cortex (DLPFC) contributes to saccade inhibition, prediction, spatial working memory, and motor learning, along with the striatum (20, 32–34). Moreover, basal ganglia circuits have been highlighted as an intermediate step between cortical eye fields and the superior colliculus (SC) (35–40).

The existence of this large and pervasive network suggests that cerebral injury, in either the acute or more chronic stage, as in neurodegeneration, has a high likelihood of affecting ocular motor control. Given the importance of ocular motor control in eye–hand coordination and the capacity to leverage ocular motor control as a marker of recovery, a better understanding of the properties of saccades poststroke may yield insights into persistently impaired eye–hand coordination. In this study, we tested eye movement control in chronic, middle cerebral artery (MCA) stroke, relative to healthy controls, in a flashed target (intentional), saccade paradigm following a similar trajectory pattern that was used to assess limb coordination in reaching studies (9, 32, 41). We hypothesized that chronic stroke subjects without obvious visual deficits on bedside testing would show abnormal saccadic control compared to healthy controls.

MATERIALS AND METHODS

The study was approved by the Institutional Review Boards of New York University and New York University School of Medicine. Informed consent was obtained according to the Declaration of Helsinki (42, 43).

Subjects

Twenty-six subjects participated in the study: 16 control (aged 54.8 ± 20.0) and 10 stroke subjects (aged 48.3 ± 15.1). Four of the stroke subjects had right hemispheric strokes and six had left hemispheric strokes (**Table 1**).

Apparatus

Subjects viewed a 21" liquid crystal display monitor at a distance 42.5 cm in a dark room; the head was stabilized in a chin + forehead rest. Saccadic eye movements were monitored using a video-based EyeLink 1000 eye tracker (SR Research, ON, Canada) sampling at 500 Hz with a spatial accuracy of 0.25–0.5°; recordings were performed monocularly in the remote/tabletop mode.

Inclusion/Exclusion Criteria

We recruited subjects with either right or left hemiparesis, meeting the following criteria: (1) age >21 years; (2) radiologically verified stroke in the MCA distribution >4 months; (3) ability to complete a full range of eye movements in horizontal and vertical directions, as assessed by the experimenter; (4) ability to complete the Fugl-Meyer Scale to define arm motor impairment (44–46); (5) willingness to complete all clinical assessments and experiments; and (6) ability to give informed consent and HIPPA certifications. Subjects were screened for visual abnormalities, as described below and were excluded if any obvious visual abnormalities were detected. The exclusion criteria were: (1) significant injury to the eye, weakness in extraocular muscles or to the visual system or vision in general, including the presence of visual field cuts or neglect; (2) significant cognitive dysfunction, as defined by a score <23 on Folstein's Mini-Mental Status Examination (47); (3) clinical depression, as defined by the Geriatric Depression Scale score >11; (4) major disability, as defined by the modified Rankin Scale >4 (48); and (5) previous neurological illness or complicated medical condition precluding the completion of the experimental protocol.

Subjects were screened to ensure that there were no confounding visual deficits on the Beery-Buktenica Developmental Test of visual–motor integration (VMI), as defined by the Beery

TABLE 1 | Clinical characteristics of stroke subjects.

Subject ID	Age (years)	Sex	H/H[a]	Stroke characteristics[b]	Chronicity (years)	Fugl-Meyer score[c]
1	55	M	R/R	L middle cerebral artery (MCA) infarct: basal ganglia	3.1	60
2	45	M	R/L	R MCA infarct: corona radiata and basal ganglia	4.9	31
3	49	M	L/R	L MCA infarct/bleed: frontal, parietal, temporal lobes and basal ganglia	4.8	24
4	25	F	R/L	R MCA infarct/bleed: frontal, parietal, temporal lobes and basal ganglia	3.6	65
5	32	F	R/L	R MCA infarct: frontal, parietal lobes and basal ganglia	7.8	49
6	68	M	R/R	L MCA infarct: frontal, parietal lobes, corona radiata and basal ganglia	9.4	51
7	71	F	R/R	L MCA infarct: parietal lobe, corona radiata and basal ganglia	10.5	59
8	41	M	R/L	R MCA infarct/bleed: frontal, temporal, occipital lobes and basal ganglia	6.1	44
9	38	M	R/R	L MCA infarct: frontal, parietal, temporal lobes and basal ganglia	7.6	28
10	59	M	R/R	L MCA infarct: corona radiata, thalamus and basal ganglia	5.3	15
Avg (SD)	48.3 (15.1)				6.3 (2.4)	42.6 (17.1)

[a]*"H/H" = handedness/hemiparesis: handedness (as assessed by Edinburgh)/hemiparesis laterality.*
[b]*"Stroke characteristics": lesion location obtained from imaging and based on detailed reports from a neuroradiologist (Yvonne W. Lui).*
[c]*"Fugl-Meyer Score": a summation of the Upper Extremity Score (out of 66), which reflects the extent of poststroke motor impairment.*

VMI (49–51), standard clinical tests for visual acuity, as defined by the Snellen chart (52), and visual field testing, assessed by confrontation testing [if in question, Goldmann or Humphrey perimetry were performed to rule out homonymous hemianopia (53)]. Hemispatial neglect was ruled out with Schenkenberg's line bisection test (54) and the single-letter cancelation test (55). Inability to bisect a straight line within 5% of the midpoint and more than three omission errors on the letter cancelation test without evidence of field deficits on testing were taken to indicate the presence of neglect (56).

Procedure

At the start of each trial, subjects were instructed to fixate a small white dot ("start position") on a computer screen with a black background. After fixation became stable (gaze velocity had fallen below 40°/s for 1250 ms), a target dot was flashed for 150 ms (**Figure 1A**). Subjects were instructed to saccade to the remembered target location as soon as possible following simultaneous offset of the target and start dots (the "go" signal). Saccade onset was defined as the moment the eyes reached a velocity of 75°/s while having moved at least 0.75°, and offset was defined as the moment gaze velocity fell below 40°/s. If the eye was in motion toward the target at the time the target was extinguished, the entire screen flashed gray to indicate that the saccade had been initiated early, and the trial was repeated. All subjects were instructed to rest between trials, as needed, to prevent fatigue.

Familiarization Saccades

Prior to making experimental saccades, subjects made 60 familiarization saccades starting from a fixation target at screen center (i.e., straight ahead) to a small target dot (0.1° radius) at a pseudo-random direction and distance. Target direction was chosen randomly and uniformly from 0° to 360°. Start-target distances were drawn from a uniform distribution (width: 1°) centered on the experimental saccade distance of 4°. That is, familiarization saccade distances were chosen randomly from the range 3.5–4.5°. Given this random selection of saccade direction and distance, familiarization targets rarely shared the same (or nearly the same) direction and distance as experimental saccades. Thus, familiarization saccades allowed us to estimate saccadic endpoint variance without providing practice with experimental saccades.

Experimental Saccades

The design of this experiment was initially based on our previous work on reaching (9), in which reaches are patterned based primarily on the target location, or on the vector, i.e., direction and extent from start to target. Here, we present results concerning the latency, kinematics and accuracy of saccades, but the experimental design reflects that earlier work. There were four possible saccade targets arranged on a 2 × 2 grid (row spacing: 4°, column spacing: 6.5°), as shown in **Figures 1A,B**. Each target was associated with four possible start positions positioned 4° away from the target at directions 30°, 150°, 210°, and 330° relative to vertical. Subjects performed two blocks of saccade trials in succession. Each block consisted of nine repetitions of the 16 start-target combinations (144 per block for a total of 288 saccades per session). In one block, saccades were grouped by movement target (**Figure 1A**) and in the other by movement vector (**Figure 1B**). In the target-grouped block, all saccades corresponding to one of the four targets were performed in random order (shown for one target in **Figure 1A**). Then, all saccades to another target were performed, etc., until all four targets' saccades were complete. In the vector-grouped block, all saccades defined by a particular movement vector (**Figure 1B**) were performed before any other movement vectors (e.g., one subject may have performed all saccades to the 30° targets, then all saccades to the 210° targets, etc., until all four vectors were completed). Note that controls were given an additional pair of target positions and two additional start positions (i.e., an additional column of two targets centered between the two columns of targets shown in **Figure 1A**, and an additional pair of start positions arranged horizontally to the left and right of each target, for a total six targets and six start positions around each target) as described by Hudson and Landy (9). Here, we pooled data across vector and target conditions when analyzing saccade metrics.

The visible target prior to each saccade was always a small dot (radius: 0.1°). However, the size of the to-be-acquired target (displayed after the saccade until the next start position was

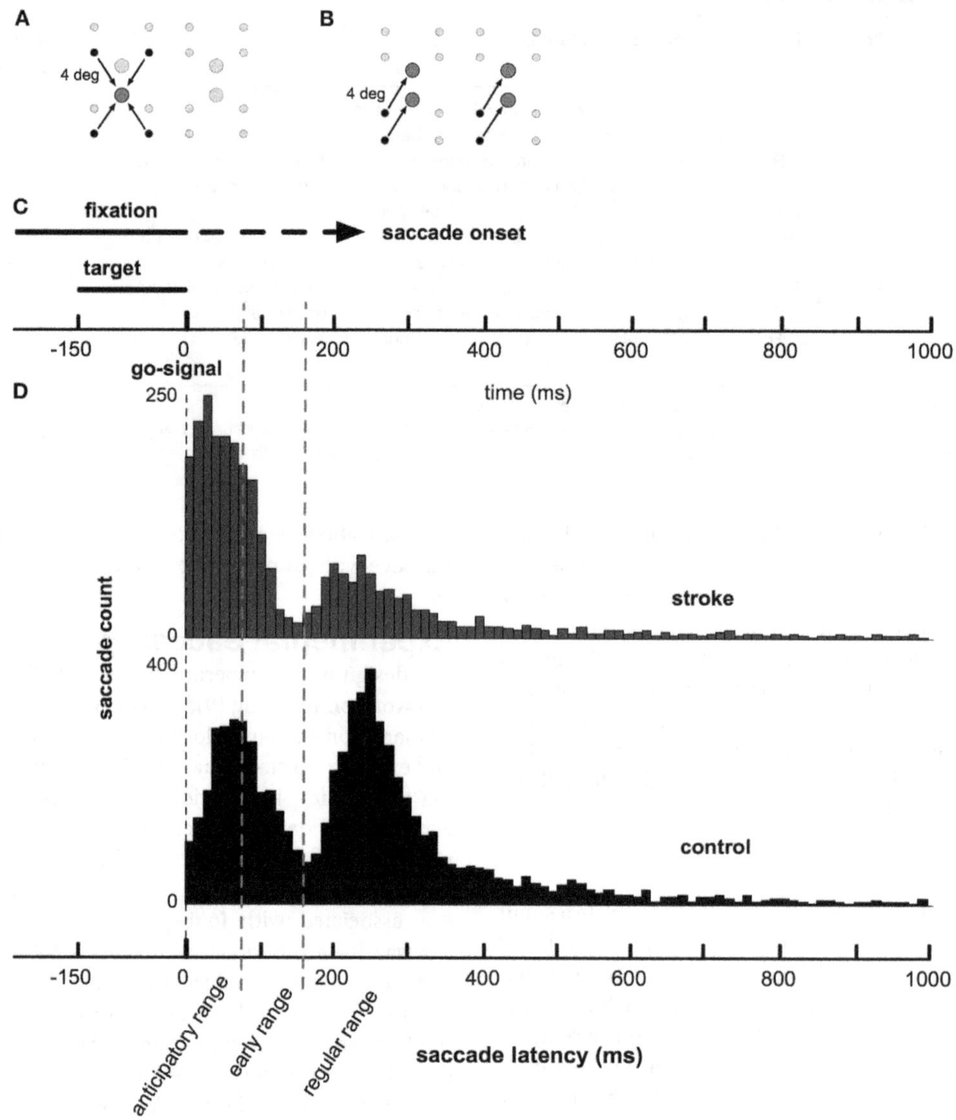

FIGURE 1 | Saccade task and timing. **(A)** Target locations (large circles) and corresponding start locations (small circles). Emphasized with arrows: one target grouping of the target-grouped condition. The set of all stimuli (four targets and corresponding start positions) is centered on the upright computer monitor. **(B)** Target locations and corresponding start locations. Emphasized with arrows: one vector grouping for the vector-grouped condition. **(C)** Presentation of fixation and saccade targets relative to the timing of saccade onset. A fixation dot was presented at the start of each trial. While the fixation remained onscreen, one of four possible targets was presented. Saccade onset was constrained to occur only after the offset of the saccade target (150 ms following its presentation). The fixation dot remained onscreen until saccade onset was detected (dashed portion of fixation line). Early saccades were rejected and those trials repeated. **(D)** Histograms of stroke (gray) and control (black) saccade latencies. Note that there were a greater number of control subjects, who completed a greater number of saccades, than for stroke subjects. Both groups show bimodal latency distributions, with both groups displaying a large early peak at between 50 and 75 ms and a smaller secondary peak near 250 ms.

fixated) was determined for each subject separately at the end of the familiarization phase of the experiment. This was done systematically to equate hit rates across subjects, and was set such that it would produce an expected hit rate of 42%. As a result, the radius of the to-be-acquired target ranged from about 0.5–1° across subjects. During the experimental saccades, when the saccade endpoint was within the bounds of the target ("target hit"), the target turned blue and a reward sound was played. When the saccade did not land within the target ("missed target"), the target turned red. The proportion of "hits" was displayed continuously at the upper right of the screen.

Calibration

Before each experimental session, subjects completed a set of center-out pursuit movements to calibrate the eye tracker to screen space. A cursor appeared at the center of the screen. Once fixated, it began to move slowly (0.8°/s) along one of the four cardinal (left, up, etc.) or four off-axis (NW, SE, etc.) directions.

The cursor stopped after moving every 2.5° from the center. When fixation on the stationary cursor was stable for 1 s, the cursor moved 2.5° again until it had stopped three times (i.e., 7.5° from center). This procedure yielded $8 \times 4 = 32$ 1-s eye-position measurements at $8 \times 3 + 1 = 25$ distinct screen positions from which spatial calibration was computed.

Statistical Analysis

Raw eye-position data were initially filtered by a 3-point median filter to remove outliers. Kinematic data traces were then obtained by first aligning data to saccade onset. Average velocity traces were computed by numerically differentiating eye position within a trial, and then averaging over trials. A second numerical differentiation prior to combining data across subjects yielded acceleration traces. Peak acceleration/deceleration and velocity were defined as the corresponding peaks of the average acceleration and velocity traces.

Analysis of temporal data (saccade latency and duration) was performed on the reciprocal of latency (in units of s^{-1}), which reduces the skew typically seen in temporal measurements, yielding more normally distributed data (57). Means and 95% confidence regions were computed on inverse-transformed data, yielding computed means that were close to the median of observed latencies and asymmetric confidence bounds when plotted in time units (s).

Two-sample *t*-tests were used to determine whether pairs of means or variances differed. Our results were unchanged if comparisons were made using Welch's *t*-test, which makes use of equations designed to account for possible heteroscedasticity and unequal sample sizes (the Welch-Satterthwaite equation for degrees of freedom). As a complement to traditional *t*-tests, we have plotted Bayesian 95% confidence regions around all computed estimates in the figures; as can be seen graphically in the corresponding figures by comparing confidence bounds, Bayesian analogues of the reported *t*-tests confirm our statistical analyses. Single proportions were compared *via* the *z*-test for equality of proportions (S_1 of N_1 vs. S_2 of N_2), where *z* is:

$$z = \frac{S_1/N_1 - S_2/N_2}{\sqrt{\left[\frac{S_1+S_2}{N_1+N_2}\right]\left(1-\left[\frac{S_1+S_2}{N_1+N_2}\right]\right)\left(\frac{1}{N_1}+\frac{1}{N_2}\right)}}.$$

Patterns in the number of saccade latencies occurring within each sub-stratification (see below) were compared via χ^2 test.

RESULTS

Saccade Timing

Distributions of saccade latencies (relative to the "go signal") were bimodal in both groups. We separated mode one (first peak) into saccades in the anticipatory range, as defined by latencies up to 80 ms, and in the "early" range, as defined by latencies between 80 and 160 ms. Mode two (second peak) included saccades in the "regular" range with latencies above 160 ms. The average timing of saccades was significantly different in stroke subjects compared to healthy control subjects. **Figure 1C** shows a schematic of the timing of the task, and **Figure 1D** displays histograms of saccade latencies. Inspection of these histograms suggests very similar latencies for the two modes in the distributions, but that the difference in the frequency distribution of saccade latency between stroke and control subjects was due to the higher number of saccades occurring in the first mode in stroke subjects and higher number of saccades in the second mode in control subjects. This pattern occurred more or less uniformly across individual subjects (raster plots, **Figure 2A**) and throughout the session (**Figure 2B**).

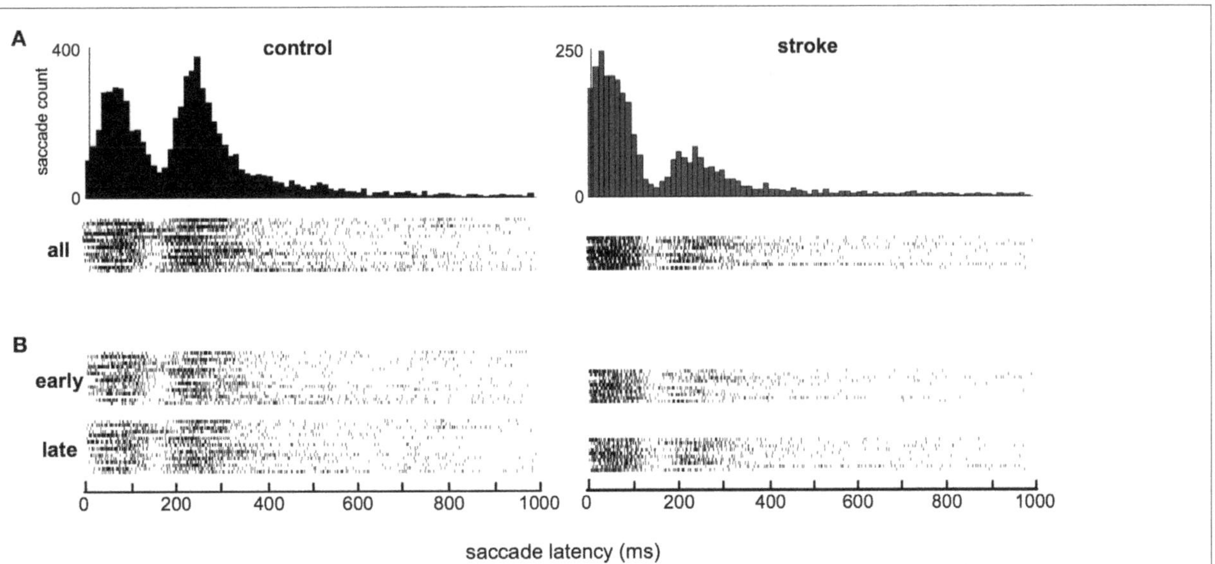

FIGURE 2 | Raster plots of individual subjects' saccade latencies. (A) All saccades. Each raster shows all saccade latencies for a single subject (16 control and 10 stroke subjects). **(B)** Saccades separated by those that occurred during the first and second halves of the session ("early" and "late"). Histograms are repeated from **Figure 1** to allow easy comparison of the high-density regions of histograms and raster plots.

The distribution of latencies from the first half of each subject's dataset was essentially identical to the pattern observed in the second half of the experiment.

Within each of the three latency ranges, we see that the overall difference in saccade latency was driven primarily by the number of saccades that fall into each of the three categories in stroke vs. control subjects. Stroke subjects displayed a disproportionate number of saccades in the anticipatory range of latencies compared to controls, whereas control subjects produced more of their saccades in the regular range compared to stroke subjects (**Figure 3A**, $\chi^2 = 895, p < 0.05$). There was no difference in the pattern of saccade latencies observed in the first and second halves of the experiment in our stroke cohort (**Figure 3B**, $\chi^2 = 1.26, p > 0.05$) or in controls ($\chi^2 = 2.35, p > 0.05$). Within each of the three ranges, there were no significant differences in saccade duration between the stroke and control cohorts (**Figure 3C**). Note that the larger number of anticipatory saccades produced by stroke subjects also resulted in a greater proportion of rejected trials due to saccades initiated prior to the "go" stimulus in stroke subjects (22.3% of all attempted saccades) vs. controls (13.8%; $z = 11.4, p < 0.05$).

Accuracy and Precision of Saccades

We separated saccade accuracy into two categories: the length of the saccade (saccade amplitude; **Figure 4A**) and the 2D distance between saccade endpoints and target center (**Figure 4B**). SDs are shown in **Figure 4C**. As expected, stroke subjects produced saccades that were more hypometric than those of controls ($t_{24} = 7.7$, $p < 0.05$), were further from the target ($t_{24} = 20.5, p < 0.05$), and were more variable ($t_{24} = 7.2$). Separating these measures based

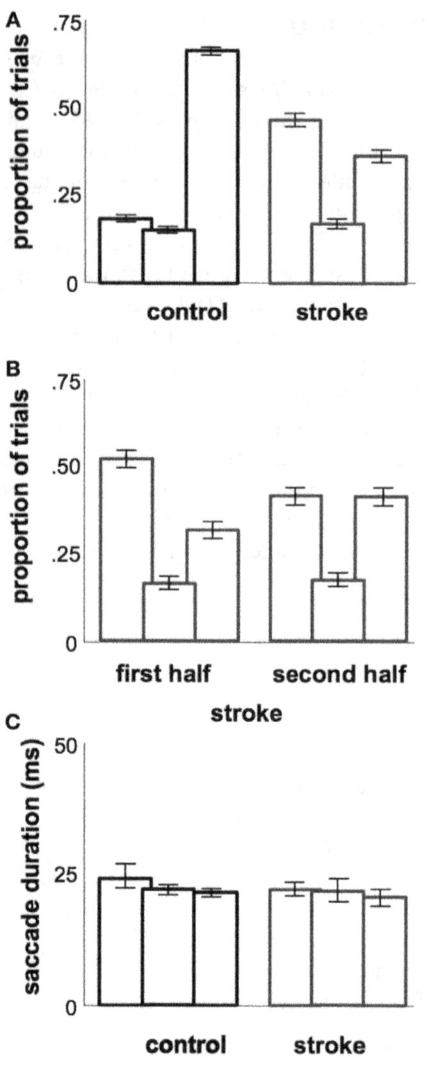

FIGURE 3 | Temporal metrics. (A) Proportions of saccades occurring in each of the three latency ranges (each triple is ordered, from left to right: anticipatory, early, regular). **(B)** Proportions of saccades occurring in each latency range, as in **(A)**, but split between the first and second halves of each stroke subject's session. **(C)** Average saccade durations occurring in each of the three latency ranges. *Error bars* (included in all plots): 95% confidence range for the mean across subjects.

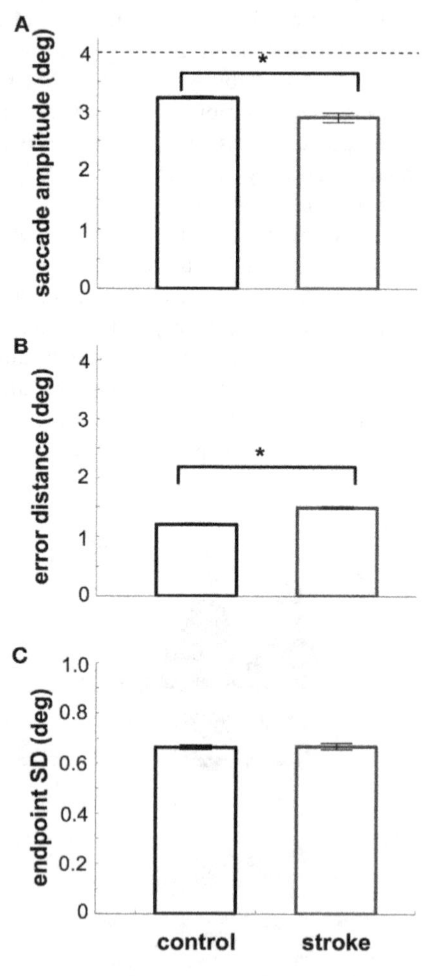

FIGURE 4 | Spatial metrics. (A) Average saccade amplitude. The dashed line indicates the distance of the target. Stroke subjects are more hypometric than controls. **(B)** Average 2D distance between saccade endpoint and target. Stroke subjects are less accurate than controls. **(C)** Endpoint SD. SD was computed assuming a symmetric error distribution. Stroke subjects show less precision of saccade endpoints (relative to their mean). *Error bars* (included in all plots): 95% confidence range for the mean across subjects.

on whether saccades latencies were in the anticipatory, early, or regular ranges, we find that saccade amplitudes of controls increase for higher saccade latencies [2.9–3.3°, $F(2,45) = 122.4$, $p < 0.05$], and a small decrease in error magnitudes for higher saccade latencies [1.5–1.2°, $F(2,45) = 269.2$, $p < 0.05$]. Finally, there was a small increase in error distance with increasing latency for stroke subjects [1.3–1.8°, $F(2,27) = 188.2$, $p < 0.05$]. There were no other latency-dependent effects in stroke subjects or for standard errors in either subject group (all $p > 0.05$).

Saccade Kinematics

Saccade velocity and acceleration profiles are typically highly stereotyped and saccade velocity profiles displayed the characteristic right-skewed shape for both groups (**Figure 5A**). However, the right-hand tail was slightly more prominent in the stroke group. This is consistent with a weaker and more prolonged deceleration phase in the velocity profile following stroke (**Figure 5B**). There was also a significant difference in acceleration profiles at the time of peak deceleration between control and stroke subjects ($t_{24} = 3.4$, $p < 0.05$).

Separation by Stroke Hemisphere or Saccade Direction

Eye movement control is lateralized and saccadic deficits may be greater for saccades made into the contralesional visual

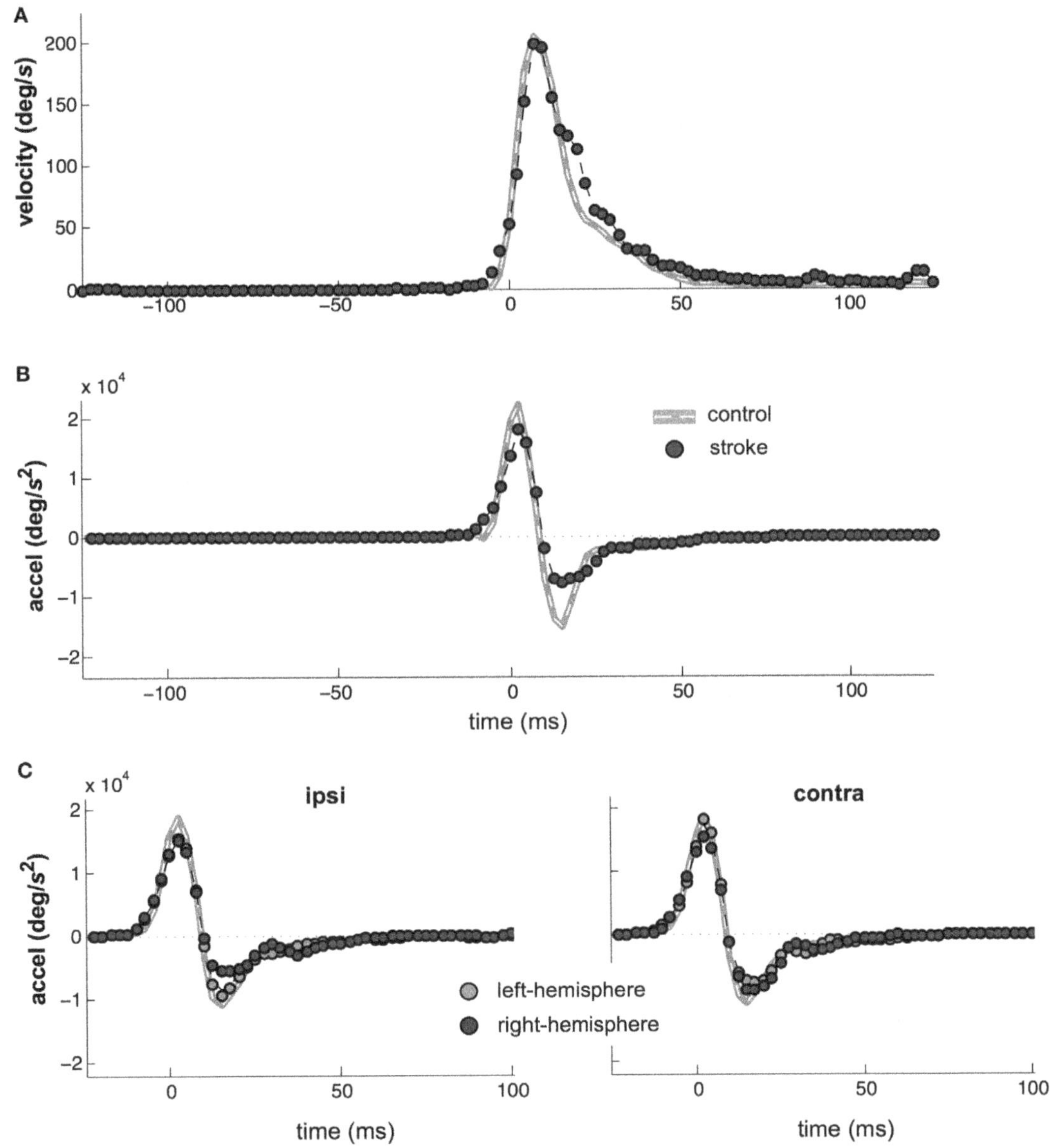

FIGURE 5 | Saccade kinematics. **(A)** Average saccade velocities of control (gray line) and stroke (circles) subjects. **(B)** Average saccade acceleration. **(C)** Average acceleration profiles separated by left- vs. right-hemisphere stroke (light- vs. dark-gray datapoints, respectively) and by whether a particular saccade was directed toward or away from the affected field (left vs. right plots, respectively). Note that all target distances were 4°, so that main sequence effects are small.

field (58, 59). Therefore, we repeated all of the above analyses separately for contralesional and ipsilesional saccades. The results were nearly identical between the contralesional and ipsilesional saccade directions. In particular, the pattern of onset latencies did not vary with saccade direction. The only significant difference occurred in the saccade kinematics, where the amplitude of the deceleration phase of the saccade waveform was asymmetrically attenuated in stroke. Although sub-stratification of this result reduced the statistical power of further testing, it appeared to be primarily the result of ipsilesional saccades in right-hemisphere stroke subjects (**Figure 5C**), as this was the subgroup in which the peak deceleration was lowest ($t_{24} = 1.94, p = 0.064$) relative to the peak deceleration in control saccades.

DISCUSSION

We have demonstrated a variety of deficits in the control of saccades after stroke in individuals with otherwise intact visual function. Most striking among these was the disproportionate number of saccades made by stroke subjects with timing in the anticipatory range (80 ms or less). Saccades in stroke subjects were also less precise (increased variance) and less accurate, compared to healthy controls. We discuss each of these deficits in turn, paying particular attention to the possibility that they may have implications for visually guided reaching and for neurodegeneration.

Saccade Latency Abnormalities: A Disinhibition Phenomenon

The shortest possible biological saccadic latency, reflecting transmission of information between retina and brainstem saccade generators and brainstem saccade generators to extraocular muscles for eye movement, is about 60 ms (60). However, the latency of typical saccades to unexpected peripheral targets is about 200 ms (32). This difference reflects decision-making and cognitive processing. In an experimental setting, saccades will often anticipate the relevant go-signal, resulting in latencies near or below the 60 ms limit. Here, we binned saccades with latencies less than or equal to 80 ms separately, and labeled them as within the "anticipatory" (61–63) range.

Although subjects were disincentivized to anticipate the go-signal based on task instructions and feedback (saccades made too early were rejected and repeated with a screen flash), such saccades were made by both groups in our task. Anticipation for the go-signal was possible because targets were shown prior to the go-signal and there was fixed timing of target onset and of go-signal. Nevertheless, the majority of saccades made by control subjects were in the regular range. In stark contrast, the majority of saccades made by stroke subjects were in the anticipatory range, perhaps suggesting an inability to suppress such saccades, rather than a purposeful decision to ignore instructions.

The inability to suppress saccades until the go signal (simultaneous offset of target and fixation cue) could represent a range of possible deficits, where at one end saccades occur reflexively in response to the target and, at the other, subjects inhibit saccades perfectly until instructed. In cerebral injury, the ability to maintain suppression or the ability to time the termination of saccade suppression may be impaired. All of these scenarios would create more saccades in the anticipatory range, as we see in our data, and should be considered inappropriate pro-saccade responses to the target. The most severe form, the complete inability to suppress a saccade to the flashed target, is not unlike the occurrence of what would be seen as inappropriate prosaccades during an anti-saccade task.

While neural control of saccades is distributed throughout a large network of cortical, subcortical, and brainstem structures (20, 32, 35–37, 39, 40, 64), the FEF, the PEF and basal ganglia play a role in intentional saccades (as in our flashed target task, as properly executed, suppressing an eye movement until the go signal). The last structure in this chain, at the convergence of the basal ganglia's multiple pathways, is the substantia nigra, which is known to have an inhibitory effect on the SC (39, 40). Studies on stroke have focused on cortical lesions affecting the ocular motor network, particularly as these neurologic insults relate directly to cortical eye fields, which exert a direct excitatory effect on the SC (3, 4, 65).

Fixation neurons in the rostral pole of the SC play a critical role in the maintenance of fixation (66), and depression of activity within these neurons releases fixation (67). Fixation-related neurons have also been identified in the substantia nigra pars reticulata (68), posterior parietal cortex (69, 70), and frontal lobes (71, 72). While it is not possible to determine the net effect on the SC in our subjects, it is possible that involvement of cortical eye fields and/or substantial basal ganglia involvement in our cohort (**Table 1**) played a role in the observed saccadic disinhibition via alteration in tonic input to the SC. This upper motor neuron-like disinhibition in ocular motor control that may be characterized here could prove beneficial in understanding the phenomenology of both acute and chronic cerebral injury, including neurodegeneration.

Speed-Accuracy Trade-off in Eye Movement Control

We observed a significant decrease in saccade amplitude (reflecting reduced saccade accuracy) and an increase in saccadic endpoint variability (reflecting reduced precision in the stroke group relative to controls). A well-known feature of motor behavior is the speed-accuracy trade-off (73). The saccadic main sequence (duration and peak velocity as a function of saccade amplitude) describes a relationship in which larger-amplitude saccades are more rapid and have longer duration. A feature of larger amplitude/faster saccades is poorer spatial accuracy; this represents the optimal trade-off in the face of signal-dependent noise inherent in ocular motor command signals (74). We found that accuracy and precision were both negatively affected in stroke. Rather than producing a consistent shift along the main sequence (i.e., toward lower peak velocities and lower amplitudes), these subjects show reduced saccadic amplitudes without a corresponding reduction in peak velocity as would be predicted by the main sequence relationship (75). However, to look at this deviation from the main sequence more closely would require a future study using a wider range of saccade magnitudes.

Implications for Rehabilitation Strategies

The difference between gross motor ability and functional motor control is a key distinction that must be made when evaluating recovery from any brain injury, including stroke, of both an acute and chronic nature, i.e., neurodegeneration. The difference between these two aspects of recovery is not in whether one can move a particular effector, but in the character of that control. In stroke subjects with residual hemiparesis, we have shown that eye movement latencies in a flashed target saccade paradigm are significantly altered in the temporal domain. These deficits in saccadic control may also affect the coupling of eye and hand movements, thereby altering functional use of the arm in individuals with stroke. After all, the integration of these systems is characterized by temporal relationships (76, 77) and small shifts in eye movement timing relative to hand-movement timing (that would typically go unnoticed during standard clinical evaluation) may alter the framework on which integrated movement plans are built (78). A clearer understanding of the synchronous and interdependent control systems directing eye and limb movements will likely be key to restoring functional ability poststroke. Furthermore, recent studies have demonstrated that eye movement execution for visually guided reaches occurs simultaneously with motor planning for arm/hand movement (79, 80). When reconciled with limb motor planning deficits in chronic stroke (81), this may create computational delays and could help explain recovery plateaus or impeded rehabilitation progress. Given that eye control precedes arm control (17, 76, 77, 82), our results highlighting dysfunctional ocular motor control may prove influential in better understanding visually guided, manual motor control. The development of strategies to rehabilitate eye movement control and ultimately to improve eye–hand coordination may be critical to the restoration of function poststroke. These ocular motor findings may also set a foundation for improved understanding in eye movement control for chronic neurodegeneration.

AUTHOR CONTRIBUTIONS

Conception and design of the study and substantial manuscript drafting: J-RR, TH, AA, PR, JR, and ML. Acquisition and analysis of data: J-RR, TH, AA, YL, JR, and ML.

ACKNOWLEDGMENTS

The authors would like to thank Dr. David S. Zee, Dr. Tamara Bushnik, and Dr. Ajax George for their thoughts, suggestions, and contributions.

FUNDING

This research was supported in part by National Institutes of Health Grants EY08266 (to MSL), HD071978 (to PR), TR000038 (to J-RR), R03 AG042379 (to J-RR, ML, and PR), and 5K12 HD001097 (to J-RR, ML, and PR).

REFERENCES

1. O'Dell MW, Lin CCD, Harrison V. Stroke rehabilitation: strategies to enhance motor recovery. *Annu Rev Med* (2009) 60:55–68. doi:10.1146/annurev.med.60.042707.104248
2. Cirstea MC, Levin MF. Compensatory strategies for reaching in stroke. *Brain* (2000) 123(Pt 5):940–53. doi:10.1093/brain/123.5.940
3. Catz A, Ron S, Ring H, Solzi P, Korczyn A. Saccadic responses in patients with hemispheric stroke. *Doc Ophthalmol* (1994) 85(3):267–74. doi:10.1007/BF01664934
4. Catz A, Ron S, Solzi P, Korczyn AD. Saccade characteristics in patients with hemispheric stroke. *J Neurol Rehabil* (1997) 11(3):175–80.
5. Pesaran B, Nelson MJ, Andersen RA. A relative position code for saccades in dorsal premotor cortex. *J Neurosci* (2010) 30(19):6527–37. doi:10.1523/JNEUROSCI.1625-09.2010
6. Dean HL, Marti D, Tsui E, Rinzel J, Pesaran B. Reaction time correlations during eye-hand coordination: behavior and modeling. *J Neurosci* (2011) 31(7):2399–412. doi:10.1523/JNEUROSCI.4591-10.2011
7. Masia L, Casadio M, Sandini G, Morasso P. Eye-hand coordination during dynamic visuomotor rotations. *PLoS One* (2009) 4(9):e7004. doi:10.1371/journal.pone.0007004
8. McRobert AP, Williams AM, Ward P, Eccles DW. Tracing the process of expertise in a simulated anticipation task. *Ergonomics* (2009) 52(4):474–83. doi:10.1080/00140130802707824
9. Hudson TE, Landy MS. Motor learning reveals the existence of multiple codes for movement planning. *J Neurophysiol* (2012) 108(10):2708–16. doi:10.1152/jn.00355.2012
10. Rizzo JR, Hudson TE, Abdou A, Rashbaum IG, George AE, Raghavan P, et al. Motor planning poststroke: impairment in vector-coded reach plans. *Physiol Rep* (2015) 3(12):e12650. doi:10.14814/phy2.12650
11. Hayhoe MM, Shrivastava A, Mruczek R, Pelz JB. Visual memory and motor planning in a natural task. *J Vis* (2003) 3(1):49–63. doi:10.1167/3.1.6
12. Ballard DH, Hayhoe MM, Li F, Whitehead SD. Hand-eye coordination during sequential tasks. *Philos Trans R Soc Lond B Biol Sci* (1992) 337(1281):331–8; discussion 8–9. doi:10.1098/rstb.1992.0111
13. Savelsbergh GJ, Williams AM, Van der Kamp J, Ward P. Visual search, anticipation and expertise in soccer goalkeepers. *J Sports Sci* (2002) 20(3):279–87. doi:10.1080/026404102317284826
14. Savelsbergh GJ, Van der Kamp J, Williams AM, Ward P. Anticipation and visual search behaviour in expert soccer goalkeepers. *Ergonomics* (2005) 48(11–14):1686–97. doi:10.1080/00140130500101346
15. Piras A, Lobietti R, Squatrito S. A study of saccadic eye movement dynamics in volleyball: comparison between athletes and non-athletes. *J Sports Med Phys Fitness* (2010) 50(1):99–108.
16. Williams AM. Perceptual skill in soccer: implications for talent identification and development. *J Sports Sci* (2000) 18(9):737–50. doi:10.1080/02640410050120113
17. Khan A, Song J, McPeek R. The eye dominates in guiding attention during simultaneous eye and hand movements. *J Vis* (2011) 11(1):9. doi:10.1167/11.1.9
18. Khan S, Leung E, Jay WM. Stroke and visual rehabilitation. *Top Stroke Rehabil* (2008) 15(1):27–36. doi:10.1310/tsr1501-27
19. Pierrot-Deseilligny C, Muri RM, Ploner CJ, Gaymard B, Rivaud-Pechoux S. Cortical control of ocular saccades in humans: a model for motricity. *Prog Brain Res* (2003) 142:3–17. doi:10.1016/S0079-6123(03)42003-7
20. Pierrot-Deseilligny C, Ploner CJ, Muri RM, Gaymard B, Rivaud-Pechoux S. Effects of cortical lesions on saccadic eye movements in humans. *Ann N Y Acad Sci* (2002) 956:216–29. doi:10.1111/j.1749-6632.2002.tb02821.x
21. Pierrot-Deseilligny C. Saccade and smooth-pursuit impairment after cerebral hemispheric lesions. *Eur Neurol* (1994) 34(3):121–34. doi:10.1159/000117025
22. Braun D, Weber H, Mergner T, Schulte-Monting J. Saccadic reaction times in patients with frontal and parietal lesions. *Brain* (1992) 115(Pt 5):1359–86. doi:10.1093/brain/115.5.1359

23. Dong W, Yan B, Johnson BP, Millist L, Davis S, Fielding J, et al. Ischaemic stroke: the ocular motor system as a sensitive marker for motor and cognitive recovery. *J Neurol Neurosurg Psychiatry* (2013) 84(3):337–41. doi:10.1136/jnnp-2012-303926
24. Anderson T. Could saccadic function be a useful marker of stroke recovery? *J Neurol Neurosurg Psychiatry* (2013) 84(3):242. doi:10.1136/jnnp-2012-304481
25. Noudoost B, Clark KL, Moore T. A distinct contribution of the frontal eye field to the visual representation of saccadic targets. *J Neurosci* (2014) 34(10):3687–98. doi:10.1523/JNEUROSCI.3824-13.2014
26. Schall JD. Neuronal activity related to visually guided saccadic eye movements in the supplementary motor area of rhesus monkeys. *J Neurophysiol* (1991) 66(2):530–58.
27. Rorie AE, Gao J, McClelland JL, Newsome WT. Integration of sensory and reward information during perceptual decision-making in lateral intraparietal cortex (LIP) of the macaque monkey. *PLoS One* (2010) 5(2):e9308. doi:10.1371/journal.pone.0009308
28. Shadlen MN, Newsome WT. Neural basis of a perceptual decision in the parietal cortex (area LIP) of the rhesus monkey. *J Neurophysiol* (2001) 86(4):1916–36.
29. Louie K, Grattan LE, Glimcher PW. Reward value-based gain control: divisive normalization in parietal cortex. *J Neurosci* (2011) 31(29):10627–39. doi:10.1523/JNEUROSCI.1237-11.2011
30. Stuphorn V, Brown JW, Schall JD. Role of supplementary eye field in saccade initiation: executive, not direct, control. *J Neurophysiol* (2010) 103(2):801–16. doi:10.1152/jn.00221.2009
31. Stuphorn V, Bauswein E, Hoffmann KP. Neurons in the primate superior colliculus coding for arm movements in gaze-related coordinates. *J Neurophysiol* (2000) 83(3):1283–99.
32. Hutton SB. Cognitive control of saccadic eye movements. *Brain Cogn* (2008) 68(3):327–40. doi:10.1016/j.bandc.2008.08.021
33. Histed MH, Pasupathy A, Miller EK. Learning substrates in the primate prefrontal cortex and striatum: sustained activity related to successful actions. *Neuron* (2009) 63(2):244–53. doi:10.1016/j.neuron.2009.06.019
34. Pasupathy A, Miller EK. Different time courses of learning-related activity in the prefrontal cortex and striatum. *Nature* (2005) 433(7028):873–6. doi:10.1038/nature03287
35. Thakkar KN, van den Heiligenberg FM, Kahn RS, Neggers SF. Frontal-subcortical circuits involved in reactive control and monitoring of gaze. *J Neurosci* (2014) 34(26):8918–29. doi:10.1523/JNEUROSCI.0732-14.2014
36. Mahamed S, Garrison TJ, Shires J, Basso MA. Stimulation of the substantia nigra influences the specification of memory-guided saccades. *J Neurophysiol* (2014) 111(4):804–16. doi:10.1152/jn.00002.2013
37. Watanabe M, Munoz DP. Effects of caudate microstimulation on spontaneous and purposive saccades. *J Neurophysiol* (2013) 110(2):334–43. doi:10.1152/jn.00046.2013
38. Gaymard B. Cortical and sub-cortical control of saccades and clinical application. *Rev Neurol (Paris)* (2012) 168(10):734–40. doi:10.1016/j.neurol.2012.07.016
39. Shires J, Joshi S, Basso MA. Shedding new light on the role of the basal ganglia-superior colliculus pathway in eye movements. *Curr Opin Neurobiol* (2010) 20(6):717–25. doi:10.1016/j.conb.2010.08.008
40. Hikosaka O, Takikawa Y, Kawagoe R. Role of the basal ganglia in the control of purposive saccadic eye movements. *Physiol Rev* (2000) 80(3):953–78.
41. Pierrot-Deseilligny C, Rivaud S, Gaymard B, Agid Y. Cortical control of memory-guided saccades in man. *Exp Brain Res* (1991) 83(3):607–17. doi:10.1007/BF00229839
42. Carlson RV, Boyd KM, Webb DJ. The revision of the declaration of Helsinki: past, present and future. *Br J Clin Pharmacol* (2004) 57(6):695–713. doi:10.1111/j.1365-2125.2004.02103.x
43. Schmidt H, Mehring S, McMillan J. Interpreting the declaration of Helsinki (2008): "must", "should" and different kinds of obligation. *Med Law* (2010) 29(4):565–91.
44. Fugl-Meyer AR, Jaasko L, Leyman I, Olsson S, Steglind S. The post-stroke hemiplegic patient. 1. A method for evaluation of physical performance. *Scand J Rehabil Med* (1975) 7(1):13–31.
45. Sanford J, Moreland J, Swanson LR, Stratford PW, Gowland C. Reliability of the Fugl-Meyer assessment for testing motor performance in patients following stroke. *Phys Ther* (1993) 73(7):447–54.
46. Wood-Dauphinee SL, Williams JI, Shapiro SH. Examining outcome measures in a clinical study of stroke. *Stroke* (1990) 21(5):731–9. doi:10.1161/01.STR.21.5.731
47. Cockrell JR, Folstein MF. Mini-mental state examination (MMSE). *Psychopharmacol Bull* (1988) 24(4):689–92.
48. van Swieten JC, Koudstaal PJ, Visser MC, Schouten HJ, van Gijn J. Interobserver agreement for the assessment of handicap in stroke patients. *Stroke* (1988) 19(5):604–7. doi:10.1161/01.STR.19.5.604
49. Malloy P, Belanger H, Hall S, Aloia M, Salloway S. Assessing visuoconstructional performance in AD, MCI and normal elderly using the Beery Visual-Motor Integration test. *Clin Neuropsychol* (2003) 17(4):544–50. doi:10.1076/clin.17.4.544.27947
50. Brown MJ. Comparison of the developmental test of Visual-Motor Integration and the Bender-Gestalt test. *Percept Mot Skills* (1977) 45(3 Pt 1):981–2. doi:10.2466/pms.1977.45.3.981
51. Breen MJ. Comparison of educationally handicapped students scores on the revised developmental test of Visual-Motor Integration and Bender-Gestalt. *Percept Mot Skills* (1982) 54(3 Pt 2):1227–30. doi:10.2466/pms.1982.54.3c.1227
52. Tannenbaum S. The eye chart and Dr. Snellen. *J Am Optom Assoc* (1971) 42(1):89–90.
53. Beck RW, Bergstrom TJ, Lichter PR. A clinical comparison of visual field testing with a new automated perimeter, the Humphrey Field Analyzer, and the Goldmann perimeter. *Ophthalmology* (1985) 92(1):77–82. doi:10.1016/S0161-6420(85)34065-4
54. Schenkenberg T, Bradford DC, Ajax ET. Line bisection and unilateral visual neglect in patients with neurologic impairment. *Neurology* (1980) 30(5):509–17. doi:10.1212/WNL.30.5.509
55. Johnston CW, Diller L. Exploratory eye movements and visual hemi-neglect. *J Clin Exp Neuropsychol* (1986) 8(1):93–101. doi:10.1080/01688638608401299
56. Suchoff IB, Kapoor N, Waxman R, Ference W. The occurrence of ocular and visual dysfunctions in an acquired brain-injured patient sample. *J Am Optom Assoc* (1999) 70(5):301–8.
57. Carpenter RH, Williams ML. Neural computation of log likelihood in control of saccadic eye movements. *Nature* (1995) 377(6544):59–62. doi:10.1038/377059a0
58. Gutteling TP, van Ettinger-Veenstra HM, Kenemans JL, Neggers SF. Lateralized frontal eye field activity precedes occipital activity shortly before saccades: evidence for cortico-cortical feedback as a mechanism underlying covert attention shifts. *J Cogn Neurosci* (2010) 22(9):1931–43. doi:10.1162/jocn.2009.21342
59. Wauschkuhn B, Verleger R, Wascher E, Klostermann W, Burk M, Heide W, et al. Lateralized human cortical activity for shifting visuospatial attention and initiating saccades. *J Neurophysiol* (1998) 80(6):2900–10.
60. Carpenter RHS. *Oculomotor Procrastination, in Eye Movements: Cognition and Visual Perception*. Hillsdale, UK: Lawrence Erlbaum (1981).
61. Klein C, Foerster F. Development of prosaccade and antisaccade task performance in participants aged 6 to 26 years. *Psychophysiology* (2001) 38(2):179–89. doi:10.1111/1469-8986.3820179
62. Ross RG, Radant AD, Young DA, Hommer DW. Saccadic eye movements in normal children from 8 to 15 years of age: a developmental study of visuospatial attention. *J Autism Dev Disord* (1994) 24(4):413–31. doi:10.1007/BF02172126
63. Sparks D, Rohrer WH, Zhang Y. The role of the superior colliculus in saccade initiation: a study of express saccades and the gap effect. *Vision Res* (2000) 40(20):2763–77. doi:10.1016/S0042-6989(00)00133-4
64. Carpenter RH. The neural control of looking. *Curr Biol* (2000) 10(8):R291–3. doi:10.1016/S0960-9822(00)00430-9
65. Machado L, Rafal RD. Control of fixation and saccades in humans with chronic lesions of oculomotor cortex. *Neuropsychology* (2004) 18(1):115–23. doi:10.1037/0894-4105.18.1.115
66. Krauzlis RJ, Dill N, Kornylo K. Activity in the primate rostral superior colliculus during the "gap effect" for pursuit and saccades. *Ann N Y Acad Sci* (2002) 956:409–13. doi:10.1111/j.1749-6632.2002.tb02842.x
67. Munoz DP, Wurtz RH. Role of the rostral superior colliculus in active visual fixation and execution of express saccades. *J Neurophysiol* (1992) 67(4):1000–2.
68. Hikosaka O, Wurtz RH. Visual and oculomotor functions of monkey substantia nigra pars reticulata. II. Visual responses related to fixation of gaze. *J Neurophysiol* (1983) 49(5):1254–67.

69. Bushnell MC, Goldberg ME, Robinson DL. Behavioral enhancement of visual responses in monkey cerebral cortex. I. Modulation in posterior parietal cortex related to selective visual attention. *J Neurophysiol* (1981) 46(4):755–72.
70. Lynch JC, Mountcastle VB, Talbot WH, Yin TC. Parietal lobe mechanisms for directed visual attention. *J Neurophysiol* (1977) 40(2):362–89.
71. Bon L, Lucchetti C. The dorsomedial frontal cortex of the macaca monkey: fixation and saccade-related activity. *Exp Brain Res* (1992) 89(3):571–80. doi:10.1007/BF00229882
72. Segraves MA, Goldberg ME. Functional properties of corticotectal neurons in the monkey's frontal eye field. *J Neurophysiol* (1987) 58(6):1387–419.
73. Abrams RA, Meyer DE, Kornblum S. Speed and accuracy of saccadic eye movements: characteristics of impulse variability in the oculomotor system. *J Exp Psychol Hum Percept Perform* (1989) 15(3):529–43. doi:10.1037/0096-1523.15.3.529
74. Harris CM, Wolpert DM. The main sequence of saccades optimizes speed-accuracy trade-off. *Biol Cybern* (2006) 95(1):21–9. doi:10.1007/s00422-006-0064-x
75. Bahill AT, Clark MR, Stark L. The main sequence, a tool for studying human eye movements. *Math Biosci* (1975) 24(3–4):191–204. doi:10.1016/0025-5564(75)90075-9
76. Lee D, Poizner H, Corcos DM, Henriques DY. Unconstrained reaching modulates eye-hand coupling. *Exp Brain Res* (2014) 232(1):211–23. doi:10.1007/s00221-013-3732-9
77. Gorbet DJ, Sergio LE. The behavioural consequences of dissociating the spatial directions of eye and arm movements. *Brain Res* (2009) 1284:77–88. doi:10.1016/j.brainres.2009.05.057
78. Kaplan J, Hier DB. Visuospatial deficits after right hemisphere stroke. *Am J Occup Ther* (1982) 36(5):314–21. doi:10.5014/ajot.36.5.314
79. Coutte A, Olivier G, Faure S, Baccino T. Preparation of forefinger's sequence on keyboard orients ocular fixations on computer screen. *Cogn Process* (2014) 15(3):415–22. doi:10.1007/s10339-014-0612-6
80. Rand MK, Stelmach GE. Effects of hand termination and accuracy requirements on eye-hand coordination in older adults. *Behav Brain Res* (2011) 219(1):39–46. doi:10.1016/j.bbr.2010.12.008
81. Raghavan P, Krakauer JW, Gordon AM. Impaired anticipatory control of fingertip forces in patients with a pure motor or sensorimotor lacunar syndrome. *Brain* (2006) 129(Pt 6):1415–25. doi:10.1093/brain/awl070
82. Song JH, McPeek RM. Eye-hand coordination during target selection in a pop-out visual search. *J Neurophysiol* (2009) 102(5):2681–92. doi:10.1152/jn.91352.2008

8

Perception of Upright: Multisensory Convergence and the Role of Temporo-Parietal Cortex

Amir Kheradmand[1,2]* and *Ariel Winnick*[1]

[1] *Department of Neurology, The Johns Hopkins University School of Medicine, Baltimore, MD, United States,* [2] *Department of Otolaryngology – Head and Neck Surgery, The Johns Hopkins University School of Medicine, Baltimore, MD, United States*

Correspondence:
Amir Kheradmand
akherad@jhu.edu

We inherently maintain a stable perception of the world despite frequent changes in the head, eye, and body positions. Such "orientation constancy" is a prerequisite for coherent spatial perception and sensorimotor planning. As a multimodal sensory reference, perception of upright represents neural processes that subserve orientation constancy through integration of sensory information encoding the eye, head, and body positions. Although perception of upright is distinct from perception of body orientation, they share similar neural substrates within the cerebral cortical networks involved in perception of spatial orientation. These cortical networks, mainly within the temporo-parietal junction, are crucial for multisensory processing and integration that generate sensory reference frames for coherent perception of self-position and extrapersonal space transformations. In this review, we focus on these neural mechanisms and discuss (i) neurobehavioral aspects of orientation constancy, (ii) sensory models that address the neurophysiology underlying perception of upright, and (iii) the current evidence for the role of cerebral cortex in perception of upright and orientation constancy, including findings from the neurological disorders that affect cortical function.

Keywords: subjective visual vertical, cerebral cortex, upright perception, Bayesian, temporo-parietal cortex, spatial orientation, orientation constancy, ocular torsion

INTRODUCTION

Spatial orientation refers to the perceptual awareness of the body position relative to the environment. While oriented to the surroundings, we maintain a stable perception of the world in upright orientation despite frequent changes in the eye, head, and body positions. Such "orientation constancy" is a key functional aspect of our spatial perception, and if disrupted the consequences can be quite debilitating due to ensuing dizziness, disorientation, and loss of balance. These symptoms are often triggered by motion or changes in the head or body positions, e.g., as in patients with vestibular dysfunction. Our perception of spatial orientation is possible because the position of the body is linked to the external environment through processing and integration of visual, vestibular, and proprioceptive information. In this process, the compensatory movement of the eyes through the vestibulo-ocular reflex is vital to maintain visual stability with changes in the head position. In frontal-eyed animals, in addition to the horizontal and vertical eye movements, lateral head tilts (i.e., with respect to gravity) lead to changes in the torsional eye position in the opposite direction of the head tilt. In humans, this ocular counter-roll (OCR) is a constrained, phylogenetically old vestibular reflex and does not match the magnitude of the head tilt (1). Such "visual-vestibular" mismatch, although sounds counter-productive, may actually represent an evolutionary advantage, as it can provide the brain with pertinent cues to quickly deconstruct perceived tilts into changes in the body position and the visual world, thus facilitating interactions with the surrounding environment. In this scheme, however, to achieve orientation constancy, the brain must be able to generate a common reference frame based on the sensory inputs that are inevitably encoded in different reference frames.

Let us examine a simple lateral head tilt more closely. In the upright position—where the vertical meridians of the eyes, head, body, and the visual world are all aligned with the gravitational vertical—maintaining upright perception is not challenging for the brain. However, as mentioned earlier, when the head is tilted and as the brain senses changes in the head position relative to gravity, OCR will only partially compensate for the amount of head tilt, typically with a low gain of about 10–25% in humans. Therefore, as a result of head tilt, the reference frames for the head, eye, and the visual world are no longer aligned along the gravitational vertical, and images become tilted on the retina (**Figure 1**). Despite separation of these individual sensory reference frames, our visual perception remains in upright orientation within a common reference frame. This perceptual constancy in upright orientation can be effectively studied by removing orienting visual cues, in which case the brain has to rely on information about the head and body positions in space and the eye position in the orbit to determine the orientation of external stimuli. A similar approach has been the basis of psychophysical experiments dating back to 1860. Around that time, Hermann Aubert, an expert in optics, used afterimages to investigate perception of vertical and horizontal line orientations in light and darkness. Using afterimages of a bright line, Aubert tilted his head with eyes closed until the afterimage was earth-horizontal. Upon opening the eyes, he found that the afterimage would deviate toward the side of the head tilt (2). George Elias Müller then investigated a range of smaller head tilts and found that the line would deviate away from the side of the head tilt (3). Müller also put forth theories to describe these perceptual errors, considering sensory contributions from the otoliths, semicircular canals, and proprioception (3). Later on, mathematical models were used to account for these findings. One of the initial quantitative models was put forth by Mittelstaedt in 1983, in which he proposed that the brain must generate an internal common reference to "*stabilize man's confidence in the stability of his world*" (4). From this perspective, he eloquently posited about discrepancies between the elements of our perception and the real world:

> ... in this facet of his subjectivity, man appears as a creature, whose mind underrates the humble services of his bodily feelings while naively taking at face value what [he] believes to see, unaware of being deceived, as it were, by the workings of a machinery which toils in the interest of survival but not in the service of truth... (4).

In recent decades, contributions of various sensory modalities to perception of upright have been studied extensively. However, currently, less is known about the neural structures and functions involved in orientation constancy. In this review, we first focus on neurobehavioral aspects of orientation constancy and describe sensory models that address the neurophysiology underlying upright perception. We then review the current evidence for the role of cerebral cortex in perception of upright and orientation

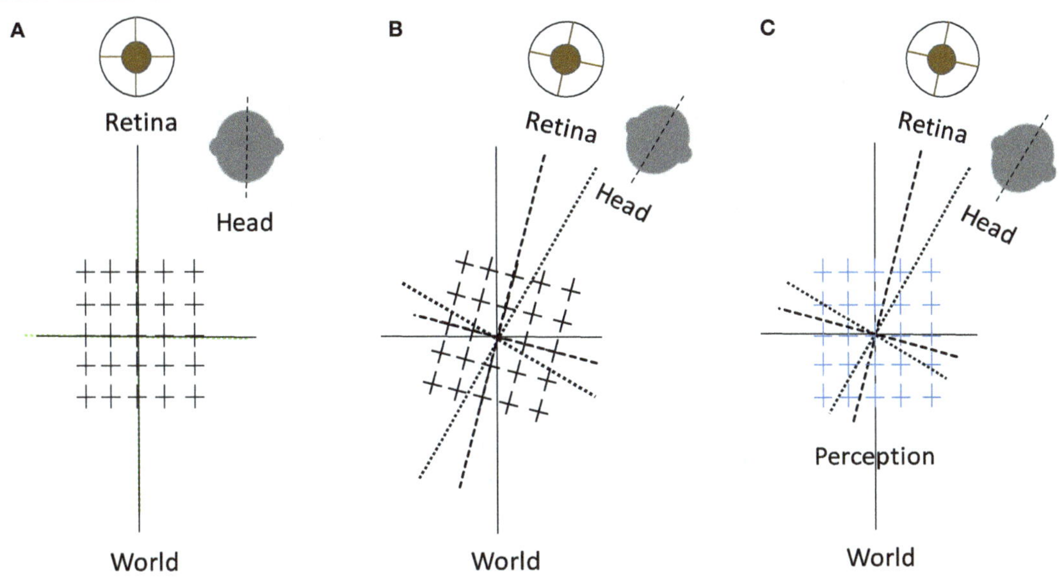

FIGURE 1 | Perception of upright and sensory reference frames: The head, eye, and the world reference frames are all aligned in upright position along the gravitational vertical **(A)**, but when the head is tilted, the ocular counter-roll only partially compensates for the amount of head tilt (gain about 10–25%), which results in a separation of the sensory reference frames that encode head-in-space and eye/retina-in-head orientations **(B)**. Despite these differences, visual perception remains in upright orientation **(C)**. Therefore, the brain—like any other sensorimotor system—must be able to integrate sensory inputs into a common reference frame to maintain a coherent perception of upright.

constancy. Finally, we outline findings from neurological disorders that impact cortical mechanisms underlying perception of upright.

NEUROBEHAVIORAL ASPECTS OF UPRIGHT PERCEPTION

Measurement Paradigms

Upright perception is typically studied by means of a psychophysical task known as the subjective visual vertical (SVV). In this task, a visual line is used to report perceived earth-vertical orientation in the absence of visual cues. Various methods have been described for SVV measurement. Some paradigms use active adjustment of the visual line stimulus, and others are based on a forced-choice task, where in each trial a visual line orientation is reported with respect to the perceived upright orientation (**Figure 2**).

Although the visual exposure in SVV paradigms is limited to a line stimulus without any other orienting cues, the line itself may affect SVV responses, especially during active adjustments (5–7). For example, the initial orientation of the line stimulus can bias upright perception in the direction of the starting line orientation, and in the opposite direction of the line movement (7–12). This bias, however, may reverse and occur as a "hysteresis" effect in the direction of the line movement when the line is presented in sequential angles in a forced-choice paradigm (6). Also, with active adjustment of the line, the upright estimate may gradually drift as a result of trial-to-trial dependency of upright adjustments and inter-correlation among consecutive SVV responses (13). In addition, the torsional position of the eyes can change in the direction of the visual line rotation, and such "torsional entrainment" may introduce biases when SVV is measured using the line rotation (14). Considering all these sources of error, a forced-choice task with a random line orientation in each trial would be the least biased method for SVV measurement, as it would remove the effects of line movement on SVV responses (15).

The length of the line stimulus can also influence SVV responses, resulting in biases in the direction of the body tilt with longer lines and in the opposite direction of the body tilt with shorter lines (16, 17). Another factor that can affect magnitude of SVV errors is the viewing distance from the visual line stimulus (18). This effect has been attributed to ocular torsion induced by changes in the vergence angle of the eyes (i.e., cycloversion). The viewing eye (i.e., monocular or binocular viewing), on the other hand, does not significantly affect SVV errors, neither in upright position nor during head tilt (6, 18).

Systematic Errors

Subjective visual vertical errors reflect challenges for the brain in maintaining a common reference frame based on sensory information encoding eye, head, and body positions. In upright position, SVV errors typically remain within 2° of earth vertical (4, 19–21). However, with lateral head or whole body tilts, there are systematic errors in the perceived upright orientation which do not correspond with the errors in perception of body tilt (4, 19, 22–25). Such inherent dissociation between the perceptions of body tilt and upright orientation is also seen with active body tilts (as opposed to passive tilts), even when the brain has access to additional proprioceptive cues or efference copy signals to encode the veridical position of the body (23).

In general, SVV errors are biased toward the direction of the body position at tilt angles greater than 60°. This finding, which reflects underestimation of upright orientation, is known as the Aubert or A-effect (**Figure 3**) (2, 4, 19, 20). At smaller tilt angles (e.g., less than 60°), however, SVV errors are often biased in the opposite direction of the body position. This finding, which reflects overestimation of upright orientation, is known as the Müller or E-effect (E for "Entgegengesetzt," German for opposite) (3, 19–21). The peak underestimation error of the A-effect is usually around 130°, and beyond this tilt angle the E-effect usually occurs again which is attributed to switching of the internal upright reference frame from the head to the feet (19, 21, 24, 26–28). Overall, the E-effect presents less consistently and less often compared with the A-effect (21, 24, 29). The variability of SVV responses also increases with the body tilts up to 120–150°, and then decreases again with the tilt angles approaching 180° (21, 26, 29–34). This pattern of SVV variability has been attributed to a tilt-dependent noise in the otolith and proprioceptive inputs (4, 21).

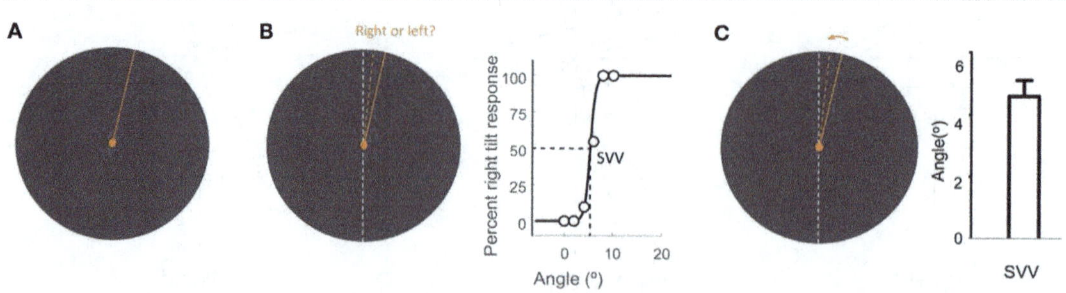

FIGURE 2 | Subjective visual vertical (SVV) measurement with the line stimulus (solid orange) presented at a random orientation in each trial **(A)**. In the forced-choice paradigm, the task is to report whether the line is tilted to the right or to the left of the perceived upright orientation (dashed orange) **(B)**. SVV is then determined by fitting a psychometric curve to the responses from all trials and is calculated as the value on the curve at which the probability of left or right responses is 50% (point of subjective equality). In the active-adjustment paradigm, the line stimulus (solid orange) is adjusted (direction shown by arrow) to the perceived upright orientation (dashed orange) **(C)**. In this paradigm, SVV is calculated as the average value from all trials. The true vertical is shown by the dashed white line **(B,C)**.

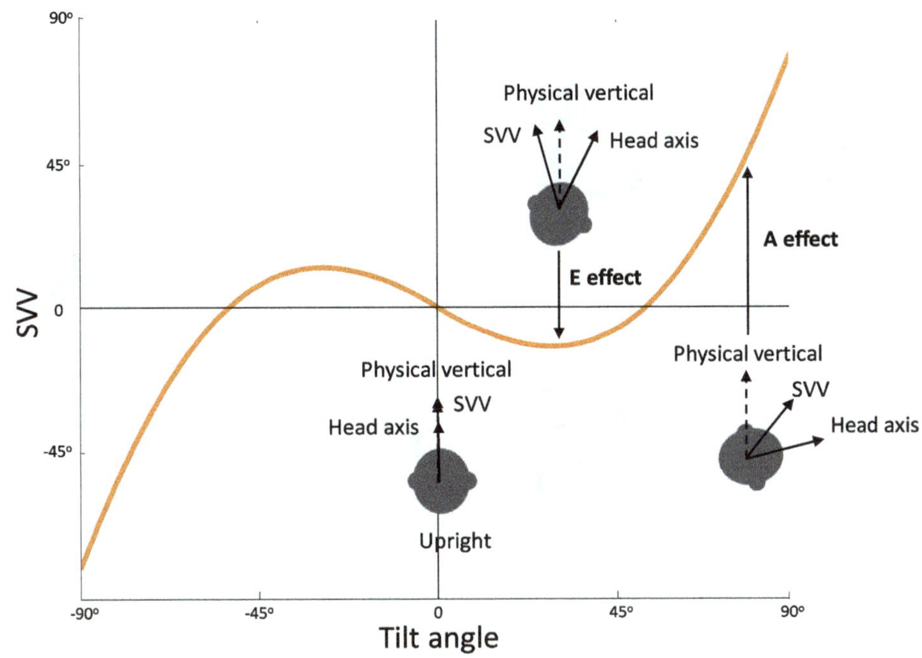

FIGURE 3 | Systematic errors of subjective visual vertical (SVV): healthy individuals typically have SVV errors within 2° of earth vertical in upright position. At large tilt angles (usually greater than 60°), SVV errors are deviated toward the tilt direction, which reflect "underestimation" of upright orientation (known as the Aubert or A-effect). At smaller tilt angles (usually less than 60°), however, SVV errors are often opposite to the tilt direction, which reflect "overestimation" of upright orientation (known as the Entgegengesetzt or E-effect).

Other Measurement Methods

Some studies have used subjective visual horizontal (SVH) instead of visual vertical measurements. The results, however, show that SVV and SVH are not invariably orthogonal to one another, especially at larger tilt angles (13, 18, 19, 35–37). In other words, errors of vertical and horizontal perception may not match at the same body tilt position and while SVV errors tend be larger in the direction of the tilt (i.e., SVV errors show larger A-effects), SVH errors tend to be larger in the opposite direction of the tilt (i.e., SVH errors show larger E-effects) (18). SVV and SVH errors have also been studied in the pitch plane, and—similar to the systematic errors in the roll plane—they reflect overestimations in the opposite direction of small pitch angles, and underestimations in the direction of large pitch angles (4, 38–40).

Another common method for measuring upright perception is with a haptic stimulus. Similar to SVV, haptic upright responses become less precise at large body tilt angles, but in some individuals they can be more accurate compared with the visual vertical responses (41–44). Also, haptic measurements tend to produce larger E-effects at smaller tilt angles (i.e., less than 60°) and may become more accurate in the supine position compared with the upright position (45–47). More importantly, the perceived haptic or postural upright can be dissociated from the visual perception of upright (48, 49). For example, while patients with unilateral vestibular loss showed significant SVV errors, their postural vertical adjustments were not different from the healthy controls (48). The disparity in the SVV and postural vertical responses in this study suggests different weights of sensory contributions to perception of upright depending on the method of measurement (e.g., haptic versus visual tasks) (49, 50). However, only few patients were included here, and the postural vertical was measured while sitting in a motor-driven chair and adjusting its orientation to the perceived upright position. In keeping with such distinct sensory contributions, haptic upright responses, in contrast to SVV, were more biased by the whole body tilt than just the head-on-body tilt in a group of healthy individuals (49).

Spatial Perception Models

In recent years, several studies have addressed neural mechanisms underlying perception of upright and the systematic errors with changes in body tilt orientation. Mittelstaedt first put forward a model in 1983 that could account for the A-effect (4). He proposed that the brain implements a computational strategy based on an internal bias signal to correct for the noisy inputs from the otolith organs (**Figure 4**). This internal signal, referred to as "the idiotropic vector," is a constant, body-fixed vector that is added to the estimated direction of gravity from the otolith inputs to determine upright orientation. At large body tilts, the effect of idiotropic vector results in a bias in upright estimates toward the body axis and thus the A-effect. According to this model, the computation of upright orientation does not influence the estimate of body tilt. Therefore, the idiotropic vector could be viewed as a computational strategy to reduce distortions in upright perception for commonly encountered small body tilts, at the expense of large A-effects for rarely encountered large body tilts.

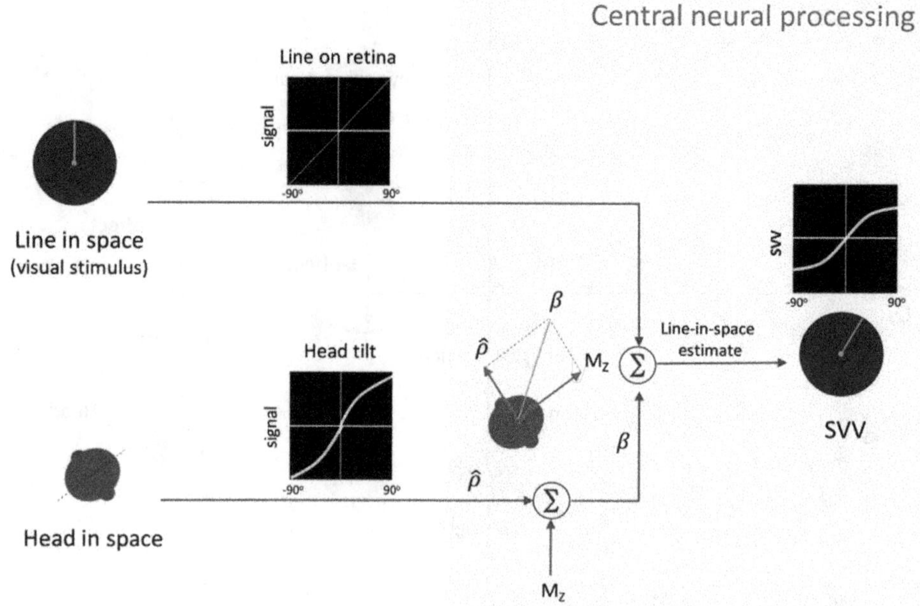

FIGURE 4 | Schematic presentation of Mittelstaedt's idiotropic vector model: visual line orientation on the retina and head tilt are the two sensory inputs in this model. The visual signal is accurate, but the head tilt signal ($\hat{\rho}$) shows increasing errors with head tilt (a range of ±90° tilt is shown in black graphs). As part of the central neural processing, vectorial summation of the head tilt signal ($\hat{\rho}$) and the head-fixed idiotropic vector (M_Z) yields the compensatory tilt signal (β). The compensatory tilt signal and the visual signal are then added to obtain an internal estimate of the upright orientation [i.e., subjective visual vertical (SVV)].

The effect of the idiotropic vector was later described within a Bayesian framework and was equated to the role of the Bayesian "prior" for processing noisy sensory signals (21, 29, 51–54). In this Bayesian spatial perception model, the upright estimate is determined by a weighted average of the existing knowledge of tilt position (i.e., the prior) and the likelihood of change in tilt position based on noisy sensory information (**Figure 5**). Since we spend most of our time in upright position, the prior for tilt position is a Gaussian distribution centered at 0° (i.e., upright position). Thus, the effect of prior could bias upright estimates and result in underestimation of true vertical at large tilt angles (i.e., the A-effect). According to the Bayesian model, the head estimate can be determined in the following relation (53):

$$\tilde{H}_S = \frac{\sigma^2_{H_{Sp}}}{\sigma^2_{H_{Sp}} + \sigma^2_{\widehat{H_S}}} \cdot H_S. \quad (1)$$

In Eq. 1, $\tilde{H}_S$ represents the final head-in-space estimate by the brain (i.e., "the posterior" in Bayesian terms), $\hat{H}_S$ the head orientation in space as measured by the head-in-space sensors, and H_S the actual head-in-space position (i.e., measured head position with respect to the direction of gravity). Among the sensory signals in the model, the head-in-space input $(\widehat{H}_S)$ is noisy (with a variance of $\sigma^2_{\widehat{H_S}}$), and thus the prior (with a small variance of $\sigma^2_{H_{Sp}}$) is taken into account to estimate the final head position $\left(\tilde{H}_S\right)$. Based on Eq. 1, the error in head estimate $\left(\mu_{\widetilde{H_S}}\right)$ is given by:

$$\mu_{\tilde{H}_S} = H_S - \tilde{H}_S = H_S - \frac{\sigma^2_{H_{Sp}}}{\sigma^2_{H_{Sp}} + \sigma^2_{\widehat{H_S}}} \cdot H_S = \frac{\sigma^2_{\widehat{H_S}}}{\sigma^2_{H_{Sp}} + \sigma^2_{\widehat{H_S}}} \cdot H_S. \quad (2)$$

De Vrijer et al. added another parameter to the Bayesian model to account for the error in estimating ocular torsion position by the brain $\left(\mu_{\widetilde{E_H}}\right)$ (**Figure 5**) (53). This "uncompensated" ocular torsion can explain the SVV error in the opposite direction of the head tilt at smaller tilt angles (i.e., the E-effect). The error in estimating ocular torsion $\left(\mu_{\widetilde{E_H}}\right)$ is determined in the following relation:

$$\mu_{\widetilde{E_H}} = \frac{\sigma^2_{\widehat{E_H}}}{\sigma^2_{E_{Hp}} + \sigma^2_{\widehat{E_H}}} \cdot \mathrm{A}\sin(H_S). \quad (3)$$

In this Eq. 3, $\hat{E}_H$ is the eye-in-head position based on sensory inputs encoding ocular torsion and E_{HP} is the prior for the eye-in-head position (with a variance $\sigma^2_{E_{Hp}}$), which is taken into account by the brain to estimate torsional eye position $\left(\tilde{E}_H\right)$. The maximum torsion amplitude is denoted by A. Since the eyes always roll in the opposite direction of the head tilt, the final error in upright perception (μ_{SVV}) can be given by subtracting Eqs 2 and 3 as below:

$$\mu_{SVV} = \mu_{\widetilde{H_S}} - \mu_{\widetilde{E_H}} = \frac{\sigma^2_{\widehat{H_S}}}{\sigma^2_{H_{Sp}} + \sigma^2_{\widehat{H_S}}} \cdot H_S - \frac{\sigma^2_{\widehat{E_H}}}{\sigma^2_{E_{Hp}} + \sigma^2_{\widehat{E_H}}} \cdot \mathrm{A}\sin(H_S). \quad (4)$$

Since this model assumes a vertical orientation of the trunk, the estimate of head-in-space $\left(\hat{H}_S\right)$ represents a combination of the otolith and proprioceptive inputs (53). Clemens et al. later proposed an update to separately account for the head and body positions using the following signals: the head orientation with respect to gravity (otoliths), body orientation in space (body

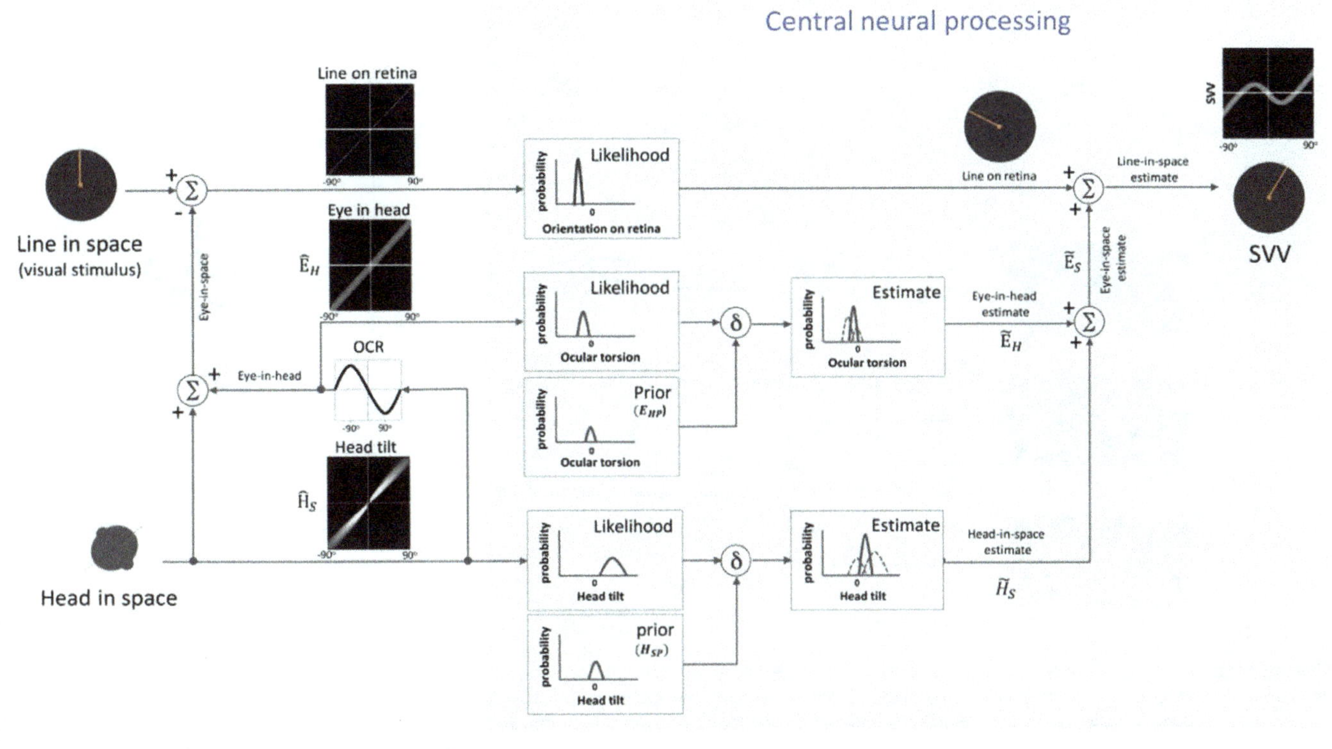

FIGURE 5 | Schematic presentation of Bayesian spatial perception model: various sensory modalities are integrated into a common spatial reference frame to determine upright orientation. A vertical line (line in space) is presented in front of a tilted observer (head in space) (a range of ±90° tilt is shown in black graphs). Signal $\hat{H}_S$, encoding head orientation in space, is accurate but contaminated by Gaussian noise. Head tilt results in ocular counter-roll (OCR) and signal $\hat{E}_H$, encoding eye-in-head orientation, is also contaminated by independent noise. As part of central neural processing, the estimates of head-in-space $(\tilde{H}_S)$ and eye-in-head $(\tilde{E}_H)$ are generated separately from the likelihoods and priors of head tilt and torsional eye position (i.e., ocular torsion). These estimates are integrated to generate eye-in-space estimate $(\tilde{E}_S)$, which is then integrated with retinal signal (line on retina) to obtain an internal estimate of the upright orientation [i.e., subjective visual vertical (SVV)].

proprioceptors), and the relative position of the head and body (neck proprioceptors) (54) (**Figure 6**). In this model, based on the optimal observer theory, the body orientation in space can be determined either "directly" using proprioceptive information from the trunk graviceptors (55–57) or "indirectly" from subtracting the signals encoding head and neck positions. Likewise, the estimate of head-in-space orientation can be obtained directly from the head position or indirectly from the body and neck proprioceptive signals. Accordingly, the optimal estimate of upright orientation is determined by integrating (1) direct information from the head position sensors (i.e., otoliths), (2) indirect information from the body and neck proprioceptors, and (3) prior information about the head and body orientations in space. The indirect sensory signals require reference frame transformation before integration with other sensory information. Thus, altogether, the final error in upright perception is calculated based on the weights of the direct and indirect information and is given by the following relation:

$$\mu_{SVV} = \left(1 - W_{HD} - W_{HI}\right)\cdot H_S - \frac{\sigma^2_{\widehat{E_H}}}{\sigma^2_{E_{Hp}} + \sigma^2_{\widehat{E_H}}}\cdot A\,\sin(H_S). \quad (5)$$

In this Eq. 5, W_{HD} represents the weight of direct sensory information, and W_{HI} represents the weight of indirect sensory information. Here, the weight of the prior (W_{HP}) works through the weights of direct and indirect sensory information, as $W_{HD} + W_{HI} + W_{HP} = 1$. Therefore, the narrower the prior distribution, the larger its relative weight compared with the weights of direct and indirect sensory information [for more details, see Ref. (54)]. In this scheme, the effect of the prior could be seen as the factor that reduces the variance of upright estimates, however, with an accuracy-precision trade-off especially at large tilt angles. Tarnutzer et al. have proposed a Bayesian model to account for the lower SVV precision at larger head tilts based on variability in the otolith inputs. In this model, the preferred directions of the otolith afferents represent different sensitivities to changes in the angle of the head tilt. Thus, an overall likelihood of head position estimate is obtained by combining the probability distributions from individual otolith afferents. In this scheme, the effectiveness of the otolith estimator—reflected by the width of the likelihood distribution—decreases at larger head tilt angles, and it is combined with the prior knowledge of the head orientation to derive the SVV estimate (21).

Multisensory Contributions

Various studies have addressed contributions of the head, neck, and trunk sensory signals to perception of upright. The findings from these studies indicate that the SVV errors are primarily

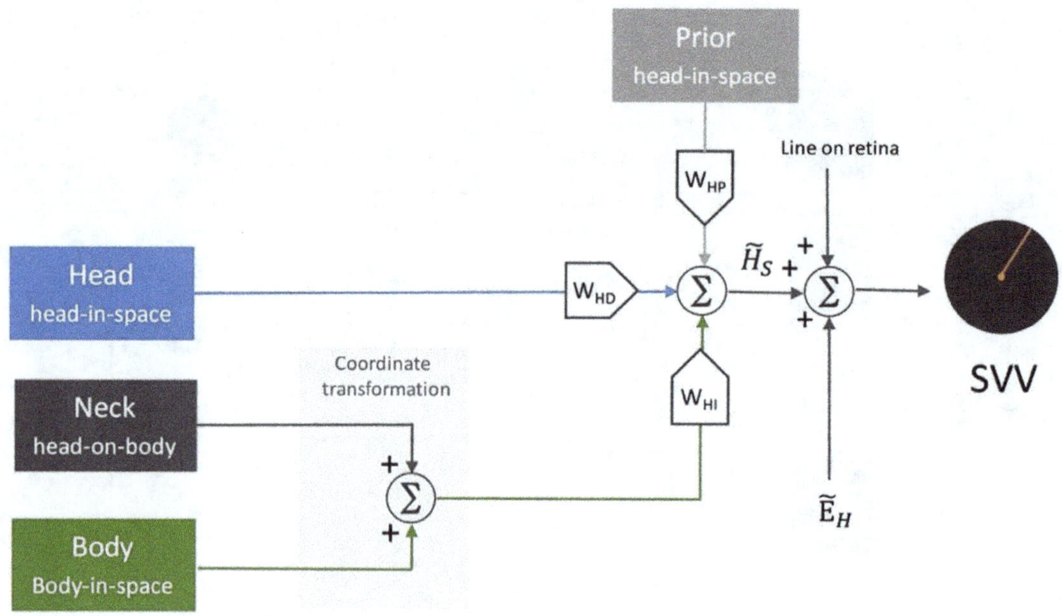

FIGURE 6 | Schematic representation of the sensory integration model: body sensors, neck sensors, and otoliths provide information about the body in-space, head-on-body, and head-in-space positions, respectively. As part of the central neural processing, the neck and body signals undergo coordinate transformation to indirectly encode head-in-space orientation. Overall, the optimal head-in-space estimate $(\tilde{H}_S)$ is obtained by the relative weights of the otolith information (W_{HD}, blue pathway), coordinate-transformed information from the body and neck sensors (W_{HI}, green pathway), and the head prior information (W_{HP}, gray pathway). The head-in-space estimate $(\tilde{H}_S)$ is then integrated with eye-in-head estimate $(\tilde{E}_H)$ and line orientation on the retina to obtain an internal estimate of the upright orientation [i.e., subjective visual vertical (SVV)].

processed in a head-in-space reference frame (30, 58–62). On the other hand, perception of body orientation is largely modulated by the proprioceptive inputs encoding trunk position, with errors that are more accurate but less precise than SVV responses (54, 55, 63–65). In line with these findings, and consistent with distinct sensory contributions to perception of body orientation from perception of upright, SVV deviations induced by galvanic vestibular stimulation (GVS) were dissociated from the errors in perception of body orientation (66).

In accordance with the multimodal sensory contributions to perception of upright, alterations in the neck, trunk, and interoceptive inputs have modulating effects on perceptual upright responses (30, 61, 67–75). For example, vibration of the neck muscles can shift SVV errors in the opposite direction of the head tilt and increase the E-effect (73, 76, 77). Thus, the brain must be able to determine upright orientation either directly, by accessing the estimate of head-in-space orientation through the sensory inputs encoding head position (e.g., otolith signals), or indirectly, through the sensory inputs encoding neck and trunk positions (54). In this context, the sensory contributions to upright perception are modulated by the body tilt position, with likely a greater weight of the head position signals (e.g., from the otoliths) around the upright position, and a substantial weight of the trunk proprioceptive signals at larger tilt angles (30, 31). Such distinct patterns of sensory contributions to perception of upright are supported by the findings in patients with vestibular and proprioceptive loss (25, 78–87). Patients with vestibular loss tend to have no E-effect at small tilt angles and more pronounced A-effects at larger tilt angles, consistent with reduced weight of head position signals and consequently relative underestimation of upright orientation (25, 80–82, 84, 86, 87). Patients with proprioceptive loss, on the other hand, have decreased A-effect consistent with reduced weight of body proprioception, and consequently relative overestimation of upright orientation (25, 88, 89).

Perception of upright has been also studied with respect to changes in body position or posture (52, 84, 90). Healthy participants lying supine had accurate SVV responses, but there were large errors in patients with vestibular loss in the supine position compared with the sitting and standing positions (84, 91). In general, SVV responses tend to be more accurate while maintaining precarious postures, where there is a risk of falling and thus a higher demand for balancing activity (e.g., standing on a beam) (92, 93). Such findings underscore the ecological aspect of upright perception in which according to the task at hand the internal estimate of upright is modulated by available sensory cues.

Systematic errors of upright perception also occur with body rotation in the roll plane, and—similar to the static roll-tilts—these dynamic errors are dissociated from the perception of the body orientation (27, 94–98). After constant-velocity roll rotations, SVV errors were transiently biased in the direction of the rotation (95–98). This "dynamic" bias was dependent on the velocity of the rotation and the final tilt position at which SVV was measured. For example, with clockwise rotations starting from the upright position, SVV errors showed a significant A-effect when the rotation stopped at large body tilt angles, whereas the errors were close to veridical when it stopped at smaller tilt angles. By contrast, with counterclockwise rotations passing through the upside-down position, SVV errors showed a significant E-effect when the rotation stopped at small tilt angles (i.e., close to the upright position), whereas the errors were close to veridical when it stopped at large tilt angles (i.e., close to the 90° tilt position) (97). This post-rotation "hysteresis" effect lasted about 1 min, suggesting that the transient bias in SVV errors was related to semicircular canal activation from the forces generated through deceleration. Perception of roll-tilt can also be induced during off-axis yaw rotation with the head upright or during on-axis yaw rotation with the head tilted on the body (99, 100). In these scenarios, rotational cues mainly from the horizontal semicircular canal stimulation affect the time course of tilt perception (101, 102). Moreover, SVV errors have been reported with the head pitched forward or backward during yaw-axis rotation. In this case, SVV errors were in the opposite direction of the rotation (same direction as the fast phase of the torsional nystagmus) and were more pronounced with the head pitched backward, consistent with a stronger effect from stimulation of the posterior semicircular canal (103).

Perception of upright has been also studied with respect to the modulating effects of visual backgrounds. Our daily environment is rich with visual cues that indicate world-horizontal and vertical orientations. In general, various visual functions (e.g., orientation discrimination, contrast detection, or visual acuity) show superior performance along the horizontal and vertical axes compared with oblique angles (e.g., 45°), which is referred to as the oblique effect (13, 20). However, visual vertical cues can have a greater effect on one's perception of spatial orientation than the perceived orientation of objects (104–107). Strong effects of visual cues on upright perception have been shown in various settings, ranging from an entire tilted furnished room to more impoverished stimuli such as a simple square frame (20, 106, 108–119). Remarkably, even the addition of a single line in the SVV paradigm can induce a visual bias in upright responses (118, 120, 121). In the case of a square frame, the visual vertical estimate is biased by the frame orientation, which is known as the rod-and-frame effect. The frame effect can be robust and, for example, significantly decrease SVV errors induced by rotating backgrounds (122, 123). This visual effect for the most part depends on the viewing distance and the head tilt position. It decreases with far viewing, indicating reduced reliability of the frame as a visual cue to upright orientation, and increases with head tilt, indicating reduced reliability of the vestibular cues to upright orientation (119, 124).

Overall, changes in the frame tilt orientation can result in periodic modulation of SVV errors by the rod-and-frame effect. Usually, frame tilts close to the perceived upright orientation result in an "attractor bias" toward the frame orientation, whereas there is a "detractor bias" at frame tilts beyond 45° and up to 90°, and no bias at frame tilts close to 90° (**Figure 7**) (118, 121, 124). This modulating effect of the frame orientation is more pronounced at larger body tilts, and it can either enhance the E-effect or decrease the A-effect depending on the body tilt orientation (105, 118, 125). The rod-and-frame effect may also vary among individuals, as some exhibit a strong frame effect (i.e., visual dependence), while others may have a weaker effect (i.e., visual independence) (126–129). A similar pattern of variability with the rod-and-frame effect has been shown in patients with vestibular loss; however, the frame effect can be asymmetrical in these patients, with reduced or even abolished visual dependence when the frame is tilted toward the healthy side, as opposed to a significant frame effect when it is tilted toward the side of vestibular loss (130). Background rotation in the roll plane (i.e., around the line of sight) can also affect upright perception and induce SVV errors in the direction of the rotation (80, 131, 132). Similar to the rod-and-frame effect, this optokinetic effect is more pronounced at larger body tilt angles and can induce a larger bias toward the side of vestibular loss (83, 133–135).

Another important factor in perception of upright is the effect of gravity on sensory modalities that encode body position (90, 136–141). As a fundamental reference for spatial orientation, the gravity vector plays a significant role in almost all aspects of our

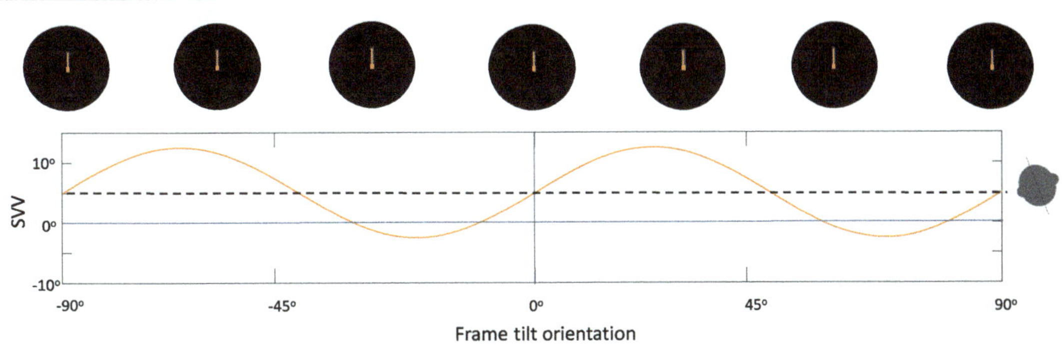

FIGURE 7 | Schematic representation of the periodic subjective visual vertical (SVV) modulation by the frame orientation (solid line) during head tilt: frame tilt orientations close to the subject's upright perception (dashed line) usually result in an "attractor bias" (i.e., toward the direction of the frame tilt), while there is a "detractor bias" at angles beyond 45° and up to 90° (i.e., away from the direction of the frame tilt). These biases caused by the frame orientation can either attenuate or accentuate SVV errors, depending on head tilt position (e.g., here 20° head tilt to the left).

balance, perception, and action. In general, gravitoinertial forces can change perceived orientation of objects, an effect that has been described as the oculogravic illusion (142). Similarly, in microgravity and weightless conditions, space crews often report visual reorientation illusions such as difficulty distinguishing between spacecraft floors, walls, and ceiling surfaces (143–146). With respect to upright perception, rotating rooms, parabolic flights, and human centrifuge have been used to study the effects of gravitoinertial forces (39, 101, 102, 140, 147–153). For example, in a centrifuge experiment, perception of tilt significantly increased late in the spaceflight duration compared with the early flight and preflight results on earth (152). This exaggerated perception of tilt also persisted into the early post-flight days. Likewise, other studies using the rod-and-frame test, optokinetic stimulation, and unilateral centrifugations (i.e., stimulating only one labyrinth at a time) have shown significant visual dependency and asymmetry in SVV responses upon returning back to the earth (146, 151, 154). These results suggest that the multisensory contributions to the internal reference for upright orientation is reduced with adaptation to microgravity. The effect of gravity on this multisensory reference is shown with gravitational forces as little as 0.15 *g* (close to the force of gravity at the moon) and up to 1.5–2 *g*, resulting in significant deviations in perception of upright (140, 148, 155, 156).

Upright Perception and Adaptation: Drift during Head Tilt

Upright perception may drift during prolonged tilts of the whole body or prolonged tilts of the head on body (15, 31, 61, 157, 158). The drift pattern is usually variable across individuals (157), but often there is a gradual change in the direction of the tilt, followed by a post-tilt bias referred to as the aftereffect (**Figure 8**) (15, 61, 157–161). When this aftereffect was studied across a wide range of body orientations, there was a "local" effect (as opposed to a "global" effect), where the post tilt bias was mainly seen in the tilt orientations adjacent to the initial, adapting position (162). For example, if the subject was initially tilted at 90°, the SVV aftereffect was more pronounced at nearby tilt angles such as 60°. Based on this finding, it was proposed that maintaining a static tilt position could bias the internal upright reference toward this adopted position, thus resulting in an aftereffect at subsequent tilt positions (162).

As mentioned earlier, ocular torsion can be a significant source of SVV errors during head tilt, due to the low OCR gain and altered orientation of the images on the retina (15, 53, 100, 103). However, neither the drift in upright perception nor the aftereffect correlate with changes in ocular torsion (15) (**Figure 8**). These findings indicate that the torsional eye position—or its driving input from the otoliths—cannot be the source of the drift or the aftereffect in perception of upright. Similar drifts have been found with haptic measurements, which also confirms that the visual error induced by ocular torsion cannot be the source of drifts in upright perception during head tilt (157, 161). Overall, SVV drifts tend to be larger and more consistent across individuals with the head-on body tilts compared with the whole body tilts (15, 157, 158, 161, 163). These findings, along with predictions from the Bayesian spatial perception model, suggest that the adaptation of neck proprioceptive inputs is the primary source of SVV drift during head tilt (15). Thus, the SVV drift is likely modulated by the position of the head relative to the body rather than the position of the

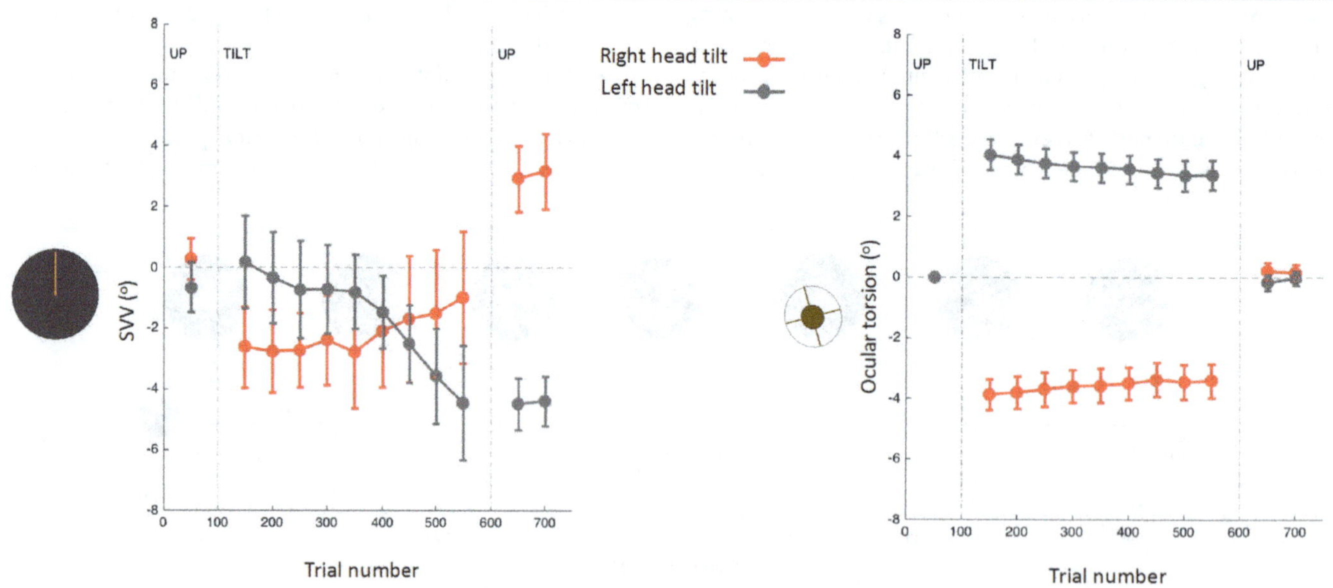

FIGURE 8 | Subjective visual vertical (SVV) and torsional eye position measured simultaneously before, during, and after prolonged head tilts (~15 min) in 12 subjects (15): data points represent SVV or ocular torsion from 100 trials during 20° head tilts to the right and left. Error bars correspond with SEM across subjects. The SVV drift is in the same direction as the head tilt, and when the head returns to upright position there is an aftereffect, also in the same direction as the head tilt. Changes in ocular torsion do not correspond to the SVV drift or aftereffect.

head or trunk relative to gravity. Visual vertical responses may also drift in upright body position, but considerably less when compared with the drift during static body tilt (13, 37). This drift attenuated when upright visual cues were present, but did not completely disappear (13).

PERCEPTION OF UPRIGHT AND CEREBRAL CORTEX

Multimodal Vestibular Cortex

Multisensory integration is a key functional aspect of neural processes involved in the perception of spatial orientation. In this context, vestibular inputs are often integrated with other sensory modalities that are incorporated into self-perception and extrapersonal spatial orientation to subserve high level cognitive and sensorimotor functions (e.g., visual and proprioceptive signals). Accordingly, graviception and orientation constancy can also be understood as functions mediated by multiple sensory modalities.

Attempts to localize vestibular function to the cerebral cortex began with the ancient descriptions of vertigo and speculations about global cerebral function (164). In recent years, electrophysiological recordings in animal studies have identified multiple cortical sites sensitive to vestibular stimulation, thus laying the groundwork for comparisons with the human cortex. The findings reveal distinct areas within the parietal and temporal cortices that receive and process vestibular inputs. These cortical areas include the parieto-insular vestibular cortex (PIVC), parts of the somatosensory cortex, the lower tip of the intraparietal sulcus, the dorsal subdivision of the middle superior temporal cortex (MSTd), the visual posterior Sylvian area (VPS), and the ventral intraparietal cortex (VIP) [for comprehensive review, see Ref. (165)]. While these vestibular areas are interconnected, there is no clear evidence that they are organized in a hierarchy similar to other sensory regions such as visual and somatosensory cortices. Direct cortical recordings suggest that PIVC is involved in the integration of vestibular and somatosensory information into a concept of "head in space" (166, 167). On the other hand, visual and vestibular signals have been recorded from MSTd, VPS, VIP, and caudal intraparietal area, with reference to heading perception or allocentric orientation in the earth-vertical direction (168–173). Note that despite the evidence for multimodal integration in these cortical areas, vestibular signals recorded from single neurons remain distinct, suggesting that sensory integration takes place through the function of a cortical network rather than individual neurons (174–176).

In human, as with primate studies, findings from cortical lesion analysis, functional imaging with caloric or galvanic stimulation (fMRI and PET), and also direct cortical stimulation point to a widely distributed multisensory vestibular system, mainly in the temporo-partieto-insular cortices [see Ref. (165) for comprehensive review]. The vestibular or combined visual-vestibular activations in these cortical regions are predominantly focused at the temporo-parietal junction (TPJ), and more specifically around the posterior parietal operculum, inferior parietal lobule, superior temporal gyrus (STG), and the junction of the intraparietal sulcus and the postcentral sulcus (177–195). Overall, the patterns of cortical activity in these studies suggest that the posterior parietal operculum is the human homologue of PIVC area in monkey, and the human homologues of VPS, VIP, and MSTd areas are within or around the inferior parietal lobule (180, 196). Note, however, that a systematic mapping of TPJ is currently lacking, and we know little about the flow of sensory information among various areas within this cortical region, or how disruption in one sensory modality may affect multisensory integration and perception of spatial orientation.

Although not addressed in animal studies, significant vestibular activation has been found in the non-dominant human cortex, i.e., the right hemisphere in right-handers and the left hemisphere in left-handers (179). Notably, the cortical mechanisms involved in spatial functions also modulate lower-level vestibular function, and a similar pattern of laterality has been shown for the cortical influence on the duration of the vestibulo-ocular reflex (i.e., the time constant) (197–199). With respect to the vestibular connections to the cerebral cortex, five distinct vestibular pathways have been identified based on functional and structural imaging analyses (200, 201). Three of these pathways run ipsilaterally, and two cross either within the pons or the midbrain. The ipsilateral pathways reach the inferior part of the insular cortex either directly or through the thalamus. Contralateral pathways run through the posterolateral thalamus to the parieto-insular cortex. In addition to connections with the brainstem, the parietal opercular regions also maintain communication with each other via an interhemispheric band of fibers passing through the antero-caudal splenium of the corpus callosum (200, 201).

Temporo-Parietal Cortex and Perception of Upright

The TPJ is a cortical hub for multiple sensory modalities, and it has been implicated in various aspects of spatial orientation including visuospatial attention, heading perception, visual gravitational motion perception, sense of embodiment, self-localization, and egocentricity (186, 187, 191, 202–213). The role of TPJ in perception of spatial orientation is especially evident from the deficits in neglect syndrome as a result of lesions involving this cortical region. Patients with neglect are unable to attend to sensory stimuli in their contralesional hemispace and also show significant contraversive deviations of upright perception in both haptic and visual tasks (214–223). These multimodal deficits in upright perception are often related to the severity of neglect symptoms and are also modulated by the head and body positions (217, 220, 224–228). In addition, abnormal visual modulation of upright perception has been reported in neglect patients. Using the rod-and-frame test, upright responses were more biased by the frame effect when it was tilted contralesionally, whereas the bias decreased when the frame was tilted toward the side of the lesion (216). Visuospatial deficits (i.e., visual extinction) have been also produced in healthy individuals by the inhibitory effect of transcranial magnetic stimulation (TMS) over the right TPJ. This transient effect, as with neglect patients,

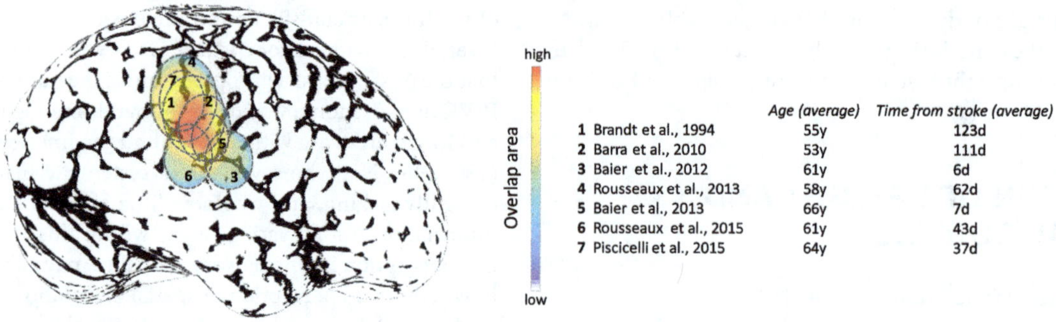

FIGURE 9 | Approximate projections of the cortical areas associated with subjective visual vertical deviation based on anatomical locations of the average lesion areas from seven studies. The color map shows the degree of overlap among cortical involvement in these studies with maximum convergence around the temporo-parietal junction. The average age of the patients in years and the average time from the stroke in days are included for each study.

was dependent on the horizontal and vertical eccentricity of the visual stimulus (229). Taken together, these findings suggest that the perception of body orientation, visuospatial awareness, and upright orientation share the same cortical networks. In this scheme, sensory processing at the TPJ would be crucial for construction of the reference frames used for both self-position and extrapersonal space transformations. In line with the multisensory role of TPJ, cortical activations within this area during visual, tactile, and vestibular sensory conflicts correspond to the perception of self-location (230–232). Accordingly, TPJ lesions are also associated with symptoms such as out-of-body experience or room tilt illusion (210, 231, 233–236). Overall, these lines of evidence indicate that TPJ is involved in generating the multisensory internal reference used by the brain to anchor "self" with respect to the surrounding environment and maintain orientation constancy especially with changes in the eye, head, and body positions.

Studies focused on the effects of brain lesions on upright perception go back as far as 1948, where SVV errors exceeding 2° were described with fronto-parietal lesions, but not occipital lesions (for comparison, note the campanile of Pisa is currently at 4°) (237). More recently, lesion studies have shown associations between cerebral cortex and abnormal upright perception in the context of hemispheric stroke (88, 221, 226, 238–242). Note that these studies have recruited patients at different post-lesion times which could affect the SVV results depending on the effect of brain adaptation following the stroke in these patients. While these studies indicate involvement of several cortical areas within and around TPJ, these lesions converge largely within the inferior parietal lobule and posterior aspect of the insular cortex (**Figure 9**). Isolated lesions within the posterior insula, however, are not associated with SVV deviations, which suggests that other cortical locations within TPJ are involved in perception of upright (243). With respect to subcortical white matter regions, lesion extensions to the superior longitudinal fascicle, inferior longitudinal fascicle, inferior occipitofrontal fascicle, and superior occipitofrontal fascicle are shown in connection with SVV deviations (239, 242). In general, lesion studies have widely reported contralesional SVV deviations, whereas only about 10% of patients may have ipsilesional SVV deviations (88, 220–222, 228, 237, 238, 240, 241, 244–248). This finding contrasts with to the SVV deviations seen with brainstem lesions, which more consistently are tilted toward the side of the lesion with caudal brainstem involvement, and away from the side of the lesion with rostral brainstem involvement (249–251). In addition, the extent of SVV deviations with cerebral cortical lesions is usually less than the SVV deviations with the brainstem or peripheral vestibular lesions (251, 252). These anatomical differences in SVV errors are likely related to the pathological changes in ocular torsion with low-level brain lesions. Such deviations in ocular torsion lead to SVV errors by directly affecting the orientation of the images on the retina. SVV errors at the level of cerebral cortex, on the other hand, are primarily linked to the neural sensory processes underlying spatial perception.

Generally, SVV errors from the right hemispheric lesions tend to be larger, long lasting, and more often associated with contralesional deviations (239, 245, 247, 248). These findings are consistent with the dominance of the right hemisphere in processing spatial information. In addition, the magnitude of SVV deviations correlates with the extent of cortical lesions, highlighting the significance of a multisensory cortical network for coherent perception of upright (88, 247). The contralesional SVV bias persists with small body tilts away from the side of the lesion, resulting in an A-effect toward the paretic side, instead of a normal E-effect in the opposite direction (88, 220, 228, 244). Such bias, however, is not present when the body is tilted toward the side of the lesion (i.e., away from the paretic side), in which case the SVV errors are comparable to normal individuals (88). It is also shown that the errors of upright perception from cortical lesions could be dissociated from perception of body position or actual postural deviations. However, patients with concurrent errors in all these domains had lesions involving the right TPJ (247, 253, 254). When measured at different body tilts, SVV and perception of body position were correlated when the body was tilted toward the side of the lesion, but such correlation was not present while tilted away from the side of the lesion (244, 255). There were also larger overestimation errors in perception of body position compared with SVV while the body was tilted away from the side of the lesion. Such dissociation between perceptions of upright and body position is consistent with different weights of sensory contributions for processing upright orientation versus body position. With respect to other axes of spatial perception, a significant backward deviation of upright responses in the pitch plane has been reported in patients with right hemisphere stroke in addition to the errors in the roll plane (222, 223).

The role of TPJ in perception of upright is also studied using non-invasive brain stimulation (256–259). We recently applied TMS in healthy participants at the right TPJ and probed its transient cortical effects on perception of upright using SVV measurements (256). The inhibitory effect of TMS at the posterior aspect of the right supramarginal gyrus (SMGp) resulted in a shift of SVV errors in the opposite direction of the head tilt (**Figure 10**). The direction of this error, induced by the focal cortical inhibition, is consistent with the "overestimation" errors reported by the cortical lesion studies [i.e., increase in E-effect; e.g., Ref. (88)]. On the other hand, when TMS was applied randomly at other cortical locations within or outside of the TPJ, there was no significant SVV deviation, suggesting a location-specific effect at SMGp. In addition, there was no change in the torsional position of the eyes despite the SVV shift at SMGp, showing that the changes in perception of upright at the level of cerebral cortex were dissociated from the changes in ocular torsion (260) (**Figure 10**). Altogether, these findings suggest that unlike subcortical regions that have direct influence over ocular torsion, TPJ is primarily involved in sensory processing. Fiori et al. also investigated the role of TPJ in upright perception using the focal inhibitory effects of TMS (257). They found that the effect of TMS at the right TPJ selectively increased SVV errors when no visual cue was provided (i.e., no visual frame during the SVV task). However, inhibition of V1–V3 and not TPJ disrupted the visual detection of a Gabor patch orientation. This functional distinction between TPJ and early visual cortex is in line with the role of TPJ in multisensory integration for perception of upright. A significant SVV shift has also been shown using transcranial direct current stimulation (tDCS) over TPJ (258). This shift was dependent on tDCS electrode placement, with SVV deviation toward the side of anode placement. There was also a rebound effect (i.e., reversal of the SVV shift) immediately after the stimulation, which lasted longer with the right cathode/left anode placement. Cortical involvement in perception of upright has also been investigated using EEG recordings (261, 262). The results suggest that early cortical activity in the lateral temporo-occipital cortex (around 100 ms post-stimulus) is important for extracting orientation features, whereas a later activation involving the temporo-occipital and parieto-occipital cortices (around 300 ms post-stimulus) reflects multisensory integration for perception of upright.

Peripheral vestibular injuries can also provide clues to the mechanisms of recovery and multisensory compensation with

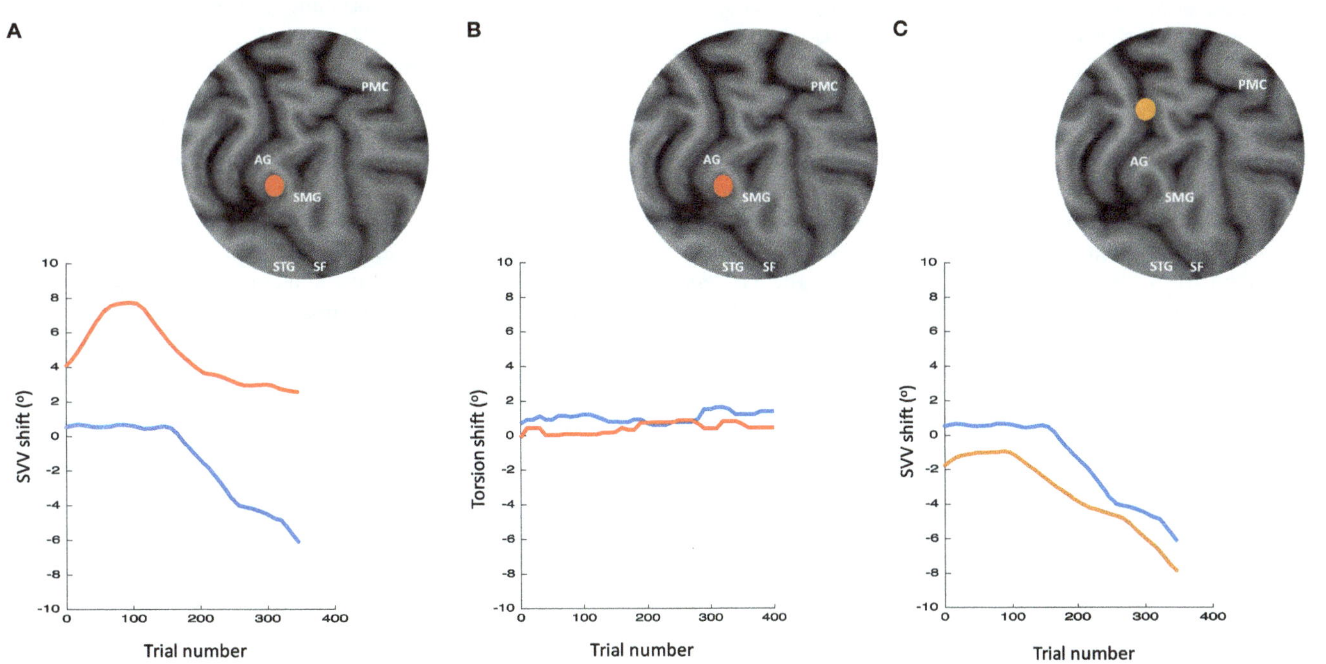

FIGURE 10 | Simultaneous subjective visual vertical (SVV) and ocular torsion recordings during prolonged left head tilt of 20° in a single subject (500 trials ~15 min) [data from Ref. (260)]: SVV shift from transcranial magnetic stimulation (TMS) at SMGp (red) is shown along with the SVV shift from the sham stimulation (i.e., no TMS) (blue) **(A)**. In both traces, there is a gradual drift over time toward the left (i.e., in the same direction as the head tilt), but the SVV shift from TMS is larger with a deviation opposite to the direction of the head tilt. Ocular torsion shift from TMS at SMGp (red) is not different form the sham stimulation (blue) **(B)**. As opposed to SMGp, SVV shift from TMS at another cortical location outside of TPJ (orange) is smaller than the sham stimulation with a deviation in the same direction as the head tilt **(C)**. PMC, primary motor cortex; SMG, supramarginal gyrus; AG, angular gyrus; STG, superior temporal gyrus; SF, Sylvian fissure.

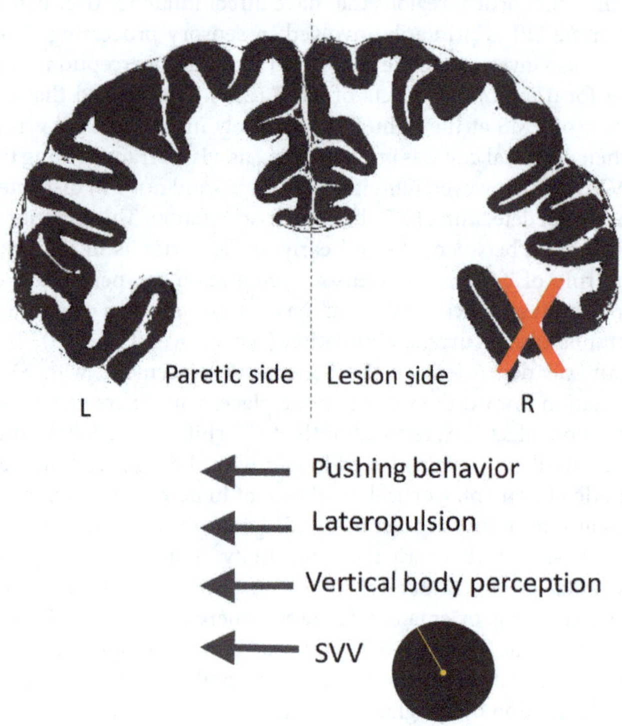

FIGURE 11 | Schematic showing the directions of subjective visual vertical (SVV) tilt and postural deviation in pusher syndrome. In these patients, SVV and postural vertical perception deviate away from the side of the lesion (X), matching the direction of postural tilt (i.e., lateropulsion) as well as the pushing behavior toward the paretic side. Therefore, patients with pushing behavior seem to actively align their body with erroneous upright and postural estimates.

respect to cortical function and upright perception. For example, it is reported that hemispheric dominance can affect the speed of recovery based on the side of peripheral vestibular injury. The recovery from the right-side vestibular loss was significantly slower than from the left-side vestibular loss in right-handers, while such difference was not found in left-handers (87). Based on this observation, it was hypothesized that the difference in the pattern of recovery in left-handers is related to a greater distribution of transcallosal connections between parietal cortices compared with right-handers (87).

Cerebral Cortical Pathology and Perception of Upright

Pathological perception of upright is widely reported with cerebral infarctions (88, 214, 220–222, 226, 228, 238–240, 244–247, 249, 253, 255, 263–285). SVV deviations in association with cortical strokes are typically found in the territory of the medial cerebral artery (MCA), mainly involving the temporal, parietal, and insular cortices. The absence of skew deviation of the eyes with these lesions suggests the affected cortical areas are primarily involved in processing sensory information (238). Notably, posterior cerebral artery infarctions, despite causing visual field defects, do not significantly alter perception of upright (238). In a sample of unilateral hemispheric infarction, the branches of the MCA resulting in SVV deviation were the temporal (mean SVV deviation about 6°), parietal (mean SVV deviation about 5°), and the deep cortical perforators (mean SVV deviation about 4°). Lesions affecting the anterior part of the internal capsule can also be associated with SVV tilt (mean SVV deviation about 3°), primarily via the lenticulostriate arteries and the anterior choroidal artery (238).

In general, hemispheric infarcts more often result in contraversive SVV deviations, while about 10% of patients may show ipsiversive SVV deviations. Pathological SVV tilts can be as large as 15°, though usually they are 5–10° and deviated leftwards as a result of right hemispheric lesions (note again that the campanile of Pisa is currently at 4°) (238, 275, 286). The range of SVV deviations in a sample of 40 patients with hemispheric stroke (time from lesions <13 weeks) was larger with the right hemispheric infarcts (−13.1° to 3.2°) compared with the left hemispheric infarcts (−3.6° to 9.3°) (228). The asymmetric hemispheric contribution to upright perception has been also shown in stroke patients with the bottom-up effects of GVS (276, 287). In these patients with right hemispheric infarcts and spatial neglect, left-cathodal but not right-cathodal galvanic stimulation significantly reduced SVV deviations, highlighting a significant cortical laterality for perception of upright. Another important factor affecting the extent and direction of SVV errors is the recovery time. Acute patients often have larger SVV errors compared with chronic patients, and such deviations often recover significantly within a few months (239, 245, 286). Patients with right hemispheric lesions also have higher variability (i.e., lower precision) in their SVV deviations (286).

Persistent SVV errors and low SVV precision are often linked to poor balance following stroke, especially in patients with the right hemispheric involvement (263, 286, 288, 289). However, perception of body orientation can be dissociated from SVV or from the actual postural deviations in these patients (63, 244, 247, 249, 253, 255, 273, 275, 277, 280–282, 290–294). For example, in a sample of 80 stroke patients reported by Perrenou et al., 34 had abnormal contralesional postural vertical tilts (i.e., deviations in posture alignment with perceived upright orientation), 44 had contralesional SVV tilts, 26 had contralesional haptic vertical tilts, and none had ipsilesional haptic or postural vertical tilts (247). Forty-one patients (52%) showed deficits in more than one modality, and 18 (22%) had transmodal contraversive deviations (i.e., SVV, postural vertical, and haptic vertical were all tilted away from the side of the lesion). In general, postural deviations in stroke patients are more closely related to the errors of postural vertical perception than to the errors of upright perception (220, 244, 247, 254, 286).

A subset of patients with cortical infarctions and postural deviations exhibit robust SVV deviations and also actively resist attempts to correct their false postural orientation back to upright position (247, 253, 265, 266, 270, 272, 274, 277, 281, 284, 294–300). This phenomenon, referred to as "pusher syndrome" (also "listing," or "lateropulsion"), is typically toward the paretic side with an incidence of approximately 5–10% among acute stroke patients (266, 278, 288). In contrast to patients with Wallenberg syndrome or thalamic astasia who pull themselves back toward upright to prevent an ipsilesional fall, pushers resist postural changes toward the non-paretic side. Patients with pusher behavior are often unable to learn to walk even with proper assistance, and their SVV errors or postural vertical deviations often last longer (275). Pushing behavior is also highly correlated with neglect symptoms and more often is associated with lesions involving the right posterior insula, STG, inferior parietal lobule, and postcentral gyrus (247, 253, 274, 278, 279, 281, 288, 297, 301, 302). In the study of Perennou et al. mentioned earlier, the patients who showed lateropulsion and pusher behavior had contraversive transmodal tilt of postural vertical, haptic vertical, and SVV (247). This finding suggests that lateropulsion and pushing behavior lie on a continuum where pushers—as opposed to those with lateropulsion only—actively align their body with their erroneous perception of upright (**Figure 11**) (247, 280, 299). When postural vertical perception was measured while standing (as opposed to sitting in other studies), pushers had large uncertainty, and, on average, ipsilesional deviation in their responses (303), showing that the postural vertical estimates can be altered by active pushing behavior while standing.

Parkinson's disease (PD) is another pathology that can affect postural control and spatial perception, due to dysfunctions involving the cortical connections with basal ganglia (304, 305). On this premise, PD measures such as trunk flexion, stance, and gait parameters have been investigated in association with SVV deviation (306–311). The postural instability in PD patients may correlate with SVV deviations, and both postural vertical perception and SVV show higher variability compared with age-matched, healthy controls (312, 313). In these patients, however, visually induced postural sway cannot be linked to the deficits in perception of upright, which suggests that the postural instability is related to abnormalities in maintaining posture rather than perceptual errors (80, 314). PD patients may also have trunk lateropulsion with the tendency for postural tilts in the direction opposite to the affected side of the body (once dubbed "scoliosis of Parkinsonism") (315). The patients with lateral trunk deviation show significantly larger SVV errors toward the trunk tilt compared with those without trunk tilt (308, 310). This lateral trunk tilt in PD has been attributed to vestibular hypofunction on the same side and described as postural imbalance syndrome with vestibular alterations or PISA (311). Patients with PISA have greater SVV deviations compared with those without the trunk tilt, either on or off of the effects of dopaminergic medications (310). Taken together, the above findings suggest that abnormal upright perception in PD patients can be linked to impaired sensorimotor processing related to corticobasal dysfunction.

Migraine syndrome can also result in visuospatial symptoms due to dysfunctions affecting neural networks from the level of brainstem to the cerebral cortex. Migraine patients with these symptoms typically complain of vertigo, dizziness, disorientation, or sense of disequilibrium, often triggered or worsened with changes in the head or body positions. This type of migraine presentation accounts for the most common cause of episodic dizziness and is classified as vestibular migraine (316–319). Patients with vestibular migraine have more pronounced postural sway compared with other types of migraine or healthy controls (320, 321). Consistent with the visuospatial symptoms in these patients, imaging analyses have found decreased gray matter volume within TPJ as well as metabolic changes in this cortical region during the attacks of vestibular migraine (322, 323). With respect to upright perception, several studies have reported SVV measurements in migraine patients (322–327). According to these studies, patients with non-vestibular migraine correctly estimate upright orientation, while those with vestibular migraine show higher variability in SVV errors compared with other headache disorders or healthy controls (319, 327–330). Patients with vestibular migraine also have reduced motion detection thresholds in the roll plane compared with non-vestibular migraine or healthy controls (331). However, currently, it is not known whether these patients with vestibular migraine also have altered perception of upright during static head or body tilts.

SUMMARY AND CONCLUSION

As a multimodal sensory reference, perception of upright represents neural processes that subserve orientation constancy. Consistent with the multisensory properties of these neural processes, several studies have described modulatory effects of gravity, visual cues, and position of the body on perception of upright. Also, various measurement paradigms have shown systematic errors of upright perception with tilting the head or body (i.e., underestimations of the true vertical orientation at large tilts and overestimations at small tilts). These errors reflect challenges for the brain in maintaining a common reference frame for upright orientation, based on the reliability of sensory signals that encode head, eye, and body positions. The computational mechanisms behind these systematic errors have been addressed using mathematical models that account for noisy sensory signals. In these models, the estimates of head, body, and ocular torsion that determine upright orientation are derived using frameworks such as Bayesian "prior" and relative weighting of sensory information.

Concerning the role of cerebral cortex in various aspect of spatial perception, animal and human studies show a widely distributed cortical network, primarily within the temporal, insular, and parietal cortices. This is not surprising considering the vital role of the information about body orientation with respect to the surrounding environment while any motor action is being contemplated. With respect to upright perception, the higher-order neural mechanisms must solve the problem of different sensory reference frames in the process of integrating various sensory information. The evidence for cortical involvement in such neural processes comes from TMS and lesion studies. The inhibitory effect of TMS at the posterior aspect of the supramarginal gyrus results in overestimation of upright orientation in the opposite direction of the head tilt. Likewise, cortical lesions involving TPJ are associated with SVV deviations primarily away from the side of the lesion. Patients with these cortical lesions may also have neglect symptoms or out-of-body experiences. Altogether, these findings suggest that perception of body orientation, visuospatial awareness, and upright orientation share the same cortical networks in which an internal reference is generated to anchor "self" with respect to the outside world and maintain orientation constancy. Currently, little is known about the flow of sensory information within these cortical networks and how disruption of one sensory modality may affect processing or integration of other sensory modalities. Future studies will have to specifically address such sensory contributions with respect to cerebral cortical involvement in perception of upright.

AUTHOR CONTRIBUTIONS

Both authors have contributed to the data gathering and writing of this manuscript.

ACKNOWLEDGMENTS

This work was supported by grants from the National Institute of Deafness and Other Communication Disorders (NIDCD); grant no. K23DC013552.

REFERENCES

1. Leigh R, Zee D. *The Neurology of Eye Movements*. 5th ed. New York: Oxford University Press (2015).
2. Aubert H. Eine scheinbare bedeutende Drehung von Objecten bei Neigung des Kopfes nach rechts oder links. *Virchows Arch Pathol Anat Physiol Klin Med* (1861) 20:381–93.
3. Müller G. Über das Aubertsche Phänomen. *Z Sinnesphysiol* (1916) 49:109–246.
4. Mittelstaedt H. A new solution to the problem of the subjective vertical. *Naturwissenschaften* (1983) 70:272–81. doi:10.1007/BF00404833
5. Baccini M, Paci M, Colletto MD, Ravenni M, Baldassi S. The assessment of subjective visual vertical: comparison of two psychophysical paradigms and age-related performance. *Atten Percept Psychophys* (2014) 76:112–22. doi:10.3758/s13414-013-0551-9
6. Kheradmand A, Gonzalez G, Otero-Millan J, Lasker A. Visual perception of upright: head tilt, visual errors and viewing eye. *J Vestib Res* (2016) 25:201–9. doi:10.3233/VES-160565
7. Pagarkar W, Bamiou D-E, Ridout D, Luxon LM. Subjective visual vertical and horizontal: effect of the preset angle. *Arch Otolaryngol Head Neck Surg* (2008) 134:394–401. doi:10.1001/archotol.134.4.394
8. Hoppenbrouwers M, Wuyts FL, Van de Heyning PH. Suppression of the E-effect during the subjective visual vertical test. *Neuroreport* (2004) 15:325–7. doi:10.1097/00001756-200402090-00023
9. Saeys W, Vereeck L, Bedeer A, Lafosse C, Truijen S, Wuyts FL, et al. Suppression of the E-effect during the subjective visual and postural vertical test in healthy subjects. *Eur J Appl Physiol* (2010) 109:297–305. doi:10.1007/s00421-010-1355-4
10. Toupet M, Van Nechel C, Grayeli AB. Subjective visual vertical tilt attraction to the side of rod presentation: effects of age, sex, and vestibular disorders. *Otol Neurotol* (2015) 36:1074–80. doi:10.1097/MAO.0000000000000771
11. Toupet M, Van Nechel C, Grayeli AB. Maturation of subjective visual vertical in children. *Otol Neurotol* (2016) 37:761–6. doi:10.1097/MAO.0000000000001044
12. Venhovens J, Meulstee J, Verhagen WIM. Static subjective visual vertical in healthy volunteers: the effects of different preset angle deviations and test-retest variability. *Neuroophthalmology* (2016) 40:113–9. doi:10.3109/01658107.2016.1156707
13. Tarnutzer AA, Fernando DP, Kheradmand A, Lasker AG, Zee DS. Temporal constancy of perceived direction of gravity assessed by visual line adjustments. *J Vestib Res* (2012) 22:41–54. doi:10.3233/VES-2011-0436
14. Mezey LE, Curthoys IS, Burgess AM, Goonetilleke SC, MacDougall HG. Changes in ocular torsion position produced by a single visual line rotating around the line of sight – visual "entrainment" of ocular torsion. *Vision Res* (2004) 44:397–406. doi:10.1016/j.visres.2003.09.026
15. Otero-Millan J, Kheradmand A. Upright perception and ocular torsion change independently during head tilt. *Front Hum Neurosci* (2016) 10:573. doi:10.3389/fnhum.2016.00573
16. Luyat M, Noël M, Thery V, Gentaz E. Gender and line size factors modulate the deviations of the subjective visual vertical induced by head tilt. *BMC Neurosci* (2012) 13:28. doi:10.1186/1471-2202-13-28
17. Wade NJ. The effect of stimulus line variations on visual orientation with head upright and tilted. *Aust J Psychol* (1969) 21:177–85. doi:10.1080/00049536908257782
18. Betts GA, Curthoys IS. Visually perceived vertical and visually perceived horizontal are not orthogonal. *Vision Res* (1998) 38:1989–99. doi:10.1016/S0042-6989(97)00401-X
19. Van Beuzekom AD, Van Gisbergen JAM. Properties of the internal representation of gravity inferred from spatial-direction and body-tilt estimates. *J Neurophysiol* (2000) 84:11–27.
20. Howard IP. *Human Visual Orientation*. New York: Wiley (1982).
21. Tarnutzer AA, Bockisch C, Straumann D, Olasagasti I. Gravity dependence of subjective visual vertical variability. *J Neurophysiol* (2009) 102:1657–71. doi:10.1152/jn.00007.2008
22. Mast F, Jarchow T. Perceived body position and the visual horizontal. *Brain Res Bull* (1996) 40:393–7; discussion 397–8. doi:10.1016/0361-9230(96)00132-3
23. Van Beuzekom AD, Medendorp WP, Van Gisbergen JAM. The subjective vertical and the sense of self orientation during active body tilt. *Vision Res* (2001) 41:3229–42. doi:10.1016/S0042-6989(01)00144-4
24. Kaptein RG, Van Gisbergen JAM. Interpretation of a discontinuity in the sense of verticality at large body tilt. *J Neurophysiol* (2004) 91:2205–14. doi:10.1152/jn.00804.2003
25. Bronstein AM. The interaction of otolith and proprioceptive information in the perception of verticality. The effects of labyrinthine and CNS disease. *Ann N Y Acad Sci* (1999) 871:324–33. doi:10.1111/j.1749-6632.1999.tb09195.x
26. Kaptein RG, Van Gisbergen JAM. Nature of the transition between two modes of external space perception in tilted subjects. *J Neurophysiol* (2005) 93:3356–69. doi:10.1152/jn.01137.2004
27. Udo de Haes HA, Schöne H. Interaction between statolith organs and semicircular canals on apparent vertical and nystagmus. Investigations on the effectiveness of the statolith organs. *Acta Otolaryngol* (1970) 69:25–31. doi:10.3109/00016487009123333
28. Mast FW. Does the world rock when the eyes roll? Allocentric orientation representation, ocular counterroll, and the subjective visual vertical. *Swiss J Psychol* (2000) 59:89–101. doi:10.1024//1421-0185.59.2.89
29. De Vrijer M, Medendorp WP, Van Gisbergen JAM. Shared computational mechanism for tilt compensation accounts for biased verticality percepts in motion and pattern vision. *J Neurophysiol* (2008) 99:915–30. doi:10.1152/jn.00921.2007
30. Alberts BBGT, Selen LPJ, Bertolini G, Straumann D, Medendorp WP, Tarnutzer AA. Dissociating vestibular and somatosensory contributions to spatial orientation. *J Neurophysiol* (2016) 116:30–40. doi:10.1152/jn.00056.2016
31. Lechner-Steinleitner S. Interaction of labyrinthine and somatoreceptor inputs as determinants of the subjective vertical. *Psychol Res* (1978) 40:65–76. doi:10.1007/BF00308464
32. Schöne H, Haes HUD. Perception of gravity-vertical as a function of head and trunk position. *Z Vergl Physiol* (1968) 60:440–4. doi:10.1007/BF00297938
33. Tarnutzer AA, Bockisch CJ, Straumann D. Head roll dependent variability of subjective visual vertical and ocular counterroll. *Exp Brain Res* (2009) 195:621–6. doi:10.1007/s00221-009-1823-4
34. Udo de Haes HAUD. Stability of apparent vertical and ocular countertorsion as a function of lateral tilt. *Percept Psychophys* (1970) 8:137–42. doi:10.3758/BF03210192
35. Jarchow T, Mast FW. The effect of water immersion on postural and visual orientation. *Aviat Space Environ Med* (1999) 70:879–86.
36. Luyat M, Gentaz E. Body tilt effect on the reproduction of orientations: studies on the visual oblique effect and subjective orientations. *J Exp Psychol Hum Percept Perform* (2002) 28:1002–11. doi:10.1037/0096-1523.28.4.1002

37. Tarnutzer AA, Fernando DP, Lasker AG, Zee DS. How stable is perceived direction of gravity over extended periods in darkness? *Exp Brain Res* (2012) 222:427–36. doi:10.1007/s00221-012-3230-5
38. Bringoux L, Tamura K, Faldon M, Gresty MA, Bronstein AM. Influence of whole-body pitch tilt and kinesthetic cues on the perceived gravity-referenced eye level. *Exp Brain Res* (2004) 155:385–92. doi:10.1007/s00221-003-1742-8
39. Carriot J, Barraud P-A, Nougier V, Cian C. Difference in the perception of the horizon during true and simulated tilt in the absence of semicircular canal cues. *Exp Brain Res* (2006) 174:158–66. doi:10.1007/s00221-006-0434-6
40. Ebenholtz SM. Perception of the vertical with body tilt in the median plane. *J Exp Psychol* (1970) 83:1–6. doi:10.1037/h0028518
41. Bauermeister M, Werner H, Wapner S. The effect of body tilt on tactual-kinesthetic perception of verticality. *Am J Psychol* (1964) 77:451–6. doi:10.2307/1421016
42. Luyat M, Gentaz E, Corte TR, Guerraz M. Reference frames and haptic perception of orientation: body and head tilt effects on the oblique effect. *Percept Psychophys* (2001) 63:541–54. doi:10.3758/BF03194419
43. Schuler JR, Bockisch CJ, Straumann D, Tarnutzer AA. Precision and accuracy of the subjective haptic vertical in the roll plane. *BMC Neurosci* (2010) 11:83. doi:10.1186/1471-2202-11-83
44. Tarnutzer AA, Bockisch CJ, Olasagasti I, Straumann D. Egocentric and allocentric alignment tasks are affected by otolith input. *J Neurophysiol* (2012) 107:3095–106. doi:10.1152/jn.00724.2010
45. Bortolami SB, Pierobon A, DiZio P, Lackner JR. Localization of the subjective vertical during roll, pitch, and recumbent yaw body tilt. *Exp Brain Res* (2006) 173:364–73. doi:10.1007/s00221-006-0385-y
46. Guerraz M, Luyat M, Poquin D, Ohlmann T. The role of neck afferents in subjective orientation in the visual and tactile sensory modalities. *Acta Otolaryngol* (2000) 120:735–8. doi:10.1080/000164800750000261
47. Lejeune L, Thouvarecq R, Anderson DI, Jouen F. Kinesthetic estimation of the main orientations from the upright and supine positions. *Acta Psychol* (2004) 117:13–28. doi:10.1016/j.actpsy.2004.05.001
48. Anastasopoulos D, Haslwanter T, Bronstein A, Fetter M, Dichgans J. Dissociation between the perception of body verticality and the visual vertical in acute peripheral vestibular disorder in humans. *Neurosci Lett* (1997) 233:151–3. doi:10.1016/S0304-3940(97)00639-3
49. Fraser LE, Makooie B, Harris LR. The subjective visual vertical and the subjective haptic vertical access different gravity estimates. *PLoS One* (2015) 10:e0145528. doi:10.1371/journal.pone.0145528
50. Gentaz E, Baud-Bovy G, Luyat M. The haptic perception of spatial orientations. *Exp Brain Res* (2008) 187:331–48. doi:10.1007/s00221-008-1382-0
51. Eggert T. *Der Einfluss orientierter Texturen auf die subjektive visuelle Vertikale und seine systemtheoretische Analyse*. Ph.D. thesis, Munich Technical University, München (1998).
52. MacNeilage PR, Banks MS, Berger DR, Bülthoff HH. A Bayesian model of the disambiguation of gravitoinertial force by visual cues. *Exp Brain Res* (2007) 179:263–90. doi:10.1007/s00221-006-0792-0
53. De Vrijer MD, Medendorp WP, Gisbergen JAMV. Accuracy-precision tradeoff in visual orientation constancy. *J Vis* (2009) 9:9. doi:10.1167/9.2.9
54. Clemens IAH, Vrijer MD, Selen LPJ, Gisbergen JAMV, Medendorp WP. Multisensory processing in spatial orientation: an inverse probabilistic approach. *J Neurosci* (2011) 31:5365–77. doi:10.1523/JNEUROSCI.6472-10.2011
55. Mittelstaedt H. Somatic versus vestibular gravity reception in man. *Ann N Y Acad Sci* (1992) 656:124–39. doi:10.1111/j.1749-6632.1992.tb25204.x
56. Mittelstaedt H. Interaction of eye-, head-, and trunk-bound information in spatial perception and control. *J Vestib Res* (1997) 7:283–302. doi:10.1016/S0957-4271(97)00027-X
57. Mittelstaedt H. Origin and processing of postural information. *Neurosci Biobehav Rev* (1998) 22:473–8. doi:10.1016/S0149-7634(97)00032-8
58. de Graaf B, Bekkering H, Erasmus C, Bles W. Influence of visual, vestibular, cervical, and somatosensory tilt information on ocular rotation and perception of the horizontal. *J Vestib Res* (1992) 2:15–30.
59. Guerraz M, Poquin D, Luyat M, Ohlmann T. Head orientation involvement in assessment of the subjective vertical during whole body tilt. *Percept Mot Skills* (1998) 87:643–8. doi:10.2466/pms.1998.87.2.643
60. Tarnutzer AA, Bockisch CJ, Straumann D. Roll-dependent modulation of the subjective visual vertical: contributions of head- and trunk-based signals. *J Neurophysiol* (2010) 103:934–41. doi:10.1152/jn.00407.2009
61. Wade NJ. Visual orientation during and after lateral head, body, and trunk tilt. *Percept Psychophys* (1968) 3:215–9. doi:10.3758/BF03212730
62. Young LR, Oman CM, Dichgans JM. Influence of head orientation on visually induced pitch and roll sensation. *Aviat Space Environ Med* (1975) 46:264–8.
63. Bisdorff AR, Wolsley CJ, Anastasopoulos D, Bronstein AM, Gresty MA. The perception of body verticality (subjective postural vertical) in peripheral and central vestibular disorders. *Brain* (1996) 119(Pt 5):1523–34. doi:10.1093/brain/119.5.1523
64. Mittelstaedt H. The role of the otoliths in perception of the vertical and in path integration. *Ann N Y Acad Sci* (1999) 871:334–44. doi:10.1111/j.1749-6632.1999.tb09196.x
65. Tarnutzer AA, Bockisch CJ, Straumann D. Visually guided adjustments of body posture in the roll plane. *Exp Brain Res* (2013) 227:111–20. doi:10.1007/s00221-013-3492-6
66. Mars F, Vercher J-L, Popov K. Dissociation between subjective vertical and subjective body orientation elicited by galvanic vestibular stimulation. *Brain Res Bull* (2005) 65:77–86. doi:10.1016/j.brainresbull.2004.11.012
67. Barbieri G, Gissot A-S, Fouque F, Casillas J-M, Pozzo T, Pérennou D. Does proprioception contribute to the sense of verticality? *Exp Brain Res* (2008) 185:545–52. doi:10.1007/s00221-007-1177-8
68. Barra J, Pérennou D, Thilo KV, Gresty MA, Bronstein AM. The awareness of body orientation modulates the perception of visual vertical. *Neuropsychologia* (2012) 50:2492–8. doi:10.1016/j.neuropsychologia.2012.06.021
69. Böhmer A, Mast F. Assessing otolith function by the subjective visual vertical. *Ann N Y Acad Sci* (1999) 871:221–31. doi:10.1111/j.1749-6632.1999.tb09187.x
70. Carriot J, Cian C, Paillard A, Denise P, Lackner JR. Influence of multisensory graviceptive information on the apparent zenith. *Exp Brain Res* (2011) 208:569–79. doi:10.1007/s00221-010-2505-y
71. Ceyte H, Cian C, Trousselard M, Barraud P-A. Influence of perceived egocentric coordinates on the subjective visual vertical. *Neurosci Lett* (2009) 462:85–8. doi:10.1016/j.neulet.2009.06.048
72. Day RH, Wade NJ. Mechanisms involved in visual orientation constancy. *Psychol Bull* (1969) 71:33. doi:10.1037/h0026872
73. McKenna GJ, Peng GCY, Zee DS. Neck muscle vibration alters visually perceived roll in normals. *J Assoc Res Otolaryngol* (2004) 5:25–31. doi:10.1007/s10162-003-4005-2
74. Riccio GE, Martin EJ, Stoffregen TA. The role of balance dynamics in the active perception of orientation. *J Exp Psychol Hum Percept Perform* (1992) 18:624–44. doi:10.1037/0096-1523.18.3.624
75. Trousselard M, Barraud P, Nougier V, Raphel C, Cian C. Contribution of tactile and interoceptive cues to the perception of the direction of gravity. *Brain Res Cogn Brain Res* (2004) 20:355–62. doi:10.1016/j.cogbrainres.2004.03.008
76. Betts GA, Barone M, Karlberg M, MacDougall H, Curthoys IS. Neck muscle vibration alters visually-perceived roll after unilateral vestibular loss. *Neuroreport* (2000) 11:2659–62. doi:10.1097/00001756-200008210-00011
77. Kawase T, Maki A, Takata Y, Miyazaki H, Kobayashi T. Effects of neck muscle vibration on subjective visual vertical: comparative analysis with effects on nystagmus. *Eur Arch Otorhinolaryngol* (2011) 268:823–7. doi:10.1007/s00405-010-1467-9
78. Alberts BBGT, Selen LPJ, Verhagen WIM, Medendorp WP. Sensory substitution in bilateral vestibular a-reflexic patients. *Physiol Rep* (2015) 3:e12385. doi:10.14814/phy2.12385
79. Bringoux L, Schmerber S, Nougier V, Dumas G, Barraud PA, Raphel C. Perception of slow pitch and roll body tilts in bilateral labyrinthine-defective subjects. *Neuropsychologia* (2002) 40:367–72. doi:10.1016/S0028-3932(01)00103-8
80. Bronstein AM, Yardley L, Moore AP, Cleeves L. Visually and posturally mediated tilt illusion in Parkinson's disease and in labyrinthine defective subjects. *Neurology* (1996) 47:651–6. doi:10.1212/WNL.47.3.651
81. Dai MJ, Curthoys IS, Halmagyi GM. Linear acceleration perception in the roll plane before and after unilateral vestibular neurectomy. *Exp Brain Res* (1989) 77:315–28. doi:10.1007/BF00274989
82. Graybiel A, Miller EF, Newsom BD, Kennedy RS. The effect of water immersion on perception of the oculogravic illusion in normal and labyrinthine-defective subjects. *Acta Otolaryngol* (1968) 65:599–610. doi:10.3109/00016486809119294

83. Lopez C, Lacour M, Ahmadi AE, Magnan J, Borel L. Changes of visual vertical perception: a long-term sign of unilateral and bilateral vestibular loss. *Neuropsychologia* (2007) 45:2025–37. doi:10.1016/j.neuropsychologia.2007.02.004
84. Lopez C, Lacour M, Léonard J, Magnan J, Borel L. How body position changes visual vertical perception after unilateral vestibular loss. *Neuropsychologia* (2008) 46:2435–40. doi:10.1016/j.neuropsychologia.2008.03.017
85. Mazibrada G, Tariq S, Pérennou D, Gresty M, Greenwood R, Bronstein AM. The peripheral nervous system and the perception of verticality. *Gait Posture* (2008) 27:202–8. doi:10.1016/j.gaitpost.2007.03.006
86. Müller JA, Bockisch CJ, Tarnutzer AA. Spatial orientation in patients with chronic unilateral vestibular hypofunction is ipsilesionally distorted. *Clin Neurophysiol* (2016) 127:3243–51. doi:10.1016/j.clinph.2016.07.010
87. Toupet M, Van Nechel C, Bozorg Grayeli A. Influence of body laterality on recovery from subjective visual vertical tilt after vestibular neuritis. *Audiol Neurootol* (2014) 19:248–55. doi:10.1159/000360266
88. Barra J, Marquer A, Joassin R, Reymond C, Metge L, Chauvineau V, et al. Humans use internal models to construct and update a sense of verticality. *Brain* (2010) 133:3552–63. doi:10.1093/brain/awq311
89. Yardley L. Contribution of somatosensory information to perception of the visual vertical with body tilt and rotating visual field. *Percept Psychophys* (1990) 48:131–4. doi:10.3758/BF03207079
90. Lopez C, Bachofner C, Mercier M, Blanke O. Gravity and observer's body orientation influence the visual perception of human body postures. *J Vis* (2009) 9:1. doi:10.1167/9.5.1
91. Luyat M, Ohlmann T, Barraud PA. Subjective vertical and postural activity. *Acta Psychol (Amst)* (1997) 95:181–93. doi:10.1016/S0001-6918(96)00015-7
92. Bray A, Subanandan A, Isableu B, Ohlmann T, Golding JF, Gresty MA. We are most aware of our place in the world when about to fall. *Curr Biol* (2004) 14:R609–10. doi:10.1016/j.cub.2004.07.040
93. Wright WG, Horak FB. Interaction of posture and conscious perception of gravitational vertical and surface horizontal. *Exp Brain Res* (2007) 182:321–32. doi:10.1007/s00221-007-0990-4
94. Correia Grácio BJ, Bos JE. Measuring dynamics of the subjective vertical and tilt using a joystick. *J Vestib Res* (2012) 22:181–9. doi:10.3233/VES-2012-0454
95. Jaggi-Schwarz K, Ortega M, Hess BJM. Reciprocal error behavior in estimated body position and subjective visual vertical. *Exp Brain Res* (2003) 150:122–5. doi:10.1007/s00221-003-1430-8
96. Jaggi-Schwarz K, Hess BJM. Influence of dynamic tilts on the perception of earth-vertical. *Exp Brain Res* (2003) 149:340–50. doi:10.1007/s00221-002-1343-y
97. Lorincz EN, Hess BJM. Dynamic effects on the subjective visual vertical after roll rotation. *J Neurophysiol* (2008) 100:657–69. doi:10.1152/jn.01248.2007
98. Vingerhoets RAA, Medendorp WP, Van Gisbergen JAM. Body-tilt and visual verticality perception during multiple cycles of roll rotation. *J Neurophysiol* (2008) 99:2264–80. doi:10.1152/jn.00704.2007
99. Clarke AH, Schönfeld U, Hamann C, Scherer H. Measuring unilateral otolith function via the otolith-ocular response and the subjective visual vertical. *Acta Otolaryngol Suppl* (2001) 545:84–7.
100. Wade SW, Curthoys IS. The effect of ocular torsional position on perception of the roll-tilt of visual stimuli. *Vision Res* (1997) 37:1071–8. doi:10.1016/S0042-6989(96)00252-0
101. Merfeld DM, Zupan LH, Gifford CA. Neural processing of gravito-inertial cues in humans. II. Influence of the semicircular canals during eccentric rotation. *J Neurophysiol* (2001) 85:1648–60.
102. Seidman SH, Telford L, Paige GD. Tilt perception during dynamic linear acceleration. *Exp Brain Res* (1998) 119:307–14. doi:10.1007/s002210050346
103. Pavlou M, Wijnberg N, Faldon ME, Bronstein AM. Effect of semicircular canal stimulation on the perception of the visual vertical. *J Neurophysiol* (2003) 90:622–30. doi:10.1152/jn.00960.2002
104. Barnett-Cowan M, Harris LR. Perceived self-orientation in allocentric and egocentric space: effects of visual and physical tilt on saccadic and tactile measures. *Brain Res* (2008) 1242:231–43. doi:10.1016/j.brainres.2008.07.075
105. Dyde RT, Jenkin MR, Harris LR. The subjective visual vertical and the perceptual upright. *Exp Brain Res* (2006) 173:612–22. doi:10.1007/s00221-006-0405-y
106. Haji-Khamneh B, Harris LR. How different types of scenes affect the subjective visual vertical (SVV) and the perceptual upright (PU). *Vision Res* (2010) 50:1720–7. doi:10.1016/j.visres.2010.05.027
107. Hussain Ismail AM, Solomon JA, Hansard M, Mareschal I. A tilt after-effect for images of buildings: evidence of selectivity for the orientation of everyday scenes. *R Soc Open Sci* (2016) 3:160551. doi:10.1098/rsos.160551
108. Asch SE, Witkin HA. Studies in space orientation; perception of the upright with displaced visual fields. *J Exp Psychol* (1948) 38:325–37. doi:10.1037/h0054121
109. Cian C, Raphel C, Barraud PA. The role of cognitive factors in the rod-and-frame effect. *Perception* (2001) 30:1427–38. doi:10.1068/p3270
110. Dyde RT, Milner AD. Two illusions of perceived orientation: one fools all of the people some of the time; the other fools all of the people all of the time. *Exp Brain Res* (2002) 144:518–27. doi:10.1007/s00221-002-1065-1
111. Fiori F, David N, Aglioti SM. Processing of proprioceptive and vestibular body signals and self-transcendence in Ashtanga yoga practitioners. *Front Hum Neurosci* (2014) 8:734. doi:10.3389/fnhum.2014.00734
112. Groen EL, Jenkin HL, Howard IP. Perception of self-tilt in a true and illusory vertical plane. *Perception* (2002) 31:1477–90. doi:10.1068/p3330
113. Howard IP, Childerson L. The contribution of motion, the visual frame, and visual polarity to sensations of body tilt. *Perception* (1994) 23:753–62. doi:10.1068/p230753
114. Jenkin HL, Dyde RT, Jenkin MR, Howard IP, Harris LR. Relative role of visual and non-visual cues in determining the direction of "up": experiments in the York tilted room facility. *J Vestib Res* (2003) 13:287–93.
115. Kupferberg A, Glasauer S, Stein A, Brandt T. Influence of uninformative visual cues on gravity perception. *Ann N Y Acad Sci* (2009) 1164:403–5. doi:10.1111/j.1749-6632.2009.03851.x
116. Mittelstaedt H. The subjective vertical as a function of visual and extraretinal cues. *Acta Psychol (Amst)* (1986) 63:63–85. doi:10.1016/0001-6918(86)90043-0
117. Tomassini A, Solomon JA, Morgan MJ. Which way is down? Positional distortion in the tilt illusion. *PLoS One* (2014) 9:e110729. doi:10.1371/journal.pone.0110729
118. Vingerhoets RA, De Vrijer M, Van Gisbergen JAM, Medendorp WP. Fusion of visual and vestibular tilt cues in the perception of visual vertical. *J Neurophysiol* (2009) 101:1321–33. doi:10.1152/jn.90725.2008
119. Zoccolotti P, Antonucci G, Goodenough DR, Pizzamiglio L, Spinelli D. The role of frame size on vertical and horizontal observers in the rod-and-frame illusion. *Acta Psychol (Amst)* (1992) 79:171–87. doi:10.1016/0001-6918(92)90031-8
120. Bjasch D, Bockisch CJ, Straumann D, Tarnutzer AA. Differential effects of visual feedback on subjective visual vertical accuracy and precision. *PLoS One* (2012) 7:e49311. doi:10.1371/journal.pone.0049311
121. Li W, Matin L. Visually perceived vertical (VPV): induced changes in orientation by 1-line and 2-line roll-tilted and pitched visual fields. *Vision Res* (2005) 45:2037–57. doi:10.1016/j.visres.2005.01.014
122. Lubeck AJA, Bos JE, Stins JF. Framing visual roll-motion affects postural sway and the subjective visual vertical. *Atten Percept Psychophys* (2016) 78:2612–20. doi:10.3758/s13414-016-1150-3
123. Pavlou M, Quinn C, Murray K, Spyridakou C, Faldon M, Bronstein AM. The effect of repeated visual motion stimuli on visual dependence and postural control in normal subjects. *Gait Posture* (2011) 33:113–8. doi:10.1016/j.gaitpost.2010.10.085
124. Alberts BBGT, de Brouwer AJ, Selen LPJ, Medendorp WP. A Bayesian account of visual-vestibular interactions in the rod-and-frame task. *eNeuro* (2016) 3. doi:10.1523/ENEURO.0093-16.2016
125. Corbett JE, Enns JT. Observer pitch and roll influence: the rod and frame illusion. *Psychon Bull Rev* (2006) 13:160–5. doi:10.3758/BF03193828
126. Bury N, Bock O. Role of gravitational versus egocentric cues for human spatial orientation. *Exp Brain Res* (2016) 234:1013–8. doi:10.1007/s00221-015-4526-z
127. Guerraz M, Poquin D, Ohlmann T. The role of head-centric spatial reference with a static and kinetic visual disturbance. *Percept Psychophys* (1998) 60:287–95. doi:10.3758/BF03206037
128. Isableu B, Ohlmann T, Cremieux J, Amblard B. Selection of spatial frame of reference and postural control variability. *Exp Brain Res* (1997) 114:584–9. doi:10.1007/PL00005667
129. Isableu B, Gueguen M, Fourré B, Giraudet G, Amorim M-A. Assessment of visual field dependence: comparison between the mechanical 3D

rod-and-frame test developed by Oltman in 1968 with a 2D computer-based version. *J Vestib Res* (2008) 18:239–47.
130. Lopez C, Lacour M, Magnan J, Borel L. Visual field dependence-independence before and after unilateral vestibular loss. *Neuroreport* (2006) 17:797–803. doi:10.1097/01.wnr.0000221843.58373.c8
131. Dichgans J, Diener HC, Brandt T. Optokinetic-graviceptive interaction in different head positions. *Acta Otolaryngol* (1974) 78:391–8. doi:10.3109/00016487409126371
132. Ward BK, Bockisch CJ, Caramia N, Bertolini G, Tarnutzer AA. Gravity dependence of the effect of optokinetic stimulation on the subject visual vertical. *J Neurophysiol* (2017) 117:1948–58. doi:10.1152/jn.00303.2016
133. Dichgans J, Held R, Young LR, Brandt T. Moving visual scenes influence the apparent direction of gravity. *Science* (1972) 178:1217–9. doi:10.1126/science.178.4066.1217
134. Goto F, Kobayashi H, Saito A, Hayashi Y, Higashino K, Kunihiro T, et al. Compensatory changes in static and dynamic subjective visual vertical in patients following vestibular schwanoma surgery. *Auris Nasus Larynx* (2003) 30:29–33. doi:10.1016/S0385-8146(02)00110-4
135. Guerraz M, Yardley L, Bertholon P, Pollak L, Rudge P, Gresty MA, et al. Visual vertigo: symptom assessment, spatial orientation and postural control. *Brain* (2001) 124:1646–56. doi:10.1093/brain/124.8.1646
136. Clark TK, Newman MC, Oman CM, Merfeld DM, Young LR. Modeling human perception of orientation in altered gravity. *Front Syst Neurosci* (2015) 9:68. doi:10.3389/fnsys.2015.00068
137. Clément G, Eckardt J. Influence of the gravitational vertical on geometric visual illusions. *Acta Astronaut* (2005) 56:911–7. doi:10.1016/j.actaastro.2005.01.017
138. Jenkin HL, Jenkin MR, Dyde RT, Harris LR. Shape-from-shading depends on visual, gravitational, and body-orientation cues. *Perception* (2004) 33:1453–61. doi:10.1068/p5285
139. Lipshits M, Bengoetxea A, Cheron G, McIntyre J. Two reference frames for visual perception in two gravity conditions. *Perception* (2005) 34:545–55. doi:10.1068/p5358
140. Mast FW. Human perception of verticality: psychophysical experiments on the centrifuge and their neuronal implications. *Jpn Psychol Res* (2000) 42:194–206. doi:10.1111/1468-5884.00146
141. Mikellidou K, Cicchini GM, Thompson PG, Burr DC. The oblique effect is both allocentric and egocentric. *J Vis* (2015) 15:24. doi:10.1167/15.8.24
142. Graybiel A. Oculogravic illusion. *AMA Arch Ophthalmol* (1952) 48:605–15. doi:10.1001/archopht.1952.00920010616007
143. Graybiel A, Kellogg RS. Inversion illusion in parabolic flight: its probable dependence on otolith function. *Aerosp Med* (1967) 38:1099–103.
144. Lackner JR. Spatial orientation in weightless environments. *Perception* (1992) 21:803–12. doi:10.1068/p210803
145. Oman CM. Human visual orientation in weightlessness. In: Harris L, Jenkin M, editors. *Levels of Perception*. New York: Springer-Verlag (2003). p. 375–98.
146. Young LR, Oman CM, Watt DG, Money KE, Lichtenberg BK. Spatial orientation in weightlessness and readaptation to earth's gravity. *Science* (1984) 225:205–8. doi:10.1126/science.6610215
147. Akin FW, Murnane OD, Pearson A, Byrd S, Kelly KJ. Normative data for the subjective visual vertical test during centrifugation. *J Am Acad Audiol* (2011) 22:460–8. doi:10.3766/jaaa.22.7.6
148. Bortolami SB, Rocca S, Daros S, DiZio P, Lackner JR. Mechanisms of human static spatial orientation. *Exp Brain Res* (2006) 173:374–88. doi:10.1007/s00221-006-0387-9
149. Bryan AS, Bortolami SB, Ventura J, DiZio P, Lackner JR. Influence of gravitoinertial force level on the subjective vertical during recumbent yaw axis body tilt. *Exp Brain Res* (2007) 183:389–97. doi:10.1007/s00221-007-1058-1
150. Carriot J, DiZio P, Nougier V. Vertical frames of reference and control of body orientation. *Neurophysiol Clin* (2008) 38:423–37. doi:10.1016/j.neucli.2008.09.003
151. Clarke AH, Schönfeld U. Modification of unilateral otolith responses following spaceflight. *Exp Brain Res* (2015) 233:3613–24. doi:10.1007/s00221-015-4428-0
152. Clément G, Moore ST, Raphan T, Cohen B. Perception of tilt (somatogravic illusion) in response to sustained linear acceleration during space flight. *Exp Brain Res* (2001) 138:410–8. doi:10.1007/s002210100706
153. Janky KL, Shepard NT. Unilateral centrifugation: utricular assessment and protocol comparison. *Otol Neurotol* (2011) 32:116–21. doi:10.1097/MAO.0b013e3181ff7549
154. Krafczyk S, Knapek M, Philipp J, Querner V, Dieterich M. Optokinetic stimulation in microgravity: torsional eye movements and subjective visual vertical. *Aviat Space Environ Med* (2003) 74:517–21.
155. de Winkel KN, Clément G, Groen EL, Werkhoven PJ. The perception of verticality in lunar and Martian gravity conditions. *Neurosci Lett* (2012) 529:7–11. doi:10.1016/j.neulet.2012.09.026
156. Harris LR, Herpers R, Hofhammer T, Jenkin M. How much gravity is needed to establish the perceptual upright? *PLoS One* (2014) 9:e106207. doi:10.1371/journal.pone.0106207
157. Tarnutzer AA, Bertolini G, Bockisch CJ, Straumann D, Marti S. Modulation of internal estimates of gravity during and after prolonged roll-tilts. *PLoS One* (2013) 8:e78079. doi:10.1371/journal.pone.0078079
158. Wade NJ. Effect of prolonged tilt on visual orientation. *Q J Exp Psychol* (1970) 22:423–39. doi:10.1080/14640747008401916
159. Gosselin G, Fagan MJ. Effects of cervical muscle fatigue on the perception of the subjective vertical and horizontal. *Springerplus* (2014) 3:78. doi:10.1186/2193-1801-3-78
160. Wade NJ, Day RH. Apparent head position as a basis for a visual aftereffect of prolonged head tilt. *Percept Psychophys* (1968) 3:324–6. doi:10.3758/BF03212477
161. Wade NJ, Day RH. Development and dissipation of a visual spatial aftereffect from prolonged head tilt. *J Exp Psychol* (1968) 76:439–43. doi:10.1037/h0025486
162. Tarnutzer AA, Bockisch CJ, Straumann D, Marti S, Bertolini G. Static roll-tilt over five minutes locally distorts the internal estimate of direction of gravity. *J Neurophysiol* (2014) 112:2672–9. doi:10.1152/jn.00540.2014
163. Day RH, Wade NJ. Involvement of neck proprioceptive system in visual after-effect from prolonged head tilt. *Q J Exp Psychol* (1968) 20:290–3. doi:10.1080/14640746808400163
164. Duque-Parra JE. Perspective on the vestibular cortex throughout history. *Anat Rec B New Anat* (2004) 280:15–9. doi:10.1002/ar.b.20031
165. Lopez C, Blanke O. The thalamocortical vestibular system in animals and humans. *Brain Res Rev* (2011) 67:119–46. doi:10.1016/j.brainresrev.2010.12.002
166. Chen A, DeAngelis GC, Angelaki DE. Macaque parieto-insular vestibular cortex: responses to self-motion and optic flow. *J Neurosci* (2010) 30:3022–42. doi:10.1523/JNEUROSCI.4029-09.2010
167. Guldin WO, Grüsser OJ. Is there a vestibular cortex? *Trends Neurosci* (1998) 21:254–9. doi:10.1016/S0166-2236(97)01211-3
168. Chen A, Gu Y, Takahashi K, Angelaki DE, Deangelis GC. Clustering of self-motion selectivity and visual response properties in macaque area MSTd. *J Neurophysiol* (2008) 100:2669–83. doi:10.1152/jn.90705.2008
169. Chen A, DeAngelis GC, Angelaki DE. Convergence of vestibular and visual self-motion signals in an area of the posterior Sylvian fissure. *J Neurosci* (2011) 31:11617–27. doi:10.1523/JNEUROSCI.1266-11.2011
170. Chen X, DeAngelis GC, Angelaki DE. Diverse spatial reference frames of vestibular signals in parietal cortex. *Neuron* (2013) 80:1310–21. doi:10.1016/j.neuron.2013.09.006
171. Chen A, Deangelis GC, Angelaki DE. Functional specializations of the ventral intraparietal area for multisensory heading discrimination. *J Neurosci* (2013) 33:3567–81. doi:10.1523/JNEUROSCI.4522-12.2013
172. Rosenberg A, Angelaki DE. Gravity influences the visual representation of object tilt in parietal cortex. *J Neurosci* (2014) 34:14170–80. doi:10.1523/JNEUROSCI.2030-14.2014
173. Vaziri S, Connor CE. Representation of gravity-aligned scene structure in ventral pathway visual cortex. *Curr Biol* (2016) 26:766–74. doi:10.1016/j.cub.2016.01.022
174. Avillac M, Denève S, Olivier E, Pouget A, Duhamel J-R. Reference frames for representing visual and tactile locations in parietal cortex. *Nat Neurosci* (2005) 8:941–9. doi:10.1038/nn1480
175. Deneve S, Latham PE, Pouget A. Efficient computation and cue integration with noisy population codes. *Nat Neurosci* (2001) 4:826–31. doi:10.1038/90541
176. Fetsch CR, Wang S, Gu Y, DeAngelis GC, Angelaki DE. Spatial reference frames of visual, vestibular, and multimodal heading signals in the dorsal subdivision of the medial superior temporal area. *J Neurosci* (2007) 27:700–12. doi:10.1523/JNEUROSCI.3553-06.2007

177. Bense S, Stephan T, Yousry TA, Brandt T, Dieterich M. Multisensory cortical signal increases and decreases during vestibular galvanic stimulation (fMRI). *J Neurophysiol* (2001) 85:886–99.
178. Bottini G, Karnath HO, Vallar G, Sterzi R, Frith CD, Frackowiak RS, et al. Cerebral representations for egocentric space: functional-anatomical evidence from caloric vestibular stimulation and neck vibration. *Brain* (2001) 124:1182–96. doi:10.1093/brain/124.6.1182
179. Dieterich M, Bense S, Lutz S, Drzezga A, Stephan T, Bartenstein P, et al. Dominance for vestibular cortical function in the non-dominant hemisphere. *Cereb Cortex* (2003) 13:994–1007. doi:10.1093/cercor/13.9.994
180. Eickhoff SB, Weiss PH, Amunts K, Fink GR, Zilles K. Identifying human parieto-insular vestibular cortex using fMRI and cytoarchitectonic mapping. *Hum Brain Mapp* (2006) 27:611–21. doi:10.1002/hbm.20205
181. Emri M, Kisely M, Lengyel Z, Balkay L, Márián T, Mikó L, et al. Cortical projection of peripheral vestibular signaling. *J Neurophysiol* (2003) 89:2639–46. doi:10.1152/jn.00599.2002
182. Fasold O, von Brevern M, Kuhberg M, Ploner CJ, Villringer A, Lempert T, et al. Human vestibular cortex as identified with caloric stimulation in functional magnetic resonance imaging. *Neuroimage* (2002) 17:1384–93. doi:10.1006/nimg.2002.1241
183. Fink GR, Marshall JC, Weiss PH, Stephan T, Grefkes C, Shah NJ, et al. Performing allocentric visuospatial judgments with induced distortion of the egocentric reference frame: an fMRI study with clinical implications. *Neuroimage* (2003) 20:1505–17. doi:10.1016/j.neuroimage.2003.07.006
184. Friberg L, Olsen TS, Roland PE, Paulson OB, Lassen NA. Focal increase of blood flow in the cerebral cortex of man during vestibular stimulation. *Brain* (1985) 108(Pt 3):609–23. doi:10.1093/brain/108.3.609
185. Janzen J, Schlindwein P, Bense S, Bauermann T, Vucurevic G, Stoeter P, et al. Neural correlates of hemispheric dominance and ipsilaterality within the vestibular system. *Neuroimage* (2008) 42:1508–18. doi:10.1016/j.neuroimage.2008.06.026
186. Kaski D, Quadir S, Nigmatullina Y, Malhotra PA, Bronstein AM, Seemungal BM. Temporoparietal encoding of space and time during vestibular-guided orientation. *Brain* (2016) 139:392–403. doi:10.1093/brain/awv370
187. Lacquaniti F, Bosco G, Indovina I, La Scaleia B, Maffei V, Moscatelli A, et al. Visual gravitational motion and the vestibular system in humans. *Front Integr Neurosci* (2013) 7:101. doi:10.3389/fnint.2013.00101
188. Lobel E, Kleine JF, Le Bihan D, Leroy-Willig A, Berthoz A. Functional MRI of galvanic vestibular stimulation. *J Neurophysiol* (1998) 80:2699–709.
189. Miyamoto T, Fukushima K, Takada T, de Waele C, Vidal P-P. Saccular stimulation of the human cortex: a functional magnetic resonance imaging study. *Neurosci Lett* (2007) 423:68–72. doi:10.1016/j.neulet.2007.06.036
190. Petit L, Beauchamp MS. Neural basis of visually guided head movements studied with fMRI. *J Neurophysiol* (2003) 89:2516–27. doi:10.1152/jn.00988.2002
191. Roberts RE, Ahmad H, Arshad Q, Patel M, Dima D, Leech R, et al. Functional neuroimaging of visuo-vestibular interaction. *Brain Struct Funct* (2017) 222:2329–43. doi:10.1007/s00429-016-1344-4
192. Schlindwein P, Mueller M, Bauermann T, Brandt T, Stoeter P, Dieterich M. Cortical representation of saccular vestibular stimulation: VEMPs in fMRI. *Neuroimage* (2008) 39:19–31. doi:10.1016/j.neuroimage.2007.08.016
193. Stephan T, Deutschländer A, Nolte A, Schneider E, Wiesmann M, Brandt T, et al. Functional MRI of galvanic vestibular stimulation with alternating currents at different frequencies. *Neuroimage* (2005) 26:721–32. doi:10.1016/j.neuroimage.2005.02.049
194. Suzuki M, Kitano H, Ito R, Kitanishi T, Yazawa Y, Ogawa T, et al. Cortical and subcortical vestibular response to caloric stimulation detected by functional magnetic resonance imaging. *Brain Res Cogn Brain Res* (2001) 12:441–9. doi:10.1016/S0926-6410(01)00080-5
195. Vallar G, Lobel E, Galati G, Berthoz A, Pizzamiglio L, Le Bihan D. A fronto-parietal system for computing the egocentric spatial frame of reference in humans. *Exp Brain Res* (1999) 124:281–6. doi:10.1007/s002210050624
196. zu Eulenburg P, Caspers S, Roski C, Eickhoff SB. Meta-analytical definition and functional connectivity of the human vestibular cortex. *Neuroimage* (2012) 60:162–9. doi:10.1016/j.neuroimage.2011.12.032
197. Arshad Q, Nigmatullina Y, Bronstein AM. Handedness-related cortical modulation of the vestibular-ocular reflex. *J Neurosci* (2013) 33:3221–7. doi:10.1523/JNEUROSCI.2054-12.2013
198. Guerraz M, Bronstein AM. Mechanisms underlying visually induced body sway. *Neurosci Lett* (2008) 443:12–6. doi:10.1016/j.neulet.2008.07.053
199. Nigmatullina Y, Hellyer PJ, Nachev P, Sharp DJ, Seemungal BM. The neuroanatomical correlates of training-related perceptuo-reflex uncoupling in dancers. *Cereb Cortex* (2013) 25:554–62. doi:10.1093/cercor/bht266
200. Dieterich M, Kirsch V, Brandt T. Right-sided dominance of the bilateral vestibular system in the upper brainstem and thalamus. *J Neurol* (2017) 264:55–62. doi:10.1007/s00415-017-8453-8
201. Kirsch V, Keeser D, Hergenroeder T, Erat O, Ertl-Wagner B, Brandt T, et al. Structural and functional connectivity mapping of the vestibular circuitry from human brainstem to cortex. *Brain Struct Funct* (2016) 221:1291–308. doi:10.1007/s00429-014-0971-x
202. Blanke O, Slater M, Serino A. Behavioral, neural, and computational principles of bodily self-consciousness. *Neuron* (2015) 88:145–66. doi:10.1016/j.neuron.2015.09.029
203. Bosco G, Carrozzo M, Lacquaniti F. Contributions of the human temporoparietal junction and MT/V5+ to the timing of interception revealed by transcranial magnetic stimulation. *J Neurosci* (2008) 28:12071–84. doi:10.1523/JNEUROSCI.2869-08.2008
204. Cazzato V, Mian E, Serino A, Mele S, Urgesi C. Distinct contributions of extrastriate body area and temporoparietal junction in perceiving one's own and others' body. *Cogn Affect Behav Neurosci* (2015) 15:211–28. doi:10.3758/s13415-014-0312-9
205. Donaldson PH, Rinehart NJ, Enticott PG. Noninvasive stimulation of the temporoparietal junction: a systematic review. *Neurosci Biobehav Rev* (2015) 55:547–72. doi:10.1016/j.neubiorev.2015.05.017
206. Hansen KA, Chu C, Dickinson A, Pye B, Weller JP, Ungerleider LG. Spatial selectivity in the temporoparietal junction, inferior frontal sulcus, and inferior parietal lobule. *J Vis* (2015) 15:15. doi:10.1167/15.13.15
207. Igelström KM, Graziano MSA. The inferior parietal lobule and temporoparietal junction: a network perspective. *Neuropsychologia* (2017). doi:10.1016/j.neuropsychologia.2017.01.001
208. Indovina I, Maffei V, Bosco G, Zago M, Macaluso E, Lacquaniti F. Representation of visual gravitational motion in the human vestibular cortex. *Science* (2005) 308:416–9. doi:10.1126/science.1107961
209. Jáuregui Renaud K. Vestibular function and depersonalization/derealization symptoms. *Multisens Res* (2015) 28:637–51. doi:10.1163/22134808-00002480
210. Lopez C, Halje P, Blanke O. Body ownership and embodiment: vestibular and multisensory mechanisms. *Neurophysiol Clin* (2008) 38:149–61. doi:10.1016/j.neucli.2007.12.006
211. Saj A, Cojan Y, Musel B, Honoré J, Borel L, Vuilleumier P. Functional neuro-anatomy of egocentric versus allocentric space representation. *Neurophysiol Clin* (2014) 44:33–40. doi:10.1016/j.neucli.2013.10.135
212. Silani G, Lamm C, Ruff CC, Singer T. Right supramarginal gyrus is crucial to overcome emotional egocentricity bias in social judgments. *J Neurosci* (2013) 33:15466–76. doi:10.1523/JNEUROSCI.1488-13.2013
213. Ventre-Dominey J. Vestibular function in the temporal and parietal cortex: distinct velocity and inertial processing pathways. *Front Integr Neurosci* (2014) 8:53. doi:10.3389/fnint.2014.00053
214. Braem B, Honoré J, Rousseaux M, Saj A, Coello Y. Integration of visual and haptic informations in the perception of the vertical in young and old healthy adults and right brain-damaged patients. *Neurophysiol Clin* (2014) 44:41–8. doi:10.1016/j.neucli.2013.10.137
215. De Renzi E, Faglioni P, Scotti G. Judgment of spatial orientation in patients with focal brain damage. *J Neurol Neurosurg Psychiatry* (1971) 34:489–95. doi:10.1136/jnnp.34.5.489
216. Funk J, Finke K, Müller HJ, Utz KS, Kerkhoff G. Visual context modulates the subjective vertical in neglect: evidence for an increased rod-and-frame-effect. *Neuroscience* (2011) 173:124–34. doi:10.1016/j.neuroscience.2010.10.067
217. Gentaz E, Badan M, Luyat M, Touil N. The manual haptic perception of orientations and the oblique effect in patients with left visuo-spatial neglect. *Neuroreport* (2002) 13:327–31. doi:10.1097/00001756-200203040-00016
218. Karnath H-O, Dieterich M. Spatial neglect – a vestibular disorder? *Brain* (2006) 129:293–305. doi:10.1093/brain/awh698
219. Karnath H-O, Rorden C. The anatomy of spatial neglect. *Neuropsychologia* (2012) 50:1010–7. doi:10.1016/j.neuropsychologia.2011.06.027
220. Kerkhoff G. Multimodal spatial orientation deficits in left-sided visual neglect. *Neuropsychologia* (1999) 37:1387–405. doi:10.1016/S0028-3932(99)00031-7

221. Kerkhoff G, Zoelch C. Disorders of visuospatial orientation in the frontal plane in patients with visual neglect following right or left parietal lesions. *Exp Brain Res* (1998) 122:108–20. doi:10.1007/s002210050497
222. Saj A, Honore J, Bernati T, Coello Y, Rousseaux M. Subjective visual vertical in pitch and roll in right hemispheric stroke. *Stroke* (2005) 36:588–91. doi:10.1161/01.STR.0000155740.44599.48
223. Utz KS, Keller I, Artinger F, Stumpf O, Funk J, Kerkhoff G. Multimodal and multispatial deficits of verticality perception in hemispatial neglect. *Neuroscience* (2011) 188:68–79. doi:10.1016/j.neuroscience.2011.04.068
224. Funk J, Finke K, Müller HJ, Utz KS, Kerkhoff G. Effects of lateral head inclination on multimodal spatial orientation judgments in neglect: evidence for impaired spatial orientation constancy. *Neuropsychologia* (2010) 48:1616–27. doi:10.1016/j.neuropsychologia.2010.01.029
225. Funk J, Finke K, Müller HJ, Preger R, Kerkhoff G. Systematic biases in the tactile perception of the subjective vertical in patients with unilateral neglect and the influence of upright vs. supine posture. *Neuropsychologia* (2010) 48:298–308. doi:10.1016/j.neuropsychologia.2009.09.018
226. Rousseaux M, Honoré J, Vuilleumier P, Saj A. Neuroanatomy of space, body, and posture perception in patients with right hemisphere stroke. *Neurology* (2013) 81:1291–7. doi:10.1212/WNL.0b013e3182a823a7
227. Saj A, Honoré J, Davroux J, Coello Y, Rousseaux M. Effect of posture on the perception of verticality in neglect patients. *Stroke* (2005) 36:2203–5. doi:10.1161/01.STR.0000182236.73502.19
228. Yelnik AP, Lebreton FO, Bonan IV, Colle FMC, Meurin FA, Guichard JP, et al. Perception of verticality after recent cerebral hemispheric stroke. *Stroke* (2002) 33:2247–53. doi:10.1161/01.STR.0000027212.26686.48
229. Cazzoli D, Müri RM, Hess CW, Nyffeler T. Horizontal and vertical dimensions of visual extinction: a theta burst stimulation study. *Neuroscience* (2009) 164:1609–14. doi:10.1016/j.neuroscience.2009.09.044
230. Arzy S, Thut G, Mohr C, Michel CM, Blanke O. Neural basis of embodiment: distinct contributions of temporoparietal junction and extrastriate body area. *J Neurosci* (2006) 26:8074–81. doi:10.1523/JNEUROSCI.0745-06.2006
231. Ionta S, Heydrich L, Lenggenhager B, Mouthon M, Fornari E, Chapuis D, et al. Multisensory mechanisms in temporo-parietal cortex support self-location and first-person perspective. *Neuron* (2011) 70:363–74. doi:10.1016/j.neuron.2011.03.009
232. Tsakiris M, Costantini M, Haggard P. The role of the right temporo-parietal junction in maintaining a coherent sense of one's body. *Neuropsychologia* (2008) 46:3014–8. doi:10.1016/j.neuropsychologia.2008.06.004
233. Blanke O, Ortigue S, Landis T, Seeck M. Neuropsychology: stimulating illusory own-body perceptions. *Nature* (2002) 419:269–70. doi:10.1038/419269a
234. Blanke O, Landis T, Spinelli L, Seeck M. Out-of-body experience and autoscopy of neurological origin. *Brain* (2004) 127:243–58. doi:10.1093/brain/awh040
235. Brandt T, Strupp M, Dieterich M. Towards a concept of disorders of "higher vestibular function". *Front Integr Neurosci* (2014) 8:47. doi:10.3389/fnint.2014.00047
236. De Ridder D, Van Laere K, Dupont P, Menovsky T, Van de Heyning P. Visualizing out-of-body experience in the brain. *N Engl J Med* (2007) 357:1829–33. doi:10.1056/NEJMoa070010
237. Bender M, Jung R. Abweichungen der subjektiven optischen Vertikalen und Horizontalen bei Gesunden und Hirnverletzten. *Eur Arch Psychiatry Clin Neurosci* (1948) 181:193–212.
238. Brandt T, Dieterich M, Danek A. Vestibular cortex lesions affect the perception of verticality. *Ann Neurol* (1994) 35:403–12. doi:10.1002/ana.410350406
239. Baier B, Suchan J, Karnath H-O, Dieterich M. Neural correlates of disturbed perception of verticality. *Neurology* (2012) 78:728–35. doi:10.1212/WNL.0b013e318248e544
240. Baier B, zu Eulenburg P, Best C, Geber C, Müller-Forell W, Birklein F, et al. Posterior insular cortex – a site of vestibular–somatosensory interaction? *Brain Behav* (2013) 3:519–24. doi:10.1002/brb3.155
241. Piscicelli C, Barra J, Davoine P, Chrispin A, Nadeau S, Pérennou D. Inter- and intra-rater reliability of the visual vertical in subacute stroke. *Stroke* (2015) 46:1979–83. doi:10.1161/STROKEAHA.115.009610
242. Rousseaux M, Braem B, Honoré J, Saj A. An anatomical and psychophysical comparison of subjective verticals in patients with right brain damage. *Cortex* (2015) 69:60–7. doi:10.1016/j.cortex.2015.04.004
243. Baier B, Conrad J, Zu Eulenburg P, Best C, Müller-Forell W, Birklein F, et al. Insular strokes cause no vestibular deficits. *Stroke* (2013) 44:2604–6. doi:10.1161/STROKEAHA.113.001816
244. Barra J, Benaim C, Chauvineau V, Ohlmann T, Gresty M, Perennou D. Are rotations in perceived visual vertical and body axis after stroke caused by the same mechanism? *Stroke* (2008) 39:3099–101. doi:10.1161/STROKEAHA.108.515247
245. Bonan IV, Leman MC, Legargasson JF, Guichard JP, Yelnik AP. Evolution of subjective visual vertical perturbation after stroke. *Neurorehabil Neural Repair* (2006) 20:484–91. doi:10.1177/1545968306289295
246. Friedmann G. The judgement of the visual vertical and horizontal with peripheral and central vestibular lesions. *Brain* (1970) 93:313–28. doi:10.1093/brain/93.2.313
247. Perennou DA, Mazibrada G, Chauvineau V, Greenwood R, Rothwell J, Gresty MA, et al. Lateropulsion, pushing and verticality perception in hemisphere stroke: a causal relationship? *Brain* (2008) 131:2401–13. doi:10.1093/brain/awn170
248. Piscicelli C, Nadeau S, Barra J, Pérennou D. Assessing the visual vertical: how many trials are required? *BMC Neurol* (2015) 15:215. doi:10.1186/s12883-015-0462-6
249. Brandt T, Dieterich M. Vestibular syndromes in the roll plane: topographic diagnosis from brainstem to cortex. *Ann Neurol* (1994) 36:337–47. doi:10.1002/ana.410360304
250. Brandt T, Dieterich M. Perceived vertical and lateropulsion: clinical syndromes, localization, and prognosis. *Neurorehabil Neural Repair* (2000) 14:1–12. doi:10.1177/154596830001400101
251. Dieterich M, Brandt T. Ocular torsion and tilt of subjective visual vertical are sensitive brainstem signs. *Ann Neurol* (1993) 33:292–9. doi:10.1002/ana.410330311
252. Hafström A, Fransson P-A, Karlberg M, Magnusson M. Idiosyncratic compensation of the subjective visual horizontal and vertical in 60 patients after unilateral vestibular deafferentation. *Acta Otolaryngol* (2004) 124:165–71. doi:10.1080/00016480410016630
253. Karnath H-O, Ferber S, Dichgans J. The origin of contraversive pushing evidence for a second graviceptive system in humans. *Neurology* (2000) 55:1298–304. doi:10.1212/WNL.55.9.1298
254. Saeys W, Vereeck L, Truijen S, Lafosse C, Wuyts FP, Van de Heyning P. Influence of sensory loss on the perception of verticality in stroke patients. *Disabil Rehabil* (2012) 34:1965–70. doi:10.3109/09638288.2012.671883
255. Barra J, Chauvineau V, Ohlmann T, Gresty M, Perennou D. Perception of longitudinal body axis in patients with stroke: a pilot study. *J Neurol Neurosurg Psychiatry* (2007) 78:43–8. doi:10.1136/jnnp.2006.089961
256. Kheradmand A, Lasker A, Zee DS. Transcranial magnetic stimulation (TMS) of the supramarginal gyrus: a window to perception of upright. *Cereb Cortex* (2015) 25:765–71. doi:10.1093/cercor/bht267
257. Fiori F, Candidi M, Acciarino A, David N, Aglioti SM. The right temporoparietal junction plays a causal role in maintaining the internal representation of verticality. *J Neurophysiol* (2015) 114:2983–90. doi:10.1152/jn.00289.2015
258. Santos-Pontelli TEG, Rimoli BP, Favoretto DB, Mazin SC, Truong DQ, Leite JP, et al. Polarity-dependent misperception of subjective visual vertical during and after transcranial direct current stimulation (tDCS). *PLoS One* (2016) 11:e0152331. doi:10.1371/journal.pone.0152331
259. Lester BD, Dassonville P. The role of the right superior parietal lobule in processing visual context for the establishment of the egocentric reference frame. *J Cogn Neurosci* (2014) 26:2201–9. doi:10.1162/jocn_a_00636
260. Otero-Millan J, Winnick A, Kheradmand A. Transcranial magnetic stimulation of supramarginal gyrus alters perception of upright without changing ocular torsion. *Soc Neurosci* (2016).
261. Corbett JE, Enns JT, Handy TC. Electrophysiological evidence for a post-perceptual influence of global visual context on perceived orientation. *Brain Res* (2009) 1292:82–92. doi:10.1016/j.brainres.2009.07.038
262. Lopez C, Mercier MR, Halje P, Blanke O. Spatiotemporal dynamics of visual vertical judgments: early and late brain mechanisms as revealed by high-density electrical neuroimaging. *Neuroscience* (2011) 181:134–49. doi:10.1016/j.neuroscience.2011.02.009
263. Baggio JAO, Mazin SSC, Alessio-Alves FF, Barros CGC, Carneiro AAO, Leite JP, et al. Verticality perceptions associate with postural control and

functionality in stroke patients. *PLoS One* (2016) 11:e0150754. doi:10.1371/journal.pone.0150754

264. Baier B, Thomke F, Wilting J, Heinze C, Geber C, Dieterich M. A pathway in the brainstem for roll-tilt of the subjective visual vertical: evidence from a lesion-behavior mapping study. *J Neurosci* (2012) 32:14854–8. doi:10.1523/JNEUROSCI.0770-12.2012
265. Bjerver K, Silfverskiöld BP. Lateropulsion and imbalance in Wallenberg's syndrome. *Acta Neurol Scand* (1968) 44:91–100. doi:10.1111/j.1600-0404.1968.tb07446.x
266. Bohannon RW. Ipsilateral pushing in stroke. *Arch Phys Med Rehabil* (1996) 77:524. doi:10.1016/S0003-9993(96)90050-7
267. Bonan IV, Guettard E, Leman MC, Colle FM, Yelnik AP. Subjective visual vertical perception relates to balance in acute stroke. *Arch Phys Med Rehabil* (2006) 87:642–6. doi:10.1016/j.apmr.2006.01.019
268. Bronstein AM, Pérennou DA, Guerraz M, Playford D, Rudge P. Dissociation of visual and haptic vertical in two patients with vestibular nuclear lesions. *Neurology* (2003) 61:1260–2. doi:10.1212/01.WNL.0000086815.22816.DC
269. Cereda C, Ghika J, Maeder P, Bogousslavsky J. Strokes restricted to the insular cortex. *Neurology* (2002) 59:1950–5. doi:10.1212/01.WNL.0000038905.75660.BD
270. Danells CJ, Black SE, Gladstone DJ, McIlroy WE. Poststroke "pushing". *Stroke* (2004) 35:2873–8. doi:10.1161/01.STR.0000147724.83468.18
271. Darling WG, Pizzimenti MA, Rizzo M. Unilateral posterior parietal lobe lesions affect representation of visual space. *Vision Res* (2003) 43:1675–88. doi:10.1016/S0042-6989(03)00179-2
272. Dieterich M, Brandt T. Wallenberg's syndrome: lateropulsion, cyclorotation, and subjective visual vertical in thirty-six patients. *Ann Neurol* (1992) 31:399–408. doi:10.1002/ana.410310409
273. Dieterich M, Brandt T. Why acute unilateral vestibular cortex lesions mostly manifest without vertigo. *Neurology* (2015) 84:1680–4. doi:10.1212/WNL.0000000000001501
274. Johannsen L, Broetz D, Naegele T, Karnath H-O. "Pusher syndrome" following cortical lesions that spare the thalamus. *J Neurol* (2006) 253:455–63. doi:10.1007/s00415-005-0025-7
275. Mansfield A, Fraser L, Rajachandrakumar R, Danells CJ, Knorr S, Campos J. Is perception of vertical impaired in individuals with chronic stroke with a history of "pushing"? *Neurosci Lett* (2015) 590:172–7. doi:10.1016/j.neulet.2015.02.007
276. Oppenländer K, Utz KS, Reinhart S, Keller I, Kerkhoff G, Schaadt A-K. Subliminal galvanic-vestibular stimulation recalibrates the distorted visual and tactile subjective vertical in right-sided stroke. *Neuropsychologia* (2015) 74:178–83. doi:10.1016/j.neuropsychologia.2015.03.004
277. Paci M, Matulli G, Megna N, Baccini M, Baldassi S. The subjective visual vertical in patients with pusher behaviour: a pilot study with a psychophysical approach. *Neuropsychol Rehabil* (2011) 21:539–51. doi:10.1080/09602011.2011.583777
278. Pedersen PM, Wandel A, Jørgensen HS, Nakayama H, Raaschou HO, Olsen TS. Ipsilateral pushing in stroke: incidence, relation to neuropsychological symptoms, and impact on rehabilitation. The Copenhagen stroke study. *Arch Phys Med Rehabil* (1996) 77:25–8. doi:10.1016/S0003-9993(96)90215-4
279. Pérennou D. Postural disorders and spatial neglect in stroke patients: a strong association. *Restor Neurol Neurosci* (2006) 24:319–34.
280. Pérennou DA, Amblard B, Leblond C, Pélissier J. Biased postural vertical in humans with hemispheric cerebral lesions. *Neurosci Lett* (1998) 252:75–8. doi:10.1016/S0304-3940(98)00501-1
281. Pérennou D, Piscicelli C, Barbieri G, Jaeger M, Marquer A, Barra J. Measuring verticality perception after stroke: why and how? *Neurophysiol Clin* (2014) 44:25–32. doi:10.1016/j.neucli.2013.10.131
282. Piscicelli C, Pérennou D. Visual verticality perception after stroke: a systematic review of methodological approaches and suggestions for standardization. *Ann Phys Rehabil Med* (2017) 60:208–16. doi:10.1016/j.rehab.2016.02.004
283. Stone SP, Halligan PW, Greenwood RJ. The incidence of neglect phenomena and related disorders in patients with an acute right or left hemisphere stroke. *Age Ageing* (1993) 22:46–52. doi:10.1093/ageing/22.1.46
284. Thömke F, Marx JJ, Iannetti GD, Cruccu G, Fitzek S, Urban PP, et al. A topodiagnostic investigation on body lateropulsion in medullary infarcts. *Neurology* (2005) 64:716–8. doi:10.1212/01.WNL.0000152040.27264.1A
285. Yang T-H, Oh S-Y, Kwak K, Lee J-M, Shin B-S, Jeong S-K. Topology of brainstem lesions associated with subjective visual vertical tilt. *Neurology* (2014) 82:1968–75. doi:10.1212/WNL.0000000000000480
286. Bonan IV, Hubeaux K, Gellez-Leman MC, Guichard JP, Vicaut E, Yelnik AP. Influence of subjective visual vertical misperception on balance recovery after stroke. *J Neurol Neurosurg Psychiatry* (2007) 78:49–55. doi:10.1136/jnnp.2006.087791
287. Saj A, Honore J, Rousseaux M. Perception of the vertical in patients with right hemispheric lesion: effect of galvanic vestibular stimulation. *Neuropsychologia* (2006) 44:1509–12. doi:10.1016/j.neuropsychologia.2005.11.018
288. Abe H, Kondo T, Oouchida Y, Suzukamo Y, Fujiwara S, Izumi S-I. Prevalence and length of recovery of pusher syndrome based on cerebral hemispheric lesion side in patients with acute stroke. *Stroke* (2012) 43:1654–6. doi:10.1161/STROKEAHA.111.638379
289. Santos-Pontelli TEG, Pontes-Neto OM, de Araujo DB, Santos AC, Leite JP. Persistent pusher behavior after a stroke. *Clinics (Sao Paulo)* (2011) 66:2169–71. doi:10.1590/S1807-59322011001200025
290. Barra J, Oujamaa L, Chauvineau V, Rougier P, Pérennou D. Asymmetric standing posture after stroke is related to a biased egocentric coordinate system. *Neurology* (2009) 72:1582–7. doi:10.1212/WNL.0b013e3181a4123a
291. Lafosse C, Kerckhofs E, Troch M, Santens P, Vandenbussche E. Graviceptive misperception of the postural vertical after right hemisphere damage. *Neuroreport* (2004) 15:887–91. doi:10.1097/00001756-200404090-00031
292. Miyai I, Mauricio RLR, Reding MJ. Parietal-insular strokes are associated with impaired standing balance as assessed by computerized dynamic posturography. *J Neurol Rehabil* (1997) 11:35–40. doi:10.1177/154596839701100106
293. Pérennou DA, Leblond C, Amblard B, Micallef JP, Rouget E, Pélissier J. The polymodal sensory cortex is crucial for controlling lateral postural stability: evidence from stroke patients. *Brain Res Bull* (2000) 53:359–65. doi:10.1016/S0361-9230(00)00360-9
294. Saj A, Honoré J, Coello Y, Rousseaux M. The visual vertical in the pusher syndrome: influence of hemispace and body position. *J Neurol* (2005) 252:885–91. doi:10.1007/s00415-005-0716-0
295. Beevor CE. Remarks on paralysis of the movements of the trunk in hemiplegia, and the muscles which are affected. *Br Med J* (1909) 1:881. doi:10.1136/bmj.1.2519.881
296. Johannsen L, Fruhmann Berger M, Karnath H-O. Subjective visual vertical (SVV) determined in a representative sample of 15 patients with pusher syndrome. *J Neurol* (2006) 253:1367–9. doi:10.1007/s00415-006-0216-x
297. Karnath H-O, Broetz D. Understanding and treating "pusher syndrome". *Phys Ther* (2003) 83:1119–25.
298. Paci M, Baccini M, Rinaldi LA. Pusher behaviour: a critical review of controversial issues. *Disabil Rehabil* (2009) 31:249–58. doi:10.1080/09638280801928002
299. Pérennou DA, Amblard B, Laassel EM, Benaim C, Hérisson C, Pélissier J. Understanding the pusher behavior of some stroke patients with spatial deficits: a pilot study. *Arch Phys Med Rehabil* (2002) 83:570–5. doi:10.1053/apmr.2002.31198
300. Punt TD, Riddoch MJ. Towards a theoretical understanding of pushing behaviour in stroke patients. *Neuropsychol Rehabil* (2002) 12:455–72. doi:10.1080/09602010244000246
301. Baier B, Janzen J, Müller-Forell W, Fechir M, Müller N, Dieterich M. Pusher syndrome: its cortical correlate. *J Neurol* (2012) 259:277–83. doi:10.1007/s00415-011-6173-z
302. Lafosse C, Kerckhofs E, Vereeck L, Troch M, Van Hoydonck G, Moeremans M, et al. Postural abnormalities and contraversive pushing following right hemisphere brain damage. *Neuropsychol Rehabil* (2007) 17:374–96. doi:10.1080/09602010601058854
303. Bergmann J, Krewer C, Selge C, Müller F, Jahn K. The subjective postural vertical determined in patients with pusher behavior during standing. *Top Stroke Rehabil* (2016) 23:184–90. doi:10.1080/10749357.2015.1135591
304. Colnat-Coulbois S, Gauchard GC, Maillard L, Barroche G, Vespignani H, Auque J, et al. Management of postural sensory conflict and dynamic balance control in late-stage Parkinson's disease. *Neuroscience* (2011) 193:363–9. doi:10.1016/j.neuroscience.2011.04.043
305. Rossi M, Soto A, Santos S, Sesar A, Labella T. A prospective study of alterations in balance among patients with Parkinson's disease. *Eur Neurol* (2009) 61:171–6. doi:10.1159/000189270

306. Azulay JP, Mesure S, Amblard B, Pouget J. Increased visual dependence in Parkinson's disease. *Percept Mot Skills* (2002) 95:1106–14. doi:10.2466/pms.2002.95.3f.1106
307. Danta G, Hilton RC. Judgment of the visual vertical and horizontal in patients with Parkinsonism. *Neurology* (1975) 25:43. doi:10.1212/WNL.25.1.43
308. Gandor F, Basta D, Gruber D, Poewe W, Ebersbach G. Subjective visual vertical in PD patients with lateral trunk flexion. *Parkinsons Dis* (2016) 2016:7489105. doi:10.1155/2016/7489105
309. Proctor F, Riklan M, Cooper IS, Teuber H-L. Judgment of visual and postural vertical by parkinsonian patients. *Neurology* (1964) 14:287–287. doi:10.1212/WNL.14.4.287
310. Scocco DH, Wagner JN, Racosta J, Chade A, Gershanik OS. Subjective visual vertical in Pisa syndrome. *Parkinsonism Relat Disord* (2014) 20:878–83. doi:10.1016/j.parkreldis.2014.04.030
311. Vitale C, Marcelli V, Furia T, Santangelo G, Cozzolino A, Longo K, et al. Vestibular impairment and adaptive postural imbalance in parkinsonian patients with lateral trunk flexion. *Mov Disord* (2011) 26:1458–63. doi:10.1002/mds.23657
312. Barnett-Cowan M, Dyde RT, Fox SH, Moro E, Hutchison WD, Harris LR. Multisensory determinants of orientation perception in Parkinson's disease. *Neuroscience* (2010) 167:1138–50. doi:10.1016/j.neuroscience.2010.02.065
313. Pereira CB, Kanashiro AK, Maia FM, Barbosa ER. Correlation of impaired subjective visual vertical and postural instability in Parkinson's disease. *J Neurol Sci* (2014) 346:60–5. doi:10.1016/j.jns.2014.07.057
314. Vaugoyeau M, Viel S, Assaiante C, Amblard B, Azulay JP. Impaired vertical postural control and proprioceptive integration deficits in Parkinson's disease. *Neuroscience* (2007) 146:852–63. doi:10.1016/j.neuroscience.2007.01.052
315. Duvoisin RC, Marsden CD. Note on the scoliosis of Parkinsonism. *J Neurol Neurosurg Psychiatry* (1975) 38:787–93. doi:10.1136/jnnp.38.8.787
316. Balaban CD. Chapter 3 – Neurotransmitters in the vestibular system. In: Furman JM, Lempert T, editors. *Handbook of Clinical Neurology Neuro-Otology*. Cambridge, MA: Elsevier (2016). p. 41–55.
317. Dieterich M, Obermann M, Celebisoy N. Vestibular migraine: the most frequent entity of episodic vertigo. *J Neurol* (2016) 263:82–9. doi:10.1007/s00415-015-7905-2
318. Furman JM, Marcus DA, Balaban CD. Vestibular migraine: clinical aspects and pathophysiology. *Lancet Neurol* (2013) 12:706–15. doi:10.1016/S1474-4422(13)70107-8
319. Lempert T, Olesen J, Furman J, Waterston J, Seemungal B, Carey J, et al. Vestibular migraine: diagnostic criteria. *J Vestib Res* (2012) 22:167.
320. Furman JM, Sparto PJ, Soso M, Marcus D. Vestibular function in migraine-related dizziness: a pilot study. *J Vestib Res* (2005) 15:327–32.
321. Teggi R, Colombo B, Bernasconi L, Bellini C, Comi G, Bussi M. Migrainous vertigo: results of caloric testing and stabilometric findings. *Headache* (2009) 49:435–44. doi:10.1111/j.1526-4610.2009.01338.x
322. Obermann M, Wurthmann S, Steinberg BS, Theysohn N, Diener H-C, Naegel S. Central vestibular system modulation in vestibular migraine. *Cephalalgia* (2014) 34:1053–61. doi:10.1177/0333102414527650
323. Shin JH, Kim YK, Kim H-J, Kim J-S. Altered brain metabolism in vestibular migraine: comparison of interictal and ictal findings. *Cephalalgia* (2014) 34:58–67. doi:10.1177/0333102413498940
324. Asai M, Aoki M, Hayashi H, Yamada N, Mizuta K, Ito Y. Subclinical deviation of the subjective visual vertical in patients affected by a primary headache. *Acta Otolaryngol* (2009) 129:30–5. doi:10.1080/00016480802032785
325. Bremova T, Caushaj A, Ertl M, Strobl R, Böttcher N, Strupp M, et al. Comparison of linear motion perception thresholds in vestibular migraine and Menière's disease. *Eur Arch Otorhinolaryngol* (2016) 273:2931–9. doi:10.1007/s00405-015-3835-y
326. Çelebisoy N, Gökçay F, Şirin H, Biçak N. Migrainous vertigo: clinical, oculographic and posturographic findings. *Cephalalgia* (2008) 28:72–7. doi:10.1111/j.1468-2982.2007.01474.x
327. Crevits L, Vanacker L, Verraes A. Patients with migraine correctly estimate the visual verticality. *Clin Neurol Neurosurg* (2012) 114:313–5. doi:10.1016/j.clineuro.2011.10.025
328. Akdal G, Özge A, Ergör G. The prevalence of vestibular symptoms in migraine or tension-type headache. *J Vestib Res* (2013) 23:101–6. doi:10.3233/VES-130477
329. Eggers SDZ, Neff BA, Shepard NT, Staab JP. Comorbidities in vestibular migraine. *J Vestib Res* (2014) 24:387–95. doi:10.3233/VES-140525
330. Kandemir A, Çelebisoy N, Köse T. Perception of verticality in patients with primary headache disorders. *J Int Adv Otol* (2014) 10:138–43. doi:10.5152/iao.2014.25
331. Lewis RF, Priesol AJ, Nicoucar K, Lim K, Merfeld DM. Dynamic tilt thresholds are reduced in vestibular migraine. *J Vestib Res* (2011) 21:323. doi:10.3233/VES-2011-0422

9

Clinical Approach to Supranuclear Brainstem Saccadic Gaze Palsies

*Alexandra Lloyd-Smith Sequeira[1], John-Ross Rizzo[1,2] and Janet C. Rucker[1,3]**

[1] Department of Neurology, New York University School of Medicine, New York, NY, United States, [2] Department of Physical Medicine and Rehabilitation, New York University School of Medicine, New York, NY, United States, [3] Department of Ophthalmology, New York University School of Medicine, New York, NY, United States

Correspondence:
Janet C. Rucker
janet.rucker@nyumc.org

Failure of brainstem supranuclear centers for saccadic eye movements results in the clinical presence of a brainstem-mediated supranuclear saccadic gaze palsy (SGP), which is manifested as slowing of saccades with or without range of motion limitation of eye movements and as loss of quick phases of optokinetic nystagmus. Limitation in the range of motion of eye movements is typically worse with saccades than with smooth pursuit and is overcome with vestibular–ocular reflexive eye movements. The differential diagnosis of SGPs is broad, although acute-onset SGP is most often from brainstem infarction and chronic vertical SGP is most commonly caused by the neurodegenerative condition progressive supranuclear palsy. In this review, we discuss the brainstem anatomy and physiology of the brainstem saccade-generating network; we discuss the clinical features of SGPs, with an emphasis on insights from quantitative ocular motor recordings; and we consider the broad differential diagnosis of SGPs.

Keywords: supranuclear, saccades, burst neuron, progressive supranuclear palsy, slow saccades

The goal of the ocular motor system is achievement of single, clear vision via maintenance of an object of visual interest on the fovea, the specialized retinal region with the greatest photoreceptor density. To achieve this, several functional classes of eye movements exist, including saccades, smooth pursuit, optokinetic nystagmus (OKN), vestibular reflexes, and vergence—each served by distinct cortical, brainstem, and cerebellar supranuclear networks. Failure of brainstem supranuclear saccade centers results in a brainstem-mediated supranuclear gaze palsy, which we refer to as a saccadic gaze palsy (SGP). We review the anatomy and physiology of brainstem immediate premotor saccade-initiating neurons and discuss SGP clinical features and its differential diagnosis. Comprehensive coverage of networks involved in saccade generation and termination is beyond the scope of this article but can be reviewed elsewhere (1).

BRAINSTEM ANATOMY AND PHYSIOLOGY OF SACCADIC GENERATORS

Saccades are rapid eye movements with which gaze is shifted to direct the fovea to objects of visual interest and explore the visual world (2, 3). Saccadic eye movements range from intentional volitional movements to reflexive involuntary movements to the quick phases of OKN. Assessment for loss of the latter is particularly helpful in early SGP detection. Saccades must be brief, most with duration less than 100 ms; they must be accurate to land the fovea on target; and they have very high velocities. Duration and velocity are a function of saccade size, with relationships referred to as and characterized by the saccade main sequences (**Figure 1A**) (4, 5). Peak velocity increases linearly for saccades smaller than 20°; however, for saccades larger than 20°, peak velocity saturates around 500°/s. These

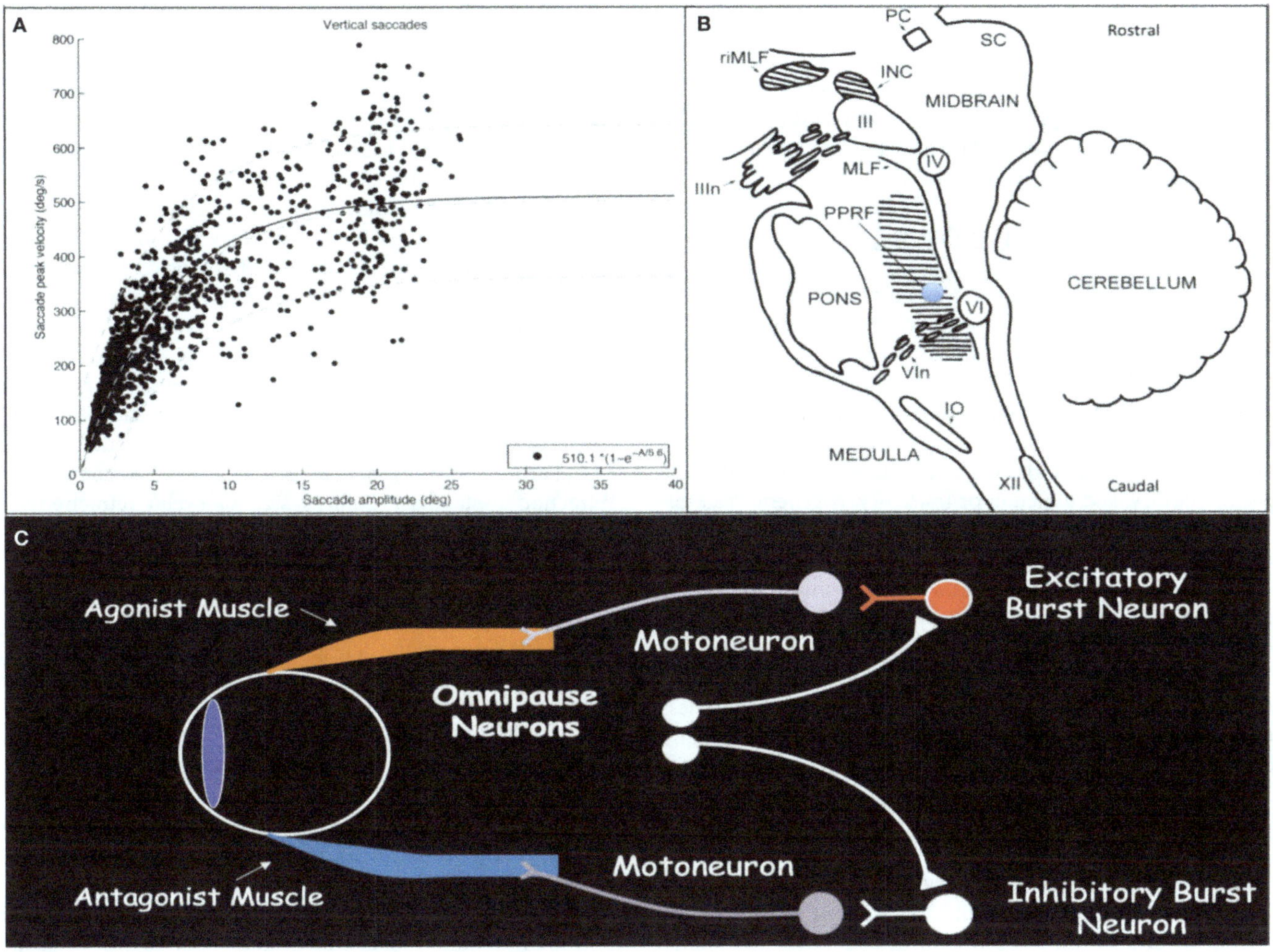

FIGURE 1 | **(A)** Main sequence plot for vertical saccades, representing the relationships between saccade amplitude and peak velocity, in a cohort of patients with concussion demonstrating normal saccadic velocities. As saccade amplitude increases, peak velocity increases in an asymptotic distribution. Light gray lines represent the 5th, 50th, and 95th percentiles, respectively, from bottom to top, in healthy disease-free controls. **(B)** Sagittal brainstem drawing showing the localization of ocular motor-related nuclei. Supranuclear burst neurons for vertical saccades are located in the midbrain in the RIMLF. The shaded region in the pons represents the PPRF, containing supranuclear burst neurons for horizontal saccades. Excitatory burst neurons are located in the region of the blue circle. Abbreviations: PC, posterior commissure; RIMLF, rostral interstitial medial longitudinal fasciculus; INC, interstitial nucleus of Cajal; SC, superior colliculus; IIIn, oculomotor nerve fascicle; III, oculomotor nucleus; IV, trochlear nucleus; MLF, medial longitudinal fasciculus; PPRF, paramedian pontine reticular formation; VI, abducens nucleus; VIn, abducens nerve rootlets; IO, inferior olive; XII, hypoglossal nerve. Drawing based on Buttner and Buttner-Ennever (6). **(C)** Schematic drawing of excitatory and inhibitory burst neurons, omnipause neurons, and their connections with agonist and antagonist extraocular muscles.

main sequence relationships allow for establishment of normal saccadic velocity ranges and are particularly helpful in the context of SGP, with which saccadic velocities become slow.

Execution of a saccade requires an initial burst of neuronal discharge, called the pulse, by excitatory burst neurons (EBNs) in the brainstem reticular formation to agonist ocular motoneurons (**Figure 1C**) (7, 8). This pulse results in vigorous contraction of the agonist muscle. The pulse is then gradually transitioned to a new tonic step innervation that maintains the eyes in the new position and is generated by neural integrators that include the medullary medial vestibular nucleus and nucleus prepositus hypoglossi for horizontal movements and the interstitial nucleus of Cajal (INC) for vertical and torsional movements (1). Simultaneous with EBN pulse firing, inhibitory burst neurons in the medullary reticular formation, caudal to the abducens nucleus, relax the antagonist muscle (9, 10). When no saccade is being generated, burst neurons are tonically inhibited by glycinergic omnipause neurons in the caudal pontine nucleus raphe interpositus (11–13).

Excitatory burst neurons for horizontal saccades are located in the paramedian pontine reticular formation (PPRF) in the pons just rostral to the abducens nucleus and, for vertical and torsional saccades, in the rostral interstitial medial longitudinal fasciculus (RIMLF) rostral to the oculomotor nucleus in the mesencephalic reticular formation, although a few are also located in the INC just caudal to the RIMLF (**Figure 1B**) (14–16). Horizontal EBNs project to ipsilateral motoneurons for ipsilateral saccades. For vertical saccades, the projection is to yoked muscle pairs (e.g., inferior rectus and superior oblique muscles for downward saccades), with bilateral projection to elevator muscles and unilateral projection to depressor muscles (17–19). RIMLF EBNs promote rapid torsional movements only ipsilaterally (e.g., the right RIMLF causes rotation of the top poles of the eyes toward the right ear) (20, 21).

CLINICAL FEATURES OF SGPs

Exam detection of SGP requires assessment not only of the static range of ocular motility, but also of dynamic eye movements in three planes. Saccades, smooth pursuit, vestibular–ocular reflexes, and OKN should be assessed horizontally and vertically (Part 1 of Video S1 in Supplementary Material). Saccades are tested by having the patient make rapid jumps with their eyes between two stationary visual targets, while noting ease of initiation, speed, accuracy, and direction or trajectory. A general "rule-of-thumb" regarding saccade speed is that one should not be able to watch the eye move through the full trajectory. If the eye can be visualized through the full trajectory of motion, the saccade is too slow. Smooth pursuit is tested by having the patient follow a slowly moving target, while observing for corrective saccades. Vestibular–ocular reflexes are tested by passive head movement while the patient fixates a central target, noting the smoothness and range of eye movements. OKN is examined by moving a striped drum or tape in front of the patient, while observing for slow following movements of the eyes and corrective saccadic quick phases. Torsional quick phases are assessed by rolling the head back and forth, bringing each ear toward each shoulder (Part 4 of Video S1 in Supplementary Material).

Saccadic gaze palsy will result in slowing of saccades horizontally or vertically (or both) with or without range limitations. Saccade slowing in isolation is evidence of SGP, even with full eye movement range. It is important to note that isolated mildly impaired eye elevation is not sufficient to diagnose SGP, as this may be seen in healthy elderly individuals as a result mechanical orbital changes (22). Some patients with selective slowing of horizontal or vertical saccades will demonstrate a curved trajectory with saccade testing (Part 3 of Video S1 in Supplementary Material). For example, in vertical SGP attempted vertical saccades may display a lateral curved trajectory, so called "round-the-house" saccades (23–26). Range deficits may also be seen during smooth pursuit, although will tend to be more severe with saccades and should be fully overcome with vestibular–ocular reflexes (Part 2 of Video S1 in Supplementary Material). This establishes the deficit as supranuclear, as vestibular–ocular supranuclear commands travel separately from saccade commands. The classic finding of OKN with SGP is loss of quick phases with a slow tonic deviation of the eyes in the direction of stimulus motion.

Pathology affecting PPRF causes horizontal SGP (Part 3 of Video S1 in Supplementary Material) (27). A unilateral lesion will cause ipsilateral conjugate gaze palsy (28). A bilateral lesion will cause horizontal conjugate gaze impairment and slowing of vertical saccades (29–32). Pathology affecting RIMLF causes vertical SGP (Part 2 of Video S1 in Supplementary Material) and affects torsional quick phases. Each RIMLF projects bilaterally to motoneurons for elevation but only unilaterally for depression, thus, RIMLF lesions theoretically have a more profound effect on downgaze. Bilateral lesions tend to cause loss of downward or all vertical saccades and abolish all torsional quick phases. The effects of unilateral lesions are less well understood. In theory, a unilateral lesion should abolish ipsilesional torsional quick phases (Part 4 of Video S1 in Supplementary Material) (33) and mildly affect downward saccades; however published reports describe more extensive deficits (34). It is likely that other structures, such as the INC, were simultaneously involved in these cases. Monocular vertical SGP is more difficult to understand, but is occasionally seen (35). A specific condition called double elevator palsy results in impairment of both elevator muscles (superior rectus and inferior oblique) in one eye. It is unclear if the lesion is supranuclear or in the oculomotor nucleus or fascicle (36, 37). A specific upgaze SGP occurs in the dorsal midbrain syndrome (e.g., Parinaud's syndrome) and is accompanied by convergence-retraction nystagmus, Collier's sign of eyelid retraction, and pupillary light-near dissociation. The SGP is likely due to involvement of projecting fibers from the INC. Classic etiologies include pineal gland neoplasms and hydrocephalus.

Patients with SGP may be visually asymptomatic, due to the symmetric nature of the deficits and lack of ocular misalignment. Diplopia and blurred vision occur more frequently when the deficit has acute onset, such as with infarction.

DIFFERENTIAL DIAGNOSIS OF SGP

Although SGP is generally very localizing, it is not pathognomonic for an EBN lesion, as saccade slowing due to dysfunction of the cerebral hemispheres, superior colliculus, and cerebellum has been reported (38–40). The differential diagnosis of brainstem SGP is quite broad, and detailed neurological evaluation with attention to associated symptoms and signs will streamline diagnostic testing and facilitate accurate diagnosis. We consider the differential in mechanistic categories, not comprehensively, but with focus on the most common and recently discovered etiologies.

Vascular

Acute-onset vertical SGP is typically due to midbrain infarction. The RIMLF is supplied by the posterior thalamo-subthalamic paramedian artery, originating from the posterior cerebral artery. A single perforating artery, the artery of Percheron, supplies both RIMLF in 20% of the population, making bilateral lesions possible from a single vessel infarct (41–43). Unilateral midbrain infarction may also cause bilateral SGP. Acute-onset horizontal SGP is typically due to pontine infarction.

In 1986, horizontal and vertical SGP following cardiac surgery was described (31). Neuropathology revealed pontine and PPRF neuronal necrosis with axonal loss and astrocytosis. Similar cases have since been described (44–49), although further pathology failed to reveal brainstem abnormalities (50), leaving injury localization and mechanism in question. Ischemic injury is considered most likely, given the temporal relationship with cardiac surgery. A recent theory proposes injury to perineural nets that surround brainstem burst neurons (51, 52).

Neurodegenerative

PSP is a neurodegenerative tauopathy. Its classic form, Richardson syndrome (53), is characterized by early falls, symmetric akinetic parkinsonism with lack of levodopa responsiveness, cognitive impairment, pseudobulbar palsy, and dysphagia. Vertical SGP is the defining characteristic, manifested early as loss of OKN quick phases (54). Excessive square wave jerks are typically present. Selective downgaze impairment is often thought representative; however, slowing of both upward and downward saccades is common and, in a cohort of 30 patients, limitation of upward range was more common (47%) than limitation of both upward and downward-range (30%), and both of the former were more common than selective downward-range limitation (23%) (55). With disease progression, horizontal saccades become affected and complete ophthalmoplegia may occur.

Additional PSP variants include, but are not limited to, corticobasal syndrome and PSP parkinsonism (53, 56), with which eye movement involvement may be subtle or occur late. While SGP with parkinsonism is highly suggestive of PSP; it is not pathognomonic, as SGP may occur in other parkinsonian conditions. In an autopsy series of 27 patients with parkinsonism and supranuclear gaze palsy, pathology was consistent with PSP in 9, Parkinson disease (PD) in 10, corticobasal degeneration in 2, multiple system atrophy in 2, Creutzfeldt–Jakob disease in 1, and Huntington disease in 1 (57). The difficulty in interpreting this study lies in the lack of details regarding eye movement features, making it impossible to differentiate between cortically mediated ocular motor apraxia and brainstem SGP. Those with PD had pathologic changes in the cortex but not in the brainstem and were unlikely to have had brainstem SGP. Saccade slowing may be seen in Lewy body dementia, corticobasal syndrome, and Huntington disease, although it tends to occur late in the disease course (58–61).

Eye movements tend to be relatively spared in amyotrophic lateral sclerosis (ALS), although some patients do exhibit SGP (62–64). In a study of 63 patients with ALS, upgaze was moderately or severely restricted in 13% (65), although it is unclear if this was due to ocular motor apraxia or brainstem SGP. Definite vertical SGP was seen in two patients with RIMLF cell loss at autopsy (62).

Metabolic/Genetic

Vertical SGP (especially downward) is a key feature of Niemann–Pick type C (NPC), present in 65% (66, 67). NPC is an autosomal-recessive illness caused by mutations in the NPC1 or NPC2 gene, in which cholesterol and lipids accumulate due to a defect in intracellular lipid trafficking. Additional features include gelastic cataplexy and hepatosplenomegaly, although in adult-onset cases, visceromegaly may be absent (68).

Gaucher disease is an autosomal-recessive sphingolipidosis caused by mutations in the GBA gene which decrease glucocerebrosidase activity (69). Gaucher type 3, the subacute neurological form, has later onset and slower progression than types 1 and 2. Horizontal SGP is characteristic, and may be the dominant feature. Additional features include myoclonic epilepsy, cerebellar ataxia, spasticity, or dementia. SGP is slowly progressive (70), and saccades have been utilized as a treatment outcome measure (71, 72).

Spinocerebellar ataxias (SCA) are due to genetic CAG-repeat expansions resulting in protein polyglutamine extension. There is substantial phenotypic overlap between mutations and mild SGP has been reported with many; however horizontal SGP with early, severe slowing of horizontal saccades is characteristic of spinocerebellar ataxia type 2 (73–77), in which saccade dysfunction is correlated with polyglutamine repeats (75).

Neoplasm

Tumors affecting the pineal gland, including pineal germinoma or teratoma, pineocytoma, pineoblastoma, glioma, or metastasis, can lead to the dorsal midbrain syndrome via compression of the midbrain tectal plate. Rarely, pineal lesions in the elderly mimic PSP (78, 79).

Paraneoplastic, Autoimmune, and Inflammatory

Ma1 and Ma2 are intracellular proteins expressed in the testes and brain (80). A study of 38 patients with anti-Ma2 encephalitis reported upward greater than downward SGP in 60% (81), some with progression to complete ophthalmoplegia. Additional ocular motor deficits include opsoclonus, ocular flutter, oculogyric crisis, nystagmus (horizontal, horizontal-torsional, and downbeat), and skew deviation. Excessive daytime sleepiness is present in a third of patients. Atypical parkinsonism occurs, thus mimicking PSP (82). It may also mimic Whipple disease with a PSP phenotype and opsoclonus or nystagmus (83).

Anti-glutamic acid decarboxylase (GAD) antibody is associated with many eye movement disorders, including downbeat and periodic alternating nystagmus, ocular flutter and opsoclonus, and ophthalmoplegia with or without stiff person syndrome (SPS) or cerebellar dysfunction (84–87). Early reports of ophthalmoplegia in SPS were attributed to myasthenia gravis and, indeed, patients may have both anti-GAD and acetylcholine receptor antibodies (88). A direct role of anti-GAD and anti-glycine receptor (GlyR) Ab in the pathology of ophthalmoplegia, as well as definitive examination findings compatible with SGP, are reported in the continuum between SPS and progressive encephalomyelitis with rigidity and myoclonus (PERM) (85, 89–93). Anti-GlyR are the hallmark antibodies associated with PERM, which is characterized by brainstem, autonomic, and spinal cord involvement (94). GAD catalyzes the conversion of glutamate to gamma-aminobutyric acid, which has a known role in saccadic premotor control at several levels, including the superior colliculus, vertical inhibitory burst neurons in the INC, and the cerebellum (16, 95, 96).

Anti-IgLON5 antibodies are associated with a novel category of neurological disease, cell surface antibody-associated neurodegeneration, at the border between autoimmune and neurodegenerative disease (97). In an analysis of the largest cohort to date of 22 patients, four syndromic types were identified: (1) sleep disorder predominant (36%), (2) bulbar predominant (27%), (3) PSP-like (25%), and (4) cognitive decline with or without chorea (14%) (98). Despite the presence of vertical SGP in some patients (99), SGP may also be horizontal and the condition differs from PSP in that parkinsonism tends to be absent with anti-IgLON5 Ab and sleep dysfunction is not a prominent PSP feature (98).

Saccadic gaze palsy is rare in demyelinating disease, but may occur as an initial demyelinating event or as an exacerbation in multiple sclerosis (76, 100, 101).

Prion Disease

Creutzfeldt–Jakob disease (CJD) can cause vertical SGP as an early or late feature and in familial or sporadic cases (102–107). SGP is typically associated with early falls and symmetric akinetic parkinsonism and, thus, mimics PSP. Clinical, radiologic, and laboratory features of CJD may be absent and PSP diagnostic criteria may be met (108), however, the course is rapidly progressive with death ensuing within 1–3 years. Familial CJD due to mutations at prion protein codons 129 and 200 on chromosome 20 has been associated with a PSP-like phenotype (102). The thalamocortical MM2 subtype, responsible for 4% of sporadic CJD cases, may underlie the PSP-like phenotype in sporadic CJD (108).

Infection

Whipple disease is a chronic infection by gram-positive bacillus *Tropheryma whipplei*. It may mimic PSP, with vertical SGP that may progress to complete ophthalmoplegia. Oculomasticatory myorhythmia is the pathognomonic, although not consistently present, finding consisting of pendular vergence oscillations and concurrent masticatory muscle contractions. Systemic features include gastrointestinal symptoms, weight loss, fever and polyarthralgia. Neurologic involvement includes cerebellar ataxia, tremor, postural instability, dystonia, myoclonus, cognitive deficits, delirium, and seizures.

CONCLUSION

Pathophysiologic understanding of brainstem mechanisms that may result in SGP is the first step in accurate identification and localization of this eye movement deficit. Chronic progressive vertical SGP is a core feature of PSP; however the differential diagnosis of SGP is broad and careful consideration must be given to the temporal course and accompanying features to ensure accurate diagnosis.

AUTHOR CONTRIBUTIONS

All authors (AL-SS, J-RR, and JR) participated in conception and organization of review, literature search, and all stages of writing—from initial draft to final product.

SUPPLEMENTARY MATERIAL

VIDEO S1 | The video contains three separate examinations: part 1. Normal examination techniques of vertical smooth pursuit, saccades, and vestibulo-ocular reflexes; part 2. A patient with a supranuclear saccadic downgaze palsy from a midbrain lesion; and part 3. A patient with spinocerebellar ataxia type 2 with slowed horizontal saccades. Part 1: Normal exam. "Normal smooth pursuit"—note the slowly moving target and smoothness of the full range of vertical pursuit without corrective saccades. "Normal saccades"—note the rapid speed and full range of vertical saccades as saccades are made to examiner command between two vertically separated targets. "Normal vestibulo-ocular reflexes"—note the full range of smooth eye movements as the participant fixates a stationary visual target in front of her while the examiner passively rotates her head in the vertical plane. Part 2. "Impaired downward pursuit"—note the full range and smoothness of excursion from midline to upgaze and back down to midline but the complete inability to pursue below the midline position. "Inability to make downward saccades"—after an initial small upward movement, note the inability of the eyes to make a saccade downward. Halfway through the clip, this patient also demonstrates stimulus-induced blepharospasm and eyelid opening apraxia. "Full downward VOR"—note the full range of downward eye movement elicited by vestibulo-ocular reflexes. This combination of range of motion deficit affecting saccades more than smooth pursuit and overcome by VOR is classic for a brainstem-mediated supranuclear gaze palsy. Part 3. "Slow horizontal saccades"—note the very slow speed of horizontal saccades with retained full range of horizontal movement in the first portion of the clip. Occasional oblique saccades are made, demonstrating the faster vertical movement first with the slower horizontal movement lagging behind. At the end of clip, note the relatively faster speed of vertical saccades. Part 4. "Normal torsional quick phases"—note both fast and slow torsional movements of the eye, invoked by rolling the head back and forth, each ear to each shoulder. "Abnormal unidirectional torsional quick phases"—in this patient with a right rostral interstitial medial longitudinal fasciculus infarction, note that in one direction, only slow torsional movements are seen and fast torsional phases are missing. This occurs when the tops poles of they eyes rotate toward the right shoulder. In the opposite direction, when the top poles of the eyes rotate toward the left shoulder, both fast and slow torsional movements are seen.

REFERENCES

1. Leigh RJ, Zee DS. *The Neurology of Eye Movements*. New York: Oxford University Press (2015).
2. Robinson DA. The mechanics of human saccadic eye movement. *J Physiol* (1964) 174:245–64. doi:10.1113/jphysiol.1964.sp007485
3. Leigh RJ, Zee DS. *The Neurology of Eye Movements*. New York: Oxford University Press (2006).
4. Boghen D, Troost BT, Daroff RB, Dell'osso LF, Birkett JE. Velocity characteristics of normal human saccades. *Invest Ophthalmol* (1974) 13:619–23.
5. Bahill AT, Clark MR, Stark L. The main sequence, a tool for studying human eye movements. *Math Biosci* (1975) 24:191–204. doi:10.1016/0025-5564(75)90075-9
6. Buttner U, Buttner-Ennever JA. Present concepts of oculomotor organization. *Prog Brain Res* (2005) 151:1–42. doi:10.1016/S0079-6123(05)51001-X
7. Van Gisbergen JA, Robinson DA, Gielen S. A quantitative analysis of generation of saccadic eye movements by burst neurons. *J Neurophysiol* (1981) 45: 417–42.
8. Sylvestre PA, Cullen KE. Quantitative analysis of abducens neuron discharge dynamics during saccadic and slow eye movements. *J Neurophysiol* (1999) 82:2612–32.
9. Strassman A, Highstein SM, Mccrea RA. Anatomy and physiology of saccadic burst neurons in the alert squirrel monkey. II. Inhibitory burst neurons. *J Comp Neurol* (1986) 249:358–80. doi:10.1002/cne.902490304
10. Scudder CA, Fuchs AF, Langer TP. Characteristics and functional identification of saccadic inhibitory burst neurons in the alert monkey. *J Neurophysiol* (1988) 59:1430–54.
11. Curthoys IS, Markham CH, Furuya N. Direct projection of pause neurons to nystagmus-related excitatory burst neurons in the cat pontine reticular formation. *Exp Neurol* (1984) 83:414–22. doi:10.1016/S0014-4886(84)90109-2
12. Buttner-Ennever JA, Cohen B, Pause M, Fries W. Raphe nucleus of the pons containing omnipause neurons of the oculomotor system in the monkey, and its homologue in man. *J Comp Neurol* (1988) 267:307–21. doi:10.1002/cne.902670302

13. Horn AK, Buttner-Ennever JA, Wahle P, Reichenberger I. Neurotransmitter profile of saccadic omnipause neurons in nucleus raphe interpositus. *J Neurosci* (1994) 14:2032–46.
14. Buttner-Ennever JA, Buttner U. A cell group associated with vertical eye movements in the rostral mesencephalic reticular formation of the monkey. *Brain Res* (1978) 151:31–47. doi:10.1016/0006-8993(78)90948-4
15. Horn AK, Buttner-Ennever JA, Suzuki Y, Henn V. Histological identification of premotor neurons for horizontal saccades in monkey and man by parvalbumin immunostaining. *J Comp Neurol* (1995) 359:350–63. doi:10.1002/cne.903590212
16. Horn AK, Helmchen C, Wahle P. GABAergic neurons in the rostral mesencephalon of the macaque monkey that control vertical eye movements. *Ann N Y Acad Sci* (2003) 1004:19–28. doi:10.1196/annals.1303.003
17. Moschovakis AK, Scudder CA, Highstein SM. Structure of the primate oculomotor burst generator. I. Medium-lead burst neurons with upward on-directions. *J Neurophysiol* (1991) 65:203–17.
18. Moschovakis AK, Scudder CA, Highstein SM, Warren JD. Structure of the primate oculomotor burst generator. II. Medium-lead burst neurons with downward on-directions. *J Neurophysiol* (1991) 65:218–29.
19. Bhidayasiri R, Plant GT, Leigh RJ. A hypothetical scheme for the brainstem control of vertical gaze. *Neurology* (2000) 54:1985–93. doi:10.1212/WNL.54.10.1985
20. Villis T, Hepp K, Schwarz U, Henn V. On the generation of vertical and torsional rapid eye movements in the monkey. *Exp Brain Res* (1989) 77:1–11.
21. Suzuki Y, Buttner-Ennever JA, Straumann D, Hepp K, Hess BJ, Henn V. Deficits in torsional and vertical rapid eye movements and shift of Listing's plane after uni- and bilateral lesions of the rostral interstitial nucleus of the medial longitudinal fasciculus. *Exp Brain Res* (1995) 106:215–32. doi:10.1007/BF00241117
22. Clark RA, Demer JL. Effect of aging on human rectus extraocular muscle paths demonstrated by magnetic resonance imaging. *Am J Ophthalmol* (2002) 134:872–8. doi:10.1016/S0002-9394(02)01695-1
23. Quinn N. The "round the houses" sign in progressive supranuclear palsy. *Ann Neurol* (1996) 40:951. doi:10.1002/ana.410400630
24. Rottach KG, Riley DE, Discenna AO, Zivotofsky AZ, Leigh RJ. Dynamic properties of horizontal and vertical eye movements in parkinsonian syndromes. *Ann Neurol* (1996) 39:368–77. doi:10.1002/ana.410390314
25. Crespi J, Brathen G, Quist-Paulsen P, Pagonabarraga J, Roig-Arnall C. Facial dystonia with facial grimacing and vertical gaze palsy with "round the houses" sign in a 29-year-old woman. *Neuroophthalmology* (2016) 40:31–4. doi:10.3109/01658107.2015.1105824
26. Eggink H, Brandsma R, Van Der Hoeven JH, Lange F, De Koning TJ, Tijssen MA. Teaching video neuroimages: the "round the houses" sign as a clinical clue for Niemann-Pick disease type C. *Neurology* (2016) 86:e202. doi:10.1212/WNL.0000000000002660
27. Johnston JL, Sharpe JA. Sparing of the vestibulo-ocular reflex with lesions of the paramedian pontine reticular formation. *Neurology* (1989) 39:876. doi:10.1212/WNL.39.6.876
28. Kommerell G, Henn V, Bach M, Lucking CH. Unilateral lesion of the paramedian pontine reticular formation. Loss of rapid eye movements with preservation of vestibulo-ocular reflex and pursuit. *Neuro Ophthlamol* (1987) 7:93–8. doi:10.3109/01658108709007435
29. Henn V, Lang W, Hepp K, Reisine H. Experimental gaze palsies in monkeys and their relation to human pathology. *Brain* (1984) 107(Pt 2):619–36. doi:10.1093/brain/107.2.619
30. Pierrot-Deseilligny C, Goasguen J, Chain F, Lapresle J. Pontine metastasis with dissociated bilateral horizontal gaze paralysis. *J Neurol Neurosurg Psychiatry* (1984) 47:159–64. doi:10.1136/jnnp.47.2.159
31. Hanson MR, Hamid MA, Tomsak RL, Chou SS, Leigh RJ. Selective saccadic palsy caused by pontine lesions: clinical, physiological, and pathological correlations. *Ann Neurol* (1986) 20:209–17. doi:10.1002/ana.410200206
32. Slavin ML. A clinicoradiographic correlation of bilateral horizontal gaze palsy and slowed vertical saccades with midline dorsal pontine lesion on magnetic resonance imaging. *Am J Ophthalmol* (1986) 101:118–20. doi:10.1016/0002-9394(86)90479-4
33. Riordan-Eva P, Faldon M, Buttner-Ennever JA, Gass A, Bronstein AM, Gresty MA. Abnormalities of torsional fast phase eye movements in unilateral rostral midbrain disease. *Neurology* (1996) 47:201–7. doi:10.1212/WNL.47.1.201
34. Ranalli PJ, Sharpe JA, Fletcher WA. Palsy of upward and downward saccadic, pursuit, and vestibular movements with a unilateral midbrain lesion: pathophysiologic correlations. *Neurology* (1988) 38:114–22. doi:10.1212/WNL.38.1.114
35. Onofrj M, Iacono D, Luciano AL, Armellino K, Thomas A. Clinically evidenced unilateral dissociation of saccades and pursuit eye movements. *J Neurol Neurosurg Psychiatry* (2004) 75:1048–50. doi:10.1136/jnnp.2003.025163
36. Jampel RS, Fells P. Monocular elevation paresis caused by a central nervous system lesion. *Arch Ophthalmol* (1968) 80:45–57. doi:10.1001/archopht.1968.00980050047008
37. Gauntt CD, Kashii S, Nagata I. Monocular elevation paresis caused by oculomotor fascicular impairment. *J Neuroophthalmol* (1995) 15:11–4. doi:10.1097/00041327-199503000-00003
38. Hikosaka O, Wurtz RH. Modification of saccadic eye movements by GABA-related substances. I. Effect of muscimol and bicuculline in monkey superior colliculus. *J Neurophysiol* (1985) 53:266–91.
39. Tusa RJ, Zee DS, Herdman SJ. Effect of unilateral cerebral cortical lesions on ocular motor behavior in monkeys: saccades and quick phases. *J Neurophysiol* (1986) 56:1590–625.
40. Takagi M, Zee DS, Tamargo RJ. Effects of lesions of the oculomotor vermis on eye movements in primate: saccades. *J Neurophysiol* (1998) 80:1911–31.
41. Percheron G. The anatomy of the arterial supply of the human thalamus and its use for the interpretation of the thalamic vascular pathology. *Z Neurol* (1973) 205:1–13.
42. Lasjaunias P, Berenstein A, Brugge KGT. *Surgical Neuroangiography*. Berlin: Springer-Verlag (2000).
43. Matheus MG, Castillo M. Imaging of acute bilateral paramedian thalamic and mesencephalic infarcts. *AJNR Am J Neuroradiol* (2003) 24:2005–8.
44. Bernat JL, Lukovits TG. Syndrome resembling PSP after surgical repair of ascending aorta dissection or aneurysm. *Neurology* (2004) 63:1141–1142; author reply 1141–1142. doi:10.1212/WNL.63.6.1141
45. Mokri B, Ahlskog JE, Fulgham JR, Matsumoto JY. Syndrome resembling PSP after surgical repair of ascending aorta dissection or aneurysm. *Neurology* (2004) 62:971–3. doi:10.1212/01.WNL.0000115170.40838.9B
46. Antonio-Santos A, Eggenberger ER. Asaccadia and ataxia after repair of ascending aortic aneurysm. *Semin Ophthalmol* (2007) 22:33–4. doi:10.1080/08820530701193275
47. Solomon D, Ramat S, Tomsak RL, Reich SG, Shin RK, Zee DS, et al. Saccadic palsy after cardiac surgery: characteristics and pathogenesis. *Ann Neurol* (2008) 63:355–65. doi:10.1002/ana.21201
48. Nandipati S, Rucker JC, Frucht SJ. Progressive supranuclear palsy-like syndrome after aortic aneurysm repair: a case series. *Tremor Other Hyperkinet Mov (N Y)* (2013) 3. doi:10.7916/D8N29VNW
49. Kim EJ, Choi KD, Kim JE, Kim SJ, Kim JS, Kim JS, et al. Saccadic palsy after cardiac surgery: serial neuroimaging findings during a 6-year follow-up. *J Clin Neurol* (2014) 10:367–70. doi:10.3988/jcn.2014.10.4.367
50. Eggers SD, Moster ML, Cranmer K. Selective saccadic palsy after cardiac surgery. *Neurology* (2008) 70:318–20. doi:10.1212/01.wnl.0000287139.01789.97
51. Eggers SD, Horn AK, Roeber S, Hartig W, Nair G, Reich DS, et al. Saccadic palsy following cardiac surgery: a review and new hypothesis. *Ann N Y Acad Sci* (2015) 1343:113–9. doi:10.1111/nyas.12666
52. Eggers SD, Horn AK, Roeber S, Hartig W, Nair G, Reich DS, et al. Saccadic palsy following cardiac surgery: possible role of perineuronal nets. *PLoS One* (2015) 10:e0132075. doi:10.1371/journal.pone.0132075
53. Williams DR, Lees AJ. Progressive supranuclear palsy: clinicopathological concepts and diagnostic challenges. *Lancet Neurol* (2009) 8:270–9. doi:10.1016/S1474-4422(09)70042-0
54. Garbutt S, Harwood MR, Kumar AN, Han YH, Leigh RJ. Evaluating small eye movements in patients with saccadic palsies. *Ann N Y Acad Sci* (2003) 1004:337–46. doi:10.1196/annals.1303.031
55. Chen AL, Riley DE, King SA, Joshi AC, Serra A, Liao K, et al. The disturbance of gaze in progressive supranuclear palsy: implications for pathogenesis. *Front Neurol* (2010) 1:147. doi:10.3389/fneur.2010.00147
56. Williams DR, De Silva R, Paviour DC, Pittman A, Watt HC, Kilford L, et al. Characteristics of two distinct clinical phenotypes in pathologically proven progressive supranuclear palsy: Richardson's syndrome and PSP-parkinsonism. *Brain* (2005) 128:1247–58. doi:10.1093/brain/awh488

57. Martin WRW, Hartlein J, Racette BA, Cairns N, Perlmutter JS. Pathologic correlates of supranuclear gaze palsy with parkinsonism. *Parkinsonism Relat Disord* (2017) 38:68–71. doi:10.1016/j.parkreldis.2017.02.027
58. Leigh RJ, Newman SA, Folstein SE, Lasker AG, Jensen BA. Abnormal ocular motor control in Huntington's disease. *Neurology* (1983) 33:1268–75. doi:10.1212/WNL.33.10.1268
59. Collewijn H, Went LN, Tamminga EP, Vegter-Van Der Vlis M. Oculomotor defects in patients with Huntington's disease and their offspring. *J Neurol Sci* (1988) 86:307–20. doi:10.1016/0022-510X(88)90107-4
60. Fearnley JM, Revesz T, Brooks DJ, Frackowiak RS, Lees AJ. Diffuse Lewy body disease presenting with a supranuclear gaze palsy. *J Neurol Neurosurg Psychiatry* (1991) 54:159–61. doi:10.1136/jnnp.54.2.159
61. de Bruin VM, Lees AJ, Daniel SE. Diffuse Lewy body disease presenting with supranuclear gaze palsy, parkinsonism, and dementia: a case report. *Mov Disord* (1992) 7:355–8. doi:10.1002/mds.870070410
62. Averbuch-Heller L, Helmchen C, Horn AK, Leigh RJ, Buttner-Ennerver JA. Slow vertical saccades in motor neuron disease: correlation of structure and function. *Ann Neurol* (1998) 44:641–8. doi:10.1002/ana.410440410
63. Ushio M, Iwasaki S, Sugasawa K, Murofushi T. Atypical motor neuron disease with supranuclear vertical gaze palsy and slow saccades. *Auris Nasus Larynx* (2009) 36:85–7. doi:10.1016/j.anl.2008.01.002
64. Donaghy C, Pinnock R, Abrahams S, Cardwell C, Hardiman O, Patterson V, et al. Slow saccades in bulbar-onset motor neurone disease. *J Neurol* (2010) 257:1134–40. doi:10.1007/s00415-010-5478-7
65. Moss HE, Mccluskey L, Elman L, Hoskins K, Talman L, Grossman M, et al. Cross-sectional evaluation of clinical neuro-ophthalmic abnormalities in an amyotrophic lateral sclerosis population. *J Neurol Sci* (2012) 314:97–101. doi:10.1016/j.jns.2011.10.016
66. Abel LA, Walterfang M, Fietz M, Bowman EA, Velakoulis D. Saccades in adult Niemann-Pick disease type C reflect frontal, brainstem, and biochemical deficits. *Neurology* (2009) 72:1083–6. doi:10.1212/01.wnl.0000345040.01917.9d
67. Salsano E, Umeh C, Rufa A, Pareyson D, Zee DS. Vertical supranuclear gaze palsy in Niemann-Pick type C disease. *Neurol Sci* (2012) 33:1225–32. doi:10.1007/s10072-012-1155-1
68. Di Lazzaro V, Marano M, Florio L, De Santis S. Niemann-Pick type C: focus on the adolescent/adult onset form. *Int J Neurosci* (2016) 126:963–71. doi:10.3109/00207454.2016.1161623
69. Stirnemann J, Belmatoug N, Camou F, Serratrice C, Froissart R, Caillaud C, et al. A review of Gaucher disease pathophysiology, clinical presentation and treatments. *Int J Mol Sci* (2017) 18:E441. doi:10.3390/ijms18020441
70. Benko W, Ries M, Wiggs EA, Brady RO, Schiffmann R, Fitzgibbon EJ. The saccadic and neurological deficits in type 3 Gaucher disease. *PLoS One* (2011) 6:e22410. doi:10.1371/journal.pone.0022410
71. Pensiero S, Accardo A, Pittis MG, Ciana G, Bembi B, Perissutti P. Saccade testing in the diagnosis and treatment of type 3 Gaucher disease. *Neurology* (2005) 65:1837. doi:10.1212/01.wnl.0000187080.74460.89
72. Schiffmann R, Fitzgibbon EJ, Harris C, Devile C, Davies EH, Abel L, et al. Randomized, controlled trial of miglustat in Gaucher's disease type 3. *Ann Neurol* (2008) 64:514–22. doi:10.1002/ana.21491
73. Zee DS, Optican LM, Cook JD, Robinson DA, Engel WK. Slow saccades in spinocerebellar degeneration. *Arch Neurol* (1976) 33:243–51. doi:10.1001/archneur.1976.00500040027004
74. Burk K, Fetter M, Abele M, Laccone F, Brice A, Dichgans J, et al. Autosomal dominant cerebellar ataxia type I: oculomotor abnormalities in families with SCA1, SCA2, and SCA3. *J Neurol* (1999) 246:789–97.
75. Velazquez-Perez L, Seifried C, Santos-Falcon N, Abele M, Ziemann U, Almaguer LE, et al. Saccade velocity is controlled by polyglutamine size in spinocerebellar ataxia 2. *Ann Neurol* (2004) 56:444–7. doi:10.1002/ana.20220
76. Rufa A, Cerase A, De Santi L, Mandala M, Nuti D, Giorgio A, et al. Impairment of vertical saccades from an acute pontine lesion in multiple sclerosis. *J Neuroophthalmol* (2008) 28:305–7. doi:10.1097/WNO.0b013e318183bd26
77. Rufa A, Federighi P. Fast versus slow: different saccadic behavior in cerebellar ataxias. *Ann N Y Acad Sci* (2011) 1233:148–54. doi:10.1111/j.1749-6632.2011.06126.x
78. Siderowf AD, Galetta SL, Hurtig HI, Liu GT. Posey and spiller and progressive supranuclear palsy: an incorrect attribution. *Mov Disord* (1998) 13:170–4. doi:10.1002/mds.870130133
79. Martins J, Moreira S, Carneiro A, Vila-Cha N. Progressive supranuclear palsy motor phenotype in a patient with pineocytoma. *Neurology* (2016) 87:340. doi:10.1212/WNL.0000000000002870
80. Lein ES, Hawrylycz MJ, Ao N, Ayres M, Bensinger A, Bernard A, et al. Genome-wide atlas of gene expression in the adult mouse brain. *Nature* (2007) 445:168–76. doi:10.1038/nature05453
81. Dalmau J, Graus F, Villarejo A, Posner JB, Blumenthal D, Thiessen B, et al. Clinical analysis of anti-Ma2-associated encephalitis. *Brain* (2004) 127:1831–44. doi:10.1093/brain/awh203
82. Adams C, Mckeon A, Silber MH, Kumar R. Narcolepsy, REM sleep behavior disorder, and supranuclear gaze palsy associated with Ma1 and Ma2 antibodies and tonsillar carcinoma. *Arch Neurol* (2011) 68:521–4. doi:10.1001/archneurol.2011.56
83. Castle J, Sakonju A, Dalmau J, Newman-Toker DE. Anti-Ma2-associated encephalitis with normal FDG-PET: a case of pseudo-Whipple's disease. *Nat Clin Pract Neurol* (2006) 2:566–572; quiz 573. doi:10.1038/ncpneuro0287
84. Tilikete C, Vighetto A, Trouillas P, Honnorat J. Anti-GAD antibodies and periodic alternating nystagmus. *Arch Neurol* (2005) 62:1300–3. doi:10.1001/archneur.62.8.1300
85. Tilikete C, Vighetto A, Trouillas P, Honnorat J. Potential role of anti-GAD antibodies in abnormal eye movements. *Ann N Y Acad Sci* (2005) 1039:446–54. doi:10.1196/annals.1325.042
86. Markakis I, Alexiou E, Xifaras M, Gekas G, Rombos A. Opsoclonus-myoclonus-ataxia syndrome with autoantibodies to glutamic acid decarboxylase. *Clin Neurol Neurosurg* (2008) 110:619–21. doi:10.1016/j.clineuro.2008.03.005
87. Dubbioso R, Marcelli V, Manganelli F, Iodice R, Esposito M, Santoro L. Anti-GAD antibody ocular flutter: expanding the spectrum of autoimmune ocular motor disorders. *J Neurol* (2013) 260:2675–7. doi:10.1007/s00415-013-7110-0
88. Thomas S, Critchley P, Lawden M, Farooq S, Thomas A, Proudlock FA, et al. Stiff person syndrome with eye movement abnormality, myasthenia gravis, and thymoma. *J Neurol Neurosurg Psychiatry* (2005) 76:141–2. doi:10.1136/jnnp.2004.036558
89. Warren JD, Scott G, Blumbergs PC, Thompson PD. Pathological evidence of encephalomyelitis in the stiff man syndrome with anti-GAD antibodies. *J Clin Neurosci* (2002) 9:328–9. doi:10.1054/jocn.2001.1014
90. Economides JR, Horton JC. Eye movement abnormalities in stiff person syndrome. *Neurology* (2005) 65:1462–4. doi:10.1212/01.wnl.0000183068.42803.33
91. Pittock SJ, Yoshikawa H, Ahlskog JE, Tisch SH, Benarroch EE, Kryzer TJ, et al. Glutamic acid decarboxylase autoimmunity with brainstem, extrapyramidal, and spinal cord dysfunction. *Mayo Clin Proc* (2006) 81:1207–14. doi:10.4065/81.9.1207
92. Oskarsson B, Pelak V, Quan D, Hall D, Foster C, Galetta S. Stiff eyes in stiff-person syndrome. *Neurology* (2008) 71:378–80. doi:10.1212/01.wnl.0000319725.22925.b4
93. Peeters E, Vanacker P, Woodhall M, Vincent A, Schrooten M, Vandenberghe W. Supranuclear gaze palsy in glycine receptor antibody-positive progressive encephalomyelitis with rigidity and myoclonus. *Mov Disord* (2012) 27:1830–2. doi:10.1002/mds.25239
94. Sarva H, Deik A, Ullah A, Severt WL. Clinical spectrum of stiff person syndrome: a review of recent reports. *Tremor Other Hyperkinet Mov (N Y)* (2016) 6:340. doi:10.7916/D85M65GD
95. Okada Y. The distribution and function of gamma-aminobutyric acid (GABA) in the superior colliculus. *Prog Brain Res* (1992) 90:249–62. doi:10.1016/S0079-6123(08)63617-1
96. Mitoma H, Song SY, Ishida K, Yamakuni T, Kobayashi T, Mizusawa H. Presynaptic impairment of cerebellar inhibitory synapses by an autoantibody to glutamate decarboxylase. *J Neurol Sci* (2000) 175:40–4. doi:10.1016/S0022-510X(00)00272-0
97. Dale RC, Ramanathan S. Cell surface antibody-associated neurodegeneration: the case of anti-IgLON5 antibodies. *Neurology* (2017) 88:1688–90. doi:10.1212/WNL.0000000000003931
98. Gaig C, Graus F, Compta Y, Hogl B, Bataller L, Bruggemann N, et al. Clinical manifestations of the anti-IgLON5 disease. *Neurology* (2017) 88:1736–43. doi:10.1212/WNL.0000000000003887
99. Bruggemann N, Wandinger KP, Gaig C, Sprenger A, Junghanns K, Helmchen C, et al. Dystonia, lower limb stiffness, and upward gaze palsy in a patient with IgLON5 antibodies. *Mov Disord* (2016) 31:762–4. doi:10.1002/mds.26608

100. Quint DJ, Cornblath WT, Trobe JD. Multiple sclerosis presenting as Parinaud syndrome. *AJNR Am J Neuroradiol* (1993) 14:1200–2.
101. Nerrant E, Tilikete C. Ocular motor manifestations of multiple sclerosis. *J Neuroophthalmol* (2017). doi:10.1097/WNO.0000000000000507
102. Bertoni JM, Label LS, Sackelleres JC, Hicks SP. Supranuclear gaze palsy in familial Creutzfeldt-Jakob disease. *Arch Neurol* (1983) 40:618–22. doi:10.1001/archneur.1983.04050090054008
103. Grant MP, Cohen M, Petersen RB, Halmagyi GM, Mcdougall A, Tusa RJ, et al. Abnormal eye movements in Creutzfeldt-Jakob disease. *Ann Neurol* (1993) 34:192–7. doi:10.1002/ana.410340215
104. Shimamura M, Uyama E, Hirano T, Murakami T, Mita S, Kitamoto T, et al. A unique case of sporadic Creutzfeldt-Jacob disease presenting as progressive supranuclear palsy. *Intern Med* (2003) 42:195–8. doi:10.2169/internalmedicine.42.195
105. Josephs KA, Tsuboi Y, Dickson DW. Creutzfeldt-Jakob disease presenting as progressive supranuclear palsy. *Eur J Neurol* (2004) 11:343–6. doi:10.1111/j.1468-1331.2004.00780.x
106. Prasad S, Ko MW, Lee EB, Gonatas NK, Stern MB, Galetta S. Supranuclear vertical gaze abnormalities in sporadic Creutzfeldt-Jakob disease. *J Neurol Sci* (2007) 253:69–72. doi:10.1016/j.jns.2006.11.010
107. Rowe DB, Lewis V, Needham M, Rodriguez M, Boyd A, Mclean C, et al. Novel prion protein gene mutation presenting with subacute PSP-like syndrome. *Neurology* (2007) 68:868–70. doi:10.1212/01.wnl.0000256819.61531.98
108. Petrovic IN, Martin-Bastida A, Massey L, Ling H, O'Sullivan SS, Williams DR, et al. MM2 subtype of sporadic Creutzfeldt-Jakob disease may underlie the clinical presentation of progressive supranuclear palsy. *J Neurol* (2013) 260:1031–6. doi:10.1007/s00415-012-6752-7

10

Eyelid Dysfunction in Neurodegenerative, Neurogenetic and Neurometabolic Disease

Ali G. Hamedani[1]* *and Daniel R. Gold*[2,3,4,5]

[1] Department of Neurology, Hospital of the University of Pennsylvania, Philadelphia, PA, United States, [2] Department of Neurology, Johns Hopkins Hospital, Baltimore, MD, United States, [3] Department of Ophthalmology, Johns Hopkins Hospital, Baltimore, MD, United States, [4] Department of Neurosurgery, Johns Hopkins Hospital, Baltimore, MD, United States, [5] Department of Otolaryngology – Head and Neck Surgery, Johns Hopkins Hospital, Baltimore, MD, United States

Correspondence:
Ali G. Hamedani
ali.hamedani@uphs.upenn.edu

Eye movement abnormalities are among the earliest clinical manifestations of inherited and acquired neurodegenerative diseases and play an integral role in their diagnosis. Eyelid movement is neuroanatomically linked to eye movement, and thus eyelid dysfunction can also be a distinguishing feature of neurodegenerative disease and complements eye movement abnormalities in helping us to understand their pathophysiology. In this review, we summarize the various eyelid abnormalities that can occur in neurodegenerative, neurogenetic, and neurometabolic diseases. We discuss eyelid disorders, such as ptosis, eyelid retraction, abnormal spontaneous and reflexive blinking, blepharospasm, and eyelid apraxia in the context of the neuroanatomic pathways that are affected. We also review the literature regarding the prevalence of eyelid abnormalities in different neurologic diseases as well as treatment strategies (**Table 1**).

Keywords: eyelid, neurodegenerative diseases, neurogenetic, blinking, blepharospasm, Parkinson, movement disorders

PTOSIS

Overview of Eyelid Elevation

During wakefulness, the muscles of eyelid elevation are tonically activated to maintain eye opening against the passive tendency of the eyelids to close, and the muscles of eyelid closure are silent except during blinks. Thus, ptosis is by definition a problem of reduced eyelid elevation rather than excess eyelid depression.

The primary muscle of upper eyelid elevation is the levator palpebrae superioris (LPS), which is innervated by the oculomotor nerve. It originates from the lesser wing of the sphenoid bone at the orbital apex, courses through the orbit superior to the superior rectus (SR) muscle, and inserts on the superior tarsal plate as well as directly on the skin of the upper eyelid, forming the lid crease. A secondary muscle (the superior tarsal muscle, also known as Müller's muscle) originates from the distal aponeurosis of the LPS and inserts on the superior tarsal plate as well. In the lower eyelid, the inferior tarsal muscle analogously inserts on the inferior tarsal plate. The tarsal muscles are both innervated by oculosympathetic nerve fibers arising from the superior cervical ganglion. The frontalis and other facial nerve-innervated muscles can indirectly affect eyelid position as well (**Figure 1**).

Several clinical measurements can aid in the localization and assessment of ptosis (1):

1. Palpebral fissure height, which is the distance between the upper and lower eyelids at rest in primary gaze and is normally at least 10 mm. This can be subdivided into the margin reflex

TABLE 1 | Summary of eyelid disorder mechanisms, associations, and treatments in neurodegenerative and neurogenetic disease.

Eyelid disorder	Mechanism(s)	Associated conditions	Treatment(s)
Ptosis	LPS weakness	CPEO spectrum, myotonic dystrophy, OPMD, congenital myasthenic syndromes, SCA28	Eyelid taping and crutches, surgical myectomy or frontalis suspension
	LPS fibrosis, dysgenesis, or dehiscence	Congenital ptosis, CFEOM	
	Oculosympathetic dysfunction	Congenital disorders of neurotransmitter synthesis	
Eyelid retraction	Dissociation between eye and eyelid position due to impaired supranuclear control of the M-group resulting in excess CCN activity	PSP, SCA3	Ocular lubrication to prevent exposure keratopathy due to increased corneal exposure
Decreased blinking	Reduced nigrocollicular pathway activity resulting in greater inhibition of spontaneous blinking	Parkinsonism (PSP > PD)	Ocular lubrication; dopaminergic therapy to treat underlying movement disorder
Increased blinking	Increased nigrocollicular pathway activity resulting in reduced inhibition of spontaneous blinking	Hyperdopaminergic disorders (e.g., HD)	Dopaminergic blockade or reduction to treat underlying movement disorder
Blepharospasm	Blink reflex hyperexcitability	Idiopathic, with or without eyelid apraxia; Meige syndrome and other dystonias; parkinsonism (PSP >> PD); SCAs	Botulinum toxin, polarized lenses, surgical myectomy (especially if comorbid eyelid apraxia) or DBS
Eyelid apraxia	Excess supranuclear LPS inhibition with or without pretarsal OO activation	Idiopathic, with or without blepharospasm; parkinsonism (PSP > MSA > PD); ALS	Botulinum toxin (specifically to pretarsal OO), eyelid crutches or goggles, trial of levodopa or other medications, rarely surgical myectomy frontalis suspension (especially if comorbid blepharospasm)

LPS, levator palpebrae superioris; CPEO, chronic progressive external ophthalmoplegia; OPMD, oculopharyngeal muscular dystrophy; CFEOM, congenital fibrosis of the extraocular muscles; SCA, spinocerebellar ataxia; CCN, central caudal nucleus; PSP, progressive supranuclear palsy; SC, superior colliculus; PD, Parkinson's disease; HD, Huntington's disease; DBS, deep brain stimulation; OO, orbicularis oculi; MSA, multiple systems atrophy; ALS, amyotrophic lateral sclerosis.

distance (MRD) 1, which is the distance between the corneal light reflex and the upper eyelid margin, and the MRD 2, which is the distance between the corneal light reflex and the lower eyelid margin.

2. Lid crease height, which is the distance between the lid crease and upper eyelid margin as measured in downgaze and is normally less than 10 mm. The most common cause of ptosis with heightened lid crease is the levator dehiscence–disinsertion syndrome (see below).
3. Eyelid excursion or levator function, which is the difference in position of the upper eyelid margin in upgaze compared to downgaze and is normally greater than or equal to 12 mm.

Of these parameters, perhaps the most useful is eyelid excursion, as it differentiates ptosis with reduced levator function from ptosis with preserved levator function. Ptosis with reduced levator function implies a lesion of the LPS or its motor control.

Ptosis due to Levator Weakness

Because it is very rich in mitochondria (2), the LPS is preferentially affected in mitochondrial myopathies. This is illustrated by the prominent ptosis that accompanies the *chronic progressive external ophthalmoplegia (CPEO)* phenotype, which can occur in isolation or in association with other mitochondrial syndromes, such as the Kearns–Sayre syndrome, sensory ataxic neuropathy with dysarthria and ophthalmoplegia, Leigh syndrome, and mitochondrial neurogastrointestinal encephalopathy among others (3). CPEO can be caused by either mitochondrial or nuclear DNA mutations (4). When the mitochondrial genome is affected by large deletions, rearrangements, or point mutations involving genes encoding for tRNA synthetases, mutations are typically somatic rather than germline, resulting in a sporadic rather than maternal pattern of inheritance. Mutations in nuclear genes can also cause CPEO and may be inherited in an autosomal dominant or recessive manner. To further complicate matters, many of these nuclear genes (e.g., OPA1) are responsible for mitochondrial homeostasis, and thus patients with inherited nuclear DNA mutations can acquire somatic mitochondrial DNA mutations over time (5). This may account for some of the phenotypic variability of these diseases. Ptosis and ophthalmoparesis may also be seen in some of the autosomal dominant spinocerebellar ataxias (SCAs) (6), particularly SCA28, which is caused by mutations in the *AFG3L2* gene (7). Interestingly, SCA28 patients have been shown to accumulate mitochondrial DNA mutations (8), suggesting a mechanism for which ptosis might appear in an otherwise purely cerebellar and pyramidal syndrome. A CPEO-like syndrome accompanied by symmetric parkinsonism has been reported in families with *c10orf2* (Twinkle) and *POLG1* mutations (9), and ptosis has also occurred in cases of early-onset Parkinson's disease (PD) due to *PARK2* mutations (10). Otherwise, ptosis is not a

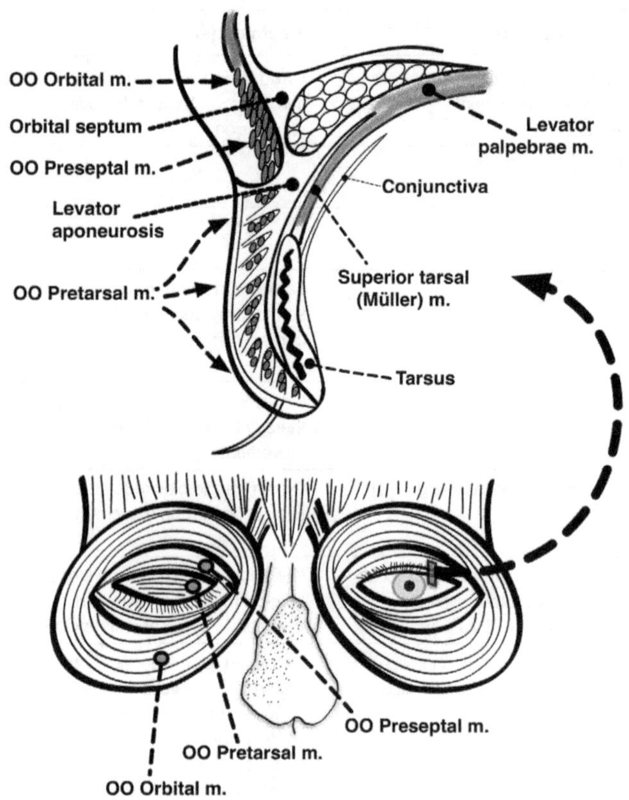

FIGURE 1 | Anatomy of the eyelids. Seen here are the major muscles of eyelid opening and closure. The levator palpebrae, which is innervated by the oculomotor nerve, inserts on the tarsus *via* the levator aponeurosis and directly on the skin of the upper eyelid. The superior tarsal muscle (also known as Muller's muscle, which is innervated by oculosympathetic fibers) originates from the levator aponeurosis and inserts on the tarsus. The orbicularis oculi (OO) is innervated by the facial nerve. It is made up of two portions: one contained within the eyelid itself (palpebral portion) and one located outside the eyelid surrounding the orbit (orbital portion). The palpebral portion of the OO can be further subdivided into preseptal and pretarsal components based on its anatomic location relative to the tarsus (Modified with permission from (154), Figure 24.5).

typical manifestation of PD or other acquired neurodegenerative disorders.

Most other inherited myopathies spare the eyelids and extraocular musculature. Notable exceptions include *oculopharyngeal muscular dystrophy (OPMD)* and *myotonic dystrophy*. The pathologic hallmark of OPMD on muscle biopsy is filamentous intranuclear inclusions composed of the misfolded polyalanine expanded *PABPN1* protein [which is similar to other trinucleotide repeat diseases such as Huntington's disease (HD)], though aggregates of dysmorphic mitochondria have also been observed (11), which may be the mechanism by which the LPS is preferentially affected. A striking feature of myotonic dystrophy is that while it is an autosomal dominant disease, the phenotype is more severe when it is inherited maternally rather than paternally, and congenital presentations are seen exclusively in the children of affected mothers (12). These observations led to the hypothesis that the pathogenesis of myotonic dystrophy may be influenced by mitochondrial factors. However, several mitochondrial DNA sequencing studies have failed to detect any variants associated with phenotype severity (13). Congenital myasthenic syndromes also frequently cause ptosis. They are caused by mutations in a number of genes involved in neuromuscular transmission, both presynaptic and postsynaptic (14).

Congenital Ptosis

Reduced levator function that is present at birth has a separate differential diagnosis, namely that of dysgenesis or fibrosis of the eyelid musculature. Isolated *congenital ptosis* is caused by dysgenesis and hypoplasia of the LPS, and typical clinical features include reduced or absent lid crease and lid lag in downgaze. Due to its shared embryologic origin with the SR, upgaze may also be affected (15). Most cases of congenital ptosis are unilateral and sporadic, but mutations in several genes have been identified in familial cases (16). Histologic examination reveals reduced muscle fiber number and fibrosis, leading many to initially suspect that the disease is primarily myopathic in pathogenesis (17). However, increasing recognition of aberrant reinnervation in these cases, including the Marcus-Gunn jaw winking phenomenon (whereby a ptotic eyelid retracts with lateral jaw movement as in sucking or chewing, suggesting innervation of the LPS by the trigeminal nerve), has led to dysinnervation-based theories, and some, therefore, group congenital ptosis with the congenital cranial dysinnervation disorders (CCDD) (18). *Congenital fibrosis of the extraocular muscles* is another CCDD that is thought to have a similar pathophysiology and produces a syndrome of ptosis and ophthalmoplegia that resembles CPEO except that it is present at birth and the ophthalmoplegia is restrictive in physiology (19). Of note, aberrant extraocular muscle innervation can produce secondary eyelid abnormalities without directly affecting the LPS. For example, in the Duane retraction syndrome, the palpebral fissure narrows during adduction not because of reduced eyelid opening or increased eyelid closure but because of simultaneous contraction of the medial and lateral recti due to dual innervation by the oculomotor nerve resulting in retraction of the globe into the orbit (20).

Mechanical Ptosis

Ptosis with preserved levator function is usually caused by a defect of the aponeurotic insertion of the LPS onto the upper eyelid. *Levator dehiscence-disinsertion syndrome* is the most common cause of acquired ptosis in adulthood and occurs when the LPS loses its insertion site on the superior tarsal plate and then reinserts on a more proximal portion of the tarsal plate or eyelid skin. This results in an abnormally increased lid crease height with preserved eyelid excursion (21). It is commonly seen with advancing age but can be accelerated by eyelid manipulation during regular contact lens use, frequent rubbing of the eyes, botulinum injection of the orbicularis oculi (OO) for the treatment of blepharospasm (22), or ocular surgery. Ptosis with preserved levator function can be inherited in relative isolation as in the autosomal dominant blepharophimosis-ptosis-epicanthus inversus syndrome (BPES) or in the setting of other craniofacial abnormalities as in trisomy 13, Turner syndrome, Noonan syndrome, Cornelia de Lange syndrome, and many of the congenital arthrogryposes (23).

As discussed later in this review, the level of tonic LPS activity depends on vertical eye position. By contrast, the superior and inferior tarsal muscles remain equally active in all directions of gaze; they are not primary eyelid elevators but instead are modulated by level of arousal and sympathetic tone. Thus, a lesion of the tarsal muscles or their oculosympathetic innervation (as in Horner's syndrome) results in mild to moderate ptosis with preserved levator function rather than the more severe ptosis with reduced levator function that is seen in true LPS weakness of neurogenic (e.g., oculomotor nerve palsy) or myogenic origin. The ptosis seen in disorders of neurotransmitter synthesis, such as tyrosine hydroxylase deficiency, aromatic L-amino acid decarboxylase deficiency, dopamine beta-hydroxylase deficiency, and brain dopamine–serotonin vesicular transport disease is thought to occur by this mechanism (24).

Treatment of Ptosis

Symptomatic treatment of ptosis is generally reserved for cases where the degree of ptosis is so great as to obscure the visual field or cause cosmetic distress. Conservative measures include temporary taping of the upper eyelids or the use of crutches attached to eyeglasses. Surgical options include shortening of the LPS, resection of the superior tarsal muscle, and frontalis suspension to elevate the entire upper eyelid complex. Other than the usual risks of any surgical procedure, the primary risk associated with surgical treatment of ptosis is incomplete eyelid closure during normal blinking and sleep (lagophthalmos) causing exposure keratopathy. Surgery should, therefore, be approached with caution especially if the muscles of eyelid closure are also weak, as in CPEO and other myopathies.

EYELID RETRACTION

Overview of Vertical Eye and Eyelid Position Coordination

To maximize protection of the cornea and tear film while avoiding obscuration of the visual field, the eyelids normally elevate in upgaze and depress in downgaze with a velocity and gain that roughly matches that of the corresponding eye movement, be it a saccade or smooth pursuit (25). A single nucleus [the central caudal nucleus (CCN) of the midbrain] is shared by both the left and right oculomotor nucleus complexes and innervates both LPS muscles; eyelid elevation is, thus, yoked between the two eyes (26). In electrophysiologic studies of primates, the CCN has a basal firing rate in primary gaze, and in upward saccades, it experiences a burst of increased firing after which its basal rate resumes (25, 27, 28). Correspondingly, in downward saccades, it experiences a pause in firing, during which the eyelid passively depresses until it reaches its target level, at which point the basal firing rate resumes. Similar firing patterns have been recorded in the SR subnucleus during vertical saccades, suggesting shared supranuclear control with the CCN (28, 29). In primates, a population of neurons called the M-group lying adjacent to the rostral interstitial nucleus of the median longitudinal fasciculus (riMLF, which generates vertical and torsional saccades) sends projections to both the CCN and the oculomotor subnuclei responsible for supraduction (namely, the SR and inferior oblique) (30). It appears to receive excitatory input from the riMLF and superior colliculus (SC) during upgaze and inhibitory input from the interstitial nucleus of Cajal (iNC) and nucleus of the posterior commissure (nPC) during downgaze (31) (**Figure 2**).

Eyelid Retraction in Midbrain Dysfunction

Disruption of these midbrain pathways is the mechanism by which central nervous system disease causes eyelid retraction. It is often accompanied by a vertical gaze palsy, as in the dorsal midbrain syndrome (also known as the *pretectal or Parinaud syndrome*, where eyelid retraction is referred to as Collier's sign) (32) and *progressive supranuclear palsy (PSP)*. Eyelid retraction in these disorders reflects a dissociation between eye position and eyelid position such that the CCN is relatively overactivated. This may be due to overstimulation of the M-group in an attempt to overcome an upgaze palsy. This hypothesis, which presumes that supranuclear input is reduced to the SR subnucleus but preserved to the CCN, is supported by the fact that eyelid retraction is often more prominent during attempted upgaze, when M-group excitation is expected to increase. Alternatively, eyelid retraction may be due to an underinhibition of the M-group by the iNC and nPC. Supportive of this hypothesis is the observation of lid lag (a failure of the eyelids to lower sufficiently during attempted downgaze, when inhibitory input to the M-group should be greatest) in some patients with eyelid retraction.

Neurodegenerative Diseases Associated With Eyelid Retraction

Eyelid retraction is seen in virtually all patients with PSP (33) and is said to result in a characteristic surprised appearance or "stare." By contrast, it has only been rarely reported in PD (34). Eyelid retraction is also a classic finding in *SCA3* (also known as *Machado-Joseph disease*); in one study, 65% of patients with SCA3 had eyelid retraction resulting in a "bulging eyes" appearance compared to less than 5% of patients with other autosomal dominant SCAs (35). Interestingly, while midbrain atrophy is the pathologic hallmark of PSP, it is rarely seen in SCA3.

Lid Nystagmus

The close relationship between vertical eye and eyelid position applies even when eye movement is involuntary, as in upbeat nystagmus (UBN). Occasionally, rhythmic movements of the eyelids can be seen without visible UBN, resulting in the so-called eyelid nystagmus or lid flutter (36). The same mechanisms by which eye and eyelid position become dissociated in eyelid retraction are probably also responsible for the absence of eye movement in eyelid nystagmus, which is often associated with midbrain ischemic and compressive lesions (37, 38). Under normal conditions, convergence increases the basal firing rate of the LPS during primary gaze, resulting in a small degree of eyelid retraction. This may explain why eyelid nystagmus can be evoked by attempted convergence (also known as Pick's sign) (39).

DECREASED BLINKING

Overview of Eyelid Closure

The primary muscle of eyelid closure is the OO, which is innervated by the facial nerve. It originates from multiple bony and connective tissue structures surrounding the medial canthus. The palpebral portion of this muscle—which can be further subdivided into pretarsal and preseptal components—is contained within the upper and lower eyelids and inserts on connective tissue structures surrounding the lateral canthus. The orbital portion of the OO lies outside the eyelids and forms a muscular ellipse encircling the orbit (1). The palpebral and orbital portions of the OO are innervated by separate populations of motor neurons within the facial nucleus (40). Other muscles of facial expression, such as the corrugator (which draws the eyebrows inferiorly and medially as in frowning), can secondarily contribute to eyelid closure as well (**Figure 1**).

Supranuclear Control of Spontaneous Blinking

Normal spontaneous blinking occurs at a rate of 15–20 blinks/min; this frequency varies considerably between individuals and is somewhat higher in women than men (41). During a blink, the LPS abruptly stops firing, and the palpebral portion (but not the orbital portion) of the OO contracts, resulting in active eyelid closure (in contrast to the passive eyelid depression that occurs during downgaze). As soon as eyelid closure is complete, the OO abruptly stops firing, basal activity of the LPS resumes and

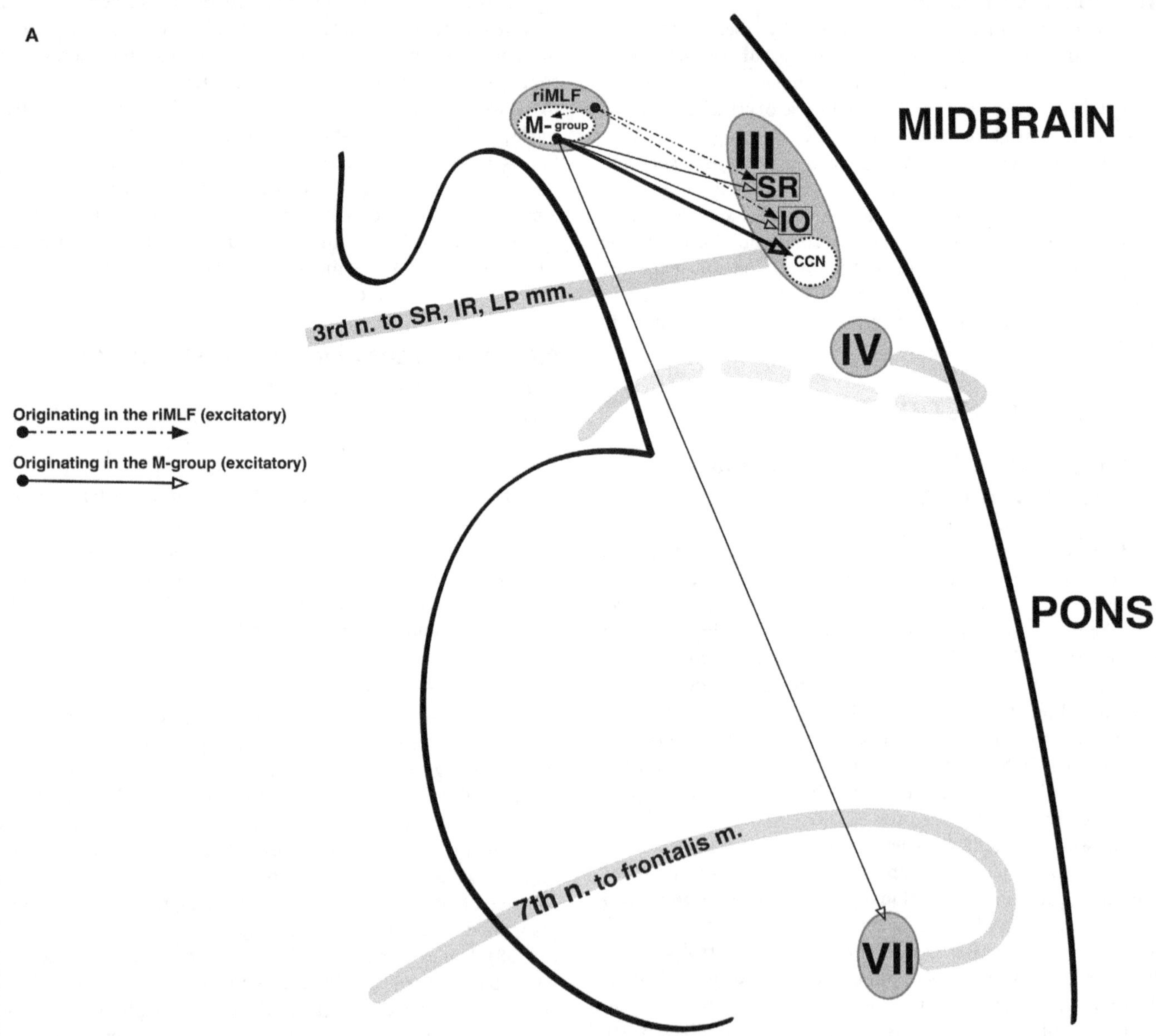

FIGURE 2 | Continued

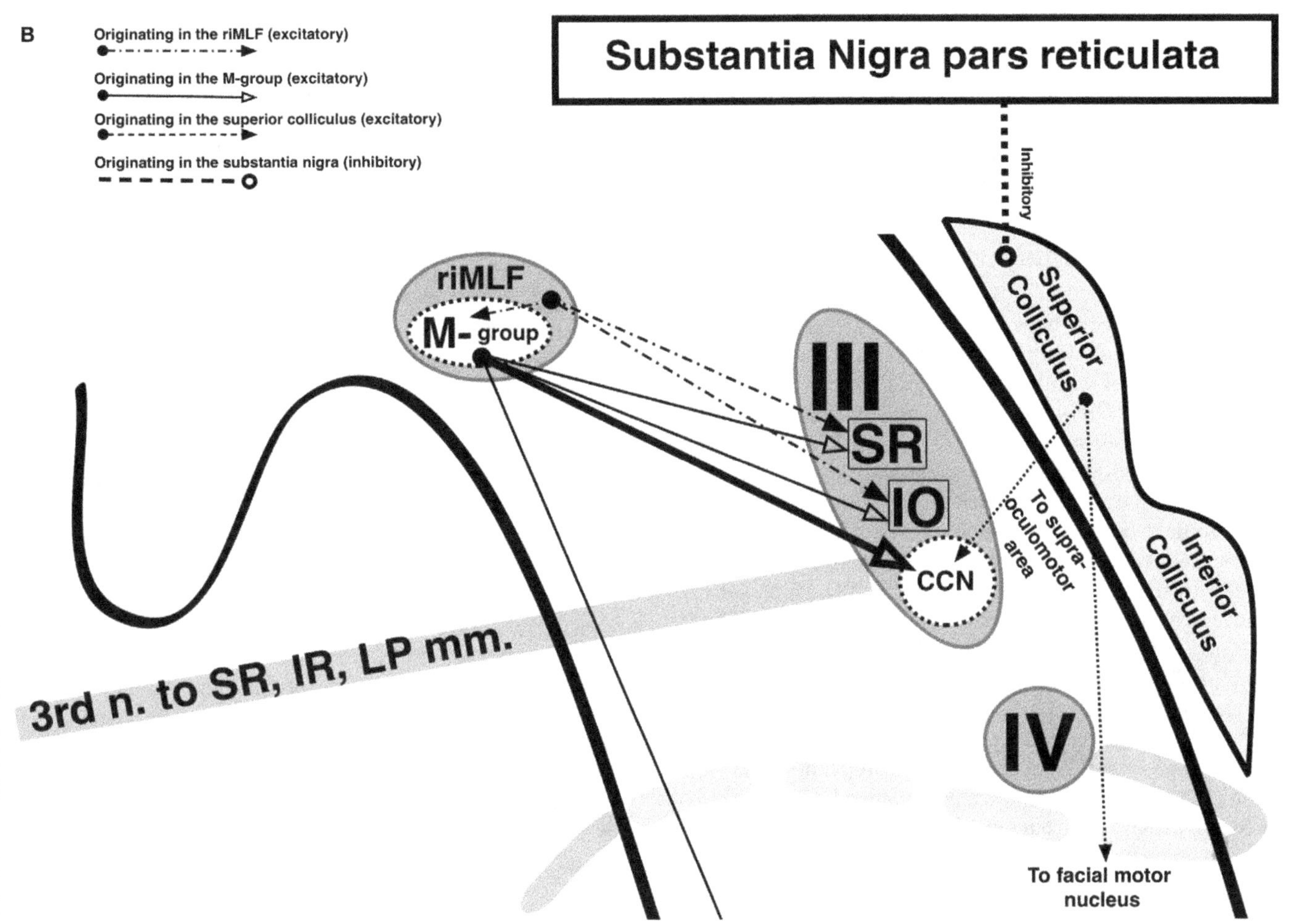

FIGURE 2 | Supranuclear control of eyelid movement. **(A)** The central caudal nucleus (CCN) of the midbrain contributes fibers to both oculomotor nerves and innervates both levator palpebrae superioris (LPS). It maintains a tonic level of activity during eye opening that transiently increased with upward eye movements and decreases with downward eye movements. During a vertical saccade, the rostral interstitial nucleus of the median longitudinal fasciculus (riMLF) is activated, and it provides excitatory input into the superior rectus (SR) and inferior oblique (IO) subnuclei of the oculomotor nerve in order to elevate the eyes. In addition, the riMLF activates the nearby M-group. The M-group provides a small amount of reinforcing excitation to the SR and IO subnuclei, but its primary excitatory output is to the CCN, resulting in an increase in firing rate which produces eyelid elevation. The M-group also synapses on the facial nucleus, presumably to provide assistance from the frontalis in eyelid elevation when needed. The opposite occurs during downgaze. Eyelid retraction in midbrain dysfunction occurs due to M-group overstimulation (in an attempt to overcome an upgaze palsy) or underinhibition (from injury to the nearby interstitial nucleus of Cajal and nucleus of the posterior commissure). **(B)** During a blink, the LPS abruptly ceases firing and the orbicularis oculi (OO), which is innervated by the facial nerve, briefly contracts. This coordination of LPS and OO activity is thought to be mediated by the superior colliculus (SC). The SC projects to the supraoculomotor area directly overlying the CCN as well as to the facial nuclei and is inhibited by the pars reticulata of the substantia nigra (SNr). In parkinsonism, there is increased activity in the SNr, which results in greater inhibition of the SC and reduced spontaneous blinking. Not shown are afferents from the trigeminal nucleus and pretectum to the SC, which mediate reflexive blinking to corneal stimulation and bright light, respectively.

the eyelid opens (42). The duration of eyelid closure in blinking must be very brief to avoid disrupting visual input. Blinking can also occur reflexively in response to various stimuli, including visual threat, bright light, tactile stimulation of the cornea or eyelids, and loud noise. With the exception of visual threat, which involves the occipital cortex, all are mediated by brainstem reflex arcs.

The anatomic pathways through which LPS and OO function is coordinated during blinking remains poorly understood, but the SC is thought to play a key role. The SC sends projections to both the facial motor nucleus and the supraoculomotor area directly overlying the CCN (43). It also receives afferent input from the trigeminal sensory nucleus (important for corneal and other trigeminally mediated blink reflexes) and dorsal midbrain (where reflexive blinking to light is mediated). Inhibitory microstimulation of the SC in primates has been shown to both suppress spontaneous blinking and increase sensitivity to blink reflexes (44, 45).

The SC is inhibited by the pars reticulata of the substantia nigra (SNr) through dopaminergic projections in the nigrocollicular pathway. The role of dopamine in promoting spontaneous blinking has been confirmed in animal studies showing an increase in blink rate with apomorphine and other dopamine agonists that is abolished in the presence of sulpiride, a dopamine receptor antagonist (46), and a correlation between dopamine level in the caudate nucleus and blink rate in animal models of MPTP-induced parkinsonism (47). Anticholinergics also increase blink rate, consistent with the hypothesis of dopamine–acetylcholine balance in the basal ganglia and the mechanistic rationale for anticholinergics in the treatment of parkinsonism (45).

Reduced Spontaneous Blinking in Parkinsonism

In *PD*, the spontaneous blink rate has been found to be roughly 30% lower than healthy controls across several studies (48, 49). Blink rate increases with both levodopa therapy (50) and deep brain stimulation (DBS) of the subthalamic nucleus (51). Rarely, PD patients may have an increased spontaneous blink rate that paradoxically decreases to normal with levodopa therapy. Typically seen in cases of advanced disease, this has been postulated by some to represent a type of "off-dystonia" (52). Blink rate is dramatically reduced in PSP to as low as 3 blinks/min, making this a feature that can help distinguish it from PD. Moreover, eyelid movements themselves are of normal amplitude and velocity in PD and are, thus, not technically bradykinetic (53); by contrast, "slow blinks" have been observed in PSP (33).

Since a major function of spontaneous blinking is to evenly distribute the tear film, reduced spontaneous blinking is associated with both subjective and objective complaints of dry eye. In one study, 63% of PD patients complained of dry eye and related symptoms, and roughly 50% had objective evidence of xerophthalmia as measured by the Schirmer or tear film build-up time tests (47). Other studies have found a significantly increased prevalence of blepharitis and meibomian gland disease in PD (54). However, these findings are confounded by autonomic dysfunction in PD and may not be solely attributable to decreased blinking and inadequate tear production. Artificial tears are often recommended, but their efficacy has not been specifically studied in this population. A trial of LipiFlow (a pulsating thermal eyepiece) compared to warm compresses for the treatment of meibomian gland dysfunction in PD is currently underway (NCT02894658) (55).

Reflexive Blinking in Parkinsonism

Given the inverse relationship between spontaneous blinking and blink reflexes, a decrease in dopamine in the SNr would be expected to enhance reflexive blinking. This manifests clinically as the glabellar reflex (trigeminally mediated blinking in response to tapping the nasion or forehead that fails to habituate, also known as Myerson's sign), which is often present in PD (56). However, the glabellar reflex is not unique to PD and is present in many other structural, metabolic, and degenerative disorders. Reflexive blinking to other stimuli such as bright light is also increased in parkinsonism, particularly in PSP, where a lack of habituation to flashing light has been found to distinguish it from PD (57).

Reflexive blinking can be studied electrophysiologically by stimulating the supraorbital nerve and recording OO activity using surface or needle electrodes (58). This elicits two responses: R1, a brief unilateral response that occurs ipsilateral to the side of stimulation with a latency of about 10 ms, and R2, a more sustained bilateral response that occurs with a latency of about 30 ms. When the LPS is recorded, there are two corresponding periods of electromyographic silence (SP1 and SP2) such that LPS and OO activity never overlap. In addition, repetitive stimulation can be performed to assess reflex excitability. This is based on the concept of prepulse inhibition—that is, through a combination of membrane refractoriness after hyperpolarization and activation of negative feedback circuits, a second stimulus elicits a weaker response compared to the first stimulus. In the case of the blink reflex, R2 is absent when the interstimulus interval is less than 200 ms, reduced by 50–60% at an interval of 500 ms, and reduced by 10–30% at an interval of 1,500 ms.

In PD patients, the R2 latency is mildly prolonged, consistent with intrinsic brainstem pathology in the early Braak stages of the disease. R2 prolongation has been shown to be greater in PD patients with dyskinesias compared to those without and in dementia with Lewy bodies compared to PD, both of which are likely a reflection of greater Lewy body burden (59, 60). More importantly, the blink reflex is hyperexcitable in PD. In one study, for example, when the supraorbital nerve was stimulated twice over a period of 250 ms, the second R2 was 84% smaller in amplitude and 50% shorter in duration compared to the first R2 among healthy controls. By contrast, PD patients off therapy had only a 60% smaller and 10% shorter second R2 response (44). Dopaminergic therapy and STN DBS in both humans (61) and animals (62) restores blink reflex excitability to normal levels. The degree of blink reflex hyperexcitability also correlates with severity of bradykinesia, rigidity, gait impairment, dysarthria, and reduced quality of life (63, 64).

INCREASED BLINKING AND BLINK-ASSISTED SACCADES

Spontaneous and Reflexive Blinking in Hyperkinetic Movement Disorders

If a hypodopaminergic state reduces spontaneous blinking and increases reflexive blinking, then a hyperdopaminergic state would be expected to increase spontaneous blinking and reduce reflexive blinking. This is indeed seen in hyperkinetic movement disorders, such as *HD*. The mean blink rate in HD patients is approximately 36 blinks/min (65), nearly double the normal rate, and up to 75% of HD patients have subjectively elevated blink rates (66). In one case of juvenile HD, excessive blinking (40 blinks/min) preceded the development of other disease manifestations by over 2 years (67). Increased spontaneous blinking is the first clinical manifestation of blepharospasm (see below) and has also been described in Wilson's disease (68). Other disorders that are thought to involve a relative excess of dopaminergic transmission and are often treated with dopamine-blocking agents, such as Tourette syndrome (69) and schizophrenia, have increased spontaneous blinking as well. The inverse relationship between spontaneous and reflexive blinking holds true in HD, as the electrophysiologic blink reflex has been shown to be underexcitable compared to normal in both symptomatic (70) and presymptomatic (71) individuals.

Relationship between Blinking and Saccades

In normal individuals, spontaneous blinks are inhibited during voluntary saccades, primarily to avoid disrupting visual input during a visually guided task. Saccades are also slower and less accurate when they are interrupted by blinks (72). However, patients with parkinsonian disorders fail to suppress blinks during voluntary saccades. In one study, normal individuals blinked an average of 15.7/min when fixating in primary gaze and 9.1/min when asked to alternate looking left and right every 5 s. By contrast, PD patients experienced a slight increase in blink rate (from 12.5 to 14.8/min), and PSP patients a substantial increase in blink rate (from 3.0 to 5.3/min) during horizontal eye movements (49). The mechanism underlying this phenomenon is not entirely known, but given that spontaneous blink rates also decrease during mental tasks requiring intense concentration, the frontal lobes are thought to play a role.

While blinks reduce the speed and accuracy of saccades, they can also be used to assist saccades in disorders of saccade initiation (also known as saccadic or ocular motor apraxia). In HD, where difficulty with saccade initiation and prolonged saccadic latency are among the earliest clinical manifestations (73, 74), the use of head thrusts and blinks is initially suppressible, but as the disease progresses, patients may be unable to initiate voluntary saccades without an obligatory blink (35% in one study) (75). Blink-assisted saccades [also termed blink-saccade synkinesis (76)] are observed in other causes of impaired saccade initiation such as the autosomal dominant SCAs, the autosomal recessive ataxias with ocular motor apraxia, ataxia-telangiectasia, congenital ocular motor apraxia, Gaucher disease, Niemann–Pick disease type C, Joubert syndrome, and others (77). During normal saccade initiation, omnipause neurons in the dorsal pons cease firing, which disinhibits excitatory burst neurons in the parapontine reticular formation (for horizontal saccades) and riMLF (for vertical and torsional saccades), resulting in a saccade. Interestingly, omnipause neuron activity is also suspended during blinks (78). If ocular motor apraxia is caused by a lack of normal supranuclear inhibition of omnipause neurons during saccade initiation, then blink-saccade synkinesis may represent an alternative method of inhibiting omnipause neurons in order to generate saccades.

BLEPHAROSPASM

Introduction to Blepharospasm

Blepharospasm is characterized by periods of involuntary, sustained, forceful eyelid closure. As it involves the co-contraction of agonist (OO) and antagonist (LPS) muscles affecting eyelid position, blepharospasm qualifies as a type of focal dystonia, and more than half of patients have a *geste antagoniste* or sensory trick that can temporarily relieve symptoms (79). It typically presents between the fourth and sixth decades of life and is more common in women than men (80). The initial clinical manifestation of blepharospasm is an increase in spontaneous blink rate that paradoxically decreases with psychomotor activation (81). Over time, blinks become increasingly forceful and prolonged, involving both the orbital and palpebral portions of the OO (sometimes termed "dystonic blinks"). Eventually, these blinks coalesce into periods of sustained eyelid closure whose frequency and duration can be so severe as to produce functional blindness (82).

Blepharospasm should not be confused with eyelid myotonia, which is characterized by impaired relaxation following voluntary or reflexive (e.g., sneezing) eyelid closure. Myotonia is seen in myotonic dystrophy as well as the non-dystrophic myotonias (e.g., myotonia congenita, paramyotonia congenita), which are caused by mutations in voltage-gated chloride and sodium channel genes and are treated with sodium channel-blocking antiepileptic drugs and the antiarrhythmic drug mexilitene (83).

Pathophysiology of Blepharospasm

It is postulated that blepharospasm represents overactivity of reflexive blinking, especially to light. Evidence for this theory comes from several observations:

1. Photophobia is an almost universal complaint in blepharospasm (84). Sun exposure has even been postulated to be a risk factor for blepharospasm given that the ratio of blepharospasm to cervical dystonia patients in movement disorders cohorts varies by season and latitude (85). Many patients report that exposure to bright light triggers spasms of eyelid closure and polarized sunglasses can be a useful adjunctive treatment (86). Ocular surface symptoms and sensitivity to tactile stimulation of the cornea and eyelids, which is also a trigger for physiologic reflexive blinking, have also been reported (87).
2. The orbital portion of the OO is normally involved in reflexive blinking but not spontaneous blinking. Given that the dystonic blinks of blepharospasm involve the orbital portion of the OO, it is suggested that they are generated *via* reflexive rather than spontaneous blinking pathways.
3. Subclinical overlap in LPS and OO activity is seen at the electromyographic level in normal reflexive blinking to light (88) but not to other stimuli. Thus, the co-contraction of these muscles in blepharospasm may represent an exaggeration of normal reflexive blinking to light.
4. The electrophysiologic blink reflex has been found to be hyperexcitable in patients with blepharospasm (89, 90). Interestingly, similar findings have been reported in patients with other focal dystonias besides blepharospasm (e.g., cervical dystonia, spasmodic dysphonia), suggesting shared pathophysiologic mechanisms (91, 92). During a *geste antagoniste*, the R2 duration shortens, but the degree of excitability does not change (93). The use of high-frequency supraorbital nerve stimulation to induce long-term depression of this reflex has been studied as a potential treatment for blepharospasm, albeit with limited success (94).

The site of pathology in blepharospasm remains unknown. The vast majority of patients have normal neuroimaging; in a single case series of 1,114 patients, only 18 (1.6%) had abnormal brain MRIs, and lesions localized to a variety of areas, including the basal ganglia, thalami, cerebellum, midbrain, and even cortex (95). Voxel-based morphometric and diffusion-tensor imaging studies have reported changes in the gray matter volume of the caudate, putamen, thalami, and cerebellum, but they have not been consistent (some reported increases, whereas others reported decreases), and it is unclear if they represent the primary site of pathology or adaptive changes in response to disease processes occurring elsewhere (96). Functional neuroimaging studies have shown hypermetabolism of a variety of cortical and deep gray matter foci, both at rest (97) and during tasks such as voluntary blinking (98), and decreased striatal dopamine binding in roughly one-third of patients (99). A case report of craniocervical blepharospasm treated with DBS found increased firing rates in the globus pallidus interna (100).

Epidemiology and Natural History of Blepharospasm

Blepharospasm may remain limited to the OO or may spread to adjacent muscles of the face, jaw, and neck, resulting in craniocervical dystonia (also known as Meige syndrome). This spread usually occurs within 5 years of blepharospasm onset (101, 102). The lifetime risk of generalization to craniocervical dystonia has been reported to be as high as 60%, though the evidence for this comes from cohort studies recruited from tertiary movement disorders centers, where the study population may not be representative of all patients with blepharospasm (103, 104). Greater age of onset, female sex, and a prior history of minor head trauma have been identified as risk factors (105). A single nucleotide polymorphism in the 3′ untranslated region of the TOR1A gene, which is the causative gene in DYT1, was also associated with a twofold increase in risk of generalization in two separate cohort studies (106). Up to 12% of patients with blepharospasm experience spontaneous remission (107). Blepharospasm may also occur in patients with parkinsonian disorders, especially PSP but occasionally multiple systems atrophy (MSA) and rarely PD. The risk of developing PSP in patients who present with blepharospasm has not been established but is likely to be low given the rarity of the condition. However, the prevalence of blepharospasm in patients with PSP is high (anywhere from 20 to 70%) (33, 108, 109). Anywhere from 5 to 30% (110) of patients with blepharospasm also have apraxia of eyelid opening (AEO) (see below); the combination of the two is especially common in PSP. Blepharospasm has also been reported in patients with autosomal dominant SCAs (6) and neurodegeneration with brain iron accumulation (111). It can be the presenting symptom of an inherited generalized dystonia (e.g., DYT1) and may be the only clinical manifestation in families with autosomal dominant focal dystonia.

Treatment of Blepharospasm

The treatment of choice for blepharospasm is chemodenervation of the OO with botulinum toxin. In addition to relieving the clinical symptoms of blepharospasm, botulinum toxin lowers the spontaneous blink rate (112) and reduces blink reflex hyperexcitability (113), presumably by reducing corneal sensory input from eye closure. In mild cases that present primarily with photophobia and increased blink frequency, polarized lenses may be useful. Some patients also report symptom improvement by wearing a tight band around the forehead, providing a constant *geste antagoniste*. Other conservative treatments that have been studied include behavioral therapy to encourage eyelid relaxation, biofeedback using EMG recording of the frontalis muscle (114), and transcranial magnetic stimulation (115). Medications that are typically used to treat other forms of dystonia (e.g., anticholinergics, baclofen, and benzodiazepines, levodopa) have been tried with mixed results. Prior to the advent of botulinum chemodenervation, surgical myectomy was routinely performed but is now reserved for the rare botulinum-resistant or intolerant patient (116). DBS has been performed in a few refractory cases with encouraging results (117).

APRAXIA OF EYELID OPENING AND CLOSURE

Overview of Voluntary Eyelid Control

The supranuclear control of voluntary eyelid elevation and depression is complex and poorly understood. Electrical stimulation of a number of frontal, temporal, parietal, and occipital lobar sites can elicit eye opening or closure, and the cortical control of eyelid position is thought to have a right hemispheric predominance (1). The impairment of voluntary eyelid motor control results in difficulty initiating voluntary eye opening and difficulty maintaining eye opening during the normal waking state. This syndrome was first described by Goldstein and Cogan in 1965, who called it "apraxia of lid opening" (118), though the use of the term apraxia has since been criticized, and other names, such as blepharocolysis, akinesia of lid opening and function, eyelid freezing, and involuntary levator palpebrae inhibition of supranuclear origin, have been proposed. Clinically, AEO consists of difficulty initiating eyelid elevation following sustained voluntary eyelid closure without evidence of involuntary OO activity. Electrophysiologically, it is characterized by the absence of LPS activity during attempted eyelid opening without concurrent palpebral or orbital OO activity as would be seen in light or forced voluntary eyelid closure, respectively. The frontalis muscle is often tonically activated in an attempt to secondarily elevate the upper eyelids. Spontaneous blinking and reflexive blinking are clinically and electrophysiologically normal, confirming that the neuromuscular apparatus of the levator palpebrae is intact and that the disorder is one of supranuclear control. PET studies have demonstrated medial frontal hypometabolism in the anterior cingulate and supplemental motor areas (119, 120).

There is evidence to suggest that at least a subset of patients with AEO may have a form of dystonia. As many as one-third of patients with AEO report a *geste antagoniste*, typically a light touch of the eyelids, that allows for temporary eye opening (121). Blepharospasm may co-exist, and AEO is occasionally unmasked by chemodenervation of the OO to treat blepharospasm, mistaken as treatment failure or ptosis due to the spread of botulinum toxin and treated with the addition of botulinum toxin to the pretarsal OO (122–124). While the OO is by definition clinically and electrophysiologically silent in AEO, selective electromyographic recordings of the pretarsal portion of the OO have revealed the presence of abnormal activity in some patients (125). Because of its technical challenges, this finding has been difficult to replicate on a larger scale, and it is unclear if these patients truly have AEO, a subtle variant of blepharospasm, or a distinct entity altogether that some have termed "OO motor persistence."

Neurodegenerative Diseases Associated With AEO

Apraxia of eyelid opening may occur in isolation or in association with an underlying neurodegenerative disorder. Of 32 patients with AEO seen at a regional referral center in Puglia, Italy, over a 10-year period, 10 were healthy, 10 had blepharospasm, 6 had PSP, and 3 had idiopathic PD (126). The number of patients with AEO who have PD may be similar to the number of patients who have PSP, but because PSP is so much rarer than idiopathic PD, the prevalence of AEO is much higher in PSP. Anywhere from 30 to 45% of patients with PSP experience AEO (127). Furthermore, AEO typically coincides with or precedes the onset of parkinsonism in PSP, whereas it is a much later manifestation of PD. AEO is also seen in MSA and corticobasal syndrome, though in the latter the underlying pathology at autopsy is one of PSP rather than true corticobasal ganglionic degeneration (128). It has also been described in cases of amyotrophic lateral sclerosis (ALS) with or without frontotemporal disease, HD, SCA2 (129), SCA3 (130), Wilson's disease, chorea-acanthocytosis, and others.

A benign unilateral AEO has been described which typically occurs on awakening and resolves after manual elevation of the affected eyelid (131). While this could represent a *geste antagoniste*, EMG studies are lacking due to the transient nature of these symptoms, and it is unclear whether this condition reflects excess OO activation or excess LPS inhibition (132). Apraxia of eyelid *closure* has also been described but is much less common. These patients constrict the corrugator and procerus muscles during attempted voluntary eyelid closure but not the OO (133); however, they are able to close their eyes normally during spontaneous and reflexive blinking. It has been reported in patients with PSP (33), HD (134), Creutzfeldt–Jakob disease, ALS (135), and acquired frontal and parietal lobe disease.

Treatment of AEO

The treatment of AEO requires a multimodal approach. Conservative measures include wearing goggles (136) or eyelid crutches (137); these serve to mechanically elevate the upper eyelid but likely also act as a *geste antagoniste*. Levodopa may improve AEO when it is isolated (138) or associated with PD (139, 140) but appears to worsen it when associated with PSP. Other medications that have been tried on a case-by-case basis include anticholinergics (141), atypical antipsychotics (142), and methylphenidate (143). Given the finding of abnormal EMG activity in the pretarsal OO in some patients with AEO, botulinum injection of the pretarsal OO is frequently performed with success (144). In cases of comorbid blepharospasm and AEO, surgical myectomy (145) or frontalis suspension (146, 147) can treat both disorders simultaneously but are generally reserved as a last resort.

The association between AEO and PD deserves special attention as it can be confounded by DBS (148). While AEO may be present in untreated PD, it can emerge or worsen after STN DBS (or posteroventral pallidotomy during the pre-DBS era) in anywhere from 2 to 31% of patients, presumably *via* the spread of current into the adjacent corticobulbar tract, particularly when higher voltages are applied to more caudal contact points. In fact, experimental low-frequency stimulation of the STN at certain voltage thresholds has been shown to induce myoclonus in the pretarsal OO (149). The weaning of levodopa following DBS may also unmask pre-existing symptoms (150). AEO usually occurs within a year of DBS implantation. An increase in spontaneous blink rate can be a harbinger of AEO during programming sessions (151). Treatment is challenging and consists of reducing voltage, increasing frequency, and administering levodopa in addition to conventional therapies. Paradoxically, some patients with AEO experience improvement with STN (151, 152) or GPi (153) DBS.

AUTHOR CONTRIBUTIONS

AH performed the primary literature review and drafted the manuscript. DG conceived of the manuscript idea and edited the manuscript.

REFERENCES

1. Liu GT, Volpe NJ, Galetta SL. *Neuro-Ophthalmology: Diagnosis and Management*. 2nd ed. Philadelphia, PA: Elsevier (2010).
2. Porter JD, Burns LA, May PJ. Morphological substrate for eyelid movements: innervation and structure of primary levator palpebrae superioris and orbicularis oculi muscles. *J Comp Neurol* (1989) 287(1):64–81. doi:10.1002/cne.902870106
3. McClelland C, Manousakis G, Lee MS. Progressive external ophthalmoplegia. *Curr Neurol Neurosci Rep* (2016) 16(6):53. doi:10.1007/s11910-016-0652-7
4. Milone M, Wong LJ. Diagnosis of mitochondrial myopathies. *Mol Genet Metab* (2013) 110(1–2):35–41. doi:10.1016/j.ymgme.2013.07.007
5. Taylor RW, Turnbull DM. Mitochondrial DNA mutations in human disease. *Nat Rev Genet* (2005) 6(5):389–402. doi:10.1038/nrg1606
6. Paulson HL. The spinocerebellar ataxias. *J Neuroophthalmol* (2009) 29(3):227–37. doi:10.1097/WNO0b013e3181b416de
7. Zuhlke C, Mikat B, Timmann D, Wieczorek D, Gillessen-Kaesbach G, Burk K. Spinocerebellar ataxia 28: novel AFG3L2 mutation in a German family with young onset, slow progression and saccadic slowing. *Cerebellum Ataxias* (2015) 2:19. doi:10.1186/s40673-015-0038-7
8. Gorman GS, Pfeffer G, Griffin H, Blakely EL, Kurzawa-Akanbi M, Gabriel J, et al. Clonal expansion of secondary mitochondrial DNA deletions associated with spinocerebellar ataxia type 28. *JAMA Neurol* (2015) 72(1):106–11. doi:10.1001/jamaneurol.2014.1753
9. Kiferle L, Orsucci D, Mancuso M, Lo Gerfo A, Petrozzi L, Siciliano G, et al. Twinkle mutation in an Italian family with external progressive ophthalmoplegia and parkinsonism: a case report and an update on the state of the art. *Neurosci Lett* (2013) 556:1–4. doi:10.1016/j.neulet.2013.09.034
10. Amboni M, Pellecchia MT, Cozzolino A, Picillo M, Vitale C, Barone P, et al. Cerebellar and pyramidal dysfunctions, palpebral ptosis and weakness as the presenting symptoms of PARK-2. *Mov Disord* (2009) 24(2):303–5. doi:10.1002/mds.22342

11. Wong KT, Dick D, Anderson JR. Mitochondrial abnormalities in oculopharyngeal muscular dystrophy. *Neuromuscul Disord* (1996) 6(3):163–6. doi:10.1016/0960-8966(95)00039-9
12. Yum K, Wang ET, Kalsotra A. Myotonic dystrophy: disease repeat range, penetrance, age of onset, and relationship between repeat size and phenotypes. *Curr Opin Genet Dev* (2017) 44:30–7. doi:10.1016/j.gde.2017.01.007
13. Poulton J, Harley HG, Dasmahapatra J, Brown GK, Potter CG, Sykes B. Mitochondrial DNA does not appear to influence the congenital onset type of myotonic dystrophy. *J Med Genet* (1995) 32(9):732–5. doi:10.1136/jmg.32.9.732
14. Engel AG, Shen XM, Selcen D, Sine SM. Congenital myasthenic syndromes: pathogenesis, diagnosis, and treatment. *Lancet Neurol* (2015) 14(4):420–34. doi:10.1016/S1474-4422(14)70201-7
15. SooHoo JR, Davies BW, Allard FD, Durairaj VD. Congenital ptosis. *Surv Ophthalmol* (2014) 59:483–92. doi:10.1016/j.survophthal.2014.01.005
16. Pavone P, Barbagallo M, Parano E, Pavone L, Souayah N, Trifiletti RR. Clinical heterogeneity in familial congenital ptosis: analysis of fourteen cases in one family over five generations. *Pediatr Neurol* (2005) 33:251–4. doi:10.1016/j.pediatrneurol.2005.03.018
17. Clark BJ, Kemp EG, Behan WM, Lee WR. Abnormal extracellular material in the levator palpebrae superioris complex in congenital ptosis. *Arch Ophthalmol* (1995) 113:1414–9. doi:10.1001/archopht.1995.01100110074028
18. Mendes S, Beselga D, Campos S, Neves A, Campos J, Carvalho S, et al. Possible rare congenital dysinnervation disorder: congenital ptosis associated with adduction. *Strabismus* (2015) 23(1):33–5. doi:10.3109/09273972.2014.999797
19. Heidary G, Engle EC, Hunter DG. Congenital fibrosis of the extraocular muscles. *Semin Ophthalmol* (2008) 23(1):3–8. doi:10.1080/08820530701745181
20. Yuksel D, Orban de Xivry JJ, Lefevre P. Review of the major findings about Duane retraction syndrome (DRS) leading to an updated form of classification. *Vision Res* (2010) 50(23):2334–47. doi:10.1016/j.visres.2010.08.019
21. Kersten RC, de Conciliis C, Kulwin DR. Acquired ptosis in the young and middle-aged adult population. *Ophthalmology* (1995) 102:924–8. doi:10.1016/S0161-6420(95)30933-5
22. Verhulst S, Smet H, De Wilde F, Tassignon MJ. Levator aponeurosis dehiscence in a patient treated with botulinum toxin for blepharospasms and eyelid apraxia. *Bull Soc Belge Ophthalmol* (1994) 252:51–3.
23. Allen RC. Genetic diseases affecting the eyelids: what should a clinician know? *Curr Opin Ophthalmol* (2013) 24:463–77. doi:10.1097/ICU.0b013e3283638219
24. Ng J, Papandreou A, Jeales SJ, Kurian MA. Monoamine neurotransmitter disorders – clinical advances and future directions. *Nat Rev Neurol* (2015) 11:567–84. doi:10.1038/nrneurol.2015.172
25. Becker W, Fuchs AF. Lid-eye coordination during vertical gaze changes in man and monkey. *J Neurophysiol* (1988) 60:1227–52.
26. Rucker JC. Normal and abnormal lid function. *Handb Clin Neurol* (2011) 102(3):403–24. doi:10.1016/B978-0-444-52903-9.00021-2
27. Fuchs AF, Becker W, Ling L, Langer TP, Kaneko CR. Discharge patterns of levator palpebrae superioris motoneurons during vertical lid and eye movements in the monkey. *J Neurophysiol* (1992) 68(1):233–43.
28. Evinger C, Shaw MD, Peck CK, Manning KA, Baker R. Blinking and associated eye movements in humans, guinea pigs, and rabbits. *J Neurophysiol* (1984) 52(2):323–39.
29. Robinson DA. Oculomotor unit behavior in the monkey. *J Neurophysiol* (1970) 33(3):393–403.
30. Horn AK, Buttner-Ennever JA, Gayde M, Messoudi A. Neuroanatomical identification of mesencephalic premotor neurons coordinating eyelid with Upgaze in the Monkey and Man. *J Comp Neurol* (2000) 420:19–34. doi:10.1002/(SICI)1096-9861(20000424)420:1<19::AID-CNE2>3.0.CO;2-D
31. Horn AK, Buttner-Ennever JA. Brainstem circuits controlling lid-eye coordination in monkeys. *Prog Brain Res* (2008) 171:87–95. doi:10.1016/S0079-6123(08)00612-2
32. Keane JR. The pretectal syndrome: 206 patients. *Neurology* (1990) 40:684–90. doi:10.1212/WNL.40.4.684
33. Friedman DI, Jankovic J, McCrary JA. Neuro-ophthalmic findings in progressive supranuclear palsy. *J Clin Neuroophthalmol* (1992) 12(2):104–9.
34. Onofrj M, Monaco D, Bonani L, Onofrj V, Bifolchetti S, Manzoli L, et al. Eyelid retraction in dementia with Lewy bodies and Parkinson's disease. *J Neurol* (2011) 258(8):1542–4. doi:10.1007/s00415-011-5942-z
35. Moro A, Munhoz RP, Arruda WO, Raskin S, Teive HA. Clinical relevance of "bulging eyes" for the differential diagnosis of spinocerebellar ataxias. *Arq Neuropsiquiatr* (2013) 71(7):428–30. doi:10.1590/0004-282X20130056
36. Milivojevic I, Bakran Z, Adamec I, Miletic Grskovic S, Habek M. Eyelid nystagmus and primary position upbeat nystagmus. *Neurol Sci* (2013) 34(8):1463–4. doi:10.1007/s10072-012-1211-x
37. Howard RS. A case of convergence evoked eyelid nystagmus. *J Clin Neuroophthal* (1986) 6(3):169–71.
38. Safran AB, Berney J, Safran E. Convergence-evoked eyelid nystagmus. *Am J Ophthalmol* (1982) 93(1):48–51.
39. Sanders MD, Hoyt WF, Daroff RB. Lid nystagmus evoked by ocular convergence: an ocular electromyographic study. *J Neurol Neurosurg Psychiatry* (1968) 31(4):368–71.
40. VanderWerf F, Brassinga P, Reits D, Aramideh M, Ongerboer de Visser B. Eyelid movements: behavioral studies of blinking in humans under different stimulus conditions. *J Neurophysiol* (2003) 89:2784–96. doi:10.1152/jn.00557.2002
41. Sforza C, Rango M, Galante D, Bresolin N, Ferrario VF. Spontaneous blinking in healthy persons: an optoelectric study of eyelid motion. *Ophthalmic Physiol Opt* (2008) 28(4):345–53. doi:10.1111/j.1475-1313.2008.00577.x
42. Esteban A, Salinero E. Reciprocal reflex activity in ocular muscles: implications in spontaneous blinking and Bell's phenomenon. *Eur Neurol* (1979) 18:157–65. doi:10.1159/000115072
43. Schmidtke N, Buttner-Ennever JA. Nervous control of eyelid function: a review of clinical, experimental, and pathological data. *Brain* (1992) 115:227–47. doi:10.1093/brain/115.1.227
44. Gnadt JW, Lu SM, Breznen B, Basso MA, Henriquez VM, Evinger C. Influence of the superior colliculus on the primate blink reflex. *Exp Brain Res* (1997) 116:389–98. doi:10.1007/PL00005767
45. Basso MA, Powers AS, Evinger C. An explanation for reflex blink hyperexcitability in Parkinson's disease. I. Superior colliculus. *J Neurosci* (1996) 16(22):7308–17.
46. Karson CN. Spontaneous eye-blink rates and dopaminergic systems. *Brain* (1983) 106:643–53. doi:10.1093/brain/106.3.643
47. Taylor JR, Elsworth JD, Lawrence MS, Sladek JR Jr, Roth RH, Redmond DE Jr. Spontaneous blink rates correlate with dopamine levels in the caudate nucleus of MPTP-treated monkeys. *Exp Neurol* (1999) 158(1):214–20. doi:10.1006/exnr.1999.7093
48. Biousse V, Skibell BC, Watts RL, Loupe DN, Drews-Botsch C, Newman NJ. Ophthalmologic features of Parkinson's disease. *Neurology* (2004) 62(2):177–80. doi:10.1212/01.WNL.0000103444.45882.D8
49. Golbe LI, Davis PH, Lepore FE. Eyelid movement abnormalities in progressive supranuclear palsy. *Mov Disord* (1989) 4(4):297–302. doi:10.1002/mds.870040402
50. Agostino R, Bologna M, Dinapoli L, Gregori B, Fabbrini G, Accornero N, et al. Voluntary spontaneous, and reflex blinking in Parkinson's disease. *Mov Disorder* (2008) 23(5):669–75. doi:10.1002/mds.21887
51. Bologna M, Fasano A, Modugno N, Fabbrini G, Berardelli A. Effects of subthalamic nucleus deep brain stimulation and L-DOPA on blinking in Parkinson's disease. *Exp Neurol* (2012) 235(1):265–72. doi:10.1016/j.expneurol.2012.02.004
52. Kimber TE, Thompson PD. Increased blink rate in advanced Parkinson's disease: a form of 'off'-period dystonia? *Mov Disord* (2000) 15(5):982–5. doi:10.1002/1531-8257(200009)15:5<982::AID-MDS1033>3.0.CO;2-P
53. Korosec M, Zidar I, Reits D, Evinger C, Vanderwerf F. Eyelid movements during blinking in patients with Parkinson's disease. *Mov Disord* (2006) 21(8):1248–51. doi:10.1002/mds.20930
54. Nowacka B, Lubinski W, Honczarenko K, Potemkowski A, Safranow K. Ophthalmological features of Parkinson's disease. Ophthalmological features of Parkinson's disease. *Med Sci Monit* (2014) 20:2243–9. doi:10.12659/MSM.890861
55. Burden S. *Lipiflow Versus Warm Compresses in Parkinson's Disease* (2016). Available from: https://clinicaltrials.gov/ct2/show/NCT02894658?term=lipiflow&rank=4

56. Brodsky H, Dat Vuong K, Thomas M, Jankovic J. Glabellar and palmomental reflexes in parkinsonian disorders. *Neurology* (2004) 63(6):1096–8. doi:10.1212/01.WNL.0000140249.97312.76
57. Kuniyoshi S, Riley DE, Zee DS, Reich SG, Whitney C, Leigh RJ. Distinguishing progressive supranuclear palsy from other forms of Parkinson's disease: evaluation of new signs. *Ann N Y Acad Sci* (2002) 956:484–6. doi:10.1111/j.1749-6632.2002.tb02862.x
58. Aramideh M, Ongerboer de Visser BW. Brainstem reflexes: electrodiagnostic techniques, physiology, normative data, and clinical applications. *Muscle Nerve* (2002) 26(1):14–30. doi:10.1002/mus.10120
59. Iriarte LM, Chacon J, Madrazo J, Chaparro P, Vadillo J. Blink reflex in dyskinetic and nondyskinetic patients with Parkinson's disease. *Eur Neurol* (1989) 29(2):67–70. doi:10.1159/000116380
60. Bonanni L, Anzellotti F, Varanese S, Thomas A, Manzoli L, Onofrj M. Delayed blink reflex in dementia with Lewy bodies. *J Neurol Neurosurg Psychiatry* (2007) 78(10):1137–9. doi:10.1136/jnnp.2006.113746
61. Costa J, Valls-Sole J, Valldeoriola F, Pech C, Rumia J. Single subthalamic nucleus deep brain stimuli inhibit the blink reflex in Parkinson's disease patients. *Brain* (2006) 129:1758–67. doi:10.1093/brain/awl143
62. Kaminer J, Thakur P, Evinger C. Effects of subthalamic deep brain stimulation on blink abnormalities of 6-OHDA lesioned rats. *J Neurophysiol* (2015) 1113(9):3038–46. doi:10.1152/jn.01072.2014
63. Iriarte LM, Chacon J, Madrazo J, Chaparro P, Vadillo J. Blink reflex in 57 parkinsonian patients with correlation between the clinical and electrophysiological parameters. *Funct Neurol* (1988) 3(2):147–56.
64. Matsumoto H, Noro H, Kaneshige Y, Chiba S, Miyano N, Motoi Y, et al. A correlation study between blink reflex habituation and clinical state in patients with Parkinson's disease. *J Neurol Sci* (1992) 107(2):155–9. doi:10.1016/0022-510X(92)90283-Q
65. Karson CN, Burns RS, LeWitt PA, Foster NL, Newman RP. Blink rates and disorders of movement. *Neurology* (1984) 34(5):677–8. doi:10.1212/WNL.34.5.677
66. Fekete R, Jankovic J. Upper facial chorea in Huntington disease. *J Clin Mov Disord* (2014) 1:7. doi:10.1186/2054-7072-1-7
67. Xing S, Chen L, Chen X, Pei Z, Zeng J, Li J. Excessive blinking as an initial manifestation of juvenile Huntington's disease. *Neurol Sci* (2008) 29(4):275–7. doi:10.1007/s10072-008-0981-7
68. Verma R, Lalla R, Patil TB. Is blinking of the eyes affected in extrapyramidal disorders? An interesting observation in a patient with Wilson disease. *BMJ Case Rep* (2012) 2012. doi:10.1136/bcr-2012-007367
69. Tharp JA, Wendelken C, Mathews CA, Marco EJ, Schreier H, Bunge SA. Tourette syndrome: complementary insights from measures of cognitive control, eyeblink rate, and pupil diameter. *Front Psychiatry* (2015) 6:95. doi:10.3389/fpsyt.2015.00095
70. Esteban A, Gimenez-Roldan S. Blink reflex in Huntington's chorea and Parkinson's disease. *Acta Neurol Scand* (1975) 52(2):145–57. doi:10.1111/j.1600-0404.1975.tb05768.x
71. De Tommaso M, Sciruicchio V, Spinelli A, Specchio N, Difruscolo O, Puca F, et al. Features of the blink reflex in individuals at risk for Huntington's disease. *Muscle Nerve* (2001) 24(11):1520–5. doi:10.1002/mus.1177
72. Rottach KG, Das VE, Wohlgemuth W, Zivotofsky AZ, Leigh RJ. Properties of horizontal saccades accompanied by blinks. *J Neurophysiol* (1998) 79(6):2895–902.
73. Lasker AG, Zee DS. Ocular motor abnormalities in Huntington's disease. *Vision Res* (1997) 37:3639–45. doi:10.1016/S0042-6989(96)00169-1
74. Golding CV, Danchaivijitr C, Hodgson TL, Tabrizi SJ, Kennard C. Identification of an oculomotor biomarker of preclinical Huntington disease. *Neurology* (2006) 67:485–7. doi:10.1212/01.wnl.0000218215.43328.88
75. Leigh RJ, Newman SA, Folstein SE, Lasker AG, Jensen BA. Abnormal ocular motor control in Huntington's disease. *Neurology* (1983l) 33(10):1268–75. doi:10.1212/WNL.33.10.1268
76. Zee DS, Chu FC, Leigh RJ, Savino PJ, Schatz NJ, Reingold DB, et al. Blink-saccade dynkinesis. *Neurology* (1983) 33(9):1233–6. doi:10.1212/WNL.33.9.1233
77. Cogan DG, Chu FC, Reingold D, Barranger J. Ocular motor signs in some metabolic diseases. *Arch Ophthalmol* (1981) 99(10):1802–8. doi:10.1001/archopht.1981.03930020676010
78. Schultz KP, Williams CR, Busettini C. Macaque pontine omnipause neurons play no direct role in the generation of eye blinks. *J Neurophysiol* (2010) 103(4):2255–74. doi:10.1152/jn.01150.2009
79. Martino D, Liuzzi D, Macerollo A, Aniello MS, Livrea P, Defazio G. The phenomenology of the *geste antagoniste* in primary blepharospasm and cervical dystonia. *Mov Disord* (2010) 25(4):407–12. doi:10.1002/mds.23011
80. Steeves TD, Day L, Dykeman J, Jette N, Pringsheim T. The prevalence of primary dystonia: a systematic review and meta-analysis. *Mov Disord* (2012) 27(14):1789–96. doi:10.1002/mds.25244
81. Bentivoglio AR, Daniele A, Albanese A, Tonali PA, Fasano A. Analysis of blink rate in patients with blepharospasm. *Mov Disord* (2006) 21(8):1225–9. doi:10.1002/mds.20889
82. Valls-Sole J, Defazio G. Blepharospasm: update on epidemiology, clinical aspects, and pathophysiology. *Front Neurol* (2016) 7:45. doi:10.3389/fneur.2016.00045
83. Matthews E, Fialho D, Tan SV, Venance SL, Cannon SC, Sternberg D, et al. The non-dystrophic myotonias: molecular pathogenesis, diagnosis, and treatment. *Brain* (2010) 133(1):9–22. doi:10.1093/brain/awp294
84. Katz BJ, Digre KB. Diagnosis, pathophysiology, and treatment of photophobia. *Surv Ophthalmol* (2016) 61(4):466–77. doi:10.1016/j.survophthal.2016.02.001
85. Molloy A, Williams L, Kimmich O, Butler JS, Beiser I, McGovern E, et al. Sun exposure is an environmental risk factor for the development of blepharospasm. *J Neurol Neurosurg Psychiatry* (2016) 87(4):420–4. doi:10.1136/jnnp-2014-310266
86. Blackburn MK, Lamb RD, Digre KB, Smith AG, Warner JE, McClane RW, et al. FL-41 tint improves blink frequency, light sensitivity, and functional limitations in patients with benign essential blepharospasm. *Ophthalmology* (2009) 116(5):997–1001. doi:10.1016/j.ophtha.2008.12.031
87. Martino D, Defazio G, Alessio G, Abbruzzese G, Girlanda P, Tinazzi M, et al. Relationship between eye symptoms and blepharospasm: a multicenter case-control study. *Mov Disord* (2005) 20:1564–70. doi:10.1002/mds.20635
88. Manning KA, Evinger C. Different forms of blinks and their two-stage control. *Exp Brain Res* (1986) 64(3):579–88. doi:10.1007/BF00340495
89. Tisch S, Limousin P, Rothwell JC, Asselman P, Quinn N, Jahanshahi M, et al. Changes in blink reflex excitability after globus pallidus internus stimulation for dystonia. *Mov Disord* (2006) 21(10):1650–5. doi:10.1002/mds.20899
90. Schwingenschuh P, Katschnig P, Edwards MJ, Teo JT, Korlipara LV, Rothwell JC, et al. The blink reflex recovery cycle differs between essential and presumed psychogenic blepharospasm. *Neurology* (2011) 76(7):610–4. doi:10.1212/WNL.0b013e31820c3074
91. Tolosa E, Montserrat L, Bayes A. Blink reflex studies in patients with focal dystonias. *Adv Neurol* (1988) 50:517–24.
92. Cohen LG, Ludlow CL, Warden M, Estegui M, Agostino R, Sedory SE, et al. Blink reflex excitability recovery curves in patients with spasmodic dysphonia. *Neurology* (1989) 39(4):572–7. doi:10.1212/WNL.39.4.572
93. Gómez-Wong E, Martí MJ, Cossu G, Fabregat N, Tolosa ES, Valls-Solé J. The 'geste antagonistique' induces transient modulation of the blink reflex in human patients with blepharospasm. *Neurosci Lett* (1998) 251(2):125–8. doi:10.1016/S0304-3940(98)00519-9
94. Kranz G, Shamim EA, Lin PT, Kranz GS, Hallet M. Long term depression-like plasticity of the blink reflex for the treatment of blepharospasm. *Mov Disord* (2013) 28(4):498–503. doi:10.1002/mds.25329
95. Khooshnoodi MA, Factor SA, Jinnah HA. Secondary blepharospasm associated with structural lesions of the brain. *J Neurol Sci* (2013) 331(102):98–101. doi:10.1016/j.jns.2013.05.022
96. Hallett M, Evinger C, Jankovic J, Stacy M; BEBRF International Workshop. Update on blepharospasm: report from the BEBRF international workshop. *Neurology* (2008) 71:1275–82. doi:10.1212/01.wnl.0000327601.46315.85
97. Zhou B, Wang J, Huang Y, Yang Y, Gong Q, Zhou D. A resting state functional magnetic resonance imaging study of patients with benign essential blepharospasm. *J Neuroophthalmol* (2013) 33(3):235–40. doi:10.1097/WNO.0b013e31828f69e5
98. Baker RS, Andersen AH, Morecraft RJ, Smith CD. A functional magnetic resonance imaging study in patients with benign essential blepharospasm. *J Neuroophthalmol* (2003) 23(1):11–5. doi:10.1097/00041327-200303000-00003

99. Horie C, Suzuki Y, Kiyosawa M, Mochizuki M, Wakakura M, Oda K, et al. Decreased dopamine D receptor binding in essential blepharospasm. *Acta Neurol Scand* (2009) 119(1):49–54. doi:10.1111/j.1600-0404.2008.01053.x
100. Foote KD, Sanchez JC, Okun MS. Staged deep brain stimulation for refractory craniofacial dystonia with blepharospasm: case report and physiology. *Neurosurgery* (2005) 56:E415. doi:10.1227/01.NEU.0000147978.67424.42
101. Abbruzzese G, Berardelli A, Girlanda P, Marchese R, Martino D, Morgante F, et al. Long-term assessment of the risk of spread in primary late-onset focal dystonia. *J Neurol Neurosurg Psychiatry* (2008) 79:392–6. doi:10.1136/jnnp.2007.124594
102. Svetel M, Pekmezovic T, Tomic A, Kresojevic N, Kostic VS. The spread of primary late-onset focal dystonia in a long-term follow up study. *Clin Neurol Neurosurg* (2015) 132:41–3. doi:10.1016/j.clineuro.2015.02.015
103. Martino D, Berardelli A, Abbruzzese G, Bentivoglio AR, Esposito M, Fabbrini G, et al. Age at onset and symptom spread in primary focal dystonia. *Mov Disord* (2012) 27(11):1447–50. doi:10.1002/mds.25088
104. Weiss EM, Hershey T, Karimi M, Racette B, Tabbal SD, Mink JW, et al. Relative risk of spread of symptoms among the focal onset dystonias. *Mov Disord* (2006) 21(8):1175–81. doi:10.1002/mds.20919
105. Defazio G, Livrea P. Epidemiology of primary blepharosmasm. *Mov Disord* (2002) 17(1):7–12. doi:10.1002/mds.1275
106. Defazio G, Matarin M, Peckham EL, Martino D, Valente EM, Singleton A, et al. The TOR1A polymorphism rs1182 and the risk of spread in primary blepharospasm. *Mov Disord* (2009) 24(4):613–6. doi:10.1002/mds.22471
107. Grandas F, Traba A, Alonso F, Esteban A. Blink reflex recovery cycle in patients with blepharospasm unilaterally treated with botulinum toxin. *Clin Neuropharmacol* (1998) 21(5):307–11.
108. Yoon WT, Chung EJ, Lee SH, Kim BJ, Lee WY. Clinical analysis of blepharospasm and apraxia of eyelid opening in patients with parkinsonism. *J Clin Neurol* (2005) 1(2):159–65. doi:10.3988/jcn.2005.1.2.159
109. Barclay CL, Lang AE. Dystonia in progressive supranuclear palsy. *J Neurol Neurosurg Psychiatry* (1997) 62(4):352–6.
110. Defazio G, Livrea P, De Salvia R, Manobianca G, Coviello V, Anaclerio D, et al. Prevalence of primary blepharospasm in a community of Puglia region, Southern Italy. *Neurology* (2001) 56(11):1579–81. doi:10.1212/WNL.56.11.1579
111. Egan RA, Weleber RG, Hogarth P, Gregory A, Coryell J, Westaway SK, et al. Neuro-ophthalmologic and electroretinographic findings in pantothenate kinase-associated neurodegeneration (formerly Hallervorden-Spatz disease). *Am J Ophthalmol* (2005) 140(2):267–74. doi:10.1016/j.ajo.2005.03.024
112. Conte A, Berardelli I, Ferrazzano G, Pasquini M, Berardelli A, Fabbrini G. Non-motor symptoms in patients with adult-onset focal dystonia: sensory and psychiatric disturbances. *Parkinsonism Relat Disord* (2016) 22:S111–4. doi:10.1016/j.parkreldis.2015.09.001
113. Quartarone A, Sant'Angelo A, Battaglia F, Bagnato S, Rizzo V, Morgante F, et al. Enhanced long-term potentiation-like plasticity of the trigeminal blink reflex circuit in blepharospasm. *J Neurosci* (2006) 26(2):716–21. doi:10.1523/JNEUROSCI.3948-05.2006
114. Surwit RS, Rotberg M. Biofeedback therapy of essential blepharospasm. *Am J Ophthalmol* (1984) 98(1):28–31. doi:10.1016/0002-9394(84)90184-3
115. Kranz G, SHamim EA, Lin PT, Kranz GS, Hallett M. Transcranial magnetic brain stimulation modulates blepharospasm: a randomized controlled study. *Neurology* (2010) 75(16):1465–71. doi:10.1212/WNL.0b013e3181f8814d
116. Pariseau B, Worley MW, Anderson RL. Myectomy for blepharospasm. *Curr Opin Ophthalmol* (2013) 24(5):488–93. doi:10.1097/ICU.0b013e3283645aee
117. Yamada K, Shinojima N, Hamasaki T, Kuratsu J. Pallidal stimulation for medically intractable blepharospasm. *BMJ Case Rep* (2016) 2016. doi:10.1136/bcr-2015-214241
118. Goldstein JE, Cogan DG. Apraxia of lid opening. *Arch Ophthalmol* (1965) 73:155–9. doi:10.1001/archopht.1965.00970030157003
119. Smith D, Ishikawa T, Dhawan V, Winterkorn JS, Eidelberg D. Lid-opening apraxia is associated with medial frontal hypometabolism. *Mov Disord* (1995) 10(3):341–4. doi:10.1002/mds.870100319
120. Suzuki Y, Kiyosawa M, Ohno N, Michizuki M, Inaba A, Mizusawa H, et al. Gluocse hypometablism in medial frontal cortex of patients with apraxia of lid opening. *Graefes Arch Clin Exp Ophthalmol* (2003) 241(7):529–34. doi:10.1007/s00417-003-0682-0
121. Defazio G, Livrea P, Lamberti P, De Salvia R, Laddomada G, Giorelli M, et al. Isolated so-called apraxia of eyelid opening: report of 10 cases and a review of the literature. *Eur Neurol* (1988) 39:204–10. doi:10.1159/000007935
122. Aramideh M, Eekhof JL, Bour LJ, Koelman JH, Speelman JD, Ongerboer de Visser BW. Electromyography and recovery of the blink reflex in involuntary eyelid closure: a comparative study. *J Neurol Neurosurg Psychiatry* (1995) 58(6):692–8.
123. Rana AQ, Kabir A, Dogu O, Patel A, Khondker S. Prevalence of blepharospasm and apraxia of eyelid opening in patients with parkinsonism, cervical dystonia, and essential tremor. *Eur Neurol* (2012) 68(5):318–21. doi:10.1159/000341621
124. Esposito M, Fasano A, Crisci C, Dubbioso R, Iodice R, Santoro L. The combined treatment with orbital and pretarsal bnotulinum toxin injections in the management of poorly responsive blepharospasm. *Neurol Sci* (2014) 35(3):397–400. doi:10.1007/s10072-013-1526-2
125. Tozlovanu V, Forget R, Iancu A, Boghen D. Prolonged orbicularis oculi activity: a major factor in apraxia of lid opening. *Neurology* (2001) 57(6):1013–8. doi:10.1212/WNL.57.6.1013
126. Lamberti P, De Mari M, Zenzola A, Aniello MS, Defazio G. Frequency of apraxia of eyelid opening in the general population and in patients with extrapyramidal disorders. *Neurol Sci* (2002) 23:S81–2. doi:10.1007/s100720200080
127. Nath U, Ben-Shiomo Y, Thomson RG, Lees AJ, Burn DJ. Clinical features oand natural history of progressive supranuclear palsy: a clinical cohort study. *Neurology* (2003) 60(6):910–6. doi:10.1212/01.WNL.0000052991.70149.68
128. Ouchi H, Toyoshima Y, Tada M, Oyake M, Aida I, Tomita I, et al. Pathology and sensitivity of current clinical criteria in corticobasal syndrome. *Mov Disord* (2014) 29(2):238–44. doi:10.1002/mds.25746
129. Kanazawa M, Thimohata T, Sato M, Onodera O, Tanaka K, Nishizawa M. Botulinum toxin A injections improve apraxia of eyelid opening without overt blepharospasm associated with neurodegenerative diseases. *Mov Disord* (2007) 22(4):597–8. doi:10.1002/mds.21367
130. Cardoso F, de Oliveira JT, Puccioni-Sohler M, Fernandes AR, de Mattos JP, Lopes-CendesI.EyeliddystoniainMachado-Josephdisease.*MovDisord*(2000) 15(5):1028–30. doi:10.1002/1531-8257(200009)15:5<1028::AID-MDS1047>3.0.CO;2-#
131. Cherian V, Foroozan R. Benign unilateral apraxia of eyelid opening. *Ophthalmology* (2010) 117(6):1265–8. doi:10.1016/j.ophtha.2009.10.032
132. Della Marca G, Losurdo A, Cordone S, Pilato F, Profice P, Testani E, et al. Teaching NeuroImages: awakening ptosis (unilateral hypnopompic eyelid palsy). *Neurology* (2013) 81(10):e71–2. doi:10.1212/WNL.0b013e3182a351e7
133. Aramideh M, Kwa IH, Brans JW, Speelman JD, Verbeeten B Jr. Apraxia of eyelid closure accompanied by denial of eye opening. *Mov Disord* (1997) 12(6):1105–8. doi:10.1002/mds.870120651
134. Bonelli RM, Niederwieser G. Apraxia of eyelid closure in Huntington's disease. *J Neural Transm* (2002) 109(2):197–201. doi:10.1007/s007020200016
135. Fukishima T, Hasegawa A, Matsubara N, Kolke R. An apraxia of eyelid closure in association with frontal lobe atrophy in a patient with amyotrophic lateral sclerosis. *Rinsho Shinkeigaku* (2007) 47(5):226–30.
136. Hirayama M, Kumano T, Aita T, Nakagawa H, Kuriyama M. Improvement of apraxia of eyelid opening by wearing goggles. *Lancet* (2000) 356(9239):1413. doi:10.1016/S0140-6736(00)02851-8
137. Ramasamy B, Rowe F, Freeman G, Owen M, Noonan C. Modified Lundie loops improve apraxia of eyelid opening. *J Neuroophthalmol* (2007) 27(1):32–5. doi:10.1097/WNO.0b013e3180334f0b
138. Dewey RB Jr, Maraganore DM. Isolated eyelid-opening apraxia: report of a new levodopa-responsive syndrome. *Neurology* (1994) 44(9):1752–4. doi:10.1212/WNL.44.9.1752
139. Yamada S, Matsuo K, Hirayama M, Sobue G. The effects of levodopa on apraxia of lid opening: a case report. *Neurology* (2004) 62(5):830–1. doi:10.1212/01.WNL.0000113751.19247.84
140. Lee KC, Finley R, Miller B. Apraxia of lid opening: dose-dependent response to carbidopa-levodopa. *Pharmacotherapy* (2004) 24(3):401–3. doi:10.1592/phco.24.4.401.33174
141. Krack P, Marion MH. "Apraxia of lid opening," a focal eyelid dystonia: clinical study of 32 patients. *Mov Disord* (1994) 9(6):610–5. doi:10.1002/mds.870090605

142. Tokisato K, Fukunaga K, Tokunaga M, Watanabe S, Nakanishi R, Yamanaga H. Aripiprazole can improve apraxia of eyelid opening in Parkinson's disease. *Intern Med* (2015) 54(23):3061–4. doi:10.2169/internalmedicine.54.4279
143. Eftekhari K, Choe CH, Vagefi MR, Gausas RE, Eckstein LA. Oral methylphenidate for the treatment of refractory facial dystonias. *Ophthal Plast Reconstr Surg* (2015) 31(3):e65–6. doi:10.1097/IOP.0000000000000079
144. Piccione F, Mancini E, Tonin P, Bizzarini M. Botulinum toxin treatment of apraxia of eyelid opening in progressive supranuclear palsy: report of two cases. *Arch Phys Med Rehabil* (1997) 78(5):525–9. doi:10.1016/S0003-9993(97)90169-6
145. Georgescu D, Vagefi MR, McMullan TF, McCann JD, Anderson RL. Upper eyelid myectomy in blepharospasm with associated apraxia of lid opening. *Am J Ophthalmol* (2008) 145(3):541–7. doi:10.1016/j.ajo.2007.10.017
146. Dressler D, Karapantzou C, Rohrbach S, Schneider S, Laskawi R. Frontalis suspension surgery to treat patients with blepharospasm and eyelid opening apraxia: long term results. *J Neural Transm* (2017) 124(2):253–7. doi:10.1007/s00702-016-1641-3
147. De Groot V, De Wilde F, Smet L, Tassignon MJ. Frontalis suspension combined with blepharoplasty as an effective treatment for blepharospasm associated with apraxia of eyelid opening. *Ophthal Plast Reconstr Surg* (2000) 16(1):34–8. doi:10.1097/00002341-200001000-00006
148. Baizabal-Carvallo JF, Jankovic J. Movement disorders induced by deep brain stimulation. *Parkinsonism Relat Disord* (2016) 25:1–9. doi:10.1016/j.parkreldis.2016.01.014
149. Tommasi G, Krack P, Fraix V, Pollak P. Effects of varying subthalamic nucleus stimulation on apraxia of lid opening in Parkinson's disease. *J Neurol* (2012) 259(1944):2592. doi:10.1007/s00415-012-6447-0
150. Umemura A, Toyoda T, Yamamoto K, Oka Y, Ishii F, Yamada K. Apraxia of eyelid opening after subthalamic deep brain stimulation may be caused by reduction of levodopa. *Parkinsonism Relat Disord* (2008) 14(8):655–7. doi:10.1016/j.parkreldis.2007.12.008
151. Weiss D, Wächter T, Breit S, Jacob SN, Pomper JK, Asmus F, et al. Involuntary eyelid closure after STN-DBS: evidence for different pathophysiological entities. *J Neurol Neurosurg Psychiatry* (2010) 81:1002–7. doi:10.1136/jnnp.2009.196691
152. Fuss G, Spiegel J, Magnus T, Moringlane JR, Becker G, Dillmann U. Improvement of apraxia of lid opening by STN-stimulation in a 70 year-old with Parkinson's disease: a case report. *Minim Invasive Neurosurg* (2004) 47(1):58–60. doi:10.1055/s-2003-812466
153. Goto S, Kihara K, Hamasaki T, Nishikawa S, Hirata Y, Ushio Y. Apraxia of lid opening is alleviated by pallidal stimulation in a patient with Parkinson's disease. *Eur J Neurol* (2000) 7(3):337–40. doi:10.1046/j.1468-1331.2000.00058.x
154. Skarf B. Normal and abnormal eyelid function. In: Miller NR, Newman NJ, Biousse V, Kerrison JB, editors. *Walsh & Hoyt's Clinical Neuro-Ophthalmology*. Philadelphia, PA: Lippincott, Williams, & Wilkins (2004). p. 1177–229.

11

Ocular Tremor in Parkinson's Disease: Discussion, Debate and Controversy

Diego Kaski[1,2] and Adolfo M. Bronstein[1,2]*

[1] *Division of Brain Sciences, Department of Neuro-Otology, Imperial College London, London, UK,* [2] *Department of Neuro-Otology, University College London, National Hospital for Neurology and Neurosurgery, London, UK*

***Correspondence:**
Diego Kaski
d.kaski@imperial.ac.uk*

The identification of ocular tremor in a small cohort of patients with Parkinson's disease (PD) had lay somewhat dormant until the recent report of a pervasive ocular tremor as a universal finding in a large PD cohort that was, however, generally absent from a cohort of age-matched healthy subjects. The reported tremor had frequency characteristics similar to those of PD limb tremor, but the amplitude and frequency of the tremor did not correlate with clinical tremor ratings. Much controversy ensued as to the origin of such a tremor, and specifically as to whether a pervasive ocular tremor was a fundamental feature of PD, or rather a compensatory eye oscillation secondary to a transmitted head tremor, and thus a measure of a normal vestibulo-ocular reflex. In this mini review, we summarize some of the evidence for and against the case for a pervasive ocular tremor in PD and suggest future experiments that may help resolve these conflicting opinions.

Keywords: eye oscillations, ocular tremor, Parkinson's disease, vestibulo-ocular reflex, head tremor

INTRODUCTION

Parkinson's disease (PD) is a neurodegenerative condition characterized by motor features including bradykinesia, rigidity, tremor, and postural instability (1) and non-motor features such as anosmia, constipation, sleep disturbance, sexual impairment, cognitive impairment, and apathy (2). While the clinical phenotype in patients with PD may vary, a majority of patients will present with clinically appreciable tremor (3). The neural correlate of PD tremor has not been fully elucidated, but its generation appears to involve supraspinal oscillators within the cerebello–thalamo–cortical network (4–6). While PD tremor affects mostly the limbs, PD patients may have tremor of the tongue, lip, or chin (7). Early writings on PD state that head tremor is not a feature of PD, a view that remains commonly accepted, and a feature that differentiates PD tremor from essential tremor (8). Nevertheless, head tremor in PD has been described. A case series of five PD patients with head tremor revealed head tremor characteristics typical of PD limb tremor, including an increase in head tremor with mental calculation, disappearance during action, dopa-responsiveness, and similar tremor frequency to limb tremor (4–6 Hz) (9). In a single patient from this series, the authors performed electrophysiological recordings showing that the limb tremor and head tremor were coherent at their fundamental frequencies. The authors further ruled out mechanical conduction of the tremor by recording electromyography from the neck and arm muscles (9). It appears then that PD tremor may occur across different body segments independently, but simultaneously. In a separate report, a single PD patient was shown to have a tongue tremor and limb tremor of equal frequency (5 Hz) (10). Finally, Hunker and Abbs examined Parkinsonian rest tremor of the lips, jaw, tongue, and index finger in three PD patients, using electromyography (11). They found uniform resting tremor frequencies across orofacial and upper limb sites (11). Given that PD tremor can manifest at multiple sites simultaneously, and be synchronized, one question is whether ocular tremor might arise as a further tremor site in PD.

The wide availability of eye-tracking devices has seen a growth of research studies exploring oculomotor control across a range of clinical conditions, including PD. An early recording of ocular oscillations in a small cohort of patients with PD failed to receive further attention until a more recent report of a "pervasive ocular tremor" that was universally present in a cohort of 112 PD patients and mostly absent in healthy controls. Magnetic head tracking in a subset of patients did not reveal any tremulous head movements, implying that the observable ocular tremor was independent of head motion. Nevertheless, given the lack of other reports of ocular fixation instability across decades of eye movement recordings in patients with Parkinsonism, the possible origin of the pervasive ocular tremor generated significant discussion and controversy.

OCULAR TREMOR IN PD

Using infrared reflectometry, Duval and Beuter first described findings of ocular tremor in three out of five patients with PD (12). Ocular oscillations were mostly uniocular (in two patients), and in these localized ipsilateral to the side of the body most affected by PD. Those three patients had ocular oscillations of similar frequency to their resting limb tremor. There was no relationship, however, between the amplitude of the eye oscillations and amplitude of resting limb tremor. In these patients with asymmetrical eye oscillations, the presence of square wave jerks in both eyes, equal in amplitude, meant that the monocular nature of the oscillation could not be attributed to an artifact of scaling between the two eyes. Patient's head was stabilized by asking patients to bite onto a wooden tongue depressor, attached to the chair on which they sat for the eye movement recordings. The authors argued that the ocular tremor was due to an "attractor effect" on movement related to the generator of the limb rest tremor, which would explain why the frequency of the ocular tremor in their three PD patients was similar to the frequency of the rest tremor of the limbs (13). Nevertheless, it is possible that such an ocular tremor may have a neural oscillator that is independent to the limb oscillator, particularly as coherence values from tremor data from each eye with rest tremor were different for two of the five PD patients. Uniocular tremor has been reported following an isolated olivary nucleus lesion (14).

"PERVASIVE OCULAR TREMOR" IN PD

Gitchel and colleagues studied the eye movements of 112 patients with idiopathic PD during steady fixation (15). They identified a continuous oscillatory fixation instability that they termed "pervasive ocular tremor" in *every* PD patient. The oscillations had an average fundamental frequency of 5.7 Hz (i.e., within the range of the limb tremor in PD; 4–7 Hz), a mean horizontal amplitude of 0.27°, and mean vertical amplitude of 0.33°. The tremor persisted for the duration of the recording, although the waveform characteristics were variable (15). **Figure 1** taken from the original manuscript shows a typical 1.2 s recording of the ocular tremor. The authors did not use head restraint but recorded head movements using a magnetic tracker in a subset of 62 PD patients and 31 controls; no head oscillation was detected in any subject.

PATHOPHYSIOLOGY OF OCULAR TREMOR

In order to try to understand the possible neural mechanism underlying the observed ocular tremor (fixation instability) in PD, one might first consider the necessary requirements of the oculomotor system to maintain steady fixation. Thus, the fixation target must rest upon the retinal fovea—an area of approximately 0.5° in diameter with the highest visual acuity (16). In addition, the image must not move more than approximately 5°/s across the retina (17), otherwise the subject would experience oscillopsia (illusory motion of the visual world). When the head is free, steady fixation thus requires the vestibulo-ocular reflex, which compensates for head movements by generating an eye movement of the same velocity but opposite direction to the head movement. If the vestibulo-ocular reflex is absent, even cardiac pulsations transmitted to the head can disrupt vision (18). When the head of a healthy subject is immobilized (e.g., with a bite bar), the subject's gaze does not in fact remain completely still but is disrupted by microtremor, microsaccades, and ocular drifts (19, 20). Therefore, could the "pervasive ocular tremor" observed in patients with PD be one of these types of eye movements?

Microtremor has a mean frequency of approximately 84 Hz and ranges from 70 to 103 Hz. Due to its high frequency and very small amplitude (1 photoreceptor width, <0.5 arcmin), microtremor does not disrupt vision (21). Microsaccades are rapid movements with frequencies of 1–2 Hz, and typically less than 1° in size. They are thought to prevent perceptual fading during fixation (22, 23). Recent work suggests that square wave intrusions, a common finding in patients with neurodegenerative movement disorders, lie on a continuum with microsaccades (24, 25). Smooth intersaccadic drifts during attempted fixation are thought to be under the control of smooth eye movements (26) and typically do not exceed 0.1°/s, unless visual feedback is removed, for example, by switching from a light to a dark environment (27). Thus, despite all these eye movements that occur during steady fixation, the SD of gaze is typically <0.2°, so while the eyes are not perfectly still, the image of interest stays mostly over the fovea, and image motion is not perceptible. Thus, given the characteristics of the "pervasive ocular tremor" in PD, they cannot be considered microtremor, microsaccades, or ocular drifts.

In contrast to these physiological "fixation ocular movements," blurred vision and oscillopsia occur when abnormal eye movements, such as acquired pendular nystagmus, cause movement of the retinal image greater than exceeds 5°/s (21). Gitchel and colleagues in fact commented that the pervasive ocular tremor observed in patients with PD was reminiscent of pendular

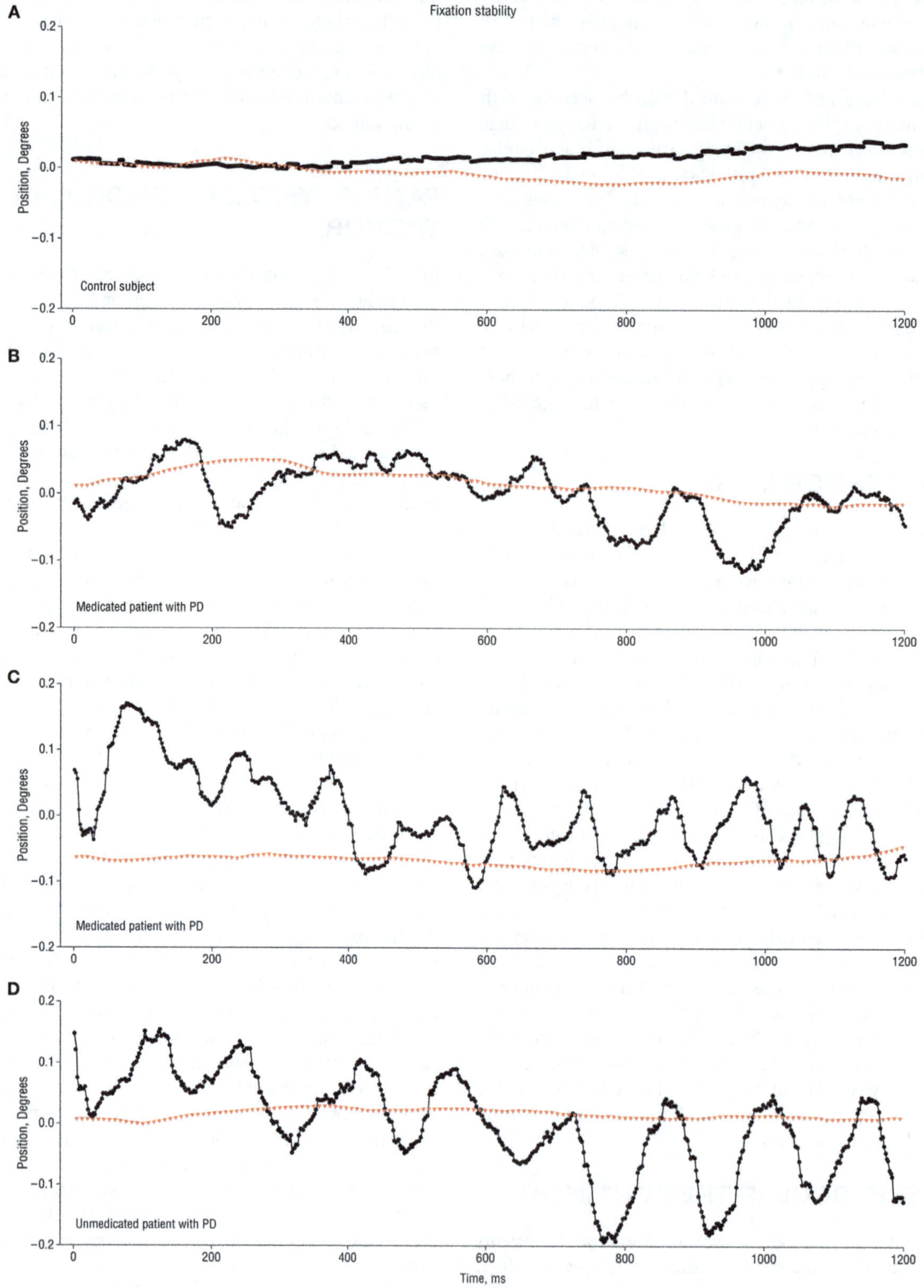

FIGURE 1 | 1.2 s recording traces of ocular tremor in patients with Parkinson's disease (PD) and healthy control [from Ref. (15) with permission]. **(A)** Eye movement recording from a control subject showing stable fixation (no ocular tremor). **(B,C)** Two different medicated PD patients showing eye oscillations of variable amplitude and approximately 6 Hz **(B)** and 10 Hz **(C)**. **(D)** Ocular tremor in an unmedicated PD patient with a larger amplitude eye oscillation of approximately 10 Hz frequency. Note the absence of any head tremor in all traces. Black circles represent horizontal eye movements, with positive values indicting rightward eye movements, and red triangles indicating rotational head movement along the azimuth.

nystagmus given the sinusoidal waveform and similar fundamental frequencies (15). They acknowledge, however, several notable differences to pendular nytsagmus, such as the smaller amplitude of the waveform they reported in their PD patients, compared to that normally seen in pendular nystagmus. Moreover, in pendular nystagmus, the phase of the oscillations is reset by saccades and this was not the case in the ocular tremor described in PD patients. Most importantly perhaps, acquired pendular nystagmus causes oscillopsia, and this was not reported by any of the PD patients studied by Gitchel et al. (15).

Finally, it is conceivable that the pervasive ocular tremor in PD stems from subtle head oscillation, inducing a normal VOR response, causing an oscillation of the eyes in response to head movement. We now summarize the evidence in support of a pervasive ocular tremor, and the evidence in support of apparent ocular tremor resulting from head oscillation (and an intact VOR).

EVIDENCE IN SUPPORT OF A PERVASIVE OCULAR TREMOR INHERENT TO PD

1. In their original description of ocular tremor in patients with PD, Duval and Beuter did not find a systematic or direct relationship between fluctuations in rest tremor of the hand and fluctuations of eye movement amplitude during ocular fixation in patients with PD (12), suggesting that the ocular tremor was independent of the limb rest tremor.
2. Duval and Beuter asked their PD subjects to bite onto a tongue depressor attached to the structure of the chair to stabilize the head during eye in space ocular movement recordings (12). The authors, however, acknowledged the possibility that head movement occurred (an accelerometer was not used to record head movements), resulting in activation of the vestibulo-ocular reflex, that could in turn explain the eye oscillations. One wonders whether asking patients to bite onto a wooden tongue depressor may itself generate a head or jaw tremor. Nevertheless, this would not explain why the oscillations were so asymmetrical between the two eyes. Moreover, the fact that all 112 PD patients in the cohort from Gitchel et al. displayed a recordable eye tremor, including unmedicated patients, suggests that ocular tremor may be a fundamental property of PD (15). Moreover, only 2 of 60 healthy controls in the study by Gitchel et al. were also found to have an ocular tremor despite no signs of Parkinsonism, one of whom then developed PD within 3 years of follow-up (15).
3. A magnetic tracker was employed to evaluate the possible contribution of head motion to the presence of the ocular tremor. The authors, however, consistently recorded no head tremor in a subset of 62 PD patients (who did, however, have ocular tremor). Electromagnetic motion recorders provide accurate displacement measures for large-amplitude, low frequency movement. Conversely, they are less accurate for low amplitude, high frequency movement, for which accelerometers are superior (28). In this light, Gitchel et al. recorded eye movements in a further subset of eight patients (29), during simultaneous head movement recording using both a triaxial accelerometer and electromagnetic tracker. They again failed to record any appreciable head tremor, despite evidence of continuous ocular tremor.
4. Indeed, ocular tremor was observed in this group of eight PD patients irrespective of whether the head was free or fixed (by mean of a head holding device and a dental impression bite plate), implying that head motion had no effect upon the presence or magnitude of the ocular tremor (29).
5. Gitchel et al. found no relationship between the amplitude of ocular tremor and clinical rating of arm tremor across their total cohort (15). This suggests that ocular tremor occurs independently of appendicular tremor and hints at a different neural generator for the tremor. Similarly, many patients from their large PD cohort had no appreciable appendicular tremor.
6. A previous study in patients with essential tremor (who often manifest head tremor) found no evidence of ocular instability, further suggesting a decorrelation between head tremor and ocular tremor (30). In this study, head tremor was assessed using a magnetic tracking device and was only apparent in two patients with ET. This is surprising given the prominent head tremor in ET patients (8).

EVIDENCE IN SUPPORT OF APPARENT OCULAR TREMOR RESULTING FROM HEAD OSCILLATION

Refuting the non-existence of a proposed clinical sign poses inherent challenges, all the more so in the case of a Parkinsonian ocular tremor that has never been observed clinically nor contributes to any visual disability in these patients. Scientific studies in small numbers of patients have suggested that the ocular tremor described in patients with PD may indeed be related to head oscillations, indicative of an intact VOR.

1. Apart from the early report by Duval and Beuter (12), and despite extensive oculographic recordings in PD, ocular tremor had not previously been described. In fact, Leigh and colleagues looked back through early oculomotor recordings in PD—using the goldstandard scleral search coil technique—and were not able to identify any evidence of ocular tremor in their studies of Parkinsonian patients over the past 30 years (31, 32), presumably because they used a chair-fixed restraint to stabilize the patients' heads (thus significantly reducing head oscillations).
2. Patients with head tremor and bilaterally *impaired VOR* have eye oscillations on fundoscopy (eye in space oscillations as there is a shift in gaze without any movement of the eyes relative to the head), termed pendular pseudonystagmus (33–35) of similar amplitude to that reported by Gitchel et al. (15). In this condition, gaze stability is negatively affected by the head tremor due to the insufficient vestibularly mediated compensatory eye movements. Patients, therefore, report oscillopsia and the clinician can observe oscillation of the fundus during ophthalmoscopy. The fact that most patients with head tremor do not report oscillopsia, nor do they show oscillation of the fundus, is testimony to how exquisitely tuned the VOR is to

generate high frequency compensatory eye movements. For this reason, a well know artifact in eye movement recordings in patients with head tremor is an apparent oscillation of the eye (eye-in-orbit as there is no shift in gaze with a normal VOR) in the oculographic trace, which is reduced during forced immobilization of the head. However, it is also known that complete immobilization of the head in human patients with significant head tremor is extremely challenging; both in patients with essential (33) and Parkinsonian tremor of the head (36), a very significant reduction of the head and eye oscillation can be obtained but complete elimination is rarely feasible.

3. Eye movements were recorded in two consecutive PD patients attending an eye movements and balance clinic. These patients also underwent simultaneous recording of head and limb movements using an android application triaxial accelerometer (36), with comparable resolution to standard axial accelerometers (37). Despite different limb tremor amplitudes in these patients, ocular oscillations were identified in both patients. These were accompanied by a recordable head tremor that had the same fundamental frequency and high coherence with both the eye oscillation and a recordable limb tremor (**Figure 2**). The eye oscillations

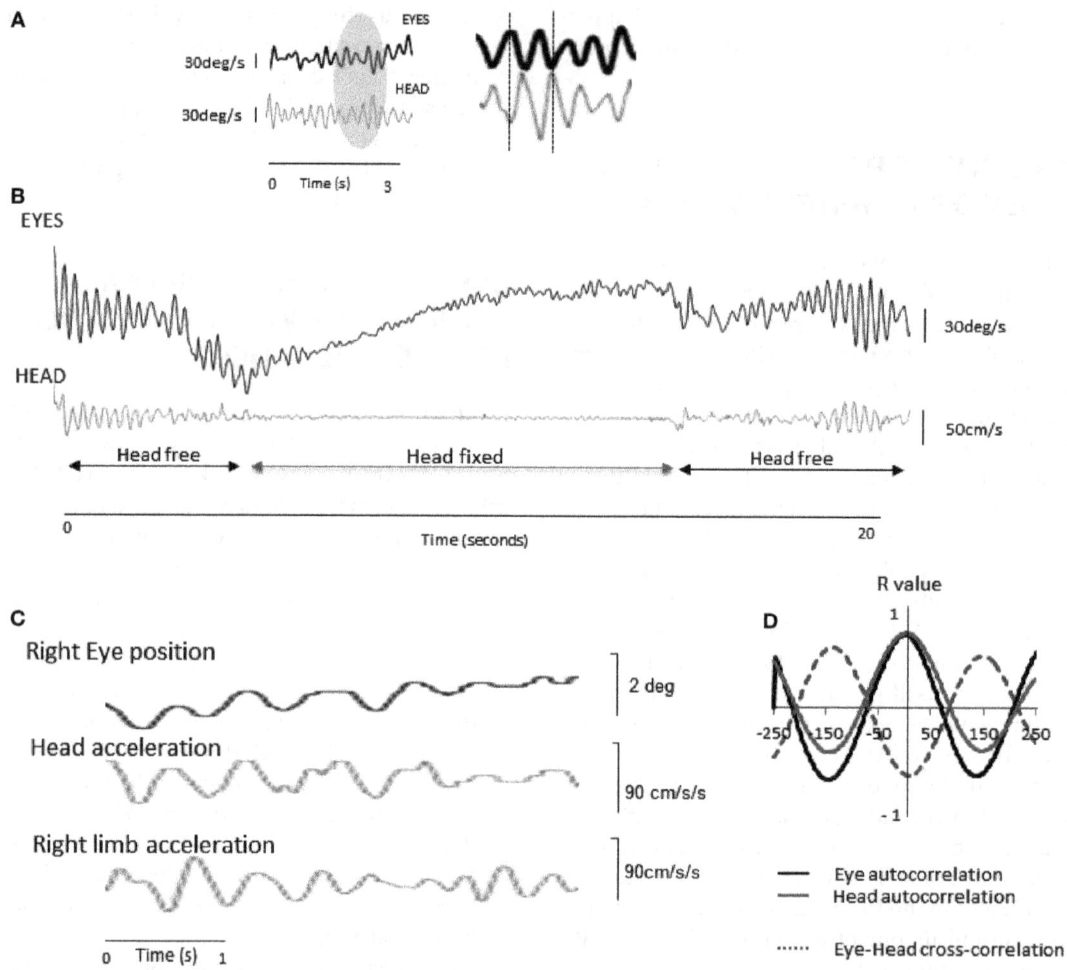

FIGURE 2 | Eye and head oscillations in two patients with Parkinson's disease (PD) [taken from Ref. (36) with permission]. **(A)** Patient 1—a 3 s recording of the eye (infrared video-oculography) and head (accelerometry) movements in a patient with PD with the head free.* To the right, a magnified view of the recordings reveals that the ocular oscillation is in antiphase to the head tremor. **(B)** When the head is physically restrained, the ocular tremor decreases in amplitude, indicating that the ocular tremor is intrinsically linked to the head tremor, and thus part of an intact VOR response. The ocular tremor is not abolished as the head can never be completely immobilized. **(C)** Raw oculographic, head, and limb tremor traces in a separate PD patient, without head restraint. The amplitude of the head and ocular tremor was smaller than in patient 1, in keeping with a smaller right limb tremor. Head tremor was not clinically visible in this patient. Head and limb oscillations were recorded from linear accelerometers. The eye and head traces appear in phase as a result of 180-degree phase shift between position (eye) and acceleration (head). **(D)** Autocorrelations for the eye and head traces and cross-correlation between the two signals over a 500-ms window for a fundamental frequency of 4.5 Hz. R values are shown in the *y* axis. *NB: In **(A)** and **(B)** head and eye traces are expressed in angular velocity units. Head acceleration values were, therefore, digitally integrated (linear acceleration to linear velocity), and corrected for eccentricity (tangential linear velocity to angular velocity, by taking into account occiput to head rotational axis distance, approximately 10 cm) using standard equations. As a leftward head rotation induces rightward occiput motion, the accelerometer trace has been inverted to correct for polarity. Finally, eye displacement recordings have been digitally differentiated (degrees to degrees/s).

were in the opposite direction (antiphase) to the head oscillation and dampened by physically restraining the head (36). This suggests that the ocular tremor is a compensatory eye movement secondary perhaps to a head tremor transmitted from the limb. The fact that these findings led to opposite conclusions to the study by Gitchel et al. raises important questions about the technical aspects of the data acquisition and patient population studied. Gitchel and colleagues used a magnetic tracker device rather than an accelerometer to record head movements; Kaski and colleagues suggest accelerometers are superior to magnetic tracking devices to record low amplitude high frequency tremor. In their follow-up study, Gitchel and colleagues used both a triaxial accelerometer and magnetic tracking device to record head tremor in eight PD patients. They found a "complete (three dimensional) lack of head movement" in these patients. Given the similarities in the accelerometers employed, the lack of head movement may relate to the use of individualized bite plates to avoid head motion. Nevertheless, such a finding remains interesting given the difficulty in achieving complete head stabilization, even with the use of bite plates, in some oculographic studies in patients with prominent head tremor (33).

4. A notable difference between the ocular tremor of PD and other known eye movements is that the pervasive ocular tremor was reportedly unaffected by "saccades, blinks, or other eye movements" (15). In contrast, every other form of ocular oscillation has been reported to be "influenced by saccades, gaze angle, convergence, or vestibular stimuli" (21). This would, therefore, suggest that the source for PD pervasive ocular tremor lies outside of the ocular motor system, such as head tremor.
5. Involuntary eye oscillations, such as in patients with acquired pendular nystagmus or downbeat nystagmus syndrome, cause troublesome oscillopsia (21). The small amplitude of the pervasive ocular tremor recorded in PD patients may have been too small to displace the fixation target from the fovea, but their high frequency would cause their root mean square velocity to exceed 5°/s, which would be expected to induce oscillopsia (38, 39). One might argue that a large root mean square retinal slip value could be accounted for by a few extreme peak values during visual fixation, whereby the majority of the eye movements are within a tolerable low-velocity range that would allow for stable vision. It has been shown, however, that root mean square velocity values of retinal slip are of clinical relevance to gaze stabilization (39).
6. A continuous eye oscillation at approximately 5 Hz and approximately 0.3° (as in "pervasive ocular tremor") should be visible during direct ophthalmoscopy (40), which amplifies the retinal image by upto a factor of 15. Indeed, ophthalmoscopy is a sensitive method for detecting eye movements (14), even as small as 0.1° [e.g., microflutter (41)]. The pervasive ocular tremor described by Gitchel et al. (15) should, therefore, be visible with an ophthalmoscope and this has never been reported in the literature. In response to this, Gitchel and colleagues oscillated a prosthetic eye using a galvanometer motor over a range of amplitudes and frequencies but did not observe oscillations of the scleral vessels at very small amplitudes (42). The properties of a prosthetic eye (and in particular the ocular media) are inherently different to the living eyeball, and therefore, further fundoscopic studies in PD patients are required to clarify this issue.
7. Duval and Beuter described uniocular tremor in patients with PD (12), which is different to the bilateral ocular tremor reported by Gitchel et al. (15). Uniocular microtremor has been seen in a patient with asymptomatic oculopalatal tremor secondary to haemorrhagic injury affecting the inferior olivary nucleus (14). This raises the question of whether the uniocular tremor described in patients with PD by Duval and Beuter had pathology affecting the inferior olivary nucleus, rather than the tremor being a fundamental feature of PD.

CLINICAL IMPLICATIONS

Because it was posited that the pervasive ocular tremor might be a clinical biomarker for PD, including in the diagnosis at the pre-symptomatic stage, it is important to scrutinize the findings of Gitchel et al. before the presence of ocular tremor gains wide acceptance as a biomarker for PD. Interestingly, electromyography has revealed rhythmical muscle activity in patients with PD despite no clinical tremor (43). This suggests that there may be a subclinical tremor in patients with PD, and that such a tremor could be transmitted to the head and manifest as an ocular tremor if the head is not fixed. Further work is needed to identify whether head tremor is indeed a ubiquitous finding in patients with PD, irrespective of clinical tremor, and whether such tremor could be identified using eye movement recordings. In such case, one would also need to find an explanation for the absence of oscillopsia in PD patients.

FUTURE DIRECTIONS

Further research from different laboratories is warranted to investigate whether patients with PD do indeed show impaired visual fixation behavior, and to systematically study the characteristics of any ocular tremor that might be detected. For such a study, eye movements should be recorded using high-resolution techniques such as scleral search coil, infrared eye tracking, or video-oculography. The head should ideally be immobilized using a custom-made bite bar, or the eye tracker should be insensitive to movements of the device with respect to the subject's head (as is available on several modern eye trackers). There should be simultaneous recording of the eyes, head, and distal limb, ensuring that the devices are appropriately calibrated, and the signals are synchronized. Tremor recording of the head and limbs should be performed using accelerometers rather than position tracking devices. Signals should, therefore, be acquired at the same sampling rate and in the same plane (e.g., yaw and pitch planes). Tremor frequency, amplitude, and coherence between tremor sites should be assessed. Such a study would benefit from including patients with a range of tremor syndromes and in PD preferably include assessments after the withdrawal of medication to exclude possible dopaminergic-related effects.

AUTHOR CONTRIBUTIONS

DK reviewed the literature and compiled the manuscript and figures. AB reviewed the literature and approved the final version of the manuscript.

REFERENCES

1. Obeso JA, Rodríguez-Oroz MC, Benitez-Temino B, Blesa FJ, Guridi J, Marin C, et al. Functional organization of the basal ganglia: therapeutic implications for Parkinson's disease. *Mov Disord* (2008) 23(Suppl 3):S548–59. doi:10.1002/mds.22062
2. Chaudhuri KR, Schapira AH. Non-motor symptoms of Parkinson's disease: dopaminergic pathophysiology and treatment. *Lancet Neurol* (2009) 8:464–74. doi:10.1016/S1474-4422(09)70068-7
3. Martin WE, Loewenson RB, Resch JA, Baker AB. Parkinson's disease. Clinical analysis of 100 patients. *Neurology* (1973) 23:783–90. doi:10.1212/WNL.23.8.783
4. Helmich RC, Hallett M, Deuschl G, Toni I, Bloem BR. Cerebral causes and consequences of Parkinsonian resting tremor: a tale of two circuits? *Brain* (2012) 135:3206–26. doi:10.1093/brain/aws023
5. Helmich RC, Janssen MJR, Oyen WJG, Bloem BR, Toni I. Pallidal dysfunction drives a cerebellothalamic circuit into Parkinson tremor. *Ann Neurol* (2011) 69:269–81. doi:10.1002/ana.22361
6. Duval C, Daneault J-F, Hutchison WD, Sadikot AF. A brain network model explaining tremor in Parkinson's disease. *Neurobiol Dis* (2015) 85:49–59. doi:10.1016/j.nbd.2015.10.009
7. Jankovic J. Parkinson's disease: clinical features and diagnosis. *J Neurol Neurosurg Psychiatry* (2008) 79:368–76. doi:10.1136/jnnp.2007.131045
8. Bain PG, Findley LJ, Thompson PD, Gresty MA, Rothwell JC, Harding AE, et al. A study of hereditary essential tremor. *Brain* (1994) 117:805–24. doi:10.1093/brain/117.4.805
9. Roze E, Coêlho-Braga MC, Gayraud D, Legrand AP, Trocello JM, Fénelon G, et al. Head tremor in Parkinson's disease. *Mov Disord* (2006) 21:1245–8. doi:10.1002/mds.20918
10. Jaulent P, Laurencin C, Robert H, Thobois S. Parkinson's disease revealed by a resting tongue tremor. *Mov Disord* (2015) 2:432–3. doi:10.1002/mdc3.12202
11. Hunker CJ, Abbs JH. Uniform frequency of parkinsonian resting tremor in the lips, jaw, tongue, and index finger. *Mov Disord* (1990) 5:71–7. doi:10.1002/mds.870050117
12. Duval C, Beuter A. Fluctuations in tremor at rest and eye movements during ocular fixation in subjects with Parkinson's disease. *Parkinsonism Relat Disord* (1998) 4:91–7. doi:10.1016/S1353-8020(98)00023-6
13. Logigian E, Hefter H, Reiners K, Freund H-J. Does tremor pace repetitive voluntary motor behavior in Parkinson's disease? *Ann Neurol* (1991) 30:172–9. doi:10.1002/ana.410300208
14. Jang L, Borruat FX. Micronystagmus of oculopalatal tremor. *Neurology* (2013) 80:e27. doi:10.1212/WNL.0b013e31827debc3
15. Gitchel GT, Wetzel PA, Baron MS. Pervasive ocular tremor in patients with Parkinson disease. *Arch Neurol* (2012) 69:1011–7. doi:10.1001/archneurol.2012.70
16. Jacobs RJ. Visual resolution and contour interaction in the fovea and periphery. *Vision Res* (1979) 19:1187–95. doi:10.1016/0042-6989(79)90183-4
17. Demer JL, Amjadi F. Dynamic visual acuity of normal subjects during vertical optotype and head motion. *Invest Ophthalmol Vis Sci* (1993) 34:1894–906.
18. Anonymous. LIVING without a balancing mechanism. *N Engl J Med* (1952) 246:458–60. doi:10.1056/NEJM195203202461207
19. Martinez-Conde S, Macknik SL. Fixational eye movements across vertebrates: comparative dynamics, physiology, and perception. *J Vis* (2008) 8:1–16. doi:10.1167/8.14.28
20. Martinez-Conde S, Macknik SL, Hubel DH. The role of fixational eye movements in visual perception. *Nat Rev Neurosci* (2004) 5:229–40. doi:10.1038/nrn1348
21. Leigh RJ, Zee DS. *The Neurology of Eye Movements*. Oxford University Press (2015). Available from: http://www.oxfordmedicine.com/view/10.1093/med/9780199969289.001.0001/med-9780199969289
22. McCamy MB, Otero-Millan J, Macknik SL, Yang Y, Troncoso XG, Baer SM, et al. Microsaccadic efficacy and contribution to foveal and peripheral vision. *J Neurosci* (2012) 32:9194–204. doi:10.1523/JNEUROSCI.0515-12.2012
23. Martinez-Conde S, Macknik SL, Troncoso XG, Dyar TA. Microsaccades counteract visual fading during fixation. *Neuron* (2006) 49:297–305. doi:10.1016/j.neuron.2005.11.033
24. Martinez-Conde S, Otero-Millan J, Macknik SL. The impact of microsaccades on vision: towards a unified theory of saccadic function. *Nat Rev Neurosci* (2013) 14:83–96. doi:10.1038/nrn3405
25. Otero-Millan J, Serra A, Leigh RJ, Troncoso XG, Macknik SL, Martinez-Conde S. Distinctive features of saccadic intrusions and microsaccades in progressive supranuclear palsy. *J Neurosci* (2011) 31:4379–87. doi:10.1523/JNEUROSCI.2600-10.2011
26. Murphy BJ, Kowler E, Steinman RM. Slow oculomotor control in the presence of moving backgrounds. *Vision Res* (1975) 15:1263–8. doi:10.1016/0042-6989(75)90172-8
27. Schneider RM, Thurtell MJ, Eisele S, Lincoff N, Bala E, Leigh RJ. Neurological basis for eye movements of the blind. *PLoS One* (2013) 8:e56556. doi:10.1371/journal.pone.0056556
28. Kaski D, Saifee TA, Buckwell D, Bronstein AM. Reply to letter-eye oscillations in Parkinson's disease relate to the vestibulo-ocular reflex. *Mov Disord* (2013) 28(6):845–6. doi:10.1002/mds.25465
29. Gitchel GT, Wetzel PA, Qutubuddin A, Baron MS. Experimental support that ocular tremor in Parkinson's disease does not originate from head movement. *Parkinsonism Relat Disord* (2014) 20:743–7. doi:10.1016/j.parkreldis.2014.03.028
30. Gitchel GT, Wetzel PA, Baron MS. Slowed saccades and increased square wave jerks in essential tremor. *Tremor Other Hyperkinet Mov (N Y)* (2013) 3. doi:10.7916/D8251GXN
31. Otero-Millan J, Schneider R, Leigh RJ, Macknik SL, Martinez-Conde S. Saccades during attempted fixation in parkinsonian disorders and recessive ataxia: from microsaccades to square-wave jerks. *PLoS One* (2013) 8:e58535. doi:10.1371/journal.pone.0058535
32. Chen AL, Riley DE, King SA, Joshi AC, Serra A, Liao K, et al. The disturbance of gaze in progressive supranuclear palsy: implications for pathogenesis. *Front Neurol* (2010) 1:147. doi:10.3389/fneur.2010.00147
33. Bronstein AM, Gresty MA, Mossman SS. Pendular pseudonystagmus arising as a combination of head tremor and vestibular failure. *Neurology* (1992) 42:1527–31. doi:10.1212/WNL.42.8.1527
34. Yen MT, Herdman SJ, Tusa RJ. Oscillopsia and pseudonystagmus in kidney transplant patients. *Am J Ophthalmol* (1999) 128:768–70. doi:10.1016/S0002-9394(99)00249-4
35. Shaikh AG, Reich S, Zee DS. Pseudonystagmus – clinical features and quantitative characteristics. *Nat Rev Neurol* (2010) 6:519–23. doi:10.1038/nrneurol.2010.103
36. Kaski D, Saifee TA, Buckwell D, Bronstein AM. Ocular tremor in Parkinson's disease is due to head oscillation. *Mov Disord* (2013) 28:534–7. doi:10.1002/mds.25342
37. Nishiguchi S, Yamada M, Nagai K, Mori S, Kajiwara Y, Sonoda T, et al. Reliability and validity of gait analysis by android-based smartphone. *Telemed J E Health* (2012) 18:292–6. doi:10.1089/tmj.2011.0132
38. Leigh RJ, Martinez-Conde S. Tremor of the eyes, or of the head, in Parkinson's disease? *Mov Disord* (2013) 28:691–3. doi:10.1002/mds.25478
39. Crane BT, Demer JL. Human gaze stabilization during natural activities: translation, rotation, magnification, and target distance effects. *J Neurophysiol* (1997) 78:2129–44.
40. Younge BR, McLaren JW, Brown WL. Retinal image stability in head tremor and nystagmus: counterintuitive observations. *J Neuroophthalmol* (2007) 27:107–14. doi:10.1097/WNO.0b013e318064e516

41. Shaikh AG, Miura K, Optican LM, Ramat S, Leigh RJ, Zee DS. A new familial disease of saccadic oscillations and limb tremor provides clues to mechanisms of common tremor disorders. *Brain* (2007) 130:3020–31. doi:10.1093/brain/awm240
42. Baron MS, Gitchel GT, Wetzel PA. Scientific data support that ocular tremor is genuine and unrelated to head movement. *Parkinsonism Relat Disord* (2014) 20:1449–50. doi:10.1016/j.parkreldis.2014.09.032
43. Shulman LM, Singer C, Bean JA, Weiner WJ. Internal tremor in patients with Parkinson's disease. *Mov Disord* (1996) 11:3–7. doi:10.1002/mds.870110103

12

Novel Eye Movement Disorders in Whipple's Disease—Staircase Horizontal Saccades, Gaze-Evoked Nystagmus and Esotropia

*Aasef G. Shaikh[1,2,3,4] and Fatema F. Ghasia[1,5]**

[1] Daroff-Dell'Osso Ocular Motility Laboratory, Cleveland VA Medical Center, Cleveland, VA, United States, [2] Department of Neurology, Case Western Reserve University, Cleveland, OH, United States, [3] Neurological Institute, University Hospitals, Cleveland, OH, United States, [4] Neurology Service, Louis Stokes, Cleveland, VA, United States, [5] Cole Eye Institute, Cleveland Clinic, Cleveland, OH, United States

***Correspondence:**
Fatema F. Ghasia
fatemaghasia@gmail.com

Whipple's disease, a rare systemic infectious disorder, is complicated by the involvement of the central nervous system in about 5% of cases. Oscillations of the eyes and the jaw, called oculo-masticatory myorhythmia, are pathognomonic of the central nervous system involvement but are often absent. Typical manifestations of the central nervous system Whipple's disease are cognitive impairment, parkinsonism mimicking progressive supranuclear palsy with vertical saccade slowing, and up-gaze range limitation. We describe a unique patient with the central nervous system Whipple's disease who had typical features, including parkinsonism, cognitive impairment, and up-gaze limitation; but also had diplopia, esotropia with mild horizontal (abduction more than adduction) limitation, and vertigo. The patient also had gaze-evoked nystagmus and staircase horizontal saccades. Latter were thought to be due to mal-programmed small saccades followed by a series of corrective saccades. The saccades were disconjugate due to the concurrent strabismus. Also, we noted disconjugacy in the slow phase of gaze-evoked nystagmus. The disconjugacy of the slow phase of gaze-evoked nystagmus was larger during monocular viewing condition. We propose that interaction of the strabismic drifts of the covered eyes and the nystagmus drift, putatively at the final common pathway might lead to such disconjugacy.

Keywords: neurodegeneration, progressive supranuclear palsy, slow saccade, parkinsonism, strabismus

INTRODUCTION

Whipple's disease is a rare systemic disorder caused by a Gram-positive bacterium *Tropheryma whippelli* (1, 2). Although malabsorption syndrome is the typical manifestation of the Whipple's disease, in 5% of cases it primarily and initially involves the central nervous system (3). Prominent cognitive symptoms including hypersomnolence had led to the identification of central nervous system Whipple as a form of "unclassifiable encephalitis" (4). In addition to robust cognitive dysfunction and hypersomnolence; complete vertical ophthalmoplegia, approximately 1 Hz convergent–divergent eye oscillations, and concurrent contractions of the masticatory muscles are the hallmark of the central nervous system Whipple's disease (5–7). The Whipple's disease can present without its classic manifestations, but with prominent parkinsonism and slowing and curved trajectories of vertical saccades (8, 9). The selective deficit of the vertical saccades in patients with Whipple's disease were attributed to the involvement of the rostral interstitial nucleus of the medial longitudinal fasciculus (riMLF), the anatomical substrate for vertical saccade generation (10). While vertical saccades in Whipple's disease are prominently affected, the horizontal saccades generated at paramedian pontine reticular formation are also often affected (8, 9).

Here, we present the quantitative study of abnormal horizontal saccades in Whipple's disease. In addition to quantitatively investigating the horizontal saccades in Whipple's disease, our study delves into the pathophysiology of series of hypometric saccades (staircase saccades) in Whipple's disease. Delineating these mechanisms will facilitate our understanding of the pathophysiology and heterogeneity of saccadic disorders. The objective measures will provide reliable and possible prodromal disease markers that will help the early differential diagnosis of disorders affecting the saccade velocity. Our Whipple's disease patient also had two other atypical features—gaze-evoked eye nystagmus and esotropia.

METHODS

Clinical Description

A 73-year-old man with a history of Whipple's disease presented for diplopia, change in gait, imbalance, memory loss, behavioral changes, and diarrhea. Cognitive examination revealed the score of 21/30 on Montreal Cognitive Assessment (MoCA, version 7.3). Examination of cranial nerves revealed vertical gaze restriction, absent vertical optokinetic nystagmus, however, vestibulo-ocular reflex was intact vertically and horizontally. The saccade latency was 276 ± 23 ms; increased compared to normal 185 ± 16 ms (*t*-test, $p < 0.01$). His horizontal saccades had multiple interruptions (staircase saccade). The saccade gain (achieved gaze-shift amplitude/desired gaze-shift amplitude) was 0.45 ± 0.16; which was significantly lower compared to normal 0.91 ± 0.02 (*t*-test, $p < 0.01$). He had 10 prism diopters of esotropia with no distance-near disparity and greater limitation of abduction than adduction. The esotropia contributed to post-saccadic drifts, which were more pronounced under monocular viewing conditions. He also had gaze-evoked nystagmus. We did not notice skew or alternating skew deviation or vertical nystagmus. The vestibulo-ocular reflex cancelation was technically difficult to perform due to increased neck tone secondary to coexisting parkinsonism. We did not get an ideal assessment of pursuit system due to overlying gaze-holding deficits. Nevertheless, our clinical impression was that the pursuit system had lower gain. He had face dystonia, but there were no rhythmic contractions of the face or the jaw. He had mild retrocollis. There was an increase in axial and appendicular tone, bradykinesia, and hypokinesia. There was pronounced shuffling of gait and reduction in arm swings on both sides. He scored 22 points on Unified Parkinson's Disease Rating Scale (axial score 10; left side 6 and right side 5). The diagnosis of Whipple's disease was established with colonoscopy and biopsy performed for the investigation of chronic diarrhea. The study revealed blunting of intestinal villi and lamina propria. There were large numbers of PAS-positive, diastase-resistant foamy macrophages. The patient had a cardiac pacemaker. Hence, brain MRI was not performed. He was then treated with intravenous ceftriaxone and has been on sulfamethoxazole.

Eye Movement Measurements

The experiment protocol adhered declaration of Helsinki, and it was approved by the Cleveland Clinic institutional review board. The subject and his legal guardian gave written informed consent for the experiment and publication of results. Binocular horizontal and vertical eye positions were captured non-invasively at 500 Hz sampling rate using video-based eye tracker (EyeLink 1000®, SR Research, ON, Canada). However, given limitation to vertical gaze, we only analyzed horizontal saccades. In monocular viewing condition, one eye was covered with the infrared permissive filter. This filter allowed infrared waves but blocked visible light waves, hence, preventing vision through the covered eye. The infrared permissive filter allowed measurement of the position of the covered eye. Technique and experimental protocol used to measure the positions of both eyes were otherwise identical for binocular and monocular viewing conditions. The details of data acquisition, signal processing, and analysis were similar as outlined in our previous studies (11–15).

RESULTS

Figure 1 illustrates an example of a visually guided saccade shifting the gaze from straight-ahead to 10° to the right and to the left in the patient with Whipple's disease and its comparison with a healthy subject. **Figure 1A** is an example of a healthy subject. In this example, the subject shifted gaze to 10° to the right side. Binocular eye positions measured during this example in healthy subject depicts uninterrupted gaze shift in 60 ms timespan (**Figure 1A**). As depicted in **Figure 1C**, the eye velocity during such gaze shift had a single peak. The right and the left eyes moved at a comparable amplitude (**Figure 1A**) and velocity (**Figure 1C**); there was no disconjugacy. **Figures 1D,G** show similar gaze shift in the patient with Whipple's disease during rightward and leftward saccades, respectively. The gaze shift in the patient took 530 ms for the right side and 535 ms for the left. The saccades were frequently interrupted as shown in an example in **Figure 1D**. During each break, the eye velocity reached 0 (**Figures 1E,H**). Such complete pause in eye movement is seen in **Figures 1D,G** and further emphasized as individual peaks and complete pause in **Figures 1E,H**. Also, the eye positions and velocities were not conjugate during such shift. The left eye had larger shift during each segment of the rightward saccade and *vice versa* for the leftward saccade. Such shifts are followed by a post-saccadic drift thereby fusing the gaze from both eyes. **Figures 1F,I** emphasize disconjugacy in the saccade amplitude.

Amplitude Velocity Relationship

As depicted in **Figures 1D–I**, the saccades in our patient are frequently interrupted, or they fall short of the target. Subsequently, there are catchup saccades that shift the eyes to reach the desired position. To quantitatively examine this phenomenology, we

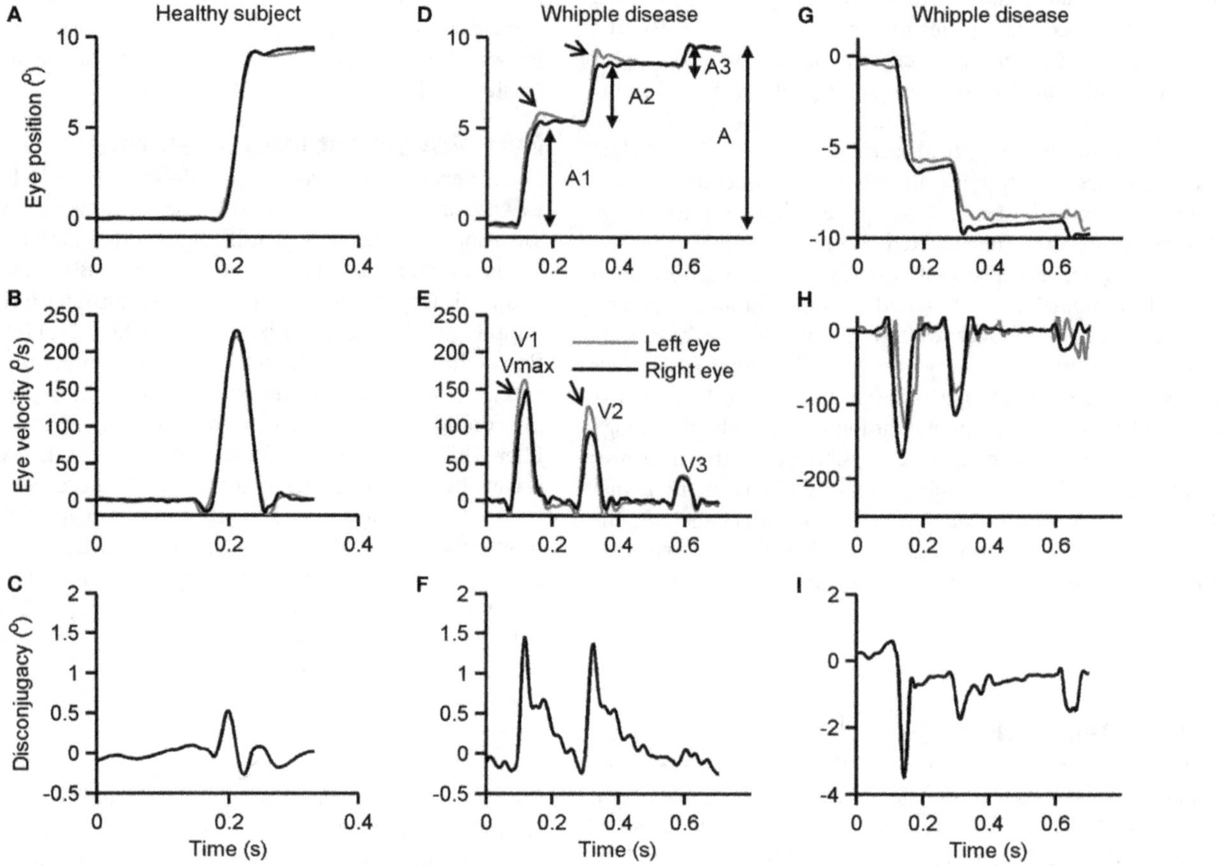

FIGURE 1 | Example of single visually guided saccade from a healthy subject **(A–C)** and its comparison in a patient with Whipple's disease. Panels **(A,D,G)** depict horizontal eye position plotted along *y*-axis while corresponding time on the *x*-axis. Panels **(B,E,H)** depict horizontal eye velocity plotted on the *y*-axis and corresponding time on the *x*-axis. Panels **(C,F,I)** illustrate the difference in right and left horizontal eye position. Arrows in panels **(D,E)** depict disconjugacy in a segmented saccade.

measured the kinematics of the visually guided horizontal saccades in patients with Whipple's disease and compared them with normal. The interruption in the visually guided saccades can be explained by three possible mechanisms. According to one mechanism, the saccade command is mal-programmed, and the executed gaze shift (saccade amplitude) is smaller than desired. As a result, the consequent saccade has smaller amplitude, as the eyes do not reach the destination; catchup saccade is further programmed to compensate for the retinal slip error. The second possibility is that the original saccade command is normally programmed, the executed eye movement starts off with appropriate amplitude and velocity matrices, but it is interrupted by the intrusive signal that imposes the breaks in the eye position hence leading to a pause in the eye movement. The third possibility is that saccade in Whipple's disease are slow in addition to being interrupted. To investigate these possibilities, we measured amplitudes and velocities of each segment of saccade (A1 and V1 in **Figures 1D,F**) as well as the desired amplitude and the maximum velocity (A and Vmax in **Figures 1D,F**). The prediction is that if saccades are programmed smaller, then their velocities (V1) are appropriately matched for the programmed amplitude (A1), hence the amplitude to velocity relationship, the main sequence, for A1 and V1 would fall within the normative range. However, the value of Vmax will be smaller for the overall amplitude (A), revealing abnormal main sequence for Vmax and A. In contrast, if saccades are normally programmed but prematurely interrupted then we expect normal amplitude to velocity relationship of the desired gaze shift and maximum velocity (Vmax and A), but velocity to amplitude relationship of staircase saccade (V1 and A1) will be above the normative range. **Figure 2A** depicts such comparison where the amplitudes of the saccade are plotted on the *x*-axis while velocities are plotted on the *y*-axis. The filled circles show Vmax to A relationship, while the open circles show V1 to A1 relationship of the segmented saccades. The amplitude to velocity relationship for segmented saccades fall along the lower margin of normative value, but the relationship of desired amplitude to velocity relationship falls below desired values. This phenomenon supports the first possibility for the pathomechanisms of abnormal horizontal saccades in Whipple's disease that is saccades are mal-programmed, their amplitude is smaller than desired, and they are followed by series of "catch-up" saccades (staircase) to accomplish the desired gaze

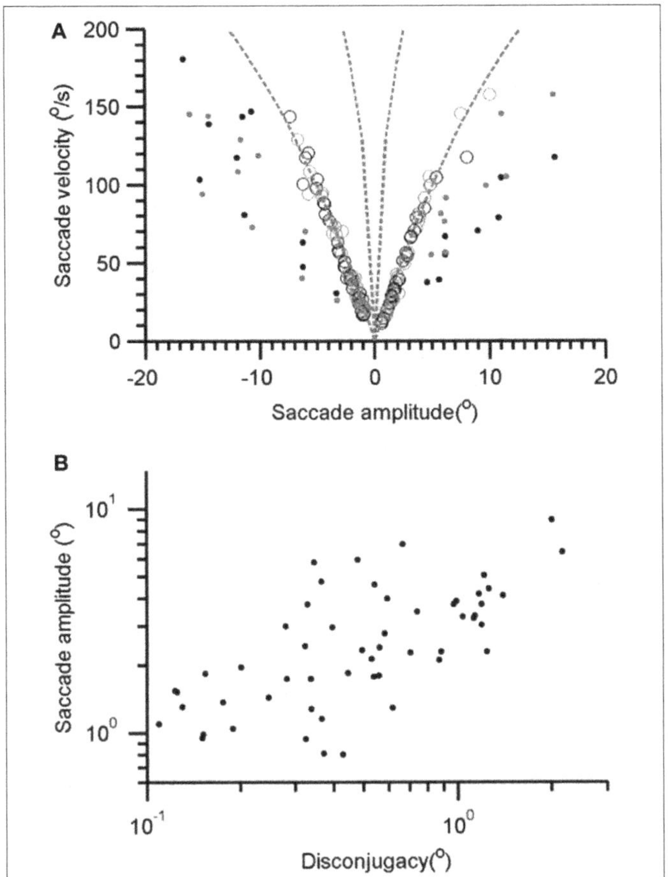

FIGURE 2 | (A) Amplitude to velocity relationship of the horizontal saccade. The open symbols depict such relationship for segmented saccade (V1 and A1 relationship, see **Figure 1C**). Filled symbols depicted the relationship of maximal velocity and desired gaze shift (Vmax and A relationship, see **Figure 1C**). Gray symbols depict rightward while black symbols are leftward saccades. **(B)** Comparison of segmented saccade amplitude and corresponding disconjugacy. Each data-point depicts one segmented saccade.

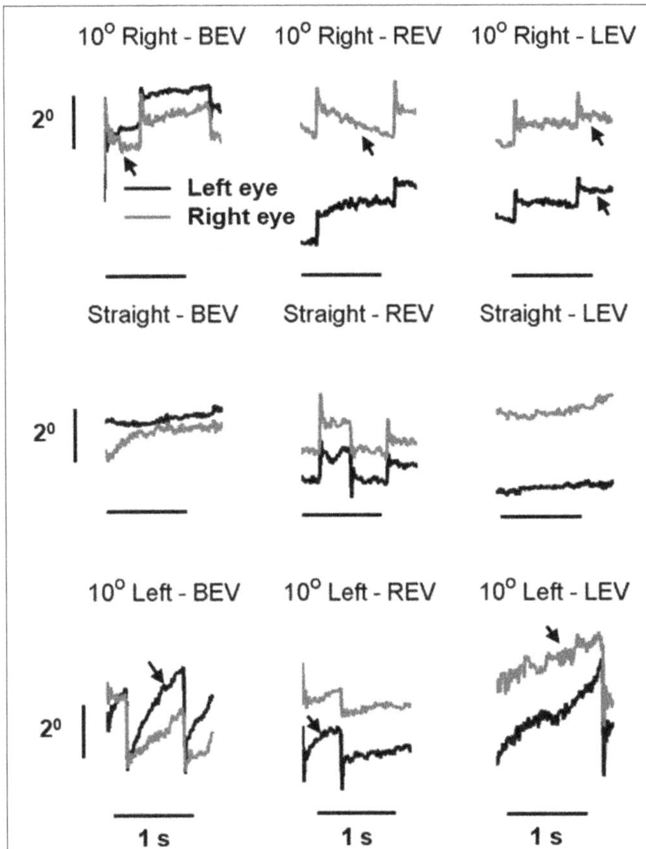

FIGURE 3 | Example of gaze-evoked nystagmus in right eye viewing, left-eye viewing, and both eyes viewing condition. Gray line is right eye while black is the left eye. Eye positions are plotted on the *y*-axis and corresponding time is plotted on the *x*-axis. The arrows depict velocity-decreasing characteristics of the nystagmus waveforms.

orientation. We found that the number of "catch-up" saccades per gaze shift ranged between 1 and 5; with a mean value of 2.7 ± 1.0.

Disconjugacy Analysis

Each segment comprising the staircase horizontal saccade was disconjugate. The disconjugacy in the staircase saccades can be explained by two possible mechanisms. One, disconjugacy is due to an uneven central command to the right and left eye in the presence of strabismus. The second possibility is that disconjugacy in the amplitude is due to the uncertain timing of putatively intrusive signal that might have led to an early break in saccade trajectory. The first possibility also predicts a systematic relationship between the saccade amplitude and the amount of disconjugacy. We compared disconjugacy (the difference between the saccade amplitude of the right and left eye) with corresponding conjugate amplitude (mean amplitude of right and left eye). There was a positive correlation, with the slope of linear fit was 2.5 and intercept was 1.27. The correlation coefficient was 0.45 (**Figure 2B**). The results suggest the amount of disconjugacy increased with increasing saccade amplitude.

Gaze-Evoked Nystagmus

Our patient also had gaze-evoked nystagmus. The slow phase of the nystagmus had velocity-decreasing waveform (arrows in **Figure 3**). The unique aspect was that the slow-phase eye velocity of the gaze-evoked nystagmus was disconjugate, more pronounced during monocular viewing condition (**Figure 3**). It is noteworthy that in addition to the drifts comprising the slow phase of the gaze-evoked nystagmus, there was a prominent post-saccadic drift of the covered eye during monocular viewing condition.

The subsequent analysis depicts the quantitative summary of kinematic properties of gaze-evoked nystagmus at various eye-in-orbit positions (**Figure 4A**). Each data-point in **Figure 4A** depicts one drift, black symbol depicts right eye, and the gray symbol is the left eye. The trend is that with rightward eye positions (positive value on the *x*-axis) show leftward drift (negative eye velocity) and *vice versa* for the leftward gaze positions. Such relationship has a slope of 0.06 and correlation coefficient of 0.31 for the right

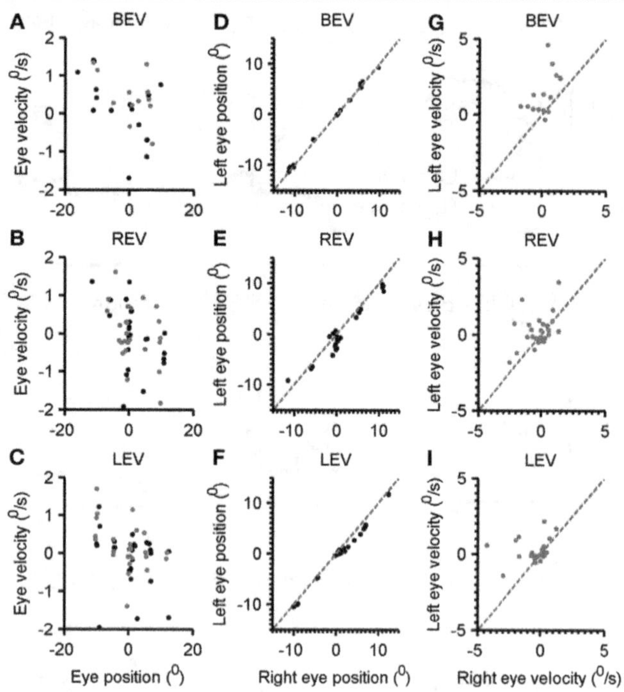

FIGURE 4 | Comparison of the eye velocity with eye position in both eyes viewing, right eye viewing, and left-eye viewing condition **(A–C)**. Gray symbols are right eye while black symbols depict the left eye. Panels **(D–F)** depict the comparison of left-eye position, and right eye position gray dashed line is an equality line. Each black symbol depicts one eccentric position. Panels **(G–I)** illustrate a comparison of left-eye velocity (*y*-axis) with the right eye velocity (*x*-axis). Each symbol depicts one drift. Gray dashed line is an equality line.

eye and 0.09 (slope) and 0.24 (correlation coefficient) for the left eye. The comparable relationship of eye velocity and amplitude was seen in right and left eye viewing conditions (**Figures 4B,C** respectively). The slope of the fitted function for the left eye during right eye viewing condition is −0.1, and for the right eye, it was −0.08. The correlation coefficient for this relation was 0.33 for the right eye and 0.2 for the left eye. During left-eye viewing condition, the slope of this relationship was −0.04 for the right eye and −0.03 for the left eye. The correlation coefficient was 0.06 and 0.09 for right and left eyes, respectively.

To assess the level of disconjugacy and the dependence of eye position, we compared the right eye position versus the left-eye position at various gaze eccentricities. As illustrated in **Figure 4D** both eyes were well aligned as all data-points (each depicting the eye position at given eccentricity) fell on the gray dashed line (equality). The slope and intercept of such relationship were 0.9 and 0.1, while the correlation coefficient was 0.99. In contrast, during right eye viewing condition the right eye position data-points frequently fell below the equality line suggesting that the right eye typically overshoots further to the right, and it normally would be followed by leftward drift (**Figure 4E**). The slope of comparison of left and right eye position in right eye viewing condition was 0.9 and intercept was 0.7; the correlation coefficient was 0.95. During left-eye viewing condition the data-point also frequently fell below the equality line suggesting that the right eye shifted further to the right (**Figure 4F**). The slope of such relationship was 0.9 and intercept was 0.8, while correlation coefficient was 0.99. It is important to note that during rightward gaze positions the disparity was larger compared to all gaze conditions. In subsequent analysis, we compared the disconjugacy in drift velocity. As illustrated in **Figure 4G**, both eye velocities were robustly uneven suggesting disconjugacy in drift velocity despite consistent eye-in-orbit orientation during eccentric gaze positions in both eyes viewing condition. The slope and intercept of such relationship were 0.05 and 1.65, while the correlation coefficient was 0.03. The comparable finding was noted during right- and left-eye viewing conditions (**Figures 4H,I**). The slope of comparison of left and right eye velocities in right eye viewing condition was 0.4 and intercept was 0.34; the correlation coefficient was 0.2. The slope of the right and left-eye velocity relationship was 0.14 and intercept was 0.28, while correlation coefficient was 0.05.

DISCUSSION

The classic features of the central nervous system Whipple's disease are pendular eye oscillations synchronized with the oscillatory jaw movements—called oculo-masticatory myorhythmia (16). Akinetic rigid forms of parkinsonism can be a manifestation of Whipple's disease (8, 9, 17, 18). These features of the central nervous system Whipple's disease can also present with slowing of vertical saccades, hence mimicking progressive supranuclear palsy (8, 9). In addition to up-gaze limitation, we found that patient with Whipple's disease also had hypometric horizontal saccades comprised of multiple interruptions (staircase saccades), gaze-evoked nystagmus, and esotropia. These features supported a likelihood of abnormal cerebellar control. In subsequent sections, we will discuss the physiology of the phenomenology seen our patient with the central nervous system Whipple's disease.

Staircase Horizontal Saccades

There are two possible mechanisms for interruptions leading to staircase saccades. According to one phenomenology, the ongoing saccades are mal-programmed; each gaze shift is associated with a lower amplitude saccade making the gaze shift smaller compared to the desired position. Subsequently, a corrective saccade is generated, but it is also mal-programmed. The consequence of such deficits is the series of multiple small saccades leading to gaze shift to the desired location. This deficit suggests dysfunction of ocular motor vermis (19, 20). The second phenomenology also suggests a deficit in the saccadic system, but here the normally programmed saccades are interrupted by external intrusive signal leading to breaks in the ongoing saccade. Accordingly, the velocity of the segmented saccades would be higher compared to their corresponding amplitude. Instead, we found low normal saccade amplitude to velocity relationship of segmented horizontal saccades. Therefore, we propose that multiple interruptions of the horizontal saccades in a patient with Whipple's disease could be due to mal-programmed saccades, favoring deficits in cerebellar control of eye movements.

We also found that each segmented saccade was associated with overshooting of one eye followed by a post-saccadic drift secondary due to esotropia as well as the pulse-step mismatch. This phenomenon led to disconjugacy in each segmented saccades followed by fusion. The amount of disconjugacy was proportional to the amplitude of the segmented saccade. Such systematic relationship between the amount of disconjugacy of the staircase and the staircase saccade amplitude is unlikely if the ongoing saccade was interrupted, but it is plausible for mal-programmed saccade. These results further supported our hypothesis that disconjugate and segmented horizontal saccades in our patient with Whipple's disease were due to mal-programmed hypometric horizontal saccade, a characteristic of cerebellar lesion causing hypometria (21, 22).

Gaze-Evoked Nystagmus

The gaze-evoked nystagmus is due to the insufficiency (leakiness) of the velocity-to-position neural integrator. Hence the direction of its slow-phase velocity reverses as the eye-in-orbit position shifts from one side of the null to the other, and the waveforms have velocity-decreasing characteristics (23, 24). Typical gaze-evoked nystagmus is seen in patients with focal or diffuse cerebellar deficit, leads to an impairment in the function of the neural integrator, and has conjugate slow phases (23). In contrast, our patient followed all characteristics of gaze-evoked nystagmus, but its slow phase was disconjugate. It is possible for the cerebellar disorder itself to cause disconjugate slow phase (19, 20, 25). However, our patient did not appear to have increased convergence tone esotropia reported in cerebellar disease patient, but had an esotropia due to horizontal gaze limitation during abduction. The difference in slow-phase velocity of the two eyes in our patient was more prominent during monocular viewing condition. We speculate that drifts of the esotropic eye that were most pronounced during monocular viewing condition interacted with the drifts that cause gaze-evoked nystagmus, possibly in the final common pathway for ocular motor control. Such interaction of post-saccadic drift and gaze-evoked nystagmus drift were more pronounced in the covered eye. Hence, we found a substantial disconjugacy in eye position and slow-phase velocity during monocular viewing condition.

In summary, unique presentation in our patient with Whipple's disease further supports possible involvement of cerebellum, in addition to the brainstem and basal ganglia. This case further suggests that the central nervous system Whipple's disease should not only be in the differential diagnosis of atypical forms of parkinsonism, such as progressive supranuclear palsy, but also multiple system atrophy. Finally, the analysis strategy proposed in this study can be used for differentiation of various disorders leading to staircase saccades, such as parkinsonian syndromes, cerebellar disorders, or deficits of brainstem saccade-generating circuits.

AUTHOR CONTRIBUTIONS

AS and FG: conceived idea, data collection, data analysis, writing, and editing manuscript.

ACKNOWLEDGMENTS

Authors thank Shivam Mittal, MD for collegial support.

FUNDING

This work was supported by grants from Knights Templar Research Foundation (FG), and Fight for Sight Foundation (FG), Blind Children's Center (FG), RPB Unrestricted grant CCLCM-CWRU, and Dystonia Medical Research Foundation/Dystonia Coalition career development award (NIH U54TR001456) (AS). Some resources used for these experiments were supported by NIH R01 EY06717 to Dr. R. John Leigh. Authors have no conflict of interests.

SUPPLEMENTARY MATERIAL

FIGURE S1 | Three panels depict 5-s long gaze-holding epochs in right, straight, and leftward gaze positions. The measurements are made during monocular viewing condition when the right eye (gray trace) was viewing. The red trace depicts (covered) left eye. Eye positions are plotted on the *y*-axis, while corresponding time is plotted on the x-axis.

REFERENCES

1. Relman DA, Schmidt TM, MacDermott RP, Falkow S. Identification of the uncultured *Bacillus* of Whipple's disease. *N Engl J Med* (1992) 327(5):293–301. doi:10.1056/NEJM199207303270501
2. Raoult D, Birg ML, La Scola B, Fournier PE, Enea M, Lepidi H, et al. Cultivation of the *Bacillus* of Whipple's disease. *N Engl J Med* (2000) 342(9):620–5. doi:10.1056/NEJM200003023420903
3. Louis ED, Lynch T, Kaufmann P, Fahn S, Odel J. Diagnostic guidelines in central nervous system Whipple's disease. *Ann Neurol* (1996) 40(4):561–8. doi:10.1002/ana.410400404
4. Van Bogaert L, Pages LRP, Labsuge R. Sur une encephalopire subaigue classable principalement oculo-facio-cervicales. *Rev Neurol* (1963) 109:443–53.
5. Knox DL, Bayless TM, Pittman FE. Neurologic disease in patients with created Whipple's disease. *Medicine* (1976) 55:467–76. doi:10.1097/00005792-197611000-00003
6. Silbert SW, Parker E, Horenstein S. Whipple's disease of the central nervous system. *Acta Neuropathol* (1976) 36(1):31–8. doi:10.1007/BF00685145
7. Pallis C, Lewis PD. *Neurology of Gastrointestinal Disease*. Amsterdam: Elsevier North-Holand Biomedical Press (1980).
8. Knox DL, Green WR, Troncoso JC, Yardley JH, Hsu J, Zee DS. Cerebral ocular Whipple's disease: a 62-year odyssey from death to diagnosis. *Neurology* (1995) 45(4):617–25. doi:10.1212/WNL.45.4.617
9. Averbuch-Heller L, Paulson GW, Daroff RB, Leigh RJ. Whipple's disease mimicking progressive supranuclear palsy: the diagnostic value of eye movement recording. *J Neurol Neurosurg Psychiatry* (1999) 66(4):532–5. doi:10.1136/jnnp.66.4.532
10. Buttner-Ennever JA, Buttner U. A cell group associated with vertical eye movements in the rostral mesencephalic reticular formation of the monkey. *Brain Res* (1978) 151(1):31–47. doi:10.1016/0006-8993(78)90948-4
11. Ghasia FF, Shaikh AG. Source of high-frequency oscillations in oblique saccade trajectory. *Exp Eye Res* (2014) 121:5–10. doi:10.1016/j.exer.2014.02.009

12. Ghasia FF, Shaikh AG. Uncorrected myopic refractive error increases microsaccade amplitude. *Invest Ophthalmol Vis Sci* (2015) 56(4):2531–5. doi:10.1167/iovs.14-15882
13. Ghasia FF, Shaikh AG, Jacobs J, Walker MF. Cross-coupled eye movement supports neural origin of pattern strabismus. *Invest Ophthalmol Vis Sci* (2015) 56(5):2855–66. doi:10.1167/iovs.15-16371
14. Shaikh AG, Otero-Millan J, Kumar P, Ghasia FF. Abnormal fixational eye movements in amblyopia. *PLoS One* (2016) 11(3):e0149953. doi:10.1371/journal.pone.0149953
15. Shaikh AG, Ghasia FF. Fixational saccades are more disconjugate in adults than in children. *PLoS One* (2017) 12(4):e0175295. doi:10.1371/journal.pone.0175295
16. Selhorst JB, Schwartz MA. Cerebral manifestations of Whipple's disease. *Mayo Clin Proc* (1988) 63(10):1057. doi:10.1016/S0025-6196(12)64926-X
17. Uldry PA, Bogousslavsky J. Partially reversible parkinsonism in Whipple's disease with antibiotherapy. *Eur Neurol* (1992) 32(3):151–3. doi:10.1159/000116813
18. Clark D, Eggenberger E. Neuro-ophthalmology of movement disorders. *Curr Opin Ophthalmol* (2012) 23(6):491–6. doi:10.1097/ICU.0b013e328358ba14
19. Takagi M, Zee DS, Tamargo RJ. Effects of lesions of the oculomotor vermis on eye movements in primate: saccades. *J Neurophysiol* (1998) 80(4):1911–31.
20. Takagi M, Tamargo R, Zee DS. Effects of lesions of the cerebellar oculomotor vermis on eye movements in primate: binocular control. *Prog Brain Res* (2003) 142:19–33. doi:10.1016/S0079-6123(03)42004-9
21. Robinson FR, Straube A, Fuchs AF. Role of the caudal fastigial nucleus in saccade generation. II. Effects of muscimol inactivation. *J Neurophysiol* (1993) 70(5):1741–58.
22. Straube A, Helmchen C, Robinson F, Fuchs A, Buttner U. Saccadic dysmetria is similar in patients with a lateral medullary lesion and in monkeys with a lesion of the deep cerebellar nucleus. *J Vestib Res* (1994) 4(5):327–33.
23. Zee DS, Yee RD, Cogan DG, Robinson DA, Engel WK. Ocular motor abnormalities in hereditary cerebellar ataxia. *Brain* (1976) 99(2):207–34. doi:10.1093/brain/99.2.207
24. Zee DS, Yamazaki A, Butler PH, Gucer G. Effects of ablation of flocculus and paraflocculus of eye movements in primate. *J Neurophysiol* (1981) 46(4):878–99.
25. Versino M, Hurko O, Zee DS. Disorders of binocular control of eye movements in patients with cerebellar dysfunction. *Brain* (1996) 119(Pt 6):1933–50. doi:10.1093/brain/119.6.1933

13

Eye Movement Abnormalities in Multiple Sclerosis: Pathogenesis, Modeling and Treatment

Alessandro Serra[1], Clara G. Chisari[2] and Manuela Matta[3]*

[1] *Neurology, Louis Stokes VA Medical Center, University Hospitals and Case Western Reserve School of Medicine, Cleveland, OH, United States,* [2] *Neurology, University of Catania, Catania, Italy,* [3] *Neurology, Ospedale San Luigi Gonzaga, Orbassano, Italy*

***Correspondence:**
Alessandro Serra
axs505@case.edu

Multiple sclerosis (MS) commonly causes eye movement abnormalities that may have a significant impact on patients' disability. Inflammatory demyelinating lesions, especially occurring in the posterior fossa, result in a wide range of disorders, spanning from acquired pendular nystagmus (APN) to internuclear ophthalmoplegia (INO), among the most common. As the control of eye movements is well understood in terms of anatomical substrate and underlying physiological network, studying ocular motor abnormalities in MS provides a unique opportunity to gain insights into mechanisms of disease. Quantitative measurement and modeling of eye movement disorders, such as INO, may lead to a better understanding of common symptoms encountered in MS, such as Uhthoff's phenomenon and fatigue. In turn, the pathophysiology of a range of eye movement abnormalities, such as APN, has been clarified based on correlation of experimental model with lesion localization by neuroimaging in MS. Eye movement disorders have the potential of being utilized as structural and functional biomarkers of early cognitive deficit, and possibly help in assessing disease status and progression, and to serve as platform and functional outcome to test novel therapeutic agents for MS. Knowledge of neuropharmacology applied to eye movement dysfunction has guided testing and use of a number of pharmacological agents to treat some eye movement disorders found in MS, such as APN and other forms of central nystagmus.

Keywords: eye movements, multiple sclerosis, internuclear ophthalmoplegia, nystagmus, pathologic saccades

INTRODUCTION

Multiple sclerosis (MS) is a common disorder of the central nervous system (CNS) that affects more than 2 million people worldwide. Once thought to be predominantly an autoimmune inflammatory disease, MS is now regarded as a complex entity characterized by inflammatory demyelinating events and a significant component of neurodegeneration that manifests as neuronal and axonal loss since the early stages of the disease. Our understanding of the disease has evolved dramatically over the years and, while MS was typically considered an immune disease targeting the white matter and due to T-cells dysfunction, it is now clear that the pathological process targets both the gray and white matter and is enacted by complex involvement and dynamics of multiple cells, including T and B-cells, macrophages, mast cells, etc. The typical variability of phenotype and disease course observed in MS, spanning from relapsing to primary or secondary progressive clinical scenarios, is probably due to different extent and combination of inflammatory and neurodegenerative processes involving various CNS areas.

Multiple sclerosis is the main cause of non-traumatic disability of young adults, and it has profound functional consequences on men and women who are often just beginning to start families and advance in their career. Disability in MS is quantified using standard scales such as the expanded disability status scale and the multiple sclerosis functional composite (1). However, such scales have limitations, especially when it comes to addressing disability arising from eye movement dysfunction, a common cause of transient or long-term impairment in MS. The presence of eye movement abnormalities correlate with greater level of disability in affected patients and generally predict a worse prognosis (2). Poor scores at automated tests of saccadic performance, such as the King-Devick (K-D) test of rapid number naming, also correlate with higher levels of disability (3). While some additional scales, such as the 25-Item National Eye Institute Visual Functioning Questionnaire and a 10-Item Neuro-Ophthalmic Supplement (4), can help track visual symptoms such as defects in binocular vision, blurred vision and diplopia, no standard evaluation includes a systematic approach for testing functional classes of eye movements in MS. Even without a formal standardized tool, an accurate bedside eye movement examination can aid or support the diagnosis of MS, for example, by providing evidence of disease dissemination in space (5). As the physiology and underlying anatomical network of eye movement control is well known from animal models and studies in humans (6), eye movement abnormalities are highly localizing to CNS structural lesions. Eye movement recording and analysis are required for more detailed quantitative characterization. One of the advantages of studying eye movements in the laboratory setting is that they can be precisely measured over time. Using such approach, for example, internuclear ophthalmoparesis has been proposed as a model for studying the effect of increased body temperature and fatigue on injured axons due to MS (7, 8).

Here, we review common eye movement disorders in MS and their pathophysiological substrate, how eye movement could be used as model or potentially marker of disease, and what treatment are currently available for ocular motor disorders encountered in MS.

EYE MOVEMENT DISORDERS IN MS

Table 1 summarizes the most common ocular motor manifestations of MS. Demyelinating lesions in the posterior fossa are a frequent cause of ocular motor dysfunction.

In the brain stem, demyelination and axonal damage of the medial longitudinal fasciculus (MLF) within the midline tegmentum of the pons (ventral to the fourth ventricle) or the midbrain (ventral to the cerebral aqueduct) results in *internuclear ophthalmoparesis (INO)*, the most common saccadic disorder observed in MS. In INO, binocular coordination (conjugacy) is disrupted with typically slowing of the adducting eye during horizontal saccades (adduction lag), best appreciated during large horizontal saccades and the fast phases of optokinetic reflex testing. On bedside examination, there could be dissociated nystagmus of the abducted eye, which actually consists of saccadic oscillations rather than true nystagmus (9). Patients with INO present with diplopia or more subtle symptoms of blurred vision and visual confusion only during head or head-on-body turns (e.g., during walking or driving) due to a transient break in binocular fusion (10). INO can be associated with skew deviation, a vertical strabismus with hypertropia on the side of the lesion, due to supranuclear disruption of the graviceptive pathways that travel through the MLF and carry utricular and vertical semicircular canals' input, or the full syndrome of ocular-tilt reaction. The latter is a combination of skew deviation, contralateral head tilt and ocular torsion, and reflects dysfunction of vestibular reactions in the roll plane (11). The role of the MLF in carrying exclusively contralateral posterior semicircular canal signals is confirmed by studies that combine MRI and the video-head-impulse test (12). Patients with unilateral INO may have vertical diplopia due to a non-evident skew deviation, which can be relieved by using a small vertical prism. Skew deviation and OTR can be seen also with lesions independent of the MLF, for example, in the cerebellum or the thalamus. Tilt of the subjective visual vertical, the inner perception of verticality, is very often found in patients with MS (13). In bilateral INO, the vertical vestibulo-ocular reflex and smooth pursuit are usually impaired, as axons in the MLF also carry vestibular and smooth pursuit signals from vestibular nuclei to midbrain nuclei concerned with vertical gaze. Convergence is typically spared in INO, unless the MLF lesion is at a higher level in the midbrain tegmentum. **Figure 1** depicts the simple network underlying binocular coordination of horizontal saccades, which is relevant to the pathophysiology of INO (6). To summarize, burst neurons lying in the paramedian pontine reticular formation (PPRF) generate a phasic velocity command called pulse, necessary to initiate the saccade, which is conveyed to two populations of neurons in the abducens nucleus: abducens motor neurons and abducens internuclear neurons. The pulse of innervation travels from abducens motor neurons along axons of the ipsilateral abducens nerve to the lateral rectus muscle, and from the abducens internuclear neurons *via* the MLF to medial rectus motoneurons in the contralateral oculomotor nucleus, which projects to the medial rectus muscle *via* the oculomotor nerve. In normal subjects, the eyes turn rapidly together as an ipsilateral conjugate saccade. Measuring of eye movements allow definition of normal limits for speed, amplitude and latency of

TABLE 1 | Eye movement disorders of multiple sclerosis.[a]

- Strabismus
  - Exotropia, especially in association with bilateral INO
  - Esotropia, commonly due to sixth nerve palsy
  - Vertical deviation, usually a skew deviation in association with INO
- Disruption of steady fixation
  - Gaze-evoked nystagmus
  - Acquired pendular nystagmus
  - Upbeat, downbeat, and torsional nystagmus
  - Positionally induced nystagmus, usually associated with vertigo
  - Saccadic intrusions and oscillations
- Impaired vestibulo-ocular responses, especially vertically associated with INO
- Impaired smooth pursuit, optokinetic, and eye-head tracking, especially vertically associated with INO
- Disorders of saccades: dysmetria, adduction slowing in INO, ocular flutter
- Horizontal gaze paresis or palsy
- Dorsal midbrain syndrome

[a]*Adapted with permission from Ref. (6).*

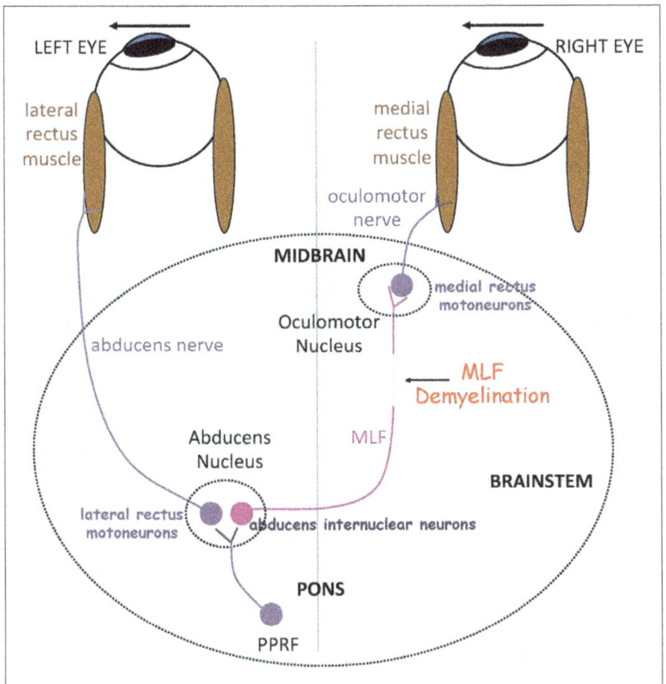

FIGURE 1 | Summary of a simple model for generating horizontal gaze shifts in INO. Premotor excitatory burst neurons lying in the paramedian pontine reticular formation (PPRF), project a pulse of innervation to the abducens nucleus (CN VI). Abducens motoneurons project the pulse of innervation *via* the sixth nerve to the right lateral rectus, which contracts rapidly to generate an abducting saccade of the left eye. Abducens internuclear neurons project the pulse of innervation, *via* the medial longitudinal fasciculus (MLF, internuclear pathway), to medial rectus motoneurons that, in turn, innervate the right medial rectus *via* the third nerve, to generate an adducting saccade of the right eye. If the MLF is demyelinated, signals are low-pass filtered and delayed, affecting the size and timing of the pulse thus causing adducting saccades of the right eye to be slow. *Adapted with permission from Ref. (6).

abducting and adducting saccades. A physiological adduction lag in the order of ~1–2 ms is generally observed in normal controls (6). Ultimately, INO in MS is due to injury of the MLF, which can no longer conduct high-frequency signals (pulse of innervation) and in turn causes slowing of the adducting eye, which in severe cases can manifest as complete paralysis.

Other brain stem syndromes encountered in MS include fascicular involvement of ocular motor cranial nerves CN III, IV, or VI, the latter sometimes as first clinical event of the disease, and nuclear syndromes such as horizontal gaze palsy, for example, if the PPRF is involved, and one-and-a-half syndrome, a combination of an ipsilateral horizontal gaze palsy with an adduction deficit on the same side. The latter can result from a lesion of the abducens nucleus and the adjacent MLF or, less commonly, from a bilateral INO combined with a unilateral abducens nerve palsy. Dorsal midbrain syndromes can also be encountered with various combinations of upward or downward saccadic gaze palsies, convergence-retraction nystagmus, and convergence impairment.

Patients with MS can present with acute central vestibular syndromes, that might be due to involvement of structures other than the intrapontine eighth nerve fascicle, including the medulla, the cerebellar peduncles, the posterior pontine tegmentum, and the midbrain (14).

The cerebellum and its connections are commonly involved by tissue damage in MS. Saccadic dysmetria is the most common disorder of saccades after INO (13), especially in relation to lesions in the cerebellar peduncles (15). Based on lesion topography, three cerebellar syndromes can be identified. Involvement of *flocculus and paraflocculus*, the so-called vestibulo-cerebellum, usually results into impaired smooth pursuit and inability to suppress the horizontal vestibulo-ocular reflex (VOR) during combined eye-head tracking (16). Gaze-evoked nystagmus (GEN) as well as downbeat nystagmus (DBN) are also found with cerebellar lesions in MS. GEN is a coarse to-and-fro eye oscillation starting with a slow centripetal drift from an eccentric position, followed by a corrective refoveating quick phase. GEN is due to a defect within the neural integrator network, a series of structures that includes the cerebellum, causing inability to hold gaze in eccentric positions (17). DBN, a spontaneous vertical eye oscillation with upward slow phases, is likely due to loss of inhibitory cerebellar control on vertical semicircular canals (18).

Lesions of the *nodulus and uvula* have been shown to cause positional nystagmus, downbeat nystagmus, and periodic alternating nystagmus. Central positional nystagmus, either downbeat or upbeat and clinically presenting as positional vertigo, has been described with demyelinating lesions in the superior cerebellar peduncle (19). Such lesions might cause positional vertigo and nystagmus through disruption of the central otolithic connections between deep cerebellar structures and the vestibular nuclei. Periodic alternating nystagmus (PAN) consists in spontaneous horizontal jerk nystagmus that reverses direction of the quick phases every 2 min. Experimentally, the ablation of the nodulus and ventral uvula in monkeys causes PAN in darkness (20). PAN is well characterized as a disorder of the "velocity storage" process, a sort of "vestibular memory" that physiologically prolongs the otherwise short-lived peripheral vestibular responses. PAN in MS has been linked to demyelination of central vestibular connections at the cerebellar peduncles (21).

Involvement of the *dorsal vermis and fastigial nuclei* typically causes saccadic dysmetria and impaired smooth pursuit, which appears "saccadic" on clinical examination. Dysmetric saccades include hypermetric saccades that overshoot the target, usually due to lesion of the fastigial nuclei, and hypometric saccades that undershoot the target, usually due to lesion of the dorsal vermis. When demyelination affects one fastigial nucleus, lesions are functionally bilateral as axons immediately cross to the contralateral nucleus. Clinically, this is evident as bilateral saccadic hypermetria.

The most common form of nystagmus found in MS is acquired pendular nystagmus (APN), which is cause of significant visual disability. Experimental studies have provided insights into the pathophyisiology of APN in MS, delineating mechanisms that translate into pharmacological treatment. Poor vision and consequent visual input delay along demyelinated visual pathways, for instance due to prior optic neuritis, may not fully explain the occurrence of the high-frequency oscillations that characterize APN. In fact, these oscillations remain unchanged in darkness when visual inputs have no influence on eye movements. Since the oscillations of APN are reset by large saccades, which produce a phase shift of the oscillation (22), it is more likely that APN originates within the neural integrator network in the brain stem and cerebellum (23). The premotor signal responsible for large saccades would basically reset the APN oscillations by silencing some neural integrator neurons that produce the nystagmus. To support this hypothesis, MS patients with APN tend to show more lesions in the paramedian pons in the region of the paramedian tract (PMT) cell groups, part of the neural integrator loop, which would consequently lose normal feedback, becoming unstable and generating the oscillations clinically evident as APN (24).

Multiple sclerosis patients may also suffer from disabling oscillopsia arising from other kind of eye oscillations, such as saccadic intrusions and oscillations, which vary as far as amplitude (e.g., square-wave jerks, macro square-wave jerks, macrosaccadic oscillations). In general, when saccadic intrusions or oscillations show an intersaccadic interval, that is a small pause of usually 200–400 msec between the saccadic to and fro movements, the most likely mechanism is an interruption of the cerebellar feedback on saccades control. On the other hand, saccadic oscillations without intersaccadic interval (e.g., ocular flutter and myoclonus) may derive from an unstable brain stem network and ultimately result from alteration of membrane properties of burst neurons (25–27).

Multiple sclerosis patients may show dysfunction of the higher order control network of eye movements. The integrity of such network can be assessed by means of several experimental paradigms. In the antisaccade task, the most widely used ocular motor test of cognitive control, one is required to inhibit an automatic saccade directed toward a visual stimulus being presented and to generate a saccade of similar amplitude in the opposite direction. A version of this test can be administered manually at bedside (28). The dorsolateral prefrontal cortex (PFC) seems to have a primary role in the inhibition of automatic, reflexive saccades otherwise initiated by the parietal eye fields. MS patients make more mistakes at the antisaccade test and generate saccades with greater latency than controls (29, 30). Such poor performance of MS may correlate also with cerebellar dysfunction as the role of the cerebellum in cognitive control is increasingly recognized (31). MS patients also make mistakes when required to generate saccades toward a remembered target, the so-called memory guided saccades, which is thought to reflect a deficit of working memory. During this task, their saccades are also inaccurate, especially when asked to execute a memorized sequence of target jumps (32). Finally, saccades made in response to predictable target jumps are usually hypometric in MS, and latencies are increased for saccades toward visual targets presented at random locations along with a visual distracter (33). These abnormalities also reflect inability to maintain inhibitory control through the PFC and its connections to thalamocorticostriatal circuits (34).

EYE MOVEMENTS AS MODEL AND MARKER OF DISEASE IN MS

Measurement and modeling of eye movements in MS has proven helpful in documenting a vast range of abnormalities and shed light onto specific pathogenic mechanisms, often providing the rationale for testing pharmacological intervention.

Internuclear ophthalmoparesis is perhaps the most useful application of eye movement measurement and modeling. INO in MS has been studied and quantified in several ways. A traditional approach, using infrared, search coil, or videooculography based techniques (6), is to compare the peak velocity, or peak acceleration, of the abducting eye versus the adducting eye during saccades. The abduction/adduction ratios of peak velocity or peak acceleration is consistently increased in patients with INO compared to normal controls (35–37). Studies have shown that mild INO may go undetected on bedside examination, which of course could have clinical implications when trying to establish a diagnosis or quantify disability (38). Another method to quantify INO is to calculate the abducting/adducting eye amplitude ratio at the time the normal abducting eye first reaches the target (first pass amplitude), and not at the end of the saccade, when a mildly affected adducting eye may eventually lands on target (39). A third method consists in plotting velocity values as a function of changes of eye position. This phase plane approach is particularly useful when attempting to distinguish true INO, for example, due to MS, from its mimickers such as a pseudo-INO due to myasthenia gravis (40). The phase plane plots show that in true INO the abducting and adducting eyes are dysconjugate from the onset of the saccade, while in pseudo-INO the initial portion of the saccade shows normal binocular coordination, only later in the movement followed by obvious dysconjugacy.

The significance of modeling INO in MS resides in the fact that the MLF is an accessible discrete pathway that lends itself as a microcosm of MS pathology, in particular demyelination and axonal loss ultimately responsible for conduction delay. INO as a reductionist model for decreased fidelity of neural conduction, has been used to study the effect of body temperature changes (Uhthoff's phenomenon) and of motor fatigue in MS. Thus, with increase in core body temperature, horizontal binocular conjugacy worsens in patients with INO (7), as it does when they are asked to make horizontal saccades continuously over several minutes (a fatigue test) (8). The approach of using eye movements to better characterize and follow over time disabling symptoms like fatigue in MS, is supported by studies showing changes of both exogenous and endogenous saccadic peak velocity, latency and amplitude in patients who report symptoms of fatigue (41, 42). The effects of ocular motor fatigue on INO can be characterized not only in terms of decreased amplitude of the saccadic pulse signal for the adducting eye but also in terms of its delayed delivery through the injured MLF (43). Both these behaviors can be reproduced by manipulating conduction gains and delays at the MLF site, within a mathematical model of the faulty circuitry responsible for INO (43).

Can INO be used as a biomarker of axonal and myelin integrity in MS? Modern applications of high-resolution MRI such as diffusion tensor imaging (DTI) techniques are able to capture architectural changes of discrete white matter tracts, including the MLF, due to myelin and axonal pathology. Coupling DTI-based neuroimaging with eye movement measurement, for example, with video oculography, may help characterize axonal integrity and myelin status and quantify tissue injury in the MLF

(44–47). With a similar approach, latency of onset of vestibulo-ocular reflex (eVOR) recorded using search-coil, was studied in relation to lesion length and DTI metrics of MLF, and was found to be more prolonged with greater extent of MLF lesions (48). This study also provided direct measurement of axonal conduction velocity within lesions involving the MLF, which was reduced below levels predicted for natively myelinated and remyelinated axons. Such approach of studying the MLF as a composite structural-functional biomarker of axonal and myelin status could be used to assess response to therapies aimed at enhancing recovery and fidelity of axonal transmission in MS. In this regard, preliminary data in three INO patients treated with the potassium channel blocker dalfampridine showed changes in horizontal saccadic conjugacy, consistent with improved transmission of the neural pulse responsible for adducting movements (49).

Can eye movements be used as a biomarker for cognitive compromise in MS? As discussed above, eye movements can be affected by dysfunction of higher-order networks that control cognition. Such abnormalities, evident mostly as errors and increased saccadic latencies at the antisaccade and memory-guided tests, may be detected in the early stages of the disease and their deterioration over time correlates with neuropsychological test scores (34). Thus, eye movements could represent a useful tool to interrogate integrity of cortical and subcortical networks, and possibly their cerebellar connections, that are involved with attention, working memory and executive function.

In summary, while Inflammatory, demyelinating, and neuro-degenerative pathology in multiple sclerosis affect both afferent and efferent visual function, the afferent visual system has been utilized to a significant larger extent as a model system for MS. A simple clinical tool such as low-contrast letter acuity testing has been shown to clearly capture visual dysfunction and visual disability in MS, and to correlate with structural changes on optical coherence tomography (OCT) and disease burden on MRI (50). The introduction of OCT has been a breakthrough in the field of MS: changes in the thickness of peripapillary retinal nerve fiber layer are felt to represent axonal damage, whereas loss of macular volume and thinning of retinal ganglion cell layer are viewed as evidence of neuronal pathology. The afferent visual system has the advantage of being probably more accessible for interrogating status and severity of disease and testing of possible agents for neuroprotection and repair in MS (51). While eye movements assessment and quantification may require special equipment and a particular clinical expertise, several studies have shown that, for instance, certain features of saccades in INO and in cognitive function, have the potential to be validated as markers of disease and treatment outcome measures.

TREATMENT OF EYE MOVEMENT DYSFUNCTION IN MS

Several pharmacological agents have been employed to treat acquired eye movement disorders, for example, pendular or downbeat nystagmus. When these disorders are secondary to multiple sclerosis, localization of causative lesions by MRI can help elucidate the pathophysiological mechanisms responsible for the eye movement impairment and drive therapeutic choices. Acquired pendular nystagmus (APN) is a classic example. As discussed above, APN is likely due to an unstable neural integrator loop, which includes the region of the paramedian tracts, where a higher disease load can be found in MS patients. Drugs that depolarize the NI cells, improving membrane stability, may reduce APN amplitude (52). Gabapentin (1,200 mg/day) and memantine (15–60 mg/day), blockers of alpha-2-delta calcium channels and glutamate receptors, respectively, reduce GABAergic inhibition of cerebellar Purkinje cells causing indirect depolarization of the cells of a key NI structure, the nucleus prepositus hypoglossi (53, 54). Downbeat nystagmus (DBN) in MS, usually caused by lesions of the cerebellar flocculus, has been shown to respond to oral clonazepam (0.5 mg 3 times daily), baclofen (10 mg 3 times daily), and gabapentin. Randomized controlled trials have shown that the potassium channel blockers

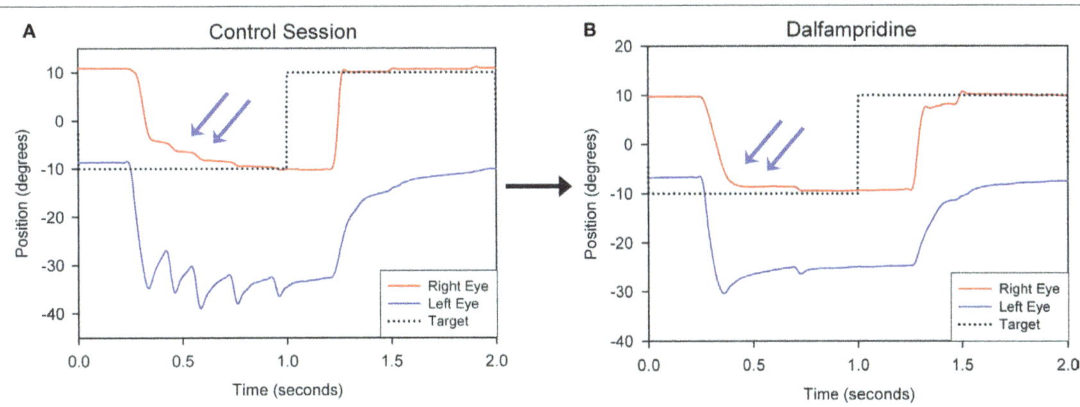

FIGURE 2 | Representative horizontal leftward saccade before **(A)** and after Dalfampridine **(B)** in one patient. **(A)** Particularly for the leftward movement the adducting eye requires several small saccades to acquire the target (arrows) and the abducting eye shows dissociated nystagmus. **(B)** The right eye requires less adducting saccades to acquire the target (arrows) and dissociated nystagmus intensity is decreased. Positive values indicate rightward movements, negative values indicate leftward movements. *Adapted with permission from Ref. (49).

3,4-diaminopyridine (3,4-DAP) had a significant effect of peak slow-phase velocity (55). 4-aminopyridine (4-AP), which restores the function of the vertical and horizontal neural integrator, should be preferred to 3,4-DAP because it crosses the blood–brain barrier more easily. Because of short half-life, a sustained release form of 4-AP such as dalfampridine (10–20 mg/day) is recommended (56–58). 4-AP has been shown effective also in upbeat nystagmus (UBN) and central positional nystagmus (59, 60), while baclofen (5–10 mg 3 times daily) can also be considered for UBN. Periodic alternating nystagmus (PAN), that could arise in MS from demyelination of central vestibular connections at the cerebellar peduncles, has been treated with oral baclofen (5–10 mg 3 times daily) in case reports. The effects of baclofen on the vestibular nuclei or vestibulocerebellum likely depend on GABA mechanisms.

Therapeutic strategies for eye movement disorders in MS may not be limited to treatment of nystagmus. Thus, as mentioned above, a study of three MS patients with chronic internuclear ophtalmoplegia (INO) showed that dalfampridine improved horizontal saccadic conjugacy, as recorded with video oculography, with one of the patients reporting actual clinical improvement of quality of vision (**Figure 2**). A double-blind placebo-controlled crossover trial of dalfampridine to treat INO and associated ocular motor fatigue due to MS is ongoing (ClinicalTrials.gov NCT02391961). Finally, non-pharmacological interventions, such as the use of base-down prisms for DBN, which is usually less intense in upward gaze, or prisms to compensate for skew deviation causing vertical diplopia in INO, should always be considered.

CONCLUSION

We have reviewed the most common eye movement disorders in MS and discussed known pathophysiological correlate for each of them. Study of eye movements in MS is particularly valuable as use of conventional and upcoming non-conventional imaging techniques coupled with eye movement recording can provide insights into mechanisms and status of disease. Eye movements abnormalities in MS are once again a promising tool with the tangible potential of serving as biomarkers of early disease, monitoring tools, and outcome measures for testing new treatments, including remyelinating agents.

AUTHOR CONTRIBUTIONS

AS: wrote draft and final version of the article, adapted, and completed table and figures. CC: and MM: critical reading, draft editing, and helped references.

FUNDING

This work was supported by Career Development Award # IK2RX001180 from the United States (U.S.) Department of Veterans Affairs, Rehabilitation Research & Development Service.

REFERENCES

1. Meyer-Moock S, Feng Y-S, Maeurer M, Dippel F-W, Kohlmann T. Systematic literature review and validity evaluation of the Expanded Disability Status Scale (EDSS) and the multiple sclerosis functional composite (MSFC) in patients with multiple sclerosis. *BMC Neurol* (2014) 4:58. doi:10.1186/1471-2377-14-58
2. Derwenskus J, Rucker JC, Serra A, Stahl JS, Downey DL, Adams NL, et al. Abnormal eye movements predict disability in MS: two-year follow-up. *Ann N Y Acad Sci* (2005) 1039:521–3. doi:10.1196/annals.1325.058
3. Moster S, Wilson JA, Galetta SL, Balcer LJ. The King-Devick (K-D) test of rapid eye movements: a bedside correlate of disability and quality of life in MS. *J Neurol Sci* (2014) 343:105–9. doi:10.1016/j.jns.2014.05.047
4. Raphael BA, Galetta KM, Jacobs DA, Markowitz CE, Liu GT, Nano-Schiavi ML, et al. Validation and test characterisitics of a 10-item neuro-ophthalmic supplement to the NEI-VFQ-25. *Am J Ophthalmol* (2006) 142:1026–35. doi:10.1016/j.ajo.2006.06.060
5. Polman CH, Reingold SC, Banwell B, Clanet M, Cohen JA, Filippi M, et al. Diagnostic criteria for multiple sclerosis: 2010 revisions to the McDonald criteria. *Ann Neurol* (2011) 69(2):292–302. doi:10.1002/ana.22366
6. Leigh RJ, Zee DS. *The Neurology of Eye Movements*. 5th ed. New York: Oxford University Press (2015).
7. Davis SL, Frohman TC, Crandall CG, Brown MJ, Mills DA, Kramer PD, et al. Modeling Uhthoff's phenomenon in MS patients with internuclear ophthalmoparesis. *Neurology* (2008) 70:1098–106. doi:10.1212/01.wnl.0000291009.69226.4d
8. Matta M, Leigh RJ, Pugliatti M, Aiello I, Serra A. Using fast eye movements to study fatigue in multiple sclerosis. *Neurology* (2009) 73(10):798–804. doi:10.1212/WNL.0b013e3181b6bbf4
9. Zee DS, Hain TC, Carl JR. Abduction nystagmus in internuclear ophthalmoplegia. *Ann Neurol* (1987) 21(4):383–8. doi:10.1002/ana.410210411
10. Mills DA, Frohman TC, Davis SL, Salter AR, McClure S, Beatty I, et al. Break in binocular fusion during head turning in MS patients with INO. *Neurology* (2008) 71:458–60. doi:10.1212/01.wnl.0000324423.08538.dd
11. Brandt T, Dieterich M. Vestibular syndromes in the roll plane: topographic diagnosis from brainstem to cortex. *Ann Neurol* (1994) 36:337–47. doi:10.1002/ana.410360304
12. Lee SH, Kim SH, Kim SS, Kang KW, Tarnutzer AA. Preferential impairment of the contralesional posterior semicircular canal in internuclear ophthalmoplegia. *Front Neurol* (2017) 8:502. doi:10.3389/fneur.2017.00502
13. Serra A, Derwenskus J, Downey DL, Leigh RJ. Role of eye movement examination and subjective visual vertical in clinical evaluation of multiple sclerosis. *J Neurol* (2003) 250:569–75. doi:10.1007/s00415-003-1038-8
14. Pula JH, Newman-Toker DE, Kattah JC. Multiple sclerosis as a cause of the acute vestibular syndrome. *J Neurol* (2013) 260:1649. doi:10.1007/s00415-013-6850-1
15. Frohman EM, Frohman TC, Fleckenstein J, Racke MK, Hawker K, Kramer PD. Ocular contrapulsion in multiple sclerosis: clinical features and pathophysiological mechanisms. *J Neurol Neurosurg Psychiatry* (2001) 70:688–92. doi:10.1136/jnnp.70.5.688
16. Sharpe JA, Goldberg HJ, Lo AW, Herishanu YO. Visual-vestibular interaction in multiple sclerosis. *Neurology* (1981) 31:427–33. doi:10.1212/WNL.31.4_Part_2.427
17. Zee DS, Yee RD, Cogan DG, Robinson DA, Engel WK. Ocular motor abnormalities in hereditary cerebellar ataxia. *Brain* (1976) 99(2):207–34. doi:10.1093/brain/99.2.207
18. Wagner JN, Glaser M, Brandt T, Strupp M. Downbeat nystagmus: aetiology and comorbidity in 117 patients. *J Neurol Neurosurg Psychiatry* (2008) 79:672–7. doi:10.1136/jnnp.2007.126284
19. Anagnostou E, Mandellos D, Limbitaki G, Papadimitriou A, Anastasopoulos D. Positional nystagmus and vertigo due to a solitary brachium conjunctivum plaque. *J Neurol Neurosurg Psychiatry* (2006) 77:790–2. doi:10.1136/jnnp.2005.084624
20. Waespe W, Cohen B, Raphan T. Dynamic modification of the vestibulo-ocular reflex by the nodulus and uvula. *Science* (1985) 228(4696):199–202. doi:10.1126/science.3871968
21. Prasad S, Galetta SL. Eye movement abnormalities in multiple sclerosis. *Neurol Clin* (2010) 28(3):641–55. doi:10.1016/j.ncl.2010.03.006
22. Das VE, Oruganti P, Kramer PD, Leigh RJ. Experimental tests of a neural-network model for ocular oscillations caused by disease of central myelin. *Exp Brain Res* (2000) 133:189–97. doi:10.1007/s002210000367
23. Kang S, Shaikh AG. Acquired pendular nystagmus. *J Neurol Sci* (2017) 375:8–17. doi:10.1016/j.jns.2017.01.033

24. Niestroy A, Rucker JC, Leigh RJ. Neuro-ophthalmologic aspects of multiple sclerosis: Using eye movements as a clinical and experimental tool. *Clin Ophthalmol* (2007) 3:267–72.
25. Ramat S, Leigh RJ, Zee DS, Optican LM. Ocular oscillations generated by coupling of brainstem excitatory and inhibitory saccadic burst neurons. *Exp Brain Res* (2005) 160(1):89–106. doi:10.1007/s00221-004-1989-8
26. Shaikh AG, Ramat S, Optican LM, Miura K, Leigh RJ, Zee DS. Saccadic burst cell membrane dysfunction is responsible for saccadic oscillations. *J Neuroophthalmol* (2008) 4:329–36. doi:10.1097/WNO.0b013e31818eb3a5
27. Shaikh AG, Zee DS, Optican LM, Miura K, Ramat S, Leigh RJ. The effects of ion channel blockers validate the conductance-based model of saccadic oscillations. *Ann N Y Acad Sci* (2011) 1233:58–63. doi:10.1111/j.1749-6632.2011.06130.x
28. Hellmuth J, Mirsky J, Heuer HW, Matlin A, Jafari A, Garbutt S, et al. Multicenter validation of a bedside antisaccade task as a measure of executive function. *Neurology* (2012) 78(23):1824–31. doi:10.1212/WNL.0b013e318258f785
29. Fielding J, Kilpatrick T, Millist L, White O. Antisaccade performance in patients with multiple sclerosis. *Cortex* (2009) 45:900–3. doi:10.1016/j.cortex.2009.02.016
30. Fielding J, Kilpatrick T, Millist L, Clough M, White O. Longitudinal assessment of antisaccades in patients with multiple sclerosis. *PLoS One* (2012) 7:e30475. doi:10.1371/journal.pone.0030475
31. Kolbe SC, Kilpatrick TJ, Mitchell PJ, White O, Egan GF, Fielding J. Inhibitory saccadic dysfunction is associated with cerebellar injury in multiple sclerosis. *Hum Brain Mapp* (2013) 28:534–7. doi:10.1002/hbm.22329
32. Fielding J, Kilpatrick T, Millist L, White O. Multiple sclerosis: cognition and saccadic eye movements. *J Neurol Sci* (2009) 277:32–6. doi:10.1016/j.jns.2008.10.001
33. Fielding J, Kilpatrick T, Millist L, White O. Control of visually guided saccades in multiple sclerosis: disruption to higher-order processes. *Neuropsychologia* (2009) 47:1647–53. doi:10.1016/j.neuropsychologia.2009.01.040
34. Fielding J, Clough M, Beh S, Millist L, Sears D, Frohman AN, et al. Ocular motor signatures of cognitive dysfunction in multiple sclerosis. *Nat Rev Neurol* (2015) 11(11):637–45. doi:10.1038/nrneurol.2015.174
35. Chen AL, Ramat S, Serra A, King SA, Leigh RJ. The role of the medial longitudinal fasciculus in horizontal gaze: tests of current hypotheses for saccade-vergence interactions. *Exp Brain Res* (2011) 208:335–43. doi:10.1007/s00221-010-2485-y
36. Flipse JP, Straathof CS, Van der Steen J, Van Leeuwen AF, Van Doorn PA, Van der Meché FG, et al. Binocular saccadic eye movements in multiple sclerosis. *J Neurol Sci* (1997) 148:53–65. doi:10.1016/S0022-510X(96)05330-0
37. Frohman EM, Frohman TC, O'Suilleabhain P, Zhang H, Hawker K, Racke MK, et al. Quantitative oculographic characterisation of internuclear ophthalmoparesis in multiple sclerosis: the versional dysconjugacy index Z score. *J Neurol Neurosurg Psychiatry* (2002) 73:51–5. doi:10.1136/jnnp.73.1.51
38. Frohman TC, Frohman EM, O'Suilleabhain P, Salter A, Dewey RB Jr, Hogan N, et al. Accuracy of clinical detection of INO in MS: corroboration with quantitative infrared oculography. *Neurology* (2003) 61:848–50. doi:10.1212/01.WNL.0000085863.54218.72
39. Frohman EM, O'Suilleabhain P, Dewey RB Jr, Frohman TC, Kramer PD. A new measure of dysconjugacy in INO: the first-pass amplitude. *J Neurol Sci* (2003) 210:65–71. doi:10.1016/S0022-510X(03)00027-3
40. Serra A, Liao K, Matta M, Leigh RJ. Diagnosing disconjugate eye movements: phase-plane analysis of horizontal saccades. *Neurology* (2008) 71:1167–75. doi:10.1212/01.wnl.0000327525.72168.57
41. Finke C, Pech LM, Sömmer C, Schlichting J, Stricker S, Endres M, et al. Dynamics of saccade parameters in multiple sclerosis patients with fatigue. *J Neurol* (2012) 259:2656–63. doi:10.1007/s00415-012-6565-8
42. Ferreira M, Pereira PA, Parreira M, Sousa I, Figueiredo J, Cerqueira JJ, et al. Using endogenous saccades to characterize fatigue in multiple sclerosis. *Mult Scler Relat Disord* (2017) 14:16–22. doi:10.1016/j.msard.2017.01.014
43. Jacobs JB, Serra A, Chisari CG, Skelly M, Matta M, Walker M, et al. Evaluation of saccades show ocular-motor fatigue in internuclear ophthalmoparesis due to multiple sclerosis. *Invest Ophthalmol Vis Sci* (2017) 58(8):755.
44. Chuang MT, Lin CC, Sung PS, Su HC, Chen YC, Liu YS. Diffusion-weighted imaging as an aid in the diagnosis of the etiology of medial longitudinal fasciculus syndrome. *Surg Radiol Anat* (2014) 36:675–80. doi:10.1007/s00276-014-1256-z
45. Fox RJ, McColl RW, Lee JC, Frohman T, Sakaie K, Frohman E. A preliminary validation study of diffusion tensor imaging as a measure of functional brain injury. *Arch Neurol* (2008) 65:1179–84. doi:10.1001/archneur.65.9.1179
46. McNulty JP, Lonergan R, Brennan PC, Evanoff MG, O'Laoide R, Ryan JT, et al. Diagnostic efficacy of conventional MRI pulse sequences in the detection of lesions causing internuclear ophthalmoplegia in multiple sclerosis patients. *Clin Neuroradiol* (2015) 25(3):233–9. doi:10.1007/s00062-014-0295-5
47. Sakaie K, Takahashi M, Dimitrov I, Togao O, Davis S, Remington G, et al. Diffusion tensor imaging the medial longitudinal fasciculus in INO: opportunities and challenges. *Ann N Y Acad Sci* (2011) 1233:307–31. doi:10.1111/j.1749-6632.2011.06156.x
48. Wang C, Paling D, Chen L, Hatton SN, Lagopoulos J, Aw ST, et al. Axonal conduction in multiple sclerosis: a combined magnetic resonance imaging and electrophysiological study of the medial longitudinal fasciculus. *Mult Scler J* (2015) 21(7):905–15. doi:10.1177/1352458514556301
49. Serra A, Skelly MM, Jacobs JB, Walker MF, Cohen JA. Improvement of internuclear ophthalmoparesis in multiple sclerosis with dalfampridine. *Neurology* (2014) 83:192–4. doi:10.1212/WNL.0000000000000567
50. Wu GF, Schwartz ED, Lei T, Souza A, Mishra S, Jacobs DA, et al. Relation of vision to global and regional brain MRI in multiple sclerosis. *Neurology* (2007) 69:2128–35. doi:10.1212/01.wnl.0000278387.15090.5a
51. Frohman EM, Costello F, Stuve O, Calabresi PA, Miller DH, Hickman SJ, et al. Modeling axonal degeneration within the anterior visual system. Implications for demonstrating neuroprotection in multiple sclerosis. *Arch Neurol* (2008) 65:26–35. doi:10.1001/archneurol.2007.10
52. Shaikh AG, Thurtell MJ, Optican LM, Leigh RJ. Pharmacological tests of hypotheses for acquired pendular nystagmus. *Ann N Y Acad Sci* (2011) 1233:320–6. doi:10.1111/j.1749-6632.2011.06118.x
53. Starck M, Albrecht H, Pöllmann W, Dieterich M, Straube A. Acquired pendular nystagmus in multiple sclerosis: an examiner-blind cross-over treatment study of memantine and gabapentin. *J Neurol* (2010) 257(3):322–7. doi:10.1007/s00415-009-5309-x
54. Thurtell MJ, Joshi AC, Leone AC, Tomsak RL, Kosmorsky GS, Stahl JS, et al. Crossover trial of gabapentin and memantine as treatment for acquired nystagmus. *Ann Neurol* (2010) 67(5):676–80. doi:10.1002/ana.21991
55. Strupp M, Teufel J, Zwergal A, Schniepp R, Khodakhah K, Feil K. Aminopyridines for the treatment of neurologic disorders. *Neurol Clin Pract* (2017) 7:65–76. doi:10.1212/CPJ.0000000000000321
56. Claassen J, Feil K, Bardins S, Teufel J, Spiegel R, Kalla R, et al. Dalfampridine in patients with downbeat nystagmus: an observational study. *J Neurol* (2013) 260:1992–6. doi:10.1007/s00415-013-6911-5
57. Ilg W, Bastian AJ, Boesch S, Burciu RG, Celnik P, Claaßen J, et al. Consensus paper: management of degenerative cerebellar disorders. *Cerebellum* (2014) 13:248–68. doi:10.1007/s12311-013-0531-6
58. Feil K, Bremova T, Muth C, Schniepp R, Teufel J, Strupp M. Update on the pharmacotherapy of cerebellar ataxia and nystagmus. *Cerebellum* (2016) 15:38–42. doi:10.1007/s12311-015-0733-1
59. Glasauer S, Kalla R, Buttner U, Strupp M, Brandt T. 4-Aminopyridine restores visual ocular motor function in upbeat nystagmus. *J Neurol Neurosurg Psychiatry* (2005) 76:451–3. doi:10.1136/jnnp.2004.045716
60. Kremmyda O, Zwergal A, la Fougere C, Brandt T, Jahn K, Strupp M. 4-Aminopyridine suppresses positional nystagmus caused by cerebellar vermis lesion. *J Neurol* (2013) 260:321–3. doi:10.1007/s00415-012-6737-6

14

Hypertrophic Olivary Degeneration and Palatal or Oculopalatal Tremor

Caroline Tilikete[1,2,3]* and Virginie Desestret[1,2,4]

[1] Neuro-Ophthalmology and Neurocognition, Hôpital Neurologique Pierre Wertheimer, Hospices Civils de Lyon, Bron, France, [2] Lyon I University, Lyon, France, [3] ImpAct Team, CRNL INSERM U1028 CNRS UMR5292, Bron, France, [4] SynatAc Team, Institut NeuroMyogène INSERM U1217/UMR CRS 5310, Lyon, France

****Correspondence:***
Caroline Tilikete
caroline.tilikete@inserm.fr

Hypertrophic degeneration of the inferior olive is mainly observed in patients developing palatal tremor (PT) or oculopalatal tremor (OPT). This syndrome manifests as a synchronous tremor of the palate (PT) and/or eyes (OPT) that may also involve other muscles from the branchial arches. It is associated with hypertrophic inferior olivary degeneration that is characterized by enlarged and vacuolated neurons, increased number and size of astrocytes, severe fibrillary gliosis, and demyelination. It appears on MRI as an increased T2/FLAIR signal intensity and enlargement of the inferior olive. There are two main conditions in which hypertrophic degeneration of the inferior olive occurs. The most frequent, studied, and reported condition is the development of PT/OPT and hypertrophic degeneration of the inferior olive in the weeks or months following a structural brainstem or cerebellar lesion. This "symptomatic" condition requires a destructive lesion in the Guillain–Mollaret pathway, which spans from the contralateral dentate nucleus *via* the brachium conjunctivum and the ipsilateral central tegmental tract innervating the inferior olive. The most frequent etiologies of destructive lesion are stroke (hemorrhagic more often than ischemic), brain trauma, brainstem tumors, and surgical or gamma knife treatment of brainstem cavernoma. The most accepted explanation for this symptomatic PT/OPT is that denervated olivary neurons released from inhibitory inputs enlarge and develop sustained synchronized oscillations. The cerebellum then modulates/accentuates this signal resulting in abnormal motor output in the branchial arches. In a second condition, PT/OPT and progressive cerebellar ataxia occurs in patients without structural brainstem or cerebellar lesion, other than cerebellar atrophy. This syndrome of progressive ataxia and palatal tremor may be sporadic or familial. In the familial form, where hypertrophic degeneration of the inferior olive may not occur (or not reported), the main reported etiologies are Alexander disease, polymerase gamma mutation, and spinocerebellar ataxia type 20. Whether or not these are associated with specific degeneration of the dentato–olivary pathway remain to be determined. The most symptomatic consequence of OPT is eye oscillations. Therapeutic trials suggest gabapentin or memantine as valuable drugs to treat eye oscillations in OPT.

Keywords: symptomatic palatal tremor, progressive ataxia and palatal tremor, pendular nystagmus, hypertrophic degeneration of inferior olive, dentato–olivary pathway, Guillain–Mollaret triangle

---

Abbreviations: HOD, hypertrophic olivary degeneration; PT, palatal tremor; OPT, oculopalatal tremor; PAPT, progressive ataxia and palatal tremor; EPT, essential palatal tremor.

INTRODUCTION

The terminology and the nosology of hypertrophic inferior olive degeneration and palatal tremor (PT) or oculopalatal tremor (OPT) has evolved over time and needs some clarification. Unilateral or bilateral hypertrophic olivary degeneration (HOD) in the medulla oblongata was first anatomically described in late nineteenth century (1). At the same time, literature focused on the observation of rhythmic PT (2) using different terms such as palatal nystagmus, palatal myoclonus, or palatal myorhythmia. It was finally classified among tremors in 1990 (3). PT is often associated with synchronous eye oscillations and such cases are termed OPT. It can also be associated with synchronous movements of the larynx, pharynx, diaphragm, and facial muscles. PT or OPT has been described in association with the anatomical observation of HOD (4). HOD was later demonstrated on MRI, where it appears as an increased T2/FLAIR signal intensity and enlargement of the inferior olive (5–7). This unique degeneration of the inferior olive most frequently develops weeks or months (8, 9) secondary to a lesion within the dentato-olivary pathway (10), originally referred to as the Guillain–Mollaret triangle (11). The lesion is most often a hemorrhagic stroke.

In 1990, Deuschl et al. suggested differentiating symptomatic PT, developing secondary to brainstem or cerebellar lesions, from essential PT (EPT) for which there is no evidence of a structural lesion (12). Patients with EPT usually have objective ear click, which is less frequent (8%) in the symptomatic form. Involvement of the tensor veli palatini muscle in EPT and of the levator veli palatini muscle in symptomatic PT might explain this clinical difference (3). However, those with symptomatic PT may also experience ear click; to distinguish forms it is of note that EPT patients neither show involvement of eye and other muscles nor evidence of structural abnormalities of the inferior olive (13). Furthermore, the etiology of EPT is heterogeneous with a considerable proportion of psychogenic cases (14) and may disappear over time (15). EPT is therefore a different disease without HOD and does not concern this review; below, PT refers to the symptomatic form.

Later on, Sperling and Herrmann (6) and then Samuel et al. (13) described a syndrome of progressive ataxia and palatal tremor (PAPT). Some of them disclose OPT. In these cases, ataxia progresses and is not the result of a monophasic illness. Sporadic and familial forms of PAPT are described. There is no visible structural causative lesion on the dentato-olivary pathway, but HOD on MRI is present in most cases. Although a specific lesion of the dendato-olivary pathway is not yet identified, PAPT could be considered as a subgroup of symptomatic PT or OPT and will therefore be described in this review.

CLINICAL FEATURES OF PT AND OPT

The first observations of synchronous rhythmical movement of the eye and palate were published 150 years ago (2). Since then, different publications have reported the clinical features of this abnormal palatal and eye movement (11, 16, 17).

Symptomatic PT is characterized by involuntary movements of the soft palate and pharynx, due to rhythmic contraction of the levator veli palatine (8, 16) (Video S1 in Supplementary Material). The movements are most commonly bilateral and symmetrical (18). In this case, the soft palate is contracted superiorly and posteriorly along with the uvula with synchronous closing of the pharynx (8). Sometimes the movement can be unilateral, the palate and uvula then being drawn to one side (17, 19). The movements are continuous, the rhythm being most frequently between 100 and 160/min (or 1.5–3 Hz) and persist during sleep (3). Patients with symptomatic PT very rarely complain of ear click (3, 18).

Oculopalatal tremor refers to the synchronous combination of PT and pendular nystagmus. Pendular nystagmus is found to be present in 30% of symptomatic PT (3), probably less frequently in case of PAPT [4 out of 28 cases in Samuel et al. (13)]. In series of patients with pendular nystagmus, up to 18% of those with HOD do not develop PT (20, 21). Patients have mainly vertical pendular oscillations of the eyes with varied combinations of torsional and horizontal components (21–24) (Video S2 in Supplementary Material). The nystagmus can sometimes take the form of convergent–divergent nystagmus (20, 25). This pendular nystagmus is of quite large mean amplitude (8°), high peak velocity (16°/s), and demonstrates irregularity (24) (**Figure 1**). It is most frequently asymmetric and dissociated in direction in the two eyes (24). While PT is mostly asymptomatic, patients with OPT complain of disturbing oscillopsia, decreased visual acuity, with deterioration of vision-specific health-related quality of life (24, 26). Other than the observed synchrony, attempts have been made to relate characteristics of the nystagmus to the associated palatal movements (22) and to the side of HOD, but the randomness of the directions, waveforms, as well as disconjugacy of nystagmus could just reflect randomly formed couplings in inferior olivary neurons (27). Furthermore, the other associated ocular motor deficit secondary to the brainstem lesion may contribute to disconjugacy of the nystagmus (28).

Other synchronous movements can be associated with palatal myoclonus, most frequently involving muscles of the gill arches: the face, the tongue, the floor of the mouth, the pharynx, the larynx, and the diaphragm (29) (Videos S1 and S2 in Supplementary Material). In some rare cases, skeletal muscle tremor, mainly of the upper limbs, may be associated (30–32). Some cases of OPT, secondary to lesion of the dentato-olivary pathway, present with focal or generalized dystonia, constituting a variant of OPT (33).

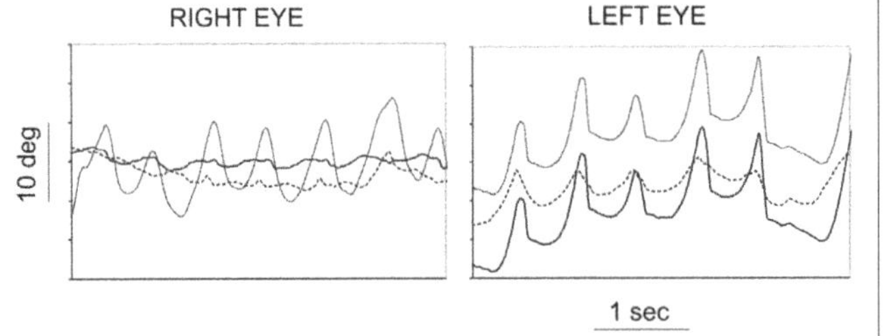

FIGURE 1 | Eye position (in degrees) traces according to time (in seconds) for right (left panel) and left (right panel) eye in an oculopalatal tremor patient. Continuous line: horizontal position, discontinuous line: vertical position, and dotted gray line: torsional position. Adapted from Ref. (24).

ETIOLOGIES

Symptomatic PT and OPT

According to the earliest described cases (2, 4, 11, 16, 17), the most common form of PT/OPT is secondary to a monophasic structural lesion of the brainstem or the cerebellum. The topography of the lesion involves the dentato-olivary pathway, part of the Guillain–Mollaret triangle (11), i.e., the pathway coming from the contralateral dentate nucleus, through the contralateral brachium conjunctivum crossing the midline, turning around the ipsilateral red nucleus, and descending in the ipsilateral central tegmental tract to the inferior olive (**Figure 2**). Central tegmental tract lesions are the most frequent and seem to be more specifically associated with OPT compared to lesions of dentate nuclei/brachium conjunctivum where only PT is observed (21, 24, 34). In these cases of symptomatic PT or OPT, the condition develops at least 1 month and up to 8 years (median between 10 and 11 months) after the occurrence of the presumed anatomical lesion (9, 13). Symptomatic PT becomes increasingly intense, reaching a peak between 5 and 24 months after lesion (35). Once established, PT or OPT persists for life, with the exception of a few patients in whom PT or OPT is reported to have disappeared completely after many years, although MRI show persistent signal change in the inferior olivary nucleus (21) (Video S3 in Supplementary Material).

The most frequent etiology of structural brainstem or cerebellar lesion is vascular and more often hemorrhagic than ischemic (11, 37). Other etiologies include brain trauma, brainstem tumors, surgical or gamma knife removal of brainstem cavernoma (38), multiple sclerosis (MS), and a broad range of other unspecific lesions [see Table 3 in Samuel et al. (13)]. It is assumed that, to be causative, this primary lesion has to be destructive, a condition that is most easily satisfied by vascular, neurosurgical, or gamma knife lesions (19).

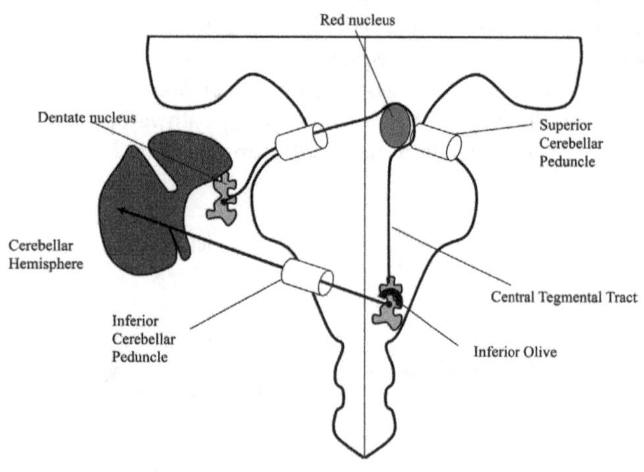

FIGURE 2 | Schematic representation of the Guillain–Mollaret triangle. The pathway coming from the contralateral dentate nucleus, through the contralateral brachium conjunctivum crosses the midline, turns around the ipsilateral red nucleus, and descends in the ipsilateral central tegmental tract to the inferior olive. Adapted from Ref. (36).

The MS cases might be further discussed. MS has been identified as a common cause of OPT, from 3 (12) to 10% (13). Mostly historical articles report cases of OPT or PT secondary to MS (39, 40). However, in MS, pendular nystagmus is much more often observed without OPT (24, 41, 42). This pendular nystagmus is of small amplitude (1°), low mean peak velocity (6°/s), high mean frequency (4–6 Hz), and is highly regular, like a sine wave (24, 41). Although confused with OPT (42), there is neither an associated PT nor HOD on MRI (24). It may be added that in historical neuropathological cases, almost all lesions are vascular in nature (11). The relatively high proportion of reported MS in PT and OPT might therefore have been overestimated. Indeed, a review of historical cases finds that they do not meet the current clinical criteria for diagnosis of MS or OPT, and neuroimaging or pathology was lacking (40, 43). Some cases seem to correspond to pendular nystagmus associated with MS, other to brainstem hemorrhage, sporadic, or familial PAPT. A notable exception is the report of two patients with clinical, biological, and MRI criteria for MS, developing OPT associated with HOD on MRI (44, 45). Although the second case was complex with history of posterior fossa tumor and radiation therapy (45), these are the only convincing observations of OPT in MS.

According to the topography of the structural lesion, other neurological manifestations may be observed in association with OPT. Patients frequently present contralateral hemiplegia, contralateral hemi-hypoesthesia or spinothalamic syndrome, ipsilateral facial palsy, ipsilateral kinetic cerebellar syndrome (24). In the case of unilateral cerebellar signs, pendular nystagmus is more pronounced in the eye on the affected side (3). Patients also frequently have a deficit in the horizontal eye movement, including fascicular abducens nerve palsy, internuclear ophthalmoplegia, one and a half syndrome, nuclear abducens syndrome (nuclear VI), or horizontal saccadic palsy (24, 41). Central vestibular manifestations have also been reported in association to OPT (46). These manifestations usually result from the primary lesion and present as a monophasic event.

Delayed and progressive worsening of extremity and gait cerebellar ataxia associated with OPT, secondary to identified structural etiologies (stroke; cavernoma; tumor and radiation therapy; subarachnoid hemorrhage; brain trauma) has also been reported (36, 47, 48). The mechanisms of OPT with delayed ataxia following brainstem lesion is not understood, although it seems to occur with larger and bilateral acute brainstem lesions (47). Hemosiderin deposition has been suggested (48), but it cannot explain the cases observed in brainstem tumors and radiotherapy. Delayed ataxia or movement disorder following a monophasic structural lesion without OPT has been reported (49, 50), which could suggest that not all progressive disorders arise from primary neurodegenerative processes (13).

Progressive Ataxia and PT

In 1985, Sperling and Herrmann (6) suggested to distinguish a syndrome associating PT, HOD, and progressive cerebellar ataxia. This entity was reported again (51), and the syndrome of progressive ataxia and palatal tremor (PAPT) was more precisely defined by Samuel et al. (13). The authors suggested differentiating sporadic PAPT from familial forms of PAPT. None of the patients have structural brainstem or cerebellar lesion, but cerebellar ataxia and cerebellar atrophy on MRI progress over years. These cases might correspond to the "degenerative" etiology suggested in older reports [see review in Samuel et al. (13)].

Sporadic PAPT

In sporadic PAPT, other than gait, trunk and limb ataxia, dysarthria, non-specific cerebellar ocular motor dysfunction is observed, such as gaze-evoked nystagmus, jerk vertical nystagmus, hypermetric saccades, and saccadic pursuit (13). All reported patients present PT. Four out of 28 patients reviewed in Samuel et al. (13) have OPT and 2 internuclear ophthalmoplegia, which indicate brainstem involvement. Patients often complain of poor vision due to oscillopsia or diplopia. Hearing loss seems to be quite frequently associated with sporadic PAPT (in four out of six patients). Other neurological manifestations are not specific. The cerebellar ataxia may precede or follow the occurrence of PT (52). Almost all patients show abnormal bilateral signal and/or HOD on MRI. There is no single theory unifying etiologies of sporadic PAPT, although some of them might be due to polymerase gamma (POLG) mutation (53, 54).

In older reports, PT and HOD has also been reported in other degenerative neurological disorders such as pathologically proven progressive supranuclear palsy (55, 56) and other undetermined neurodegenerative diseases (57). The nosology of these cases, presenting with progressive neurological deficit, other than cerebellar ataxia, needs to be clarified.

Familial PAPT

Familial PAPT is more complex than sporadic PAPT and may include a variety of etiologies. They are associated with marked brainstem and cervical cord atrophy with corticospinal tract findings, and the olivary MRI abnormalities may be lacking (13). Three main known etiologies may be considered: Alexander disease, POLG mutation, and spinocerebellar ataxia type 20 (SCA20).

Alexander disease is one of the most reported known etiologies of familial progressive neurological disorder associated with PT (57–61). Alexander disease is a leukodystrophy, that is pathologically characterized by the presence of Rosenthal fibers, and that is caused by mutations in the gene encoding glial fibrillary acidic protein on chromosome 17q21 (62) and present as a progressive neurological disorder that can occur in an infantile, juvenile, or adult form (59). It usually results from *de novo* mutations, with autosomal dominant inheritance in future generations (59). In juvenile and adult forms, the patients exhibit palatal myoclonus, spastic tetraparesia, mild cerebellar dysfunction, and associated ocular motor abnormalities (60). There is no description of HOD in large series of adult-onset Alexander disease (63), but one recent case with a phenotype of PAPT presented inferior olive hypertrophia (64). In only one case, associated "ocular myoclonus" was described (60).

Recent observations of PT or OPT with HOD, or HOD without clinical manifestations of PT or OPT have been reported in association with POLG mutation (53, 54, 65). Mutations of the mitochondrial DNA (mtDNA) encoded by the POLG gene are an important cause of pediatric and adult-onset mitochondrial disease. In adults, they are associated with multiple mtDNA deletions leading to a wide spectrum of dominant and recessive progressive neurological disorders, often described as syndromes, such as progressive external ophthalmoplegia, Alpers syndrome, sensory ataxic neuropathy, dysarthria and ophthalmoparesis (65, 66). POLG mutation should also be considered in patients with PAPT or progressive ataxia with inferior olive hypersignal (54), even in sporadic cases, and even without other frequently associated neurological signs such as sensory neuronopathy associated with weakness of ocular, pharyngeal, axial, and/or limb muscles (66).

Autosomal dominant SCA20 is a rare spinocerebellar ataxia characterized by a slowly progressive ataxia and dysarthria; two-thirds of those affected also display PT ("myoclonus") with increased inferior olivary T2 signal (67). In these patients, CT scan shows dentate calcification, without concomitant pallidal calcification. The locus of genetic mutation overlaps that of spinocerebellar ataxia type 5 on chromosome 11, but the phenotypes are very different (68). More recently, a single case of adult-onset GM2-gangliosidosis type II (Sandhoff disease) presenting PT and cerebellar ataxia has been reported, although inferior olive signal was not described (69).

Toxic HOD

There are few reports of reversible inferior olive MRI hypersignal among diffuse MRI changes associated with toxic-induced encephalopathy, such as metronidazole (70). Although none of them was associated with the clinical syndrome of PT or OPT, toxic lesions have a predilection for dentate nuclei and brainstem tegmentum, suggesting reversible lesion of the Guillain–Mollaret triangle (70). One case of reversible PT induced by fluoxetine has been reported, although HOD on MRI is not mentioned (71).

NEUROPATHOLOGY OF THE DEGENERATIVE HYPERTROPHIC INFERIOR OLIVARY NUCLEUS

Histological features of degenerative olivary hypertrophy had been previously reported by numerous authors, mainly in old French publications (1, 4, 11, 31, 72, 73). On postmortem pathological observations, they described macroscopic hypertrophy of the inferior olives associated with neuron swelling with vacuolation (so-called "fenestrated neurons"), bizarre nerve cell shape, severe fibrillary gliosis, and demyelination of the olive white matter (**Figure 3**). These pathological hallmarks have been thought to result from transynaptic degeneration secondary to a lesion of the ipsilateral central tegmental tract or the contralateral dentate nucleus. More recent immunohistochemical studies identified various changes in the neurons, their neurites, and presynaptic terminals confirming this hypothesis (74, 75). The main finding is a decreased synaptophysin immunoreactivity confirming the presynaptic abnormalities linked to deafferentation (75). In 1981, Goto and Kaneko published a neuropathological study of eight cases of pontine hemorrhage involving unilaterally or bilaterally central tegmental tracts with different

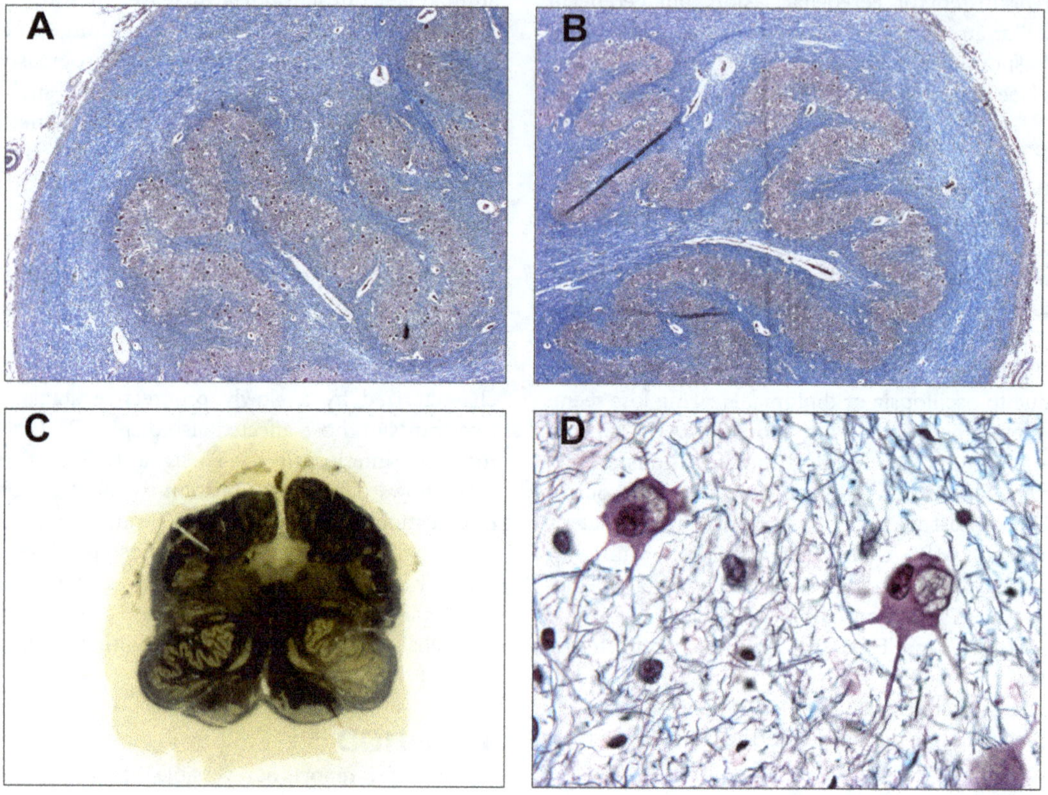

FIGURE 3 | Pathological features of degenerative inferior olive hypertrophy. Hypertrophic inferior olive **(A)** compared to contralateral side **(B)** (Bodian Luxol, X200). Note the mild demyelination of the surrounding white matter. **(C)** Coronal section of the medulla oblongata showing hypertrophy of the left inferior olive (Loyez stain). **(D)** Swelled and vacuolated nerve cells ("fenestrated neurons") observed in the hypertrophic inferior olive [from **(A)**, Bodian Luxol, X400]. Courtesy of Charles Duyckaerts and Franck Bielle, Escourolle's Lab, Pitie-Salpetriere Hospital, Paris, France. Adapted from Ref. (51).

survival periods (76). This study demonstrated six neuropathological stages: (1) no olivary changes (<24 h after onset); (2) degeneration of the olivary amiculum (periphery of the olive, at 2–7 days or more); (3) mild olivary enlargement with neuronal hypertrophy and no glial reaction (at about 3 weeks); (4) culminant hypertrophy of both neurons and astrocytes (at about 8.5 months); (5) olivary pseudohypertrophy with neuronal dissolution (at about 9.5 months and later); and (6) olivary atrophy with neuronal disappearance (after a few years).

Degenerative olivary hypertrophy is predominantly observed in patients with manifest damage of the dentato–olivary pathway (4, 11, 31, 37, 73, 77). It is predominantly but not always associated with PT/OPT, more specifically following head injury (37). All these neuropathological studies agree with the hypothesis of a unique feature of olivary hypertrophy related to transneuronal degeneration in response to deafferentation following dentato–olivary pathway lesion.

Most interestingly, the only pathological study of PAPT with HOD revealed a unique tau pathology (78). This case showed symmetrical unspecific inferior olivary hypertrophy, without focal brainstem lesion. Strikingly, insoluble tau deposits were exclusively found in some infratentorial neurons, in particular in the inferior olives. Combination of primary tauopathy and secondary degenerative changes in the olives suggested to the authors that "primary degenerative process affecting a portion of olivary neurons could trigger retrograde degeneration of the *dentato-olivary* fibers, which might cause secondary (deafferentation type) hypertrophic degeneration in other olivary neurons, perhaps through loss of axon collaterals." Such a hypothesis of a primary focal tauopathy leading to deafferentation-induced hypertrophic degeneration finds an echo with the observations of HOD in patients with pathologically-proven supranuclear palsy tauopathy (56, 57).

RADIOLOGICAL FEATURES

Hypertrophic Olivary Degeneration

The historical observations of neuropathological changes in the inferior olive found their radiological correlates in the observation of increased signal intensity and enlargement of the inferior olive seen on proton density-weighted and T2/FLAIR MRI (6, 7, 79) (**Figure 4**). The term HOD was then also conventionally used to define these abnormal signals on MRI, even if there is only hypersignal (5, 80). The temporal evolution of these abnormal signals follows pathological changes (81, 82). The hypersignal appears around 1 month after the ictus and persists, while hypertrophy is not usually observed until 6 months after ictus and resolves at approximately 3–4 years after ictus (5) (**Figure 5**). In some

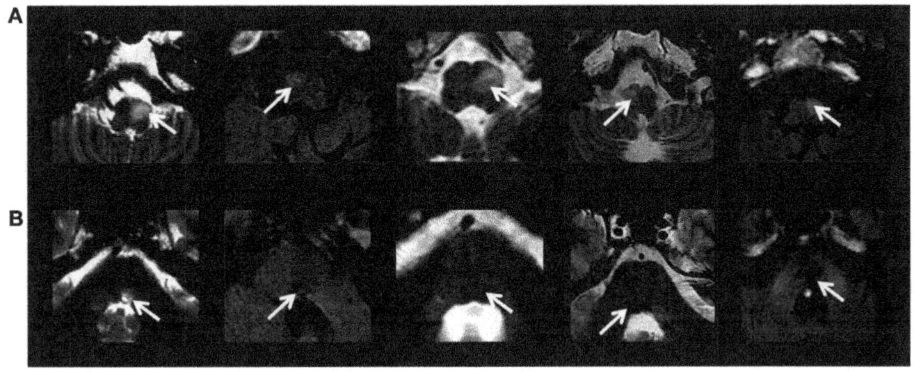

FIGURE 4 | Axial FLAIR or T2 MRI (1.5-T GE scanners) at **(A)** inferior olive level and **(B)** midpontine tegmentum level in five patients with symptomatic oculopalatal tremor. White arrows in **(A)** indicate the abnormal inferior olive hypersignal and in **(B)** the causative lesion. Adapted from Ref. (24).

cases, the MRI hypersignal may also return to normal (13, 83). HOD on MRI is unilateral or bilateral in case of symptomatic PT and bilateral in case of PAPT (84, 85). It may also be lacking in familial PAPT (7, 13). In symptomatic PT, HOD usually appears contralateral in case of cerebellar lesion and ipsilateral in case of lateralized central tegmental tract lesion (5, 21, 85). It may precede the clinical manifestations of PT or OPT (80) and even be observed without the development of PT (86). In symptomatic OPT, dissociated pendular nystagmus seems to predict unilateral HOD on MRI with accuracy, while symmetric pendular nystagmus is associated with either unilateral or bilateral HOD (21). Finally, radiological cases of idiopathic HOD without any structural lesion in the Guillain–Mollaret triangle, neither PT, OPT, or PAPT are described (87).

Cerebral Metabolism Imaging

There is discordance in cerebral metabolism imaging; one study found inferior olive hypermetabolism (88), and the other one that used statistical parametric mapping, failed to show metabolic changes in the inferior olive (34).

Cerebellar Changes Associated With HOD

MRI of the cerebellum in patients with symptomatic PT found atrophic changes suggesting a degenerative process involving the dentate nucleus and the cerebellar cortex on the side opposite to the HOD (89). Degeneration of cerebellar cortex secondary to HOD has already been discussed in some neuropathological studies (90).

PHYSIOPATHOLOGY OF PT/OPT ASSOCIATED WITH HOD

The main accepted explanation of PT or OPT associated with the development of HOD is that the abnormal inferior olive plays a significant role in PT/OPT (4). First of all, the HOD would develop secondary to dentato-olivary pathway lesion at least for the symptomatic forms, due to a denervation mechanism (77). Normal inferior olivary neurons can generate spontaneous oscillations and are electrically coupled by dendrodendritic gap junctions (91, 92). In case of dentato-olivary pathway lesion, denervated olivary neurons released from inhibitory inputs would enlarge and develop sustained synchronized oscillations (91). Animal models of HOD show the development of spikes on denervated inferior olivary neurons, supporting electrotonic coupling through gap junctions (93). In this hypothesis, inferior olive would be the oscillator of palatal and/or ocular tremor. This is further supported by the observation of disturbed cerebellar function (motor learning) in patients with SPT (94, 95) and the temporal relationship of the development of HOD and the clinical symptoms. This is finally further supported by the observation of inferior olivary nucleus hypermetabolism (86). However, the main criticism against the involvement of inferior olive as part of the mechanism for OPT is the observation of decreased hypertrophy of inferior olive in time while OPT persists, or other observations showing absent inferior olivary nucleus hypermetabolism (34) in patients, and functional imaging showing synchronous decreased cerebellar activity and OPT with clonazepam, but no decrease of inferior olive activity (96). Some authors suggested that inferior olive could be involved in the development of PT/OPT but not in maintaining the symptoms (35).

A fascinating recent model suggested both the implication of inferior olive oscillator generating spike trains at 1–2 Hz and cerebellar modulation/amplification of the motor output (27, 97) (**Figure 6**). In this model of pendular nystagmus in OPT, the synchronized signal from the inferior olive reaches *via* climbing fibers Purkinje cells and the deep cerebellar nuclei including vestibular nuclei. In turn, the signal in the vestibular nuclei projects indirectly to the Purkinje cells, *via* a mossy fiber/granule cells-parallel fiber. The repeated inferior olive pulses would create periodic climbing and parallel fiber inputs to Purkinje cells at approximately the same time and create a learning signal back to the vestibular nuclei, contributing to smoothing and amplifying pulse (27). While this model seems to reproduce many of the aspects of OPT and specifically the 1–2 Hz irregular oscillation, it cannot prove that both inferior olive and cerebellum are necessary to explain it.

The topography of this tremor involving structures corresponding embryologically to the first to fifth branchial arches has received less interest. In 1949, Stern suggested that PT would be

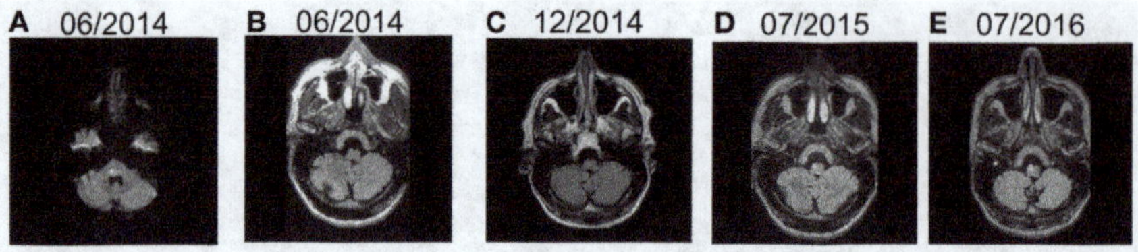

FIGURE 5 | Temporal evolution of right-sided inferior olive hypersignal in a patient with symptomatic oculopalatal tremor. The patient presented a right-sided pontine tegmental lesion in June 2014 seen on the diffusion MRI scan **(A)**, and the medulla showed no abnormal hypersignal on FLAIR MRI **(B)**. Subsequently, right inferior olive hypersignal was observed 6 months later **(C)**, with increasing signal 1 year later **(D)** and right inferior olive hypertrophy was observed 2 years later **(E)**.

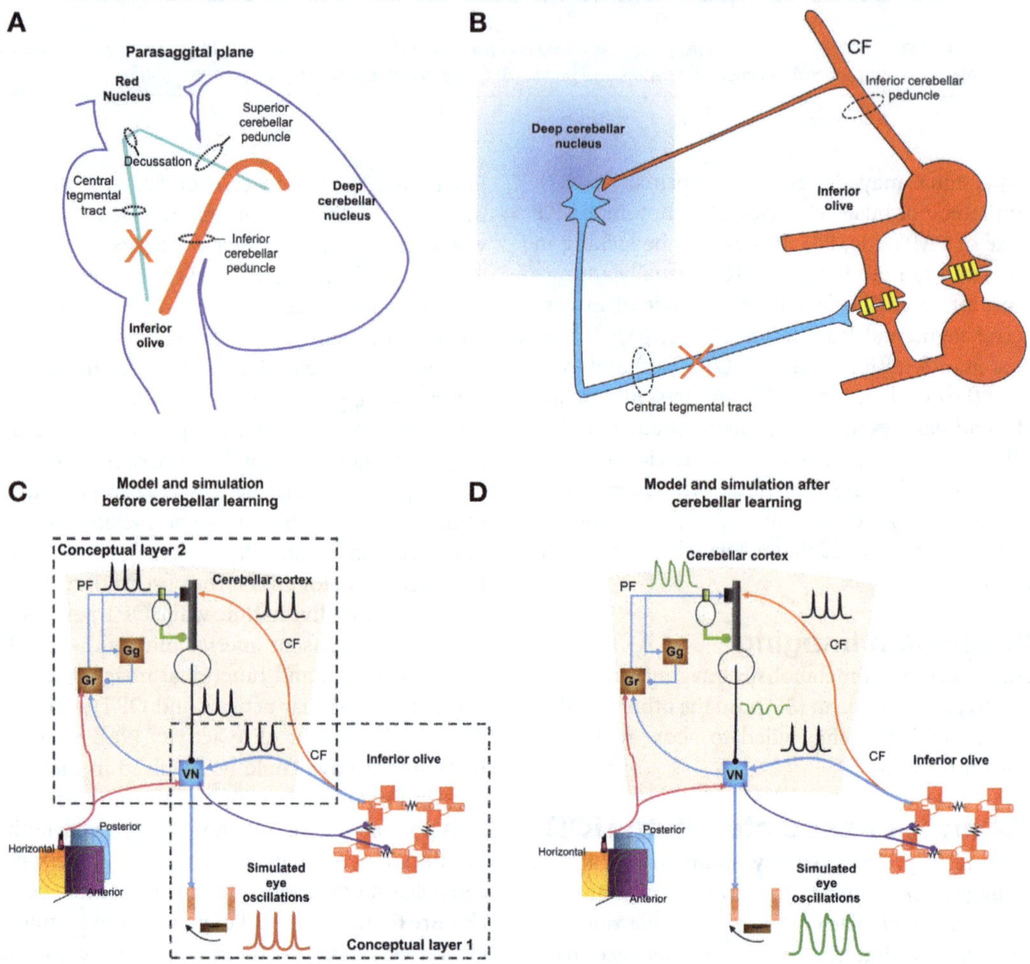

FIGURE 6 | Schematic representation of the Guillain–Mollaret triangle formed by connections between the deep cerebellar nuclei and contralateral inferior olive, which pass near the red nucleus **(A)**. The conduction strength through the dendrodendritic gap junctions (schematized with yellow connexon channels; DD) between adjacent inferior olivary neurons are inhibited by projections from the deep cerebellar nuclei (blue projection) **(B)**. Lesions in the Guillain–Mollaret triangle [red X in **(A,B)**] also result in hypertrophy of inferior olive neurons causing development of abnormal soma-somatic gap junction. Schematic representation of a model for classical delay conditioning **(C,D)**. Model and traces from simulations after inferior olive hypertrophy but before cerebellar learning **(C)**. Inferior olive and cerebellar modules after hypertrophy and learning **(D)**. Lower left corner shows icon for semicircular canals **(C,D)**. Simulated membrane potentials (black), eye oscillations (magenta). CF, climbing fibers; PF, parallel fibers; DD, dendrodendritic gap junction; SS, soma-somatic gap junction; Gr, granule cell layer; IN, interneurons; PC, Purkinje neurons [(27) with permission for reproduction of material].

the human homolog of a primitive accessory respiratory reflex in gill-breathing vertebrates, leading to the hypothesis of recurrence of an archaic phenomenon (98). The limitation to the branchial arches muscles suggested to authors that the central tegmental tract lesion causes hypersensitivity of the nucleus ambiguous that innervate branchial muscles (99). However, this does not properly explain how 1–2 Hz oscillation develop in the arches, while Shaikh's model does.

TREATMENT

Therapeutic trials have been mainly performed on acquired pendular nystagmus, which is the most symptomatic consequence of OPT. The most rigorous treatment trials in acquired pendular nystagmus (due to MS or OPT) led to the proposal of gabapentin or memantine as valuable drugs (26, 100–104). Only one study specifically tested gabapentin, memantine, and baclofen in a group of six patients with acquired pendular nystagmus in OPT with a significant effect of gabapentin and memantine on reduction of nystagmus amplitude and frequency irregularity (102). We have also observed sustained decrease of nystagmus velocity in some patients (**Figure 7**). Another study found marked improvement of both eye and palate movements as well as complaints by patients (including audible clicks) with trihexyphenidyl; however, patients with PT following a structural lesion, EPT, and MS, but not those with OPT, were included (105). There have been suggestions of testing drugs that reduce electrotonic coupling among hypertrophied inferior olive neurons by blocking connexons like quinine, carbenoxolone, or mefloquine (27), but no study has since been published. Botulinum toxin has been tested on pendular nystagmus in OPT with variable success (106) and in clicking tinnitus in PT (107).

In a different approach, bilateral deep brain stimulation of the red nucleus in one patient with OPT (and failure of medical treatment) was tested (108). This study failed to show any improvement of eye oscillation. The failure of this intervention may be explained by erroneous interpretation of mechanism of OPT. The hypothesis was to interfere with the rhythmicity of the olivocerebellar circuit, but the target was the afferent dentato-olivary pathway within the red nucleus region.

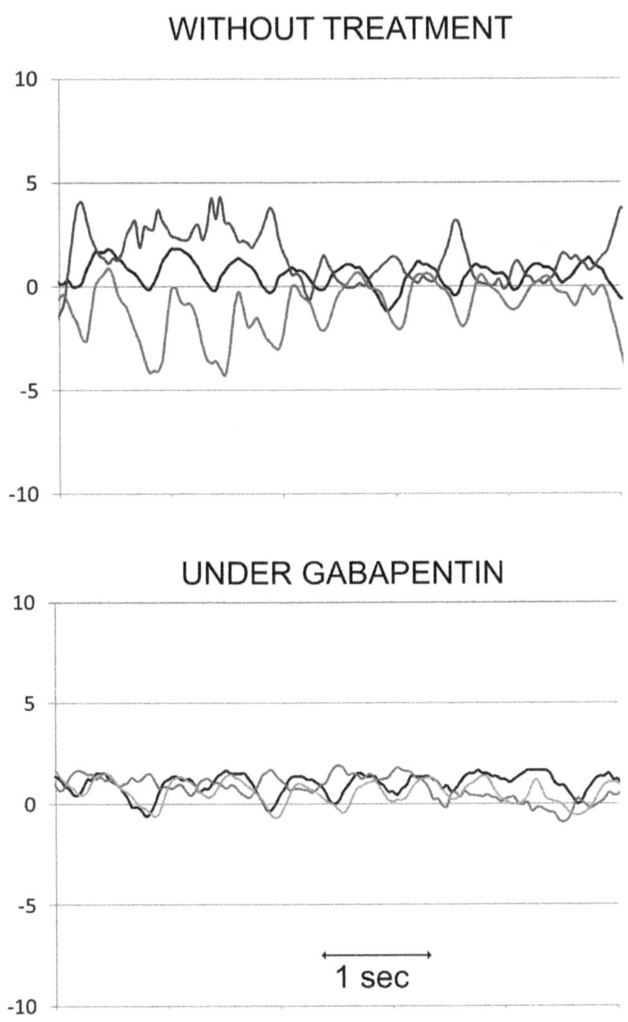

FIGURE 7 | Eye position (in degrees) traces over time (in seconds) in one oculopalatal tremor patient, without treatment (upper panel) and under gabapentin (lower panel). Dark line: horizontal position, gray line: vertical position, and light gray line: torsional position. Note the decrease in nystagmus amplitude, mainly in the torsional plane, under gabapentin.

AUTHOR CONTRIBUTIONS

Both CT and VD contributed to conception or design of the work; drafting the work and revising; final approval of the version to be published; and the agreement to be accountable for all aspects of the work in ensuring that questions related to the accuracy or integrity of any part of the work are appropriately investigated and resolved.

ACKNOWLEDGMENTS

We gratefully acknowledge Dr. Franck Bielle and Prof. Charles Duyckaerts for their pathological expertise and for providing microphotographs of postmortem cases (Raymond Escourolle Laboratory, La Salpetriere Hospital, Paris, France). We gratefully acknowledge Philip Robinson for English language editing (Direction de la Recherche Clinique, Hospices Civils de Lyon).

SUPPLEMENTARY MATERIAL

VIDEO S1 | Palatal and chin tremor. This 30-year-old patient presented an acute pontine hemorrhagic stroke resulting in left hemiplegia and right facial palsy. Three months later, he complained of oscillopsia. T2 MRI showed pontine hemorrhagic scar. In addition to pendular nystagmus (not shown), synchronous left-sided palatal and chin tremor around 1 Hz frequency can be observed in this video. T2 MRI showed left-sided hypertrophic olivary degeneration at medullar level.

VIDEO S2 | Ocular and upper lip tremor. This 29-year-old patient presented an acute hemorrhagic pontine stroke. He presented with right-sided hemiplegia, left-sided facial palsy, dysarthria, and left-sided gaze palsy. A few months later, he complained of oscillopsia. The video shows binocular incongruent 1.6 Hz pendular nystagmus, and left upper lip synchronous tremor. There was also palatal tremor (not shown). MRI found left-sided hypertrophic olivary degeneration.

VIDEO S3 | Decrease of pendular nystagmus with time in a patient with symptomatic oculopalatal tremor (OPT). OPT was diagnosed in 2012 but occurred a few weeks after surgical treatment of bleeding brainstem cavernoma in 2010. During follow-up, the patient described a decrease in oscillopsia and observation disclosed great decrease in nystagmus in 2016, without any pharmacological treatment.

REFERENCES

1. Oppenheim H. Über ein bei Krankheitsprocessen in der hinteren Schadelgrube beobachtetes symptom. *Neurol Zbl* (1889) 8:132–4.
2. Spencer HR. Pharyngeal and laryngeal "nystagmus". *Lancet* (1886) 2:702. doi:10.1016/S0140-6736(01)78357-2
3. Deuschl G, Toro C, Valls-Sole J, Zeffiro T, Zee DS, Hallett M. Symptomatic and essential palatal tremor. 1. Clinical, physiological and MRI analysis. *Brain* (1994) 117(Pt 4):775–88. doi:10.1093/brain/117.4.775
4. Van Bogaert L, Bertrand I. Sur les myoclonies associées synchrones et rythmiques par lésion en foyer du tronc cérébral. *Rev Neurol* (1928) 1(2):203.
5. Goyal M, Versnick E, Tuite P, Cyr JS, Kucharczyk W, Montanera W, et al. Hypertrophic olivary degeneration: metaanalysis of the temporal evolution of MR findings. *AJNR Am J Neuroradiol* (2000) 21(6):1073–7.
6. Sperling MR, Herrmann C Jr. Syndrome of palatal myoclonus and progressive ataxia: two cases with magnetic resonance imaging. *Neurology* (1985) 35(8):1212–4. doi:10.1212/WNL.35.8.1212
7. Yokota T, Hirashima F, Furukawa T, Tsukagoshi H, Yoshikawa H. MRI findings of inferior olives in palatal myoclonus. *J Neurol* (1989) 236(2):115–6. doi:10.1007/BF00314408
8. Dubinsky RM, Hallett M. Palatal myoclonus and facial involvement in other types of myoclonus. *Adv Neurol* (1988) 49:263–78.
9. Matsuo F, Ajax ET. Palatal myoclonus and denervation supersensitivity in the central nervous system. *Ann Neurol* (1979) 5(1):72–8. doi:10.1002/ana.410050111
10. Lapresle J, Hamida MB. The dentato-olivary pathway. Somatotopic relationship between the dentate nucleus and the contralateral inferior olive. *Arch Neurol* (1970) 22(2):135–43. doi:10.1001/archneur.1970.00480200041004
11. Guillain G, Mollaret P. Deux cas de myoclonies synchrones et rythmées vélo-pharyngo-laryngo-oculo-diaphragmatiques: le problème anatomique et physiologique. *Rev Neurol* (1931) 2:545–66.
12. Deuschl G, Mischke G, Schenck E, Schulte-Monting J, Lucking CH. Symptomatic and essential rhythmic palatal myoclonus. *Brain* (1990) 113(Pt 6):1645–72. doi:10.1093/brain/113.6.1645
13. Samuel M, Torun N, Tuite PJ, Sharpe JA, Lang AE. Progressive ataxia and palatal tremor (PAPT): clinical and MRI assessment with review of palatal tremors. *Brain* (2004) 127(Pt 6):1252–68. doi:10.1093/brain/awh137
14. Zadikoff C, Lang AE, Klein C. The 'essentials' of essential palatal tremor: a reappraisal of the nosology. *Brain* (2006) 129(Pt 4):832–40. doi:10.1093/brain/awh684
15. Jacobs L, Newman RP, Bozian D. Disappearing palatal myoclonus. *Neurology* (1981) 31(6):748–51. doi:10.1212/WNL.31.6.748
16. Leshin N, Stone TT. Continuous rhythmic movements of the palate, pharynx and larynx. *Arch Neurol Psychiat* (1931) 31:1236.
17. Riley HA, Brock S. Rhythmic myoclonus of the muscles of the palate, pharynx, larynx and other regions. *Arch Neurol Psychiat* (1933) 29:726. doi:10.1001/archneurpsyc.1933.02240100045004
18. Deuschl G, Toro C, Hallett M. Symptomatic and essential palatal tremor. 2. Differences of palatal movements. *Mov Disord* (1994) 9(6):676–8. doi:10.1002/mds.870090615
19. Lapresle J. Rhythmic palatal myoclonus and the dentato-olivary pathway. *J Neurol* (1979) 220(4):223–30. doi:10.1007/BF00314146
20. Gresty MA, Ell JJ, Findley LJ. Acquired pendular nystagmus: its characteristics, localising value and pathophysiology. *J Neurol Neurosurg Psychiatry* (1982) 45(5):431–9. doi:10.1136/jnnp.45.5.431
21. Kim JS, Moon SY, Choi KD, Kim JH, Sharpe JA. Patterns of ocular oscillation in oculopalatal tremor: imaging correlations. *Neurology* (2007) 68(14):1128–35. doi:10.1212/01.wnl.0000258665.37827.f6
22. Nakada T, Kwee IL. Oculopalatal myoclonus. *Brain* (1986) 109(Pt 3):431–41. doi:10.1093/brain/109.3.431
23. Talks SJ, Elston JS. Oculopalatal myoclonus: eye movement studies, MRI findings and the difficulty of treatment. *Eye* (1997) 11(Pt 1):19–24. doi:10.1038/eye.1997.4
24. Tilikete C, Jasse L, Pelisson D, Vukusic S, Durand-Dubief F, Urquizar C, et al. Acquired pendular nystagmus in multiple sclerosis and oculopalatal tremor. *Neurology* (2011) 76(19):1650–7. doi:10.1212/WNL.0b013e318219fa9c
25. Galvez-Ruiz A, Roig C, Muñoz S, Arruga J. Convergent-divergent nystagmus as a manifestation of oculopalatal tremor. *Neuroophthalmology* (2011) 35(5–6):276–9. doi:10.3109/01658107.2011.609606
26. Thurtell MJ, Joshi AC, Leone AC, Tomsak RL, Kosmorsky GS, Stahl JS, et al. Crossover trial of gabapentin and memantine as treatment for acquired nystagmus. *Ann Neurol* (2010) 67(5):676–80. doi:10.1002/ana.21991
27. Shaikh AG, Hong S, Liao K, Tian J, Solomon D, Zee DS, et al. Oculopalatal tremor explained by a model of inferior olivary hypertrophy and cerebellar plasticity. *Brain* (2010) 133(Pt 3):923–40. doi:10.1093/brain/awp323
28. Leigh RJ, Zee DS. *The Neurology of Eye Movement*. 5th ed. New York: Oxford University Press (2015).
29. Borruat FX. Oculopalatal tremor: current concepts and new observations. *Curr Opin Neurol* (2013) 26(1):67–73. doi:10.1097/WCO.0b013e32835c60e6
30. Alstadhaug KB. Oculopalatal and cerebellar limb tremor due to hypertrophic olivary degeneration. *Eur J Neurol* (2007) 14(5):e6–7. doi:10.1111/j.1468-1331.2007.01719.x
31. Guillain G, Thurel R. Myoclonies vélo-pharyngo-laryngo-oculo-diaphragmatiques associées a des myoclonies synchrones squelettiques. *Rev Neurol* (1932) 2:677–84.
32. Nagaoka M, Narabayashi H. Palatal myoclonus – its remote influence. *J Neurol Neurosurg Psychiatry* (1984) 47(9):921–6. doi:10.1136/jnnp.47.9.921
33. Shaikh AG, Ghasia FF, DeLong MR, Jinnah HA, Freeman A, Factor SA. Ocular palatal tremor plus dystonia – new syndromic association. *Mov Disord Clin Pract* (2015) 2(3):267–70. doi:10.1002/mdc3.12193
34. Moon SY, Cho SS, Kim YK, Kim SE, Kim JH, Kim JS. Cerebral glucose metabolism in oculopalatal tremor. *Eur J Neurol* (2008) 15(1):42–9. doi:10.1111/j.1468-1331.2007.01997.x
35. Nishie M, Yoshida Y, Hirata Y, Matsunaga M. Generation of symptomatic palatal tremor is not correlated with inferior olivary hypertrophy. *Brain* (2002) 125(Pt 6):1348–57. doi:10.1093/brain/awf126
36. Tilikete C, Hannoun S, Nighoghossian N, Sappey-Marinier D. Oculopalatal tremor and severe late-onset cerebellar ataxia. *Neurology* (2008) 71(4):301. doi:10.1212/01.wnl.0000318287.29513.6d
37. Jellinger K. Hypertrophy of the inferior olives. Report on 29 cases. *Z Neurol* (1973) 205(2):153–74. doi:10.1007/BF00316018
38. Yun JH, Ahn JS, Park JC, Kwon DH, Kwun BD, Kim CJ. Hypertrophic olivary degeneration following surgical resection or gamma knife radiosurgery of brainstem cavernous malformations: an 11-case series and a review of literature. *Acta Neurochir* (2013) 155(3):469–76. doi:10.1007/s00701-012-1567-y
39. Chokroverty S, Barron KD. Palatal myoclonus and rhythmic ocular movements: a polygraphic study. *Neurology* (1969) 19(10):975–82. doi:10.1212/WNL.19.10.975
40. Dereux MJ. Myoclonies vélo-pharyngo-laryngées et oculaires chez un malade atteint de sclérose en plaques. *Rev Neurol* (1938) 69:135–8.
41. Itoh Y, Sakata E. Acquired pendular oscillation after brain-stem hemorrhage. *Acta Otolaryngol Suppl* (1989) 468:205–8. doi:10.3109/00016488909139046
42. Lopez LI, Bronstein AM, Gresty MA, Du Boulay EP, Rudge P. Clinical and MRI correlates in 27 patients with acquired pendular nystagmus. *Brain* (1996) 119(Pt 2):465–72. doi:10.1093/brain/119.2.465
43. Tranchant C, Bhatia KP, Marsden CD. Movement disorders in multiple sclerosis. *Mov Disord* (1995) 10(4):418–23. doi:10.1002/mds.870100403
44. Revol A, Vighetto A, Confavreux C, Trillet M, Aimard G. [Oculo-palatal myoclonus and multiple sclerosis]. *Rev Neurol* (1990) 146(8–9):518–21.
45. Sudhakar P, Parmar H, Cornblath WT. Oculopalatal tremor in multiple sclerosis with spontaneous resolution. *Neurol Clin Pract* (2012) 2(3):255–7. doi:10.1212/CPJ.0b013e31826af275
46. Tarnutzer AA, Palla A, Marti S, Schuknecht B, Straumann D. Hypertrophy of the inferior olivary nucleus impacts perception of gravity. *Front Neurol* (2012) 3:79. doi:10.3389/fneur.2012.00079
47. Eggenberger E, Cornblath W, Stewart DH. Oculopalatal tremor with tardive ataxia. *J Neuroophthalmol* (2001) 21(2):83–6. doi:10.1097/00041327-200106000-00003
48. Kumar N, Eggers SD, Milone M, Keegan BM. Acquired progressive ataxia and palatal tremor: importance of MRI evidence of hemosiderin deposition and vascular malformations. *Parkinsonism Relat Disord* (2011) 17(7):565–8. doi:10.1016/j.parkreldis.2011.04.018

49. Louis ED, Lynch T, Ford B, Greene P, Bressman SB, Fahn S. Delayed-onset cerebellar syndrome. *Arch Neurol* (1996) 53(5):450–4. doi:10.1001/archneur.1996.00550120016004

50. Scott BL, Jankovic J. Delayed-onset progressive movement disorders after static brain lesions. *Neurology* (1996) 46(1):68–74. doi:10.1212/WNL.46.1.68

51. Leger JM, Duyckaerts C, Brunet P. Syndrome of palatal myoclonus and progressive ataxia: report of a case. *Neurology* (1986) 36(10):1409–10. doi:10.1212/WNL.36.10.1409-a

52. de Jong FJ, Boon AJ. Progressive ataxia and palatal tremor – two cases with an unusual clinical presentation and course. *Parkinsonism Relat Disord* (2012) 18(7):904–5. doi:10.1016/j.parkreldis.2012.04.002

53. Mongin M, Delorme C, Lenglet T, Jardel C, Vignal C, Roze E. Progressive ataxia and palatal tremor: think about POLG mutations. *Tremor Other Hyperkinet Mov (N Y)* (2016) 6:382. doi:10.7916/D86M36RK

54. Nicastro N, Ranza E, Antonarakis SE, Horvath J. Pure progressive ataxia and palatal tremor (PAPT) associated with a new polymerase gamma (POLG) mutation. *Cerebellum* (2016) 15(6):829–31. doi:10.1007/s12311-015-0749-6

55. Hanihara T, Amano N, Takahashi T, Itoh Y, Yagishita S. Hypertrophy of the inferior olivary nucleus in patients with progressive supranuclear palsy. *Eur Neurol* (1998) 39(2):97–102. doi:10.1159/000007915

56. Suyama N, Kobayashi S, Isino H, Iijima M, Imaoka K. Progressive supranuclear palsy with palatal myoclonus. *Acta Neuropathol* (1997) 94(3):290–3. doi:10.1007/s004010050706

57. Kulkarni PK, Muthane UB, Taly AB, Jayakumar PN, Shetty R, Swamy HS. Palatal tremor, progressive multiple cranial nerve palsies, and cerebellar ataxia: a case report and review of literature of palatal tremors in neurodegenerative disease. *Mov Disord* (1999) 14(4):689–93. doi:10.1002/1531-8257(199907)14:4<689::AID-MDS1022>3.0.CO;2-8

58. de Yebenes JG, Vazquez A, Rabano J, de Seijas EV, Urra DG, Obregon MC, et al. Hereditary branchial myoclonus with spastic paraparesis and cerebellar ataxia: a new autosomal dominant disorder. *Neurology* (1988) 38(4):569–72. doi:10.1212/WNL.38.4.569

59. Howard KL, Hall DA, Moon M, Agarwal P, Newman E, Brenner M. Adult-onset Alexander disease with progressive ataxia and palatal tremor. *Mov Disord* (2008) 23(1):118–22. doi:10.1002/mds.21774

60. Schwankhaus JD, Parisi JE, Gulledge WR, Chin L, Currier RD. Hereditary adult-onset Alexander's disease with palatal myoclonus, spastic paraparesis, and cerebellar ataxia. *Neurology* (1995) 45(12):2266–71. doi:10.1212/WNL.45.12.2266

61. Thyagarajan D, Chataway T, Li R, Gai WP, Brenner M. Dominantly-inherited adult-onset leukodystrophy with palatal tremor caused by a mutation in the glial fibrillary acidic protein gene. *Mov Disord* (2004) 19(10):1244–8. doi:10.1002/mds.20161

62. Li R, Johnson AB, Salomons G, Goldman JE, Naidu S, Quinlan R, et al. Glial fibrillary acidic protein mutations in infantile, juvenile, and adult forms of Alexander disease. *Ann Neurol* (2005) 57(3):310–26. doi:10.1002/ana.20406

63. Graff-Radford J, Schwartz K, Gavrilova RH, Lachance DH, Kumar N. Neuroimaging and clinical features in type II (late-onset) Alexander disease. *Neurology* (2014) 82(1):49–56. doi:10.1212/01.wnl.0000438230.33223.bc

64. Sebesto JR, van Gerpen JA. Teaching video neuroimages: palatal tremor in adult-onset Alexander disease. *Neurology* (2016) 86(24):e252. doi:10.1212/WNL.0000000000002763

65. Kinghorn KJ, Kaliakatsos M, Blakely EL, Taylor RW, Rich P, Clarke A, et al. Hypertrophic olivary degeneration on magnetic resonance imaging in mitochondrial syndromes associated with POLG and SURF1 mutations. *J Neurol* (2013) 260(1):3–9. doi:10.1007/s00415-012-6564-9

66. Tchikviladze M, Gilleron M, Maisonobe T, Galanaud D, Laforet P, Durr A, et al. A diagnostic flow chart for POLG-related diseases based on signs sensitivity and specificity. *J Neurol Neurosurg Psychiatry* (2015) 86(6):646–54. doi:10.1136/jnnp-2013-306799

67. Storey E. *Spinocerebellar Ataxia Type 20*. Pagon RA, Adam MP, Ardinger HH, Wallace SE, Amemiya A, Bean LJH, et al., editors. Seattle, WA: University of Washington (2007).

68. Storey E, Knight MA, Forrest SM, Gardner RJ. Spinocerebellar ataxia type 20. *Cerebellum* (2005) 4(1):55–7. doi:10.1080/14734220410019048

69. Pretegiani E, Rosini F, Federighi P, Cerase A, Dotti MT, Rufa A. Pendular nystagmus, palatal tremor and progressive ataxia in GM2-gangliosidosis. *Eur J Neurol* (2015) 22(6):e67–9. doi:10.1111/ene.12661

70. Seok JI, Yi H, Song YM, Lee WY. Metronidazole-induced encephalopathy and inferior olivary hypertrophy: lesion analysis with diffusion-weighted imaging and apparent diffusion coefficient maps. *Arch Neurol* (2003) 60(12):1796–800. doi:10.1001/archneur.60.12.1796

71. Bharucha KJ, Sethi KD. Complex movement disorders induced by fluoxetine. *Mov Disord* (1996) 11(3):324–6. doi:10.1002/mds.870110318

72. Lapresle J, Ben Hamida M. Correspondance somatotopique, secteur par secteur, des dégénérescences de l'olive bulbaire consécutives à des lésions limitées du noyau dentelé contro-latéral. *Rev Neurol* (1965) 113(4):439–48.

73. Marie P, Foix C. Sur la dégénération pseudo-hypertrophique de l'olive bulbaire. *Rev Neurol* (1913) 26:48–52.

74. Ogawa K, Kamei S, Ichihara K, Uehara K, Suzuki Y, Uchihara T, et al. Immunohistochemical study of pseudohypertrophy of the inferior olivary nucleus. *Clin Neuropathol* (2014) 33(1):68–75. doi:10.5414/NP300594

75. Ogawa K, Mizutani T, Uehara K, Minami M, Suzuki Y, Uchihara T. Pathological study of pseudohypertrophy of the inferior olivary nucleus. *Neuropathology* (2010) 30(1):15–23. doi:10.1111/j.1440-1789.2009.01033.x

76. Goto N, Kaneko M. Olivary enlargement: chronological and morphometric analyses. *Acta Neuropathol* (1981) 54(4):275–82. doi:10.1007/BF00697000

77. Gauthier JC, Blackwood W. Enlargement of the inferior olivary nucleus in association with lesions of the central tegmental tract or dentate nucleus. *Brain* (1961) 84(3):341–61. doi:10.1093/brain/84.3.341

78. Mari Z, Halls AJM, Vortmeyer A, Zhukareva V, Kunihiro U, Lee VM, et al. Clinico-pathological correlation in progressive ataxia and palatal tremor: a novel tauopathy. *Mov Disord Clin Pract* (2014) 50–6. doi:10.1002/mdc3.12014

79. Pierot L, Cervera-Pierot P, Delattre JY, Duyckaerts C, Chiras J, Brunet P. Palatal myoclonus and inferior olivary lesions: MRI-pathologic correlation. *J Comput Assist Tomogr* (1992) 16(1):160–3.

80. Yokota T, Tsukagoshi H. Olivary hypertrophy precedes the appearance of palatal myoclonus. *J Neurol* (1991) 238(7):408. doi:10.1007/BF00319861

81. Birbamer G, Buchberger W, Felber S, Aichner F. MR appearance of hypertrophic olivary degeneration: temporal relationships. *AJNR Am J Neuroradiol* (1992) 13(5):1501–3.

82. Revel MP, Mann M, Brugieres P, Poirier J, Gaston A. MR appearance of hypertrophic olivary degeneration after contralateral cerebellar hemorrhage. *AJNR Am J Neuroradiol* (1991) 12(1):71–2.

83. Yanagisawa T, Sugihara H, Shibahara K, Kamo T, Fujisawa K, Murayama M. Natural course of combined limb and palatal tremor caused by cerebellar-brain stem infarction. *Mov Disord* (1999) 14(5):851–4. doi:10.1002/1531-8257(199909)14:5<851::AID-MDS1022>3.0.CO;2-G

84. Hirono N, Kameyama M, Kobayashi Y, Udaka F, Mezaki T, Abe K, et al. MR demonstration of a unilateral olivary hypertrophy caused by pontine tegmental hematoma. *Neuroradiology* (1990) 32(4):340–2. doi:10.1007/BF00593060

85. Uchino A, Hasuo K, Uchida K, Matsumoto S, Tsukamoto Y, Ohno M, et al. Olivary degeneration after cerebellar or brain stem haemorrhage: MRI. *Neuroradiology* (1993) 35(5):335–8. doi:10.1007/BF00588362

86. Robin JJ, Alcala H. Olivary hypertrophy without palatal myoclonus associated with a metastatic lesion to the pontine tegmentum. *Neurology* (1975) 25(8):771–5. doi:10.1212/WNL.25.8.771

87. Gu CN, Carr CM, Kaufmann TJ, Kotsenas AL, Hunt CH, Wood CP. MRI findings in nonlesional hypertrophic olivary degeneration. *J Neuroimaging* (2015) 25(5):813–7. doi:10.1111/jon.12267

88. Dubinsky RM, Hallett M, Di Chiro G, Fulham M, Schwankhaus J. Increased glucose metabolism in the medulla of patients with palatal myoclonus. *Neurology* (1991) 41(4):557–62. doi:10.1212/WNL.41.4.557

89. Kim SJ, Lee JH, Suh DC. Cerebellar MR changes in patients with olivary hypertrophic degeneration. *AJNR Am J Neuroradiol* (1994) 15(9):1715–9.

90. Anderson JR, Treip CS. Hypertrophic olivary degeneration and Purkinje cell degeneration in a case of long-standing head injury. *J Neurol Neurosurg Psychiatry* (1973) 36(5):826–32. doi:10.1136/jnnp.36.5.826

91. Manor Y, Rinzel J, Segev I, Yarom Y. Low-amplitude oscillations in the inferior olive: a model based on electrical coupling of neurons with heterogeneous channel densities. *J Neurophysiol* (1997) 77(5):2736–52.

92. Sotelo C, Llinas R, Baker R. Structural study of inferior olivary nucleus of the cat: morphological correlates of electrotonic coupling. *J Neurophysiol* (1974) 37(3):541–59.

93. Ruigrok TJ, de Zeeuw CI, Voogd J. Hypertrophy of inferior olivary neurons: a degenerative, regenerative or plasticity phenomenon. *Eur J Morphol* (1990) 28(2–4):224–39.
94. Deuschl G, Toro C, Valls-Sole J, Hallett M. Symptomatic and essential palatal tremor. 3. Abnormal motor learning. *J Neurol Neurosurg Psychiatry* (1996) 60(5):520–5. doi:10.1136/jnnp.60.5.520
95. Shaikh AG, Wong AL, Optican LM, Zee DS. Impaired motor learning in a disorder of the inferior olive: is the cerebellum confused? *Cerebellum* (2017) 16(1):158–67. doi:10.1007/s12311-016-0785-x
96. Yakushiji Y, Otsubo R, Hayashi T, Fukuchi K, Yamada N, Hasegawa Y, et al. Glucose utilization in the inferior cerebellar vermis and ocular myoclonus. *Neurology* (2006) 67(1):131–3. doi:10.1212/01.wnl.0000223837.52895.2e
97. Hong S, Leigh RJ, Zee DS, Optican LM. Inferior olive hypertrophy and cerebellar learning are both needed to explain ocular oscillations in oculopalatal tremor. *Prog Brain Res* (2008) 171:219–26. doi:10.1016/S0079-6123(08)00631-6
98. Stern MM. Rhythmic palatopharyngeal myoclonus. *J Nerv Ment Dis* (1949) 109:48–53. doi:10.1097/00005053-194901000-00006
99. Kane SA, Thach WT. *Palatal Myoclonus and Function of the Inferior Olive: Are They Related?* Strat P, editor. Berlin: Springer (1989).
100. Averbuch-Heller L, Tusa RJ, Fuhry L, Rottach KG, Ganser GL, Heide W, et al. A double-blind controlled study of gabapentin and baclofen as treatment for acquired nystagmus. *Ann Neurol* (1997) 41(6):818–25. doi:10.1002/ana.410410620
101. Bandini F, Castello E, Mazzella L, Mancardi GL, Solaro C. Gabapentin but not vigabatrin is effective in the treatment of acquired nystagmus in multiple sclerosis: how valid is the GABAergic hypothesis? *J Neurol Neurosurg Psychiatry* (2001) 71(1):107–10. doi:10.1136/jnnp.71.1.107
102. Shaikh AG, Thurtell MJ, Optican LM, Leigh RJ. Pharmacological tests of hypotheses for acquired pendular nystagmus. *Ann N Y Acad Sci* (2011) 1233:320–6. doi:10.1111/j.1749-6632.2011.06118.x
103. Starck M, Albrecht H, Pollmann W, Dieterich M, Straube A. Acquired pendular nystagmus in multiple sclerosis: an examiner-blind cross-over treatment study of memantine and gabapentin. *J Neurol* (2010) 257(3):322–7. doi:10.1007/s00415-009-5309-x
104. Starck M, Albrecht H, Pollmann W, Straube A, Dieterich M. Drug therapy for acquired pendular nystagmus in multiple sclerosis. *J Neurol* (1997) 244(1):9–16. doi:10.1007/PL00007728
105. Jabbari B, Rosenberg M, Scherokman B, Gunderson CH, McBurney JW, McClintock W. Effectiveness of trihexyphenidyl against pendular nystagmus and palatal myoclonus: evidence of cholinergic dysfunction. *Mov Disord* (1987) 2(2):93–8. doi:10.1002/mds.870020202
106. Repka MX, Savino PJ, Reinecke RD. Treatment of acquired nystagmus with botulinum neurotoxin A. *Arch Ophthalmol* (1994) 112(10):1320–4. doi:10.1001/archopht.1994.01090220070025
107. Penney SE, Bruce IA, Saeed SR. Botulinum toxin is effective and safe for palatal tremor: a report of five cases and a review of the literature. *J Neurol* (2006) 253(7):857–60. doi:10.1007/s00415-006-0039-9
108. Wang D, Sanchez J, Foote KD, Sudhyadhom A, Bhatti MT, Lewis S, et al. Failed DBS for palliation of visual problems in a case of oculopalatal tremor. *Parkinsonism Relat Disord* (2009) 15(1):71–3. doi:10.1016/j.parkreldis.2008.01.020

15

Vestibular Deficits in Neurodegenerative Disorders: Balance, Dizziness and Spatial Disorientation

*Thomas Cronin, Qadeer Arshad and Barry M. Seemungal**

Division of Brain Sciences, Department of Medicine, Charing Cross Hospital, London, United Kingdom

***Correspondence:**
Barry M. Seemungal
b.seemungal@imperial.ac.uk

The vestibular system consists of the peripheral vestibular organs in the inner ear and the associated extensive central nervous system projections—from the cerebellum and brainstem to the thalamic relays to cortical projections. This system is important for spatial orientation and balance, both of critical ecological importance, particularly for successful navigation in our environment. Balance disorders and spatial disorientation are common presenting features of neurodegenerative diseases; however, little is known regarding central vestibular processing in these diseases. A ubiquitous aspect of central vestibular processing is its promiscuity given that vestibular signals are commonly found in combination with other sensory signals. This review discusses how impaired central processing of vestibular signals—typically in combination with other sensory and motor systems—may account for the impaired balance and spatial disorientation in common neurodegenerative conditions. Such an understanding may provide for new diagnostic tests, potentially useful in detecting early disease while a mechanistic understanding of imbalance and spatial disorientation in these patients may enable a vestibular-targeted therapy for such problems in neurodegenerative diseases. Studies with state of the art central vestibular testing are now much needed to tackle this important topic.

Keywords: vestibular system, vestibular perception, neurodegeneration, spatial disorientation, balance

INTRODUCTION

The peripheral vestibular apparatus transduces head acceleration, both angular and linear acceleration (including gravity being equivalent to a physical linear acceleration), and functionally speaking plays an important role in the control of eye movement, posture, gait, and egocentric perception. The vestibular end-organ consists of the otolith organs—which transduce linear acceleration; and the semi-circular canals which transduce angular acceleration. From there the signal pass to the vestibular nerve, the brainstem and cerebellar circuits, vestibular thalamic projections, vestibulospinal projections, and finally the vestibular cortical network. Functionally, the vestibular system senses self-motion ("am I moving") and spatial orientation ("where am I now"), with the neuroanatomical correlates mediating these vestibular sensations being distinct.

Vestibular, visual, and proprioceptive sensory input is integrated in the brain and used to subsequently adjust the outgoing motor response to maintain balance, posture, and gaze stabilization. Vestibular dysfunction—arising from peripheral or central components of the vestibular system—may manifest as illusory self-motion (dizziness/vertigo) and spatial disorientation, which in turn can impair balance.

The overall prevalence of vestibular dysfunction in adults aged over 40 in the USA is 35%, representing 69 million individuals (1). Specifically, patients with vestibular dysfunction are at significantly greater risk of falls, involving both symptomatic and asymptomatic patient groups (1). Resultantly, vestibular dysfunction has a major impact on mortality, morbidity, health-care resources (1), and socioeconomic productivity (2).

The vestibular system is phylogenetically one of the oldest of all of the sensory systems (3) and the earliest to mature during development (4) and, thus, presents a potentially pertinent area of study in the context of neurodegeneration. For instance, work in Alzheimer's disease (AD) demonstrates areas of neuronal degeneration in phylogenetically older neurones (5).

With an aging population, we are facing a rise of both vestibular disorders and neurodegenerative conditions. Dizziness and imbalance are important in neurodegenerative disease due to their association with falls. In addition, detection of dizziness and imbalance, and specific vestibular testing may have a potential role in the identification of neurodegeneration, especially in the initial stages of the disease process. For future treatments in neurodegenerative disorders to be most effective, earlier detection is likely to be vital to restrict neuronal loss.

In this review, we will focus on dizziness, imbalance, and spatial disorientation in relation to the neurodegenerative conditions of AD, progressive supranuclear palsy (PSP), frontotemporal dementia (FTD), motor neurone disease (MND), multiple system atrophy (MSA), and Parkinson's disease (PD). In doing so, we demonstrate how detecting central and even peripheral vestibular pathology is important for the diagnosis and management of these conditions.

ALZHEIMER'S DISEASE

Alzheimer's disease is a from of dementia that typically presents with memory disturbance. It is characterized by beta-amyloid deposition in the brain, neurofibrillary tangles, and neuronal death. Imbalance is a little recognized feature of AD (6, 7), despite the condition carrying a high risk of falls (8) and gait abnormalities (9). Up to third of newly diagnosed AD patients complain of spatial disorientation (10), with wandering, for instance, a frequent symptom of AD (11).

Patients with AD are also three times more likely to experience a fracture compared to age-matched controls (12), and 47% have been observed to fall over the course of 1 year (13). Moreover, falls have been suggested to precede detectable cognitive changes in AD patients. A prospective study of presumptive preclinical AD patients found a higher rate of falls compared to aged-matched controls (14).

Nakamagoe et al. evaluated balance in individuals with AD and healthy aged-matched controls, using an eyes-closed stepping test. They reported that AD subjects were significantly more likely to move and turn than stay in the same position after 50 steps (7). Furthermore, stabilometry (objective study of body sway during quiet standing) testing has been demonstrated to be significantly altered in AD patients across measures of antero-posterior sway, latero-lateral sway, and area of confidence ellipsis, worsening in each parameter when eyes were closed. In particular, the authors identified a strong correlation between impairment in the anterior–posterior sway component for the AD subjects and reduced cognitive scores (6). This has led some researchers to suggest balance disturbance is the leading cause of falls in patients with AD (7).

Further insights into the cause of falls in AD patients have been identified by provoking compensatory postural adjustments through virtual reality (15). Patients with AD demonstrated slower response times to adjusting body position in response to changing visual stimuli, with this effect pronounced in the AD group with a history of falls. The AD faller group was also shown to have abnormal postural correction, reflecting worse inherent postural stability. Postural control was also related to higher cognitive processing, with the authors concluding that falls may result in AD patients from insufficient cognitive resources to control posture. Indeed, dual-task gait testing (assessing gait while performing a challenging cognitive task) in patients with mild cognitive impairment who went on to develop dementia showed a reduced gait performance relative to those who did not (16), with future study addressing this paradigm in other neurodegenerative disorders (17).

This follows from work performed by Barra and colleagues that used spatial and verbal tasks in conjunction with a balance task performed in young healthy adults which found an increase incidence of falls during spatial-task performance. The authors concluded that cognitive performance was maintained at the expense of balance, transgressing the "posture first" principle (18). Note, other studies have suggested a principle of "posture first" in older adults and "cognition first" in younger adults (19); however, exactly why, when, and what causes this change in strategy remains obscure.

A core brain area implicated in spatial orientation is the hippocampus (20), with this area being among the earliest regions to degenerate during the course of AD (21). Aside from a few studies within humans (22, 23), the evidence for a major role of the vestibular system in hippocampal function has come from animal studies involving vestibular stimulation or lesions (24–27). Further, in a study by Brandt et al., they demonstrated that in patients with bilateral vestibular loss, major atrophy of the hippocampus that correlated with impairments on spatial memory tasks (23). This association has led some to speculate on causal relationship between peripheral vestibular loss and AD (28, 29). Namely, anterograde degeneration, in which destruction of lower structures, i.e., peripheral vestibular apparatus, leads to degeneration of their higher projection zones, i.e., vestibular projections and the hippocampus (28). However, there is no empirical epidemiological evidence to support peripheral vestibular loss as a risk factor for AD.

A related but distinct question is the role of the hippocampus in vestibular cortical processing. Over the last four decades, animal experimentalists have demonstrated the remarkable properties of a group of cells in the hippocampus—place cells—that effectively indicate the position of the animal within its environment (30). These cells' indication of spatial position are updated by vestibular input, especially in the dark, and indeed, vestibular ablation renders these cellular systems permanently dysfunctional (31), indicating that the integrity of the peripheral vestibular system is obligatory for these spatial guidance systems.

A key concept in place cell functions (and head direction cells that provide a compass like indication of head angular orientation) is the conversion of inertial signals of motion to position—a function called path integration (30). Two recent human lesion studies, however, found no effect of hippocampal lesions upon path integration function (32, 33). Instead, lesions, due to stroke, in the temporoparietal junction (TPJ) (33) have been shown to impair vestibular-guided spatial orientation. It follows that AD may affect spatial orientation by its effect on vestibular cortical regions such as the TPJ.

Perhaps more important is the impact upon cortical networks with multimodal imaging studies showing a consistent disruption in AD (34). Given the evidence of a widespread vestibular brain network involved in the vestibular perception of self-motion (35, 36), it can be expected that pathological changes associated with AD are likely to impact upon this neural system.

PROGRESSIVE SUPRANUCLEAR PALSY

PSP is a pathologically defined disease underpinned by the accumulation of hyperphosphorylated tau throughout the brain, as well as in distinctive regions. Its clinical phenotype is however variable. PSP often presents with falls early in the course of the disease (37, 38). The midbrain is affected early on in the disease course (39). Although the vestibular nuclei (primarily in the pontomedullary junction) show loss of neurones at autopsy (40), the angular VOR (dependent on the semi-circular canal system and producing eye rotations to compensate for head angular rotation) is relatively maintained until later stages of the disease course (41), inferring preserved canalicular projections. In contrast, failure of saccular projections to the vestibular nuclei result (39) in markedly impaired linear (translational) VOR—a function reliant upon the otolithic sacculus and utriculus (42). This otolihic dysfunction corresponds clinically with the impaired ability of PSP patients' convergence and near viewing of a target, and may also reflect damage to the interstitial nucleus of Cajal (43, 39).

The hypothesis of saccular projection impairment is further supported by vestibular-evoked myogenic potentials (VEMPs) testing in patients with PSP. cVEMPs consist of inhibitory potentials recorded from the sternocleidomastoid ("cervical" VEMP—cVEMP) in response to loud sounds, and are used in the testing of vestibulospinal reflexes. During movement, otolithic inputs are integral for producing the vestibulospinal reflexes that adjust muscle tone so that stable posture can be maintained. Depending on bone or air sound conduction, saccular afferents can be preferentially activated through cVEMPs, with this being the case in the latter conduction (44). In contrast, oVEMPs uses the inferior oblique muscle of the eye ("ocular" VEMP—oVEMP) to measure utricular function (45). Liao and colleagues found a significant reduction of cVEMP amplitude in PSP patients compared to age-matched healthy control group, with air sound conduction, inferring impaired function of the saccular pathways (42). They concluded that since the pathways mediating cVEMPs synapse in the lateral vestibular nuclei, this was not necessarily an inevitable feature of degenerative brainstem disease, but rather a specific sign in PSP.

Accordingly, the impaired ability to adjust vestibular reflexes for translational motion through the environment may be one component in the postural defect in PSP (42). However, how much this contributes to postural instability and falls in comparison to other factors is yet to be elucidated. Indeed, findings of impaired proprioceptive sensory inputs in PSP indicate it is likely to be an abnormality in central sensory integration, rather than a sole vestibular deficit (46). Dale et al. performed postural stability tasks on PSP patients versus healthy controls, finding patients with PSP had an inability to perceive backward tilt of the surface or body. Proposals for future study are focusing on the association between the VOR, postural deficits and falls in PSP (47).

Chen et al. have related this possible PSP pathogenesis ecologically to the bipedal upright locomotion (39). They proposed that PSP may owe its selective set of disturbances of eye movements and balance due to restricted involvement of a recently developed neural system that deals with erect permanent bipedal locomotion, the main components of which lie in the midbrain. Nevertheless, a distinct neural system for bipedalism is contentious, and furthermore, permanent bipedalism can be considered an adaptation of what is common—intermittent bipedalism, and whether a neural system between these states is distinct would be a further level of speculation. It is unclear whether PSP affects primates, although recent neuropathological analysis of cynomolgus monkeys found the cytopathology and distribution of tau deposits resemble those of PSP (48).

Additional vestibular mechanisms that may contribute to postural instability in PSP may include the vestibulo-collic reflex, which stabilizes the head on the body. PSP patients often show head turns opposite to the direction of intended gait due to over activity of the vestibulocollic reflex (49), which has been notionally attributed to the involvement of the brainstem reticular nuclei (50).

Computerized posturography testing can differentiate early PSP from early PD (51) and age-matched controls (52). Ondo and colleagues utilized the sensory organization test (SOT), where subjects are asked to stand still under a variety of altered sensory conditions (51). The SOT parameter that best differentiated PSP and PD was when both visual and proprioceptive inputs were deprived, leading the authors to conclude there was a vestibular pattern of dysfunction.

The limit of stability test (LOS) was also found to be abnormal in PSP (51, 52). LOS measures path sway, time, and distance traveled by the patient's center of gravity from an initial starting point to eight different points (51). The backward direction score was identified as being most severely affected, which is consistent with the higher frequency of falls in the backward direction in PSP patients (52). Of note, preservation in scores for the left (non-dominant side—with testing being performed on right sided dominant individuals) and forward-left (non-dominant forward diagonal) directions were reported (52) and may reflect the distribution of central PSP pathology.

This backward fall phenomenon may draw comparison with "Tumarkin" drop attacks ("otolithic crises") found in a subset of Meniere's disease patients. Tumarkin falls occur without warning and without loss of consciousness, with a stereotyped direction, bearing similarities to falls in PSP. The pathophysiology of Tumarkin drop attacks is felt to be caused by a burst of neural impulses from the otolithic organs to the vestibulospinal pathways, triggering the fall (53). Indeed, cVEMP testing in Tumarkin patients has demonstrated which were more likely to be elevated or absent thresholds compared to the patient's unaffected ear, implicating the involvement of the saccule in these patients (54). Similarly, as mentioned earlier, cVEMP measurements are also found to be abnormal in PSP (42), although this is likely to implicate saccular projections, rather than peripheral dysfunction as in Tumarkin attacks. Furthermore, falls in PSP are likely to be multifactorial, with axial rigidity also likely contributing to the nature of PSP falls (55).

Studied techniques to improve balance in PSP have involved audio-biofeedback (56). This consists of adding artificial sensory information that informs the brain about actual body posture and movements. In a study of eight patients with PSP, significant improvements in the Berg Balance Scale (which involves 14 different balance tasks) were observed after 6 weeks.

FRONTOTEMPORAL DEMENTIA

Frontotemporal dementia is characteristically a pre-senile dementia that presents with a progression deterioration of personality, social interaction, and cognition. Studied measures of gait and balance have been found to be abnormal in FTD when compared with controls (57). The limit of stability and dynamic balance testing were impaired in patients with FTD. In comparison, spatial orientation has been found to be relatively intact in FTD individuals (58). Tu and colleagues investigated spatial orientation using a novel virtual supermarket task to compare patients with AD and FTD. Subjects watched a sequence of videos from a first-person perspective moving through a virtual supermarket and were commanded to preserve orientation to an initial starting point. Analyses revealed significantly impaired spatial orientation in AD, compared to FTD patient groups, and was able to discriminate the two groups to a high degree at presentation.

Voxel-based morphometry, a neuroimaging analysis technique to investigate focal differences in brain anatomy, was also performed on the subjects, identifying significantly greater atrophy in medial parietal and retrosplenial regions for AD patients compared to FTD patients. The authors went on to speculate that the retrosplenial region plays a crucial role in spatial orientation (58).

Nakamagoe et al. performed caloric and visual suppression testing on 14 patients with FTD (59). In healthy subjects, vestibular-nystagmus induced by the caloric test can be suppressed by visual fixation (i.e., visual suppression) and impaired visual fixation is typically indicative of a central pathology (i.e., cerebellum, brainstem and cerebral cortex). It was found that FTD participants typically had an impaired visual suppression compared to controls. Further analysis was performed according to clinical features of the FTD patients, indicating that visual suppression of the VOR was significantly more altered in FTD patients with gait disturbance. The authors concluded that damage to the vestibular cortex, which they related to the inferior parietal lobule, might be responsible for the impairment of visual suppression in FTD patients. However, one caveat to this interpretation would be the identification of a discrete vestibular cortex, rather than the notion of distributed central projections of vestibular information in various cortical networks (60, 61).

MOTOR NEURONE DISEASE

Motor neurone disease is a progressive disorder in which degeneration of the upper and lower motor neurons leads to progressive weakness of bulbar, limb, and trunk muscles. As a result, falls are common in patients with MND, with a prospective longitudinal cohort study of MND patients showing an annual incidence of 64% (62). Interestingly, a study of head and other physical trauma injury in patients with MND, demonstrated a higher risk of injury compared to controls in the first year after diagnosis that subsequently reverted back to the level in the control group 1 year after diagnosis (63). In addition, with many MND patients reporting unsteadiness and fear of falling early in the course of the disease (64), this may suggest other factors as well muscle weakness may be contributing to falls in MND.

Sanjak et al. used SOT in computerized posturgraphy to assess vestibular deficits in patients who were ambulatory with MND compared to healthy controls (64). They found that MND subjects in the normative range in clinical mobility displayed distinct impairment in equilibrium testing and an increased number of falls during conditions of altered support surface, when vision was absent or sway-referenced, in comparison with healthy controls, suggesting a vestibular pattern of impairment. The authors hypothesized that cerebellar involvement in MND may result in this particular pattern of vestibular deficit since the peripheral function was preserved in these patients. Nonetheless, caution is required on the interpretation of SOT in such patients, when factors such as inherent muscle weakness and spasticity may also lead to postural instability and increased body sway, independent of vestibular dysfunction.

Vestibular-evoked myogenic potential measurement has also been performed on patients with MND, showing no abnormalities in patients in the early stages of the disease (65). Additional assessment of the vestibular system in MND has found abnormalities in visual suppression (66) and caloric testing (67). Ohki et al. found abnormalities of visual suppression in two out of nine patients with early stages of MND (66), which is indicative of cerebellum pathology.

MULTIPLE SYSTEM ATROPHY

Multiple system atrophy is an a oligodendrogliopathy characterized by prominent alpha-synuclein inclusions, resulting in neuronal death, which manifests clinically with autonomic failure, ataxia, and parkinsonism. Balance and gait are also frequently found to be disturbed in MSA (68), and symptom assessment scales focusing on these parameters are important for the evaluation of patients in early stages of MSA (69).

It is typically classified into a cerebellar predominant (MSA-C) and parkinsonism predominant (MSA-P) subtypes. Lee and Koh retrospectively identified the clinical features of 20 MSA-C patients, with disequilibrium (50%) and dizziness (15%) the most common initial presentation (38). For 21 MSA-P patients, tremor was the most frequent symptom (19%), while dizziness was found in 10%. Similarly, Sakakibara and Hirumab found 60% (9/15) of patients with MSA-C reported dizziness on head-turning (70).

Falls are frequent in MSA (71), and abnormalities in VEMPs for MSA patients have been associated with an increased risk of falling (72).

It is important to note, however, due to the frequent finding of orthostatic hypotension, identifying vestibular-related dizziness and balance impairment can be a challenge (73, 74). Nevertheless, vestibular function testing in MSA is abnormal (72, 75), pathological studies at autopsy show neuronal loss in the vestibular nuclei (76) and neuroimaging demonstrate degeneration in flocculus and nodulus in the cerebellum of MSA patients (70).

Impaired VOR suppression on visual fixation has also been identified in MSA (70, 77, 78). Indeed, its use as has been put forward as a method of distinguishing PD from MSA (78). Despite this assertion, abnormalities have been found in the cerebellum of PD patients (79), and impaired VOR suppression has been documented in such patients (80).

PARKINSON'S DISEASE

Parkinson's disease is broadly classified as a "movement disorder" but encompasses a wide variety of motor and non-motor symptoms, which results from the irreversible loss of dopaminergic neurones. Postural instability is one of the most disabling features in PD. Using computerized posturography integrated with a virtual reality system to analyze LOS, patients with PD were found to have a reduced LOS area and greater postural sway compared with healthy subjects (81). The deterioration in postural control was significantly associated with major risk of falls. Additionally, the manipulation of sensory input on the subjects was suggestive of reduced use of vestibular information to maintain postural control. Moreover, computerized posturography using SOT in patients with PD also demonstrated impaired processing of vestibular information (82, 83), with additional study indicating this was independent from the stage of the disease (84).

Perturbation of proprioceptive information in PD patients found no reweighting of vestibular inputs (85), which contrasts when performed in healthy subjects (86), with authors concluding that the issue of postural control in PD lay not in the ability to generate movement but the inability to perceive movement. However, this conclusion, neglects the issue of impaired anticipatory postural adjustments found in PD, while the sensory evaluation performed was limited to visual, vestibular, and proprioceptive stimulation.

Functional neuroimaging of PD patients has demonstrated reduced neuronal activity in the cingulate sulcus visual area (87), where vestibular and optic inputs are integrated (88), as well as showing reduced activation of this area is associated with increased disease severity (87). Therefore, a deficit of central sensory processing in PD is implied.

Vestibular-evoked myogenic potential responses in PD patients have been linked to the motor and non-motor symptoms (89). Specifically, impaired cVEMP testing in PD patients has been shown to be correlated significantly to contralateral rigidity, bradykinesia severity, ipsilateral dyskinesia scores, as well as sleep, mood, and memory impairment. Indeed, cVEMP testing in PD patients compared to aged-matched controls has been frequently found to be abnormal (72, 90, 91). This reflects potential brainstem pathology among PD patients, which links previous study of pathological changes in the vestibular nuclei of PD patients (92), and disrupted connections between vestibular nuclei and the dorsal raphe nuclei (93). Additional mechanisms for this may include the reduced effect of dopamine on the excitability of vestibular nuclei found in PD patients (94).

Peripheral ipsilateral vestibular paresis has been associated with lateral trunk deviation (Pisa syndrome) in patients with PD (95). In addition, the perception of the subjective visual vertical (the ability of a person to perceive earth-vertical with respect to gravity) has been demonstrated to be deviated in PD patients with lateral trunk flexion (96). Gandor and colleagues produced a similar finding in PD patients, and discussed that altered verticality perception in PD may reflect a central vestibular processing deficit (97).

The symptom of freezing of gait (FOG) in PD has also been related to the vestibular system. Huh et al. evaluated PD patients with FOG, PD patients without FOG, and aged-matched healthy controls using the SOT (98). PD patients with FOG showed worse postural sensory processing compared to those without FOG and a particular inability to use vestibular information. The authors attributed this with abnormal central processing of vestibular signals in PD. However, a causal relationship between FOG and impaired vestibular processing based on these results cannot yet be established until future research analyzing the imaging correlates of postural sensory deficits in PD patients with FOG is undertaken.

The brain area implicated in FOG is the pedunculopontine nucleus (PPN) (99). Direct projections to the PPN from vestibular nuclei have been confirmed in primates (100), and vestibular stimuli in macaque monkeys enhance the activity of the PPN neurones (101). PPN deep brain stimulation (DBS) in PD reduces falls (102). We showed that PPN DBS in PD patients showed improved vestibular perceptual thresholds (103). Paradoxically, PPN stimulation worsened sway in these patient in the dark. Although this could imply worse postural control, a strategy of increased postural movement to improve sensory feedback could provide additional information to the vestibular system to help control balance. The recent developments in new DBS targets in improving balance control in PD provide a fertile ground for future study and therapeutic approaches, e.g., recently studies of PPN stimulation in PSP patients has showed promising results (104).

Similarly, targeted vestibular rehabilitation and therapy in PD has received attention, demonstrating improved postural control and balance performance (105–108). Stimulation of the vestibulospinal tract through proprioceptive disturbance and visual suppression improved double stance gait performance in patients with PD compared to those receiving standard physiotherapy (109). Moreover, in a single patient study, repeated caloric stimulation produced improvement in assessment scores for motor and non-motor symptoms of PD, which was sustained at 5-month follow-up (110). Yet, vestibular rehabilitation tended represents different techniques in different studies illustrating it as a potentially disparate practice. Furthermore, small number studies and frequent lack of randomization and comparator impair meaningful results.

Galvanic vestibular stimulation, involving transcranial direct current stimulation, can stimulate and inhibit vestibular afferents. Its use in PD patients has demonstrated improvement of postural instability (111, 112) and motor performance (113, 114). Similarly, stochastic vestibular stimulation, which uses subthreshold electrical noise has demonstrated improvements in postural control for PD patients (115, 116). These are, however, small number studies with limited follow-up of patients.

CONCLUSION

This review highlights the role of vestibular function and dysfunction, in a number of neurodegenerative diseases, with a particular focus on the central vestibular system. Permanent bipedal locomotion is a hallmark of the human species, and is critically dependent upon the integration and processing of multiple sensory information (i.e., visual proprioceptive and vestibular sensory inputs), notwithstanding the requisite peripheral function. As a result, only limited neurodegeneration in central vestibular areas may result in significant clinical manifestations, especially imbalance and falls. Some of the disease areas discussed illustrate genuine advances in our understanding of neurodegenerative conditions, which can aid diagnostic and treatment strategies. A deeper mechanistic understanding of the role of the dysfunction of central vestibular systems in neurodegenerative disease is, therefore, much warranted.

Presently vestibular testing in neurodegenerative disease all too often focuses on peripheral (i.e., canal and otolith) function. Rather, testing should explore additional deficits in the central vestibular circuits. Indeed, state of the art exploration of central vestibular deficits is much warranted to provide a deeper mechanistic understanding of how balance and spatial disorientation so frequently arises in neurodegenerative disease.

AUTHOR CONTRIBUTIONS

All authors listed have made substantial, direct, and intellectual contribution to the work and approved it for publication.

FUNDING

This work was supported by the Medical Research Council, the Imperial Health Charity, and the NIHR Imperial Biomedical Research Centre.

REFERENCES

1. Agrawal Y, Carey JP, Della Santina CC, Schubert MC, Minor LB. Disorders of balance and vestibular function in US adults: data from the National Health and Nutrition Examination Survey, 2001-2004. *Arch Intern Med* (2009) 169(10):938–44. doi:10.1001/archinternmed.2009.66
2. Bronstein AM, Golding JF, Gresty MA, Mandala M, Nuti D, Shetye A, et al. The social impact of dizziness in London and Siena. *J Neurol* (2010) 257:183–90. doi:10.1007/s00415-009-5287-z
3. Romer AS. *The Vertebrate Body*. London: WB Saunders Company (1950).
4. Nandi R, Luxon LM. Development and assessment of the vestibular system. *Int J Audiol* (2008) 47(9):566–77. doi:10.1080/14992020802324540
5. Lyness SA, Zarow C, Chui HC. Neuron loss in key cholinergic and aminergic nuclei in Alzheimer disease: a meta-analysis. *Neurobiol Aging* (2003) 24(1):1–23. doi:10.1016/S0197-4580(02)00057-X
6. Leandri M, Cammisuli S, Cammarata S, Baratto L, Campbell J, Simonini M, et al. Balance features in Alzheimer's disease and amnestic mild cognitive impairment. *J Alzheimer Dis* (2009) 16(1):113–20. doi:10.3233/JAD-2009-0928
7. Nakamagoe K, Fujimiya S, Koganezawa T, Kadono K, Shimizu K, Fujizuka N, et al. Vestibular function impairment in Alzheimer's disease. *J Alzheimer Dis* (2015) 47(1):185–96. doi:10.3233/JAD-142646
8. Perttila NM, Öhman H, Strandberg TE, Kautiainen H, Raivio M, Laakkonen ML, et al. How do community-dwelling persons with Alzheimer disease fall falls in the FINALEX study. *Dement Geriatr Cogn Dis Extra* (2017) 7(2):195–203. doi:10.1159/000477394
9. Annweiler C, Beauchet O, Bartha R, Wells JL, Borrie MJ, Hachinski V, et al. Motor cortex and gait in mild cognitive impairment: a magnetic resonance spectroscopy and volumetric imaging study. *Brain* (2013) 136(3):859–71. doi:10.1093/brain/aws373
10. Guariglia CC, Nitrini R. Topographical disorientation in Alzheimer's disease. *Arq Neuropsiquiatr* (2009) 67(4):967–72. doi:10.1590/S0004-282X2009000600001
11. Alzheimer's Association. 2016 Alzheimer's disease facts and figures. *Alzheimer Dement* (2016) 12(4):459–509. doi:10.1016/j.jalz.2016.03.001
12. Buchner DM, Larson EB. Falls and fractures in patients with Alzheimer-type dementia. *JAMA* (1987) 257:1492–5. doi:10.1001/jama.1987.03390110068028
13. Allan LM, Ballard CG, Rowan EN, Kenny RA. Incidence and prediction of falls in dementia: a prospective study in older people. *PLoS One* (2009) 4:e5521. doi:10.1371/journal.pone.0005521
14. Stark SL, Roe CM, Grant EA, Hollingsworth H, Benzinger TL, Fagan AM, et al. Preclinical Alzheimer disease and risk of falls. *Neurology* (2013) 81(5):437–43. doi:10.1212/WNL.0b013e31829d8599
15. Gago MF, Yelshyna D, Bicho E, Silva HD, Rocha L, Lurdes Rodrigues M, et al. Compensatory postural adjustments in an oculus virtual reality environment and the risk of falling in Alzheimer's disease. *Dement Geriatr Cogn Dis Extra* (2016) 6(2):252–67. doi:10.1159/000447124
16. Montero-Odasso MM, Sarquis-Adamson Y, Speechley M, Borrie MJ, Hachinski VC, Wells J, et al. Association of dual-task gait with incident dementia in mild cognitive impairment: results from the gait and brain study. *JAMA Neurol* (2017). doi:10.1001/jamaneurol.2017.0643
17. Montero-Odasso M, Pieruccini-Faria F, Bartha R, Black SE, Finger E, Freedman M, et al. Motor phenotype in neurodegenerative disorders: gait and balance platform study design protocol for the ontario neurodegenerative research initiative (ONDRI). *J Alzheimer Dis* (2017):1–5. doi:10.3233/JAD-170149
18. Barra J, Bray A, Sahni V, Golding JF, Gresty MA. Increasing cognitive load with increasing balance challenge: recipe for catastrophe. *Exp Brain Res* (2006) 174(4):734–45. doi:10.1007/s00221-006-0519-2
19. Berger L, Bernard-Demanze L. Age-related effects of a memorizing spatial task in the adults and elderly postural control. *Gait Posture* (2011) 33:300–2. doi:10.1016/j.gaitpost.2010.10.082
20. Maguire EA, Frackowiak RS, Frith CD. Recalling routes around London: activation of the right hippocampus in taxi drivers. *J Neurosci* (1997) 17(18):7103–10.
21. Braak H, Braak E. Neuropathological stageing of Alzheimer-related changes. *Acta Neuropathol* (1991) 82(4):239–59. doi:10.1007/BF00308809

22. Vitte E, Derosier C, Caritu Y, Berthoz A, Hasboun D, Soulie D. Activation of the hippocampal formation by vestibular stimulation: a functional magnetic resonance imaging study. *Exp Brain Res* (1996) 112(3):523–6. doi:10.1007/BF00227958
23. Brandt T, Schautzer F, Hamilton DA, Brüning R, Markowitsch HJ, Kalla R, et al. Vestibular loss causes hippocampal atrophy and impaired spatial memory in humans. *Brain* (2005) 128(11):2732–41. doi:10.1093/brain/awh617
24. Horii A, Takeda N, Mochizuki T, Okakura-Mochizuki K, Yamamoto Y, Yamatodani A. Effects of vestibular stimulation on acetylcholine release from rat hippocampus: an in vivo microdialysis study. *J Neurophysiol* (1994) 72:605–11.
25. Sharp PE, Blair HT, Etkin D, Tzanetos DB. Influences of vestibular and visual motion information on the spatial firing patterns of hippocampal place cells. *J Neurosci* (1995) 15(Pt 1):173–89.
26. Russell NA, Horii A, Smith PF, Darlington CL, Bilkey DK. Lesions of the vestibular system disrupt hippocampal theta rhythm in the rat. *J Neurophysiol* (2006) 96(4–14):10. doi:10.1152/jn.00953.2005
27. Tai SK, Ma J, Ossenkopp KP, Leung LS. Activation of immobility-related hippocampal theta by cholinergic septohippocampal neurons during vestibular stimulation. *Hippocampus* (2012) 22(4):914–25. doi:10.1002/hipo.20955
28. Previc FH. Vestibular loss as a contributor to Alzheimer's disease. *Med Hypotheses* (2013) 80:360–7. doi:10.1016/j.mehy.2012.12.023
29. Harun A, Oh ES, Bigelow RT, Studenski S, Agrawal Y. Vestibular impairment in dementia. *Otol Neurotol* (2016) 37(8):1137–42. doi:10.1097/MAO.0000000000001157
30. Eichenbaum H, Dudchenko P, Wood E, Shapiro M, Tanila H. The hippocampus, memory, and place cells: is it spatial memory or a memory space? *Neuron* (1999) 23:209–26. doi:10.1016/S0896-6273(00)80773-4
31. Stackman RW, Clark AS, Taube JS. Hippocampal spatial representations require vestibular input. *Hippocampus* (2002) 12(3):291–303. doi:10.1002/hipo.1112
32. Kim S, Sapiurka M, Clark RE, Squire LR. Contrasting effects on path integration after hippocampal damage in humans and rats. *Proc Natl Acad Sci U S A* (2013) 110(12):4732–7. doi:10.1073/pnas.1300869110
33. Kaski D, Quadir S, Nigmatullina Y, Malhotra P, Bronstein AM, Seemungal BM. Temporoparietal encoding of space and time during vestibular-guided orientation. *Brain* (2016) 139(Pt 2):392–403. doi:10.1093/brain/awv370
34. Zhao X, Liu Y, Wang X, Liu B, Xi Q, Guo Q, et al. Disrupted small-world brain networks in moderate Alzheimer's disease: a resting-state fMRI study. *PLoS One* (2012) 7(2012):e33540. doi:10.1371/journal.pone.0033540
35. Seemungal BM. The cognitive neurology of the vestibular system. *Curr Opin Neurol* (2014) 27(1):125–32. doi:10.1097/WCO.0000000000000060
36. Nigmatullina Y, Hellyer PJ, Nachev P, Sharp DJ, Seemungal BM. The neuroanatomical correlates of training-related perceptuo-reflex uncoupling in dancers. *Cereb Cortex* (2015) 25(2):554–62. doi:10.1093/cercor/bht266
37. Cherchi M. Infrequent causes of disequilibrium in the adult. *Otolaryngol Clin North Am* (2011) 44:405–14. doi:10.1016/j.otc.2011.01.011
38. Lee SW, Koh SB. Clinical features and disability milestones in multiple system atrophy and progressive supranuclear palsy. *J Mov Disord* (2012) 5(2):42–7. doi:10.14802/jmd.12010
39. Chen AL, Riley DE, King SA, Joshi AC, Serra A, Liao K, et al. The disturbance of gaze in progressive supranuclear palsy: implications for pathogenesis. *Front Neurol* (2010) 1:147. doi:10.3389/fneur.2010.00147
40. Steele JC, Richardson JC, Olszewski J. Progressive supranuclear palsy. A heterogeneous degeneration involving the brain stem, basal ganglia and cerebellum with vertical gaze and pseudobulbar palsy, nuchal dystonia and dementia. *Arch Neurol* (1964) 10:333–59. doi:10.1001/archneur.1964.00460160003001
41. Das VE, Leigh RJ. Visual–vestibular interaction in progressive supranuclear palsy. *Vision Res* (2000) 40:2077–208110. doi:10.1016/S0042-6989(00)00046-8
42. Liao K, Wagner J, Joshi A, Estrovich I, Walker MF, Strupp M, et al. Why do patients with PSP fall? Evidence for abnormal otolith responses. *Neurology* (2008) 70:802–9. doi:10.1212/01.wnl.0000304134.33380.1e
43. Kokkoroyannis T, Scudder CA, Balaban CD, Highstein SM, Moschovakis AK. Anatomy and physiology of the primate interstitial nucleus of Cajal. 1. Efferent projections. *J. Neurophysiol* (1996) 75:725–73.
44. Rosengren SM, Welgampola MS, Colebatch JG. Vestibular evoked myogenic potentials: past, present and future. *Clin Neurophysiol* (2010) 121:636–51. doi:10.1016/j.clinph.2009.10.016
45. Welgampola MS, Carey JP. Waiting for the evidence: VEMP testing and the ability to differentiate utricular versus saccular function. *Otolaryngol Head Neck Surg* (2010) 143(2):281. doi:10.1016/j.otohns.2010.05.024
46. Dale ML, Horak FB, Wright WG, Schoneburg BM, Nutt JG, Mancini M. Impaired perception of surface tilt in progressive supranuclear palsy. *PLoS One* (2017) 12(3):e0173351. doi:10.1371/journal.pone.0173351
47. Srulijes K, Mack DJ, Klenk J, Schwickert L, Ihlen EA, Schwenk M, et al. Association between vestibulo-ocular reflex suppression, balance, gait, and fall risk in ageing and neurodegenerative disease: protocol of a one-year prospective follow-up study. *BMC Neurol* (2015) 15:192. doi:10.1186/s12883-015-0447-5
48. Uchihara T, Endo K, Kondo H, Okabayashi S, Shimozawa N, Yasutomi Y, et al. Tau pathology in aged cynomolgus monkeys is progressive supranuclear palsy/corticobasal degeneration-but not Alzheimer disease-like -Ultrastructural mapping of tau by EDX. *Acta Neuropathol Commun* (2016) 4:118. doi:10.1186/s40478-016-0385-5
49. Bisdorff AR, Bronstein AM, Wolsley C, Lees AJ. Torticollis due to disinhibition of the vestibulo-collic reflex in a patient with Steele–Richardson–Olszewski syndrome. *Mov Disord* (1997) 12:328–36. doi:10.1002/mds.870120311
50. Murdin L, Bronstein AM. Head deviation in progressive supranuclear palsy: enhanced vestibulo-collic reflex or loss of resetting head movements? *J Neurol* (2009) 256:1143–5. doi:10.1007/s00415-009-5090-x
51. Ondo W, Warrior D, Overby A, Calmes J, Hendersen N, Olson S, et al. Computerized posturography analysis of progressive supranuclear palsy: a case-control comparison with Parkinson's disease and healthy controls. *Arch Neurol* (2000) 57:1464–9. doi:10.1001/archneur.57.10.1464
52. Ganesan M, Pasha SA, Pal PK, Yadav R, Gupta Direction A. specific preserved limits of stability in early progressive supranuclear palsy: a dynamic posturographic study. *Gait Posture* (2012) 35:625–9. doi:10.1016/j.gaitpost.2011.12.012
53. Ishiyama G, Ishiyama A, Baloh RW. Drop attacks and vertigo secondary to a non-Meniere otologic cause. *Arch Neurol* (2003) 60(1):71–5. doi:10.1001/archneur.60.1.71
54. Timmer FC, Zhou G, Guinan JJ, Kujawa SG, Herrmann BS, Rauch SD. Vestibular evoked myogenic potential (VEMP) in patients with Ménière's disease with drop attacks. *Laryngoscope* (2006) 116(5):776–9. doi:10.1097/01.mlg.0000205129.78600.27
55. Tarnutzer AA, Newman-Toker DE. Fits, faints, funny turns, and falls in the differential diagnosis of the dizzy patient. In: Bronstein A, editor. *Oxford Textbook of Vertigo and Imbalance*. Oxford University Press (2013). 321 p.
56. Nicolai S, Mirelmann A, Herman T, Zijlstra A, Mancini M, Becker C, et al. Improvement of balance after audio-biofeedback. A 6-week intervention study in patients with progressive supranuclear palsy. *Z Gerontol Geriatr* (2010) 43(4):224–8. doi:10.1007/s00391-010-0125-6
57. Velayutham SG, Chandra SR, Bharath S, Shankar RG. Quantitative balance and gait measurement in patients with frontotemporal dementia and Alzheimer diseases: a pilot study. *Indian J Psychol Med* (2017) 39(2):176–82. doi:10.4103/0253-7176.203132
58. Tu S, Wong S, Hodges JR, Irish M, Piguet O, Hornberger Lost M. in spatial translation – a novel tool to objectively assess spatial disorientation in Alzheimer's disease and frontotemporal dementia. *Cortex* (2015) 67:83–94. doi:10.1016/j.cortex.2015.03.016
59. Nakamagoe K, Kadono K, Koganezawa T, Takiguchi M, Terada M, Yamamoto F, et al. Vestibular impairment in frontotemporal dementia syndrome. *Dement Geriatr Cogn Dis Extra* (2016) 6(2):194–204. doi:10.1159/000445870
60. Brandt T, Dieterich M. The vestibular cortex: its locations, functions, and disorders. *Ann N Y Acad Sci* (1999) 871(1):293–312. doi:10.1111/j.1749-6632.1999.tb09193.x
61. Guldin WO, Akbarian S, Grüsser OJ. Cortico-cortical connections and cytoarchitectonics of the primate vestibular cortex: a study in squirrel monkeys (*Saimiri sciureus*). *J Comp Neurol* (1992) 326(3):375–401. doi:10.1002/cne.903260306
62. Brooks BR, Li J, Huang W, Anderson FA, Miller RG, Mitsumoto H. Epidemiology of falls in amyotrophic lateral sclerosis patients: analysis of cross-sectional and prospective cohorts in the ALS CARE registry. *Annals of Neurology*; (Vol. 62). 2007 Jan 1; Hoboken, NJ, USA: Wiley-Liss (2007). p. S23–4.
63. Turner MR, Abisgold J, Yeates DGR, Talbot K, Goldacre MJ. Head and other physical trauma requiring hospitalization is not a significant risk factor

in the development of ALS. *J Neurol Sci* (2010) 288:45–8. doi:10.1016/j.jns.2009.10.010
64. Sanjak M, Hirsch MA, Bravver EK, Bockenek WL, Norton HJ, Brooks BR. Vestibular deficits leading to disequilibrium and falls in ambulatory amyotrophic lateral sclerosis. *Arch Phys Med Rehabil* (2014) 95:1933–9. doi:10.1016/j.apmr.2014.05.024
65. Kilic S, Gazioglu S, Serap-Zengin K, Dübüş HÜ, Boz C. Cervical vestibular evoked myogenic potential to air-conducted sound in early amyotrophic lateral sclerosis. *Clin Neurophysiol* (2012) 42:119–23. doi:10.1016/j.neucli.2012.01.001
66. Ohki M, Kanayama R, Nakamura T, Okuyama T, Kimura Y, Koike Y. Ocular abnormalities in amyotrophic lateral sclerosis. *Acta Otolaryngol Suppl* (1994) 511:138–42. doi:10.3109/00016489409128318
67. Steinmetz EF, Lebo CP, Norris FH Jr. Electronystagmographic findings in motor neuron disease. *Laryngoscope* (1974) 84:281–9. doi:10.1288/00005537-197402000-00010
68. Geser F, Seppi K, Stampfer-Kountchev M, Köllensperger M, Diem A, Ndayisaba JP, et al. The European multiple system atrophy-study group (EMSA-SG). *J Neural Transm* (2005) 112:1677–86. doi:10.1007/s00702-005-0328-y
69. Matsushima M, Yabe I, Oba K, Sakushima K, Mito Y, Takei A, et al. Comparison of different symptom assessment scales for multiple system atrophy. *Cerebellum* (2016) 15:190–200. doi:10.1007/s12311-015-0686-4
70. Sakakibaraa R, Hirumab K, Uchiyama T, Hattori T. Head-turning dizziness in multiple system atrophy. *Parkinsonism Relat Disord* (2004) 10(4):255–6. doi:10.1016/j.parkreldis.2004.02.005
71. Abdo WF, Borm GF, Munneke M, Verbeek MM, Esselink RAJ, Bloem BR. Ten steps to identify atypical parkinsonism. *J Neurol Neurosurg Psychiatry* (2006) 77(12):1367–9. doi:10.1136/jnnp.2006.091322
72. Venhovens J, Meulstee J, Bloem BR, Verhagen WIM. Neurovestibular analysis and falls in Parkinson's disease and atypical parkinsonism. *Eur J Neurosci* (2016) 43:1636–46. doi:10.1111/ejn.13253
73. Drachman DA. A 69-year-old man with chronic dizziness. *JAMA* (1998) 280:2111–8. doi:10.1001/jama.280.24.2111
74. Mathias CJ, Mallipeddi R, Bleasdale-Barr K. Symptoms associated with orthostatic hypotension in pure autonomic failure and multiple system atrophy. *J Neurol* (1999) 246:893–8. doi:10.1007/s004150050479
75. Wang SR, Young YH. Multiple system atrophy manifested as dizziness and imbalance: a report of two cases. *Eur Arch Otorhinolaryngol* (2003) 260:404–7. doi:10.1007/s00405-003-0595-x
76. Wenning GK, Tison F, Ben Shlomo Y, Daniel SE, Quinn NP. Multiple system atrophy: a review of 203 pathologically proven cases. *Mov Disord* (1997) 12:133–47. doi:10.1002/mds.870120203
77. Anderson T, Luxon L, Quinn N, Daniel S, Marsden CD, Bronstein A. Oculomotor function in multiple system atrophy: clinical and laboratory features in 30 patients. *Mov Disord* (2008) 23:977–84. doi:10.1002/mds.21999
78. Rascol O, Sabatini U, Fabre N, Senard JM, Simonetta-Moreau M, Montastruc JL, et al. Abnormal vestibuloocular reflex cancellation in multiple system atrophy and progressive supranuclear palsy but not in Parkinson's disease. *Mov Disord* (1995) 10:163–70.
79. Wu T, Hallett M. The cerebellum in Parkinson's disease. *Brain* (2013) 136(3):696–709. doi:10.1093/brain/aws360
80. Halmagyi GM, Gresty MA. Clinical signs of visual-vestibular interaction. *J Neurol Neurosurg Psychiatry* (1979) 42(10):934–9. doi:10.1136/jnnp.42.10.934
81. Doná F, Aquino CC, Gazzola JM, Borges V, Silva SM, Ganança FF, et al. Changes in postural control in patients with Parkinson's disease: a posturographic study. *Physiotherapy* (2016) 102:272–9. doi:10.1016/j.physio.2015.08.009
82. Rossi-Izquierdo M, Basta D, Rubio-Rodríguez JP, Santos-Pérez S, Ernst A, Sesar-Ignacio Á, et al. Is posturography able to identify fallers in patients with Parkinson's disease? *Gait Posture* (2014) 40:53–7. doi:10.1016/j.gaitpost.2014.02.003
83. Colnat-Coulbois S, Gauchard GC, Maillard L, Barroche G, Vespignani H, Auque J, et al. Management of postural sensory conflict and dynamic balance control in late-stage Parkinson's disease. *Neuroscience* (2011) 193:363–9. doi:10.1016/j.neuroscience.2011.04.043
84. Rossi M, Soto A, Santos S, Sesar A, Labella T. A prospective study of alterations in balance among patients with Parkinson's disease. Protocol of the postural evaluation. *Eur Neurol* (2009) 61:171–6. doi:10.1159/000189270
85. Hwang S, Agada P, Grill S, Kiemel T, Jeka JJ. A central processing sensory deficit with Parkinson's disease. *Exp Brain Res* (2016) 234:2369–79. doi:10.1007/s00221-016-4642-4
86. Hwang S, Agada P, Kiemel T, Jeka JJ. Dynamic reweighting of three modalities for sensor fusion. *PLoS One* (2014) 9:e88132. doi:10.1371/journal.pone.0088132
87. Putcha D, Ross RS, Rosen ML, Norton DJ, Cronin-Golomb A, Somers DC, et al. Functional correlates of optic flow motion processing in Parkinson's disease. *Front Integr Neurosci* (2014) 8:57. doi:10.3389/fnint.2014.00057
88. Cardin V, Smith AT. Sensitivity of human visual and vestibular cortical regions to egomotion-compatible visual stimulation. *Cerebral Cortex* (2010) 20(8):1964–73. doi:10.1093/cercor/bhp268
89. Shalash AS, Hassan DM, Elrassas HH, Salama MM, Méndez-Hernández E, Salas-Pacheco JM, et al. Auditory- and vestibular-evoked potentials correlate with motor and non-motor features of Parkinson's disease. *Front Neurol* (2017) 8:55. doi:10.3389/fneur.2017.00055
90. Pollak L, Prohorov T, Kushnir M, Rabey M. Vestibulocervical reflexes in idiopathic Parkinson disease. *Neurophysiol Clin* (2009) 39:235–40. doi:10.1016/j.neucli.2009.07.001
91. de Natale ER, Ginatempo F, Paulus KS, Manca A, Mercante B, Pes GM, et al. Paired neurophysiological and clinical study of the brainstem at different stages of Parkinson's Disease. *Clin Neurophysiol* (2015) 126:1871–8. doi:10.1016/j.clinph.2014.12.017
92. Seidel K, Mahlke J, Siswanto S, Kruger R, Heinsen H, Auburger G, et al. The brainstem pathologies of Parkinson's disease and dementia with Lewy bodies. *Brain Pathol* (2015) 25:121–35. doi:10.1111/bpa.12168
93. Halberstadt AL, Balaban CD. Selective anterograde tracing of the individual serotonergic and nonserotonergic components of the dorsal raphe nucleus projection to the vestibular nuclei. *Neuroscience* (2007) 147:207–23. doi:10.1016/j.neuroscience.2007.03.049
94. Pötter-Nerger M, Reich MM, Colebatch JG, Deuschl G, Volkmann J. Differential effect of DOPA and subthalamic stimulation on vestibular activity in Parkinson's disease. *Mov Disord* (2012) 27:1268–75. doi:10.1002/mds.25061
95. Vitale C, Marcelli V, Furia T, Santangelo G, Cozzolino A, Longo K, et al. Vestibular impairment and adaptive postural imbalance in parkinsonian patients with lateral trunk flexion. *Mov Disord* (2011) 26:1458–63. doi:10.1002/mds.23657
96. Scocco DH, Wagner JN, Racosta J, Chade A, Gershanik OS. Subjective visual vertical in Pisa syndrome. *Parkinsonism Relat Disord* (2014) 20(8):878–83. doi:10.1016/j.parkreldis.2014.04.030
97. Gandor F, Basta D, Gruber D, Poewe W, Ebersbach G. Subjective visual vertical in PD patients with lateral trunk flexion. *Parkinsons Dis* (2016) 2016:7489105. doi:10.1155/2016/7489105
98. Huh YE, Hwang S, Kim K, Chung WH, Youn J, Cho JW. Postural sensory correlates of freezing of gait in Parkinson's disease. *Parkinsonism Relat Disord* (2016) 25:72–7. doi:10.1016/j.parkreldis.2016.02.004
99. Fling BW, Cohen RG, Mancini M, Nutt JG, Fair DA, Horak FB. Asymmetric pedunculopontine network connectivity in parkinsonian patients with freezing of gait. *Brain* (2013) 136:2405–18. doi:10.1093/brain/awt172
100. Hazrati LN, Parent A. Projection from the deep cerebellar nuclei to the pedunculopontine nucleus in the squirrel monkey. *Brain Res* (1992) 585:267–71. doi:10.1016/0006-8993(92)91216-2
101. Aravamuthan BR, Angelaki DE. Vestibular responses in the macaque pedunculopontine nucleus and central mesencephalic reticular formation. *Neuroscience* (2012) 223:183–99. doi:10.1016/j.neuroscience.2012.07.054
102. Moro E, Hamani C, Poon Y-Y, Al-Khairallah T, Dostrovsky JO, Hutchison WD, et al. Unilateral pedunculopontine stimulation improves falls in Parkinson's disease. *Brain* (2010) 133(1):215–24. doi:10.1093/brain/awp261
103. Yousif N, Bhatt H, Bain PG, Nandi D, Seemungal BM. The effect of pedunculopontine nucleus deep brain stimulation on postural sway and vestibular perception. *Eur J Neurol* (2016) 23(3):668–70. doi:10.1111/ene.12947
104. Rowe J, Khan A, Romanowski C, Isaac C, Khan S, Mair R, et al. Clinical experience with pedunculopontine nucleus stimulation in conditions with nigrostriatal disconnection. *World Neurosurg* (2016) 89:9–18. doi:10.1016/j.wneu.2015.11.054
105. Acarer A, Karapolat H, Celebisoy N, Ozgen G, Colakoglu Z. Is customized vestibular rehabilitation effective in patients with Parkinson's? *NeuroRehabilitation* (2015) 37(2):255–62. doi:10.3233/NRE-151258

106. Basta D. Efficacy of a vibrotactile neurofeedback training in stance and gait conditions for the treatment of balance deficits: a double-blind, placebo-controlled multicenter study. *Otol Neurotol* (2011) 32:1492–9. doi:10.1097/MAO.0b013e31823827ec
107. Zeigelboim BS, Klagenberg KF, Teive HA, Munhoz RP, Martins-Bassetto J. Vestibular rehabilitation: clinical benefits to patients with Parkinson disease. *Arq Neuropsiquiatr* (2009) 67(2A):219–23. doi:10.1590/S0004-282X2009000200009
108. Rossi-Izquierdo M, Soto-Varela A, Santos-Perez S, Sesar-Ignacio A, Labella-Caballero T, Rossi-Izquierdo M, et al. Vestibular rehabilitation with computerised dynamic posturography in patients with Parkinson's disease: improving balance impairment. *Disabil Rehabil* (2009) 31(23):1907–16. doi:10.1080/09638280902846384
109. Tramontano M, Bonnì S, Martino Cinnera A, Giacomo K, Cinnera MA, Tramontano M, et al. Blindfolded balance training in patients with Parkinson's disease: a sensory-motor strategy to improve the gait. *Parkinsons Dis* (2016) 2016:7536862.
110. Wilkinson D, Podlewska A, Sakel M. A durable gain in motor and non-motor symptoms of Parkinson's disease following repeated caloric vestibular stimulation: a single-case study. *NeuroRehabilitation* (2016) 38(2):179–82. doi:10.3233/NRE-161308
111. Kataoka H, Okada Y, Kiriyama T, Kita Y, Nakamura J, Morioka S, et al. Can postural instability respond to galvanic vestibular stimulation in patients with Parkinson's disease? *J Mov Disord* (2016) 9(1):40–3. doi:10.14802/jmd.15030
112. Okada Y, Kita Y, Nakamura J, Kataoka H, Kiriyama T, Ueno S, et al. Galvanic vestibular stimulation may improve anterior bending posture in Parkinson's disease. *Neuroreport* (2015) 26:405–10. doi:10.1097/WNR.0000000000000360
113. Lee S, Kim DJ, Svenkeson D, Parras G, Oishi MMK, McKeown MJ. Multifaceted effects of noisy galvanic vestibular stimulation on manual tracking behavior in Parkinson's disease. *Front Syst Neurosci* (2015) 9:5. doi:10.3389/fnsys.2015.00005
114. Pan W, Soma R, Kwak S, Yamamoto Y. Improvement of motor functions by noisy vestibular stimulation in central neurodegenerative disorders. *J Neurol* (2008) 255:1657–61. doi:10.1007/s00415-008-0950-3
115. Samoudi G, Jivegård M, Mulavara AP, Bergquist F. Effects of stochastic vestibular galvanic stimulation and LDOPA on balance and motor symptoms in patients with Parkinson's disease. *Brain Stimulat* (2015) 8(3):474–80. doi:10.1016/j.brs.2014.11.019
116. Pal S, Rosengren SM, Colebatch JG. Stochastic galvanic vestibular stimulation produces a small reduction in sway in Parkinson's disease. *J Vestib Res* (2009) 19:137–42. doi:10.3233/VES-2009-0360

16

Saccadic Impairments in Patients with the Norrbottnian Form of Gaucher's Disease Type 3

Josefine Blume[1]*, Stanislav Beniaminov[1], Cecilia Kämpe Björkvall[2], Maciej Machaczka[3] and Per Svenningsson[1]*

[1] Section of Neurology, Department of Clinical Neuroscience, Center for Molecular Medicine, Karolinska Institute, Stockholm, Sweden, [2] Hematology Center Karolinska, Department of Medicine at Huddinge, Karolinska Institutet, Karolinska University Hospital Huddinge, Stockholm, Sweden, [3] Department of Medicine, Sunderby Regional Hospital of Norrbotten County, Luleå, Sweden

***Correspondence:**
Josefine Blume
josefine.blume@ki.se;
Per Svenningsson
per.svenningsson@ki.se

Background: Chronic neuronopathic Gaucher's disease type 3 (GD3) is relatively frequent in northern Sweden. Besides multiple other neurological symptoms, horizontal gaze palsy or oculomotor apraxia is common in GD3.

Objective: To characterize the saccades in patients with Norrbottnian GD3 with respect to their neurological and cognitive status using a computer-based eye-tracking technique.

Methods: Horizontal and vertical reflexive saccades as well as antisaccades of nine GD3 patients [4M/5F; 41.1 ± 11.0 years; modified severity scoring tool (mSST): 9.3 ± 5.4; Montreal Cognitive Assessment (MoCA): 24.0 ± 4.2] and age-matched controls were analyzed using EyeBrain T2, a head-mounted binocular eye tracker. Systematic clinical assessment included the mSST, a valid tool for monitoring the neurological progression in GD3 and MoCA.

Results: In Norrbottnian GD3 patients, gain, peak, and average velocity (107.5°/s ± 41.8 vs. 283.9°/s ± 17.0; $p = 0.0009$) of horizontal saccades were reduced compared to healthy controls (HCs). Regarding vertical saccades, only the average velocity of downward saccades was decreased (128.6°/s ± 63.4 vs. 244.1°/s ± 50.8; $p = 0.004$). Vertical and horizontal saccadic latencies were increased (294.3 ms ± 37.0 vs. 236.5 ms ± 22.4; $p = 0.005$) and the latency of horizontal reflexive saccades was correlated with the mSST score ($R^2 = 0.80$; $p = 0.003$). The latency of antisaccades showed association to MoCA score ($R^2 = 0.70$; $p = 0.009$). GD3 patients made more errors in the antisaccade task (41.5 ± 27.6% vs. 5.2 ± 5.8%; $p = 0.005$), and the error rate tended to correlate with the cognitive function measured in MoCA score ($p = 0.06$).

Conclusion: The mean age of 41 years of our GD3 cohort reflects the increased life expectancy of patients in the Norrbottnian area compared to other GD3 cohorts. Marked impairment of horizontal saccades was evident in all patients, whereas vertical saccades showed distinct impairment of downward velocity. Latency of reflexive saccades was associated with the severity of neurological symptoms. Increased latency and error rate in the antisaccade task were linked to cognitive impairment. The assessment of saccades provides markers for neurological and neuropsychological involvement in Norrbottnian GD3.

Keywords: Gaucher's disease, Norrbottnian form, saccades, eye movements, antisaccades

INTRODUCTION

Gaucher's disease (GD) is the most common lysosomal storage disorder resulting from glucocerebrosidase (GBA) deficiency, caused by homozygote mutations in the GBA gene. Clinical manifestations are organomegaly, hematological complications, and neurological symptoms (1). The neuronopathic forms of GD emerge either acute in early childhood (GD2) or chronic Gaucher's disease type 3 (GD3). A subtype of chronic neuronopathic phenotype is called Norrbottnian type, referring to its relatively high prevalence of 1:17,500 inhabitants of Norrbotten, a northern part of Sweden (2). The missense mutation L444P (c.1448T>C) is frequent among these patients (3). Despite the same genetic cause, the clinical course of the disease differs between individuals. The symptom burden is highly variable and can include horizontal supranuclear gaze palsy, ataxia, spastic paresis, cognitive impairment, and seizures (4). Enzyme replacement therapy is effective concerning the hematological and visceral manifestations. However, it has no favorable effect on the neurological outcome (5).

Impairment of eye movements is a common feature in lysosomal storage disorders and assessment of saccades may be a useful diagnostic tool. Different patterns of saccade impairment allow to relate pathology in the corresponding brain regions that, in turn, may allow to distinguish neurological conditions from similar symptoms with different pathophysiological substrate. For instance, patients with late-onset Tay–Sachs disease show characteristic transient decelerations and premature termination of saccades (6), whereas vertical supranuclear gaze palsy is a key clinical feature in patients with Niemann–Pick type C disease (7). In GD2 and GD3, horizontal gaze palsy or oculomotor apraxia is common and may even be the initial complain (8). Saccade analysis provides a marker for neurological involvement in GD and was already used as an outcome measurement in treatment studies (9). In a 4-year follow up of 15 GD3 patients with a median age of 15.7 years, saccade velocity was reduced and horizontal saccadic latency was increased and showed deterioration over time (10).

In this cross-sectional study, we used a computer-based eye-tracking technique to characterize the saccades in Norrbottnian GD3 patients with respect to a systematic assessment of their neurological and cognitive status. To our knowledge, this is the first study to evaluate saccades in Norrbottnian GD3 patients.

MATERIALS AND METHODS

Nine GD3 patients were recruited from among the affected patients at Norrbotten and examined at Sunderby Hospital in Luleå. Age- and sex-matched healthy controls (HCs) were examined at Karolinska University Hospital, Stockholm. The study was approved by the local research ethics committee and all participants provided written informed consent in accordance with the Declaration of Helsinki. Systematic clinical assessment was performed using the modified severity scoring tool (mSST) (11), a valid tool for monitoring neurological progression in GD3 which includes 12 items. For cognitive assessment, the Montreal Cognitive Assessment (MoCA) was used.

Eye movements were analyzed using EyeBrain T2® (medical device with CE label for clinical use Class IIa, ISO 9001, ISO 13485), a head-mounted binocular eye tracker with an acquisition speed of 300 Hz. Data were acquired for both eyes by presenting stimuli on a 22 inches wide screen 60 cm away. A chin rest minimized head movement during recording. MeyeParadigm® 2.1 was used to present series of stimuli and capture data. For each paradigm, a series of 12 stimuli was given after standardized verbal instructions. Paradigms included reflexive saccades with fixed target amplitudes in a horizontal (20°) and vertical (12°) step task, horizontal gap task (20°), and horizontal antisaccades (20°). The stimuli appeared outward from a central target position for a fixed period of 1,000 ms. The gap task was included to assess the rate of express saccades. For detailed information about the paradigms and parameter definition, see Data Sheet S1 in Supplementary Material.

Results are presented as mean and SD. Between group comparisons with a two-tailed significance level of 0.05 were performed using Mann–Whitney U test. Pearson correlation and least square regression were done to correlate quantitative variables. We refrained from multivariate regression because of small sample size.

RESULTS

In clinical examination, seven of the nine patients showed signs of oculomotor apraxia with delayed onset and slowness of horizontal saccades. In three individuals, distinct horizontal gaze palsy was present. In one of them, impairment of vertical eye movements was found additionally. This patient scored highest in the mSST score also and was excluded from further saccade analysis due to severe gaze palsy (patient 9). Demographic data, clinical signs, and scores are listed in **Table 1**.

Saccade examination using EyeBrain revealed impairment of horizontal saccades in all patients (**Table 2**). Average and peak velocity as well as saccadic gain of horizontal saccades were significantly decreased in GD3 patients compared to HCs (**Figure 1**). **Figure 2** demonstrates an exemplary set of horizontal saccades of patient 5 and the age-matched HC. Since peak velocity of a saccade linearly depends on its gain for saccade amplitudes up to 20°, we illustrated the saccadic main sequence for the same patient and control additionally (**Figure 2**). Two severely affected individuals (patients 2 and 8) showed sustained lateral gaze with a loss of saccadic step phase and unilateral horizontal gaze palsy with markedly decreased saccade amplitudes. Solely in these two patients, the abduction–adduction ratio of average velocity was elevated over 1.0 to 1.69 and 1.6, respectively.

As shown in **Table 2**, the gain of vertical saccades remained normal. Downward saccades were slower than upward saccades in all patients without reaching statistical significance. The average velocity of downward saccades was significantly decreased compared to HCs, whereas no difference was found in upward saccades.

Saccade latency was prolonged compared to HCs in all paradigms, horizontal and vertical (**Table 2**). Latency of horizontal reflexive saccades was significantly associated with the mSST

TABLE 1 | Demographic data, clinical signs, and scores.

Patient	Age	Sex	Mutation	Therapy/ age	Modified severity scoring tool	Montreal cognitive assessment	Epilepsy/age of onset	Abnormal gaze	Cerebellar signs	Pyramidal signs	Extrapyramidal signs
1	50	F	L444P/L444P	ERT	5.5	26	N	Y	N	Y	N
2	43	F	L444P/L444P	Allo-BMT/9	17	19	Y/23	Y	Y	Y	Y
3	31	F	L444P/L444P	Allo-BMT/2	8.5	25	Y/16	Y	N	Y	Y
4	51	M	L444P/L444P	ERT	14	26	Y/45	Y	Y	Y	N
5	28	M	L444P/L444P	ERT	12	24	Y/17	Y	Y	N	N
6	38	F	L444P/L444P	ERT	1	26	N	N	N	N	N
7	23	M	L444P/A341T	ERT	1	30	N	N	N	Y	N
8	56	F	L444P/L444P	ERT	11.5	25	N	Y	Y	Y	N
9	50	M	L444P/L444P	ERT	13	15	N	Y	Y	Y	N
Mean	41.1	56% F	100/89%	78% ERT	9.3 ± 5.4	24.0 ± 4.2	44% Y/25.25	78% Y	56% Y	78% Y	22% Y

TABLE 2 | Saccade characteristics of Gaucher's disease type 3 (GD3) patients and controls.

	GD3 patients	Controls	p
Age	40.0 ± 11.2	40.0 ± 10.9	1
Sex (female/male)	5/3	5/3	1
Latency (ms)			
Step horizontal	294.3 ± 36.9	236.5 ± 22.4	**0.005****
Step downward	293.8 ± 45.0	235.5 ± 22.4	**0.004****
Step upward	301.5 ± 71.3	229.1 ± 16.7	**0.002****
Gap horizontal	255.7 ± 51.3	211.4 ± 25.4	0.05
Antisaccades	271.3 ± 37.6	231.2 ± 20.9	**0.01***
Gain			
Step horizontal	0.85 ± 0.08	0.94 ± 0.03	**0.01***
Step downward	0.87 ± 0.08	0.96 ± 0.07	0.09
Step upward	0.86 ± 0.12	0.90 ± 0.03	0.7
Gap horizontal	0.81 ± 0.14	0.96 ± 0.01	**0.0002*****
Average velocity (°/s)			
Step horizontal	107.5 ± 41.8	283.9 ± 17.0	**0.0009*****
Step downward	128.6 ± 63.4	244.1 ± 50.8	**0.004****
Step upward	178.5 ± 78.5	215.6 ± 66.1	0.3
Gap horizontal	103.5 ± 47.5	273.7 ± 28.3	**0.0009*****
Peak velocity (°/s)			
Step horizontal	226.7 ± 58.7	519.7 ± 50.5	**0.0009*****
Step downward	345.9 ± 195.4	455.3 ± 102.5	0.1
Step upward	393.1 ± 148.3	410.3 ± 113.5	0.9
Gap horizontal	203.0 ± 68.4	484.7 ± 66.5	**0.0009*****
Antisaccades error rate	41.5 ± 27.6%	5.2 ± 5.8%	**0.005****
Number of express saccades	2.0 ± 2.1	1.4 ± 2.1	0.6

*The significance level was established as: *p ≤ 0.05, **p ≤ 0.01, ***p ≤ 0.001. Significant results (p < 0.05) in bold.*

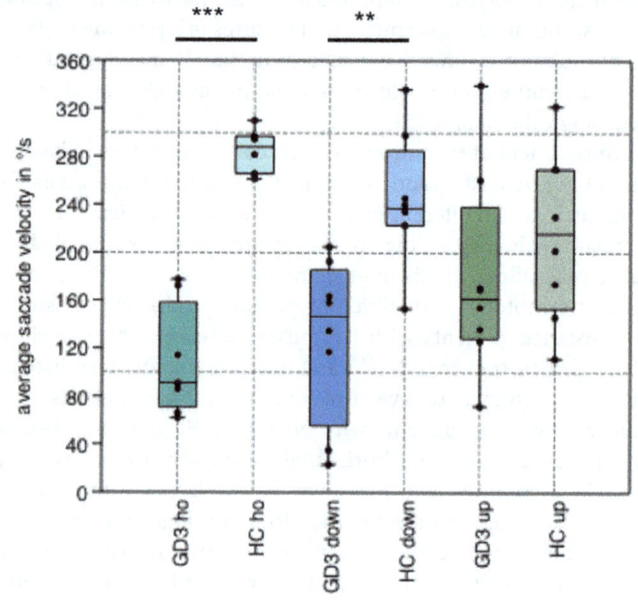

FIGURE 1 | Boxplot of average saccade velocity. Boxplot showing the average saccade velocity of horizontal (ho), downward (down), and upward (up) saccades in the step paradigm. Gaucher's disease type 3 (GD3) patients performed horizontal ($p = 0.0009$) and downward ($p = 0.004$) saccades in significantly reduced velocity compared to healthy controls (HCs), whereas there was no difference in upward saccades ($p = 0.3$).

score (step: $R^2 = 0.80$; $p = 0.003$; gap: $R^2 = 0.73$; $p = 0.007$; **Figure 3**). The gap effect (12) was detectable in patients ($p = 0.01$) and controls ($p = 0.02$). We found no difference in the rates of express or anticipated saccades.

Montreal Cognitive Assessment and mSST score were associated in a bivariate linear regression model ($R^2 = 0.60$; $p = 0.02$), while both showed no association to age ($p = 0.5$ and $p = 0.2$, respectively). The antisaccade latency was associated with MoCA score ($R^2 = 0.70$; $p = 0.009$), but not to age ($p = 0.5$). GD3 patients made more errors in the antisaccade task than HCs. The antisaccade error rate showed significant correlation to age ($R^2 = 0.54$; $p = 0.04$) and tended to correlate with mSST scores ($R^2 = 0.50$; $p = 0.052$) and to MoCA score ($R^2 = 0.47$; $p = 0.06$).

DISCUSSION

In this paper, we describe the characteristics of saccades in nine patients with Norrbottnian type GD3 with respect to their neurological and cognitive status for the first time. Impairment of horizontal gaze is the most frequent neurological feature in GD3 and, indeed, was found in all patients when assessed using a computer-based eye-tracking technique. The mean age of 41 years in our GD3 cohort reflects the increased life expectancy and milder course of the disease in patients from the Norrbottnian area compared to other GD3 cohorts.

In Norrbottnian GD3 patients, gain and velocity were clearly abnormal in horizontal saccades compared to healthy

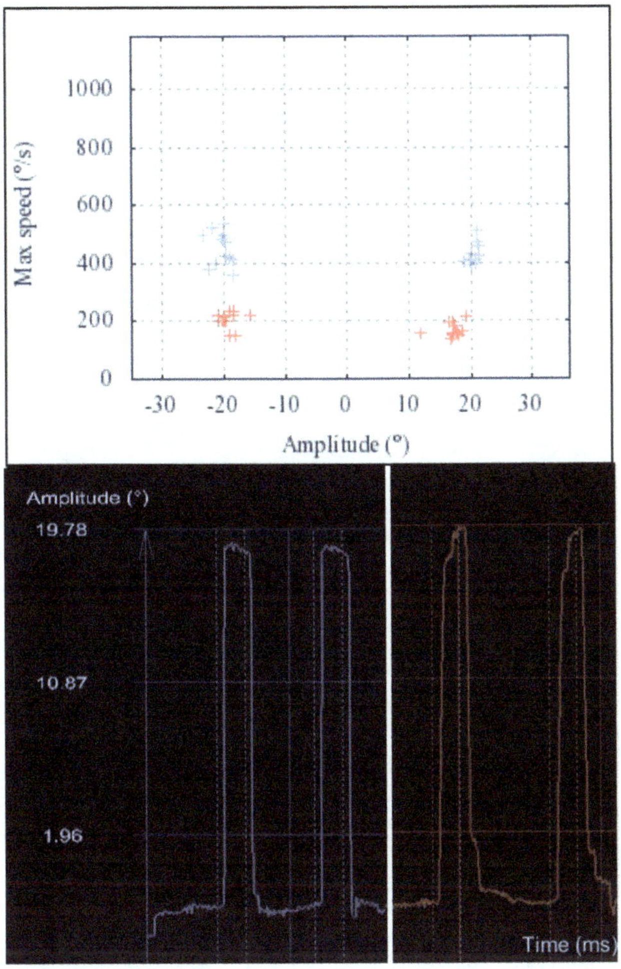

FIGURE 2 | Main sequence of horizontal saccades. Upper: the main sequence illustrates the linear dependency of peak velocity and amplitude of a saccade. The main sequences of 20° horizontal saccades are shown for one Gaucher's disease type 3 (GD3) patient (red) and one healthy control (HC) (blue). Lower: representative raw recordings of two exemplary horizontal saccades for the same GD3 patient (red, right) and HC (blue, left). The broken lines represent the appearance and disappearance of the 20° lateral stimulus. The GD3 saccades show longer duration, with decreased average velocity. Additionally, the gain of the first saccade is mildly reduced and one correction saccade is needed to reach the target.

individuals. Regarding vertical saccades, only average velocity of downward saccades was decreased while upward saccades appeared normal, besides prolonged latency. The distinct impairment of downward saccades is a feature in other neurodegenerative diseases with predominant impairment of vertical gaze like Niemann–Pick type C (13) and progressive supranuclear palsy as well. However, the pathophysiological mechanisms underlying the differential effects on midbrain pathways for downward and upward saccade generation in these diseases are not fully understood. Reduced velocity of horizontal saccades is caused by affection of the premotor burst neurons in the ipsilateral paramedian pontine reticular formation, whereas slowing of vertical saccades indicates a subsequent involvement of the rostral interstitial medial longitudinal fascicle (14), which may be caused by spreading of GD3 pathology in advanced stages of the disease. Here, additional involvement of omnipause neurons in the raphe interpositus nucleus may lead to further slowing of both horizontal and vertical saccades.

Two patients with severe neurological symptoms showed sustained lateral gaze and an increased abduction/adduction velocity ratio, which may indicate additional involvement of internuclear neurons or the medial longitudinal fasciculus that link the ipsilateral abducens nucleus to the contralateral oculomotorius nucleus. Horizontal saccadic hypometria may be caused by spreading of GD3 pathology to neuronal integrator cells in cerebellar dorsal vermis or nucleus prepositus hypoglossi (14). The exact evolution of neuropathological changes in GD3 in relation to the clinical course is still unknown. Brains of advanced stage GD3 patients showed widespread perivascular Gaucher cells as well as gliosis and neuronal cell loss in brainstem and cerebellum (15). However, no clear accentuation of neuropathological changes was found in the pons.

The delayed initiation of saccades, measured as prolonged latency, led to the term oculomotor apraxia in GD (6). Horizontal saccadic latency was associated with the severity of neurological symptoms measured in mSST in our cohort. An increased latency reflects alterations in the oculomotor processing above the brainstem level, e.g., cortical dysfunction affecting the frontal or parietal eye field (14). The severity of neurological involvement, especially the presence of epilepsy, may be caused by more wide-ranging Gaucher pathology in supratentorial areas. A study using diffusion-weighted magnetic resonance imaging in 13 infantile neuronopathic GD2 patients demonstrated reduced diffusion coefficient (ADC) values in cortical temporal, cortical and subcortical frontal regions, corticospinal tract, cerebellum, and midbrain compared to HCs (16), suggesting extensive alterations of tissue integrity in these regions. In our study, four of the nine patients suffered from epilepsy, mostly focal dyscognitive seizures beginning in adolescent or in adulthood, but no progressive myoclonic epilepsy. Patients with epilepsy showed significantly longer latencies of horizontal saccades, but no difference in their velocity compared to patients without epilepsy. However, an influence of the antiepileptic treatment on saccade performance is possible. On the other hand, patients with epilepsy were more affected by GD3 in several ways, showed more ataxia, extrapyramidal signs, and spasticity, which suggest more severe involvement of higher brain areas. Furthermore, the differences to HCs in all saccade parameters remained significant when only GD3 patients without epilepsy were included in the analysis.

The performance in the antisaccade task is associated with functional and imaging markers of executive function in healthy individuals and several neurodegenerative diseases (17). In our GD3 cohort, antisaccade errors tended to be associated with the cognitive function measured in MoCA. Additionally, the antisaccade latency correlated with MoCA, but not to mSST score or age and may be an age-independent marker for supratentorial involvement in GD3. As antisaccades are known to reflect frontal-based functions, a more focused assessment of executive tasks in a larger sample of patients could be helpful to prove our findings.

In summary, our results strengthen the findings of former studies of eye movements in GD (8) and provide additional evidence

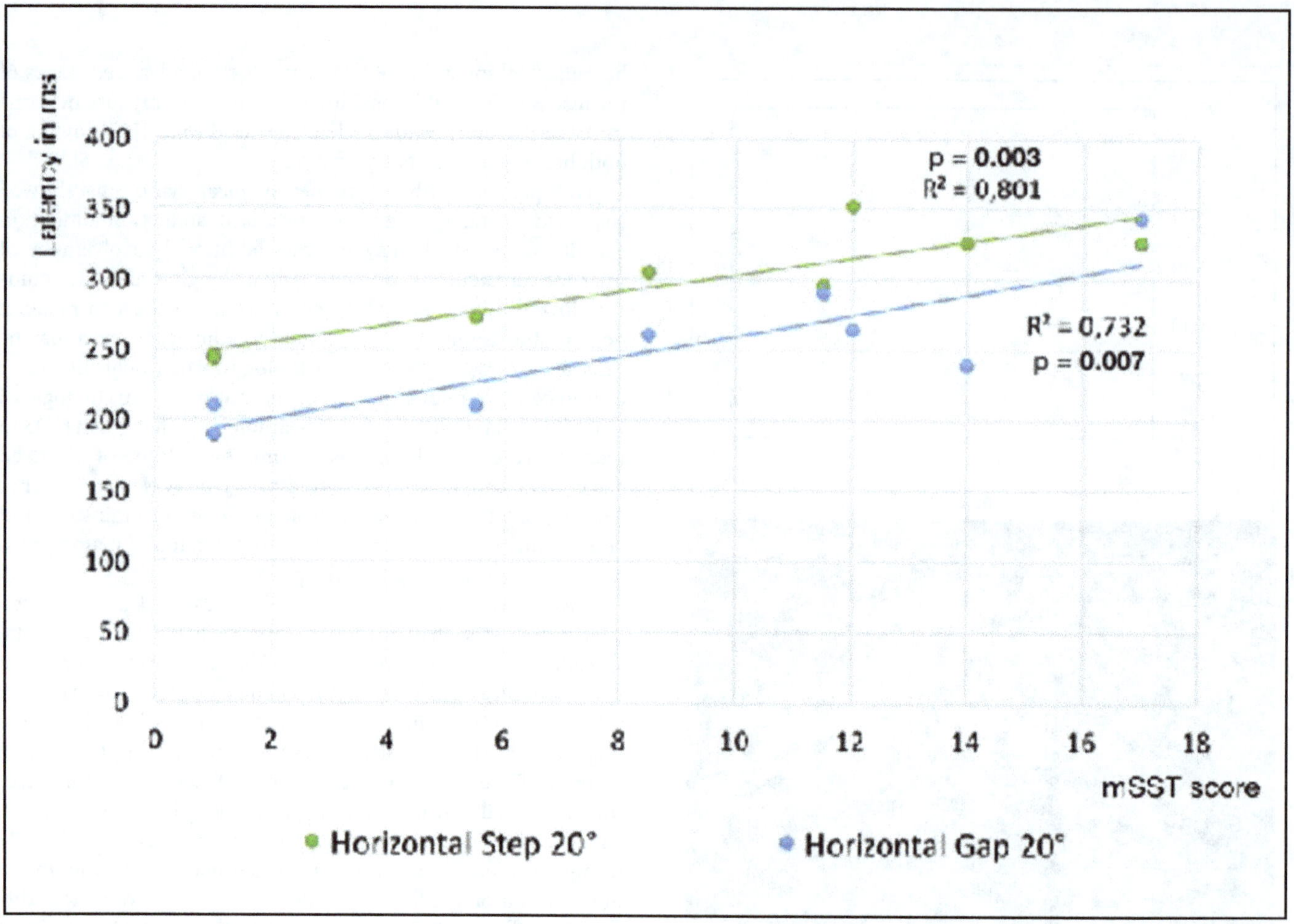

FIGURE 3 | Slope of reflexive saccade latency vs. Gaucher's disease type 3 clinical score. Linear regression slopes of saccade latency vs. modified severity scoring tool (mSST) for horizontal saccades in the step and gap paradigm. The association is significant for both paradigms (step: $R^2 = 0.83$; $p = 0.003$; gap: $R^2 = 0.73$; $p = 0.007$). Comparing the latencies of both paradigms, a gap effect was detectable ($p = 0.01$).

that saccadic impairment reflects neurological and neuropsychological involvement in GD3, including the Norrbottnian type.

AUTHOR CONTRIBUTIONS

Conception of the study and substantial manuscript drafting: JB and PS. Acquisition of data: JB, PS, CB, MM, and SB. Analysis of data: JB, PS, and SB.

ACKNOWLEDGMENTS

The authors would like to thank the study subjects of this project.

FUNDING

Funding was obtained from the Strat Neuro program at Karolinska Institutet. PS is a Wallenberg Clinical Scholar.

REFERENCES

1. Cox TM. Gaucher disease: clinical profile and therapeutic developments. *Biologics* (2010) 4:299–313. doi:10.2147/BTT.S7582
2. Erikson A. Gaucher disease-Norrbottnian type (III). Neuropaediatric and neurobiological aspects of clinical patterns and treatment. *Acta Paediatr Scand Suppl* (1986) 326:1–42. doi:10.1111/j.1651-2227.1986.tb14936.x
3. Dahl N, Lagerström M, Erikson A, Pettersson U. Gaucher disease type III (Norrbottnian type) is caused by a single mutation in exon 10 of the glucocerebrosidase gene. *Am J Hum Genet* (1990) 47:275–8.
4. Machaczka M, Paucar M, Björkvall CK, Smith NJ, Cox TM, Forsgren L, et al. Novel hyperkinetic dystonia-like manifestation and neurological disease course of Swedish Gaucher patients. *Blood Cells Mol Dis* (2016). doi:10.1016/j.bcmd.2016.10.011
5. Altarescu G, Hill S, Wiggs E, Jeffries N, Kreps C, Parker CC, et al. The efficacy of enzyme replacement therapy in patients with chronic neuronopathic Gaucher's disease. *J Pediatr* (2001) 138:539–47. doi:10.1067/mpd.2001.112171
6. Rucker JC, Shapiro BE, Han YH, Kumar AN, Garbutt S, Keller EL, et al. Neuro-ophthalmology of late-onset Tay-Sachs disease (LOTS). *Neurology* (2004) 63(10):1918–26. doi:10.1212/01.WNL.0000144275.76658.F4
7. Salsano E, Umeh C, Rufa A, Pareyson D, Zee DS. Vertical supranuclear gaze palsy in Niemann-Pick type C disease. *Neurol Sci* (2012) 33(6):1225–32. doi:10.1007/s10072-012-1155-1

8. Gross-Tsur V, Har-Even Y, Gutman I, Amir N. Oculomotor apraxia: the presenting sign of Gaucher disease. *Pediatr Neurol* (1989) 5(2):128–9. doi:10.1016/0887-8994(89)90042-8
9. Schiffmann R, Fitzgibbon EJ, Harris C, DeVile C, Davies EH, Abel L, et al. Randomized, controlled trial of miglustat in Gaucher's disease type 3. *Ann Neurol* (2008) 64(5):514–22. doi:10.1002/ana.21491
10. Benko W, Ries M, Wiggs EA, Brady RO, Schiffmann R, Fitzgibbon EJ. The saccadic and neurological deficits in type 3 Gaucher disease. *PLoS One* (2011) 6(7):e22410. doi:10.1371/journal.pone.0022410
11. Davies EH, Mengel E, Tylki-Szymanska A, Kleinotiene G, Reinke J, Vellodi A. Four-year follow-up of chronic neuronopathic Gaucher disease in Europeans using a modified severity scoring tool. *J Inherit Metab Dis* (2011) 34:1053–9. doi:10.1007/s10545-011-9347-z
12. Saslow MG. Effects of components of displacement-step stimuli upon latency for saccadic eye movement. *J Opt Soc Am* (1967) 57(8):1024–9. doi:10.1364/JOSA.57.001024
13. Abel LA, Bowman EA, Velakoulis D, Fahey MC, Desmond P, Macfarlane MD, et al. Saccadic eye movement characteristics in adult Niemann-Pick Type C disease: relationships with disease severity and brain structural measures. *PLoS One* (2012) 7(11):e50947. doi:10.1371/journal.pone.0050947
14. Ramat S, Leigh RJ, Zee DS, Optican LM. What clinical disorders tell us about the neural control of saccadic eye movements. *Brain* (2007) 130(Pt 1):10–35. doi:10.1093/brain/awl309
15. Winkelman MD, Banker BQ, Victor M, Moser HW. Non-infantile neuronopathic Gaucher's disease: a clinicopathologic study. *Neurology* (1983) 33(8):994–1008. doi:10.1212/WNL.33.8.994
16. Abdel Razek AA, Abd El-Gaber N, Abdalla A, Fathy A, Azab A, Rahman AA. Apparent diffusion coefficient vale of the brain in patients with Gaucher's disease type II and type III. *Neuroradiology* (2009) 51(11):773–9. doi:10.1007/s00234-009-0548-1
17. Mirsky JB, Heuer HW, Jafari A, Kramer JH, Schenk AK, Viskontas IV, et al. Anti-saccade performance predicts executive function and brain structure in normal elders. *Cogn Behav Neurol* (2011) 24(2):50–8. doi:10.1097/WNN.0b013e318223f6c6

17

Effects of Deep Brain Stimulation on Eye Movements and Vestibular Function

Aasef G. Shaikh[1,2*], *Chrystalina Antoniades*[3], *James Fitzgerald*[3,4] *and Fatema F. Ghasia*[2,5]

[1] *Department of Neurology, University Hospitals, Case Western Reserve University, Cleveland, OH, United States,* [2] *Daroff-Dell'Osso Ocular Motility Laboratory, Cleveland VA Medical Center, Cleveland, OH, United States,* [3] *NeuroMetrology Lab, Nuffield Department of Clinical Neurosciences, University of Oxford, Oxford, United Kingdom,* [4] *Nuffield Department of Surgical Sciences, University of Oxford, Oxford, United Kingdom,* [5] *Cole Eye Institute, Cleveland Clinic, Cleveland, OH, United States*

Correspondence:
Aasef G. Shaikh
aasefshaikh@gmail.com

Discovery of inter-latching circuits in the basal ganglia and invention of deep brain stimulation (DBS) for their modulation is a breakthrough in basic and clinical neuroscience. The DBS not only changes the quality of life of hundreds of thousands of people with intractable movement disorders, but it also offers a unique opportunity to understand how the basal ganglia interacts with other neural structures. An attractive yet less explored area is the study of DBS on eye movements and vestibular function. From the clinical perspective such studies provide valuable guidance in efficient programming of stimulation profile leading to optimal motor outcome. From the scientific standpoint such studies offer the ability to assess the outcomes of basal ganglia stimulation on eye movement behavior in cognitive as well as in motor domains. Understanding the influence of DBS on ocular motor function also leads to analogies to interpret its effects on complex appendicular and axial motor function. This review focuses on the influence of globus pallidus, subthalamic nucleus, and thalamus DBS on ocular motor and vestibular functions. The anatomy and physiology of basal ganglia, pertinent to the principles of DBS and ocular motility, is discussed. Interpretation of the effects of electrical stimulation of the basal ganglia in Parkinson's disease requires understanding of baseline ocular motor function in the diseased brain. Therefore we have also discussed the baseline ocular motor deficits in these patients and how the DBS changes such functions.

Keywords: Parkinson's disease, tremor, dystonia, neuromodulation, saccade, pursuit, gaze holding

INTRODUCTION

Deep brain stimulation (DBS) is the standard of care in treatment of movement disorders including Parkinson's disease (PD), essential tremor, and dystonia. In addition to the compelling clinical benefits seen in the over 100,000 movement disorders patients treated worldwide, DBS also offers an opportunity to study the effects of electrical stimulation of the basal ganglia on the physiology of motor, sensory, or cognitive systems. The focus of this review is to discuss the effects of DBS of globus pallidus internus (GPi), subthalamic nucleus (STN), and thalamus on ocular motor and vestibular functions. While interpreting the effects of DBS on any aspect of physiology, it is critical to appreciate that such surgery is by definition performed on diseased brains and the effects of stimulation are conflated with the effects of the condition being treated. Nevertheless with a good understanding of the baseline eye movement abnormalities in the patient population concerned, and suitable healthy controls where needed, it is possible to gain insights into normal physiology, disease pathophysiology, and how DBS affects them (1).

HOW DOES DBS WORK?

Although DBS can dramatically improve the motor symptoms of PD, essential tremor, and dystonia, its physiological mechanism of action remains unclear. Because stimulation and lesional surgery at the same sites produce similar beneficial effects in PD, it was previously believed that DBS produced a "physiological ablation" of the target. This is consistent with a simple physiological model of the basal ganglia and PD, where symptoms are due to increased activity of the STN and GPi. It was, therefore, hypothesized that DBS improves clinical symptoms by suppressing the *outflow* of the basal ganglia.

This simple view is no longer tenable, but the mechanism of action of DBS remains poorly understood with several possible explanations (2–4). Stimulation almost certainly causes neuronal excitation, most likely of axons, which have lower firing thresholds than neuronal somata. The consequence of this is likely not to be simply the up-regulation or down-regulation of one or more nuclei, but rather the disruption of some form of pathological network activity. Contemporary studies suggest hyper-synchronization of spontaneous neural activity as a cause of tremor and rigidity. It follows that de-synchronization of such activity might resolve these symptoms. De-synchronization is possible by lesioning the parts of hyper-synchronized circuit (e.g., pallidotomy or thalamotomy), or electrically stimulating (thereby suppressing) the circuit (e.g., DBS) (5, 6). Another possible type of pathological activity is "neural noise" due to excessive random firing, as is seen in the medium spiny neurons of the striatum in PD. Such noise can interfere with information flow within the basal ganglia and it has been suggested that pallidal DBS might act to dampen the noise (7).

APPLIED ANATOMY, PHYSIOLOGY, AND PATHOPHYSIOLOGY OF BASAL GANGLIA IN OCULAR MOTOR CONTROL

The frontal eye field (FEF), supplementary eye field (SEF), dorsolateral prefrontal cortex (DLPFC), and the parietal eye fields project to the basal ganglia, which then relay this input to the superior colliculus (8, 9). The cortical areas project to the caudate nucleus which sends direct inhibitory fibers to the substantia nigra pars reticulata (SNr) and an indirect projection to the STN via the external segment of the globus pallidus (**Figure 1A**) [The figure modified with permission from (10)]. The SNr maintains tonic GABAergic inhibition on the superior colliculus (11, 12); timely and transient cessation of such inhibitory control leads to timely saccade initiation (9, 13, 14). Lesions of the caudate nucleus decrease the velocity and the amplitude of saccades (15). Pharmacological inhibition of the SNr after muscimol injection results in saccadic intrusions and contralaterally directed spontaneous saccades (16). Electrical stimulation of the SNr results in reduced latency and hypometric memory or visually guided saccades (17). In pathological states such as PD, the superior colliculus remains in an inhibited state due to hyperactivity of the SNr (See thick arrow **Figure 1B**) [the figure modified with permission from (10)].

EYE MOVEMENT ABNORMALITIES IN PD

PD is a common neurodegenerative disorder with a complex and variable mixture of clinical features including slowness of movements (bradykinesia), resting tremor, shuffling gait, mask-like facies, and increased muscle tone. A wide range of eye movement abnormalities have been reported in PD, affecting smooth pursuit, vergence, fixation, saccades, and gaze holding (10, 18–23). Abnormalities in smooth pursuit eye movements include a reduction in the eye velocity relative to target movement, i.e., decreased smooth pursuit gain. The reduction in gain worsens as the disease progresses (21). Insufficiency of both convergence and divergence has been described (24–26). A reduction in smooth pursuit gain, mild restriction in upgaze (27), and convergence insufficiency is also seen in elderly who are otherwise healthy, but is more marked in PD. Subjects with PD have saccadic intrusions during attempted steady gaze fixation, followed by return; these movements are called square-wave jerks (10, 20, 28). While square-waves [see **Figures 2A,C**; the figure reproduced with permission from (10)] are often notable in healthy individuals (29), their hypometric characteristic followed by a catch up saccade, just like hypometric visually guided saccades (see **Figure 2B**), ("staircase square-waves") is a unique feature of PD [see **Figures 2A,D**; the figure reproduced with permission from (10)].

Several studies have shown abnormalities in visually guided saccades in subjects with PD. Visually guided prosaccades (saccades toward a novel target) show increased latency (30–34), which progresses over time. Analyzing the distribution of latencies over multiple trials can help in the differential diagnosis of PD and other parkinsonian syndromes (35). Surprisingly, treatment with levodopa, despite alleviating motor symptoms, further increases latency (36). Patients with PD also often have difficulty in inhibiting the reflexive prosaccadic response or initiating a voluntary response in the opposite direction during the antisaccade task. This leads to a higher than normal antisaccadic error rate (AER) (37, 38).

Saccades in parkinsonian patients show an increased prevalence of hypometria, compared to healthy controls (10, 22). Asymmetry of hypometria can be seen in subjects with asymmetric PD, the saccades being more hypometric on the more symptomatic side (39). Series of hypometric saccades that ultimately leads to shift the gaze to its target appears like a "staircase" (40, 41). While staircases increase the time taken to reach the target of interest, this does not imply reduction in the saccade velocity (10). Although there is increased variability in the peak velocity, only the subjects with advanced PD have saccade slowing (21, 28, 42). Correlation between eye movement abnormalities and freezing of gait has also been observed in PD

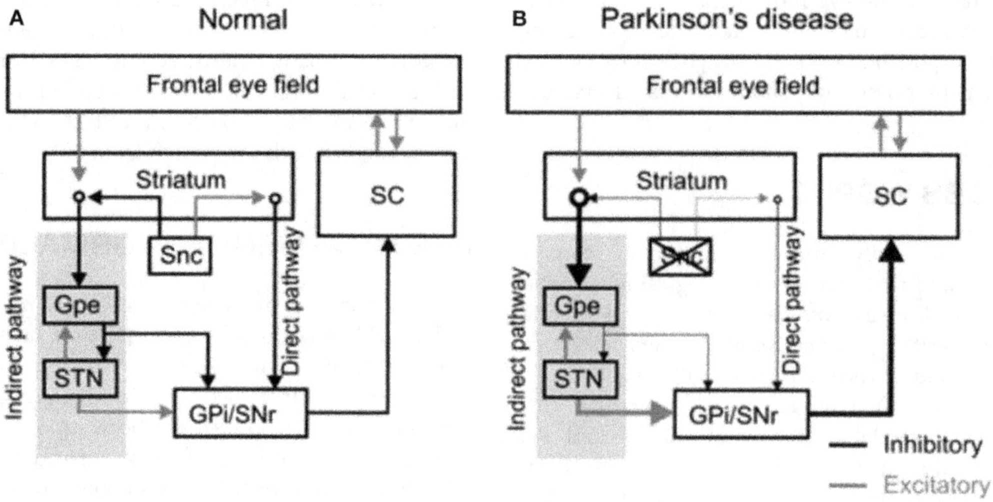

FIGURE 1 | Diagram summarizes organization of the basal ganglia nuclei and their projections. **(A)** The substantia nigra pars compacta (Snc) sends excitatory and inhibitory projections to the striatum. Latter subsequently projects to the basal ganglia outflow nuclei—the globus pallidum internus (GPi) and substantia nigra pars reticulata (SNr) via, parallel, direct and indirect pathways. The direct pathway neurons in the striatum receive excitatory projections from the SNc and sends direct inhibitory projections to GPi and SNr, while inhibitory projections from SNc are sent to the striatal indirect pathway. The indirect pathway, via globus pallidum externus (GPe) and subthalamic nucleus (STN), influences the SNr and GPi. As a result of these connections the dopaminergic neuronal degeneration, as seen in Parkinson's disease, leads to disinhibition of GPi and SNr. Such dysinhibtion leads to inappropriate inhibition of the superior colliculus (SC) (relative thickness of the arrows represents the strength of projection **(B)**. [Figure and corresponding legend modified with permission from (10)].

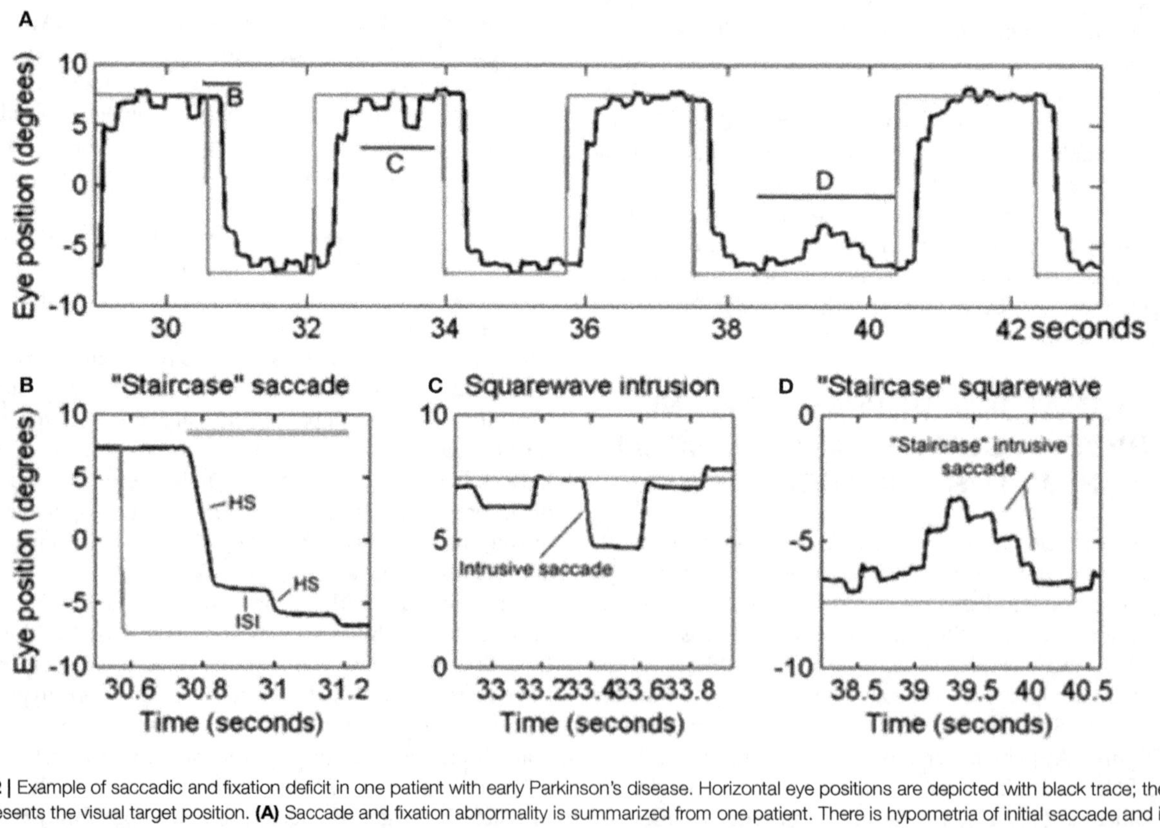

FIGURE 2 | Example of saccadic and fixation deficit in one patient with early Parkinson's disease. Horizontal eye positions are depicted with black trace; the gray trace represents the visual target position. **(A)** Saccade and fixation abnormality is summarized from one patient. There is hypometria of initial saccade and it is then followed by several hypometric corrective saccades (HS). Latter brings the gaze to the target. Horizontal lines in **(A)** depict the portion of the eye movement trace that is temporally zoomed in **(B–D)**. Thick, horizontal, gray line is the target acquisition time. **(C)** Depicts an example of square-wave jerk (SWJ), while **(D)** shows "staircase" square-wave jerk. ISI, inter-saccadic interval. [Figure and legend reproduced with permission from (10)].

(20, 43, 44). PD patients with freezing of gait have increased antisaccade latency and variability in the saccade velocity and accuracy (44).

EFFECTS OF DBS ON SACCADES

DBS is known to influence some saccade abnormalities; for example, prosaccade latency is reduced by the STN or GPi DBS (45–47). DBS is unique in doing this: both levodopa treatment and lesional surgery do the opposite, despite the fact that both of these treatments produce symptomatic improvement. This is further evidence that the physiological mechanism of action of DBS is not simply a physiological ablation. The STN not only facilitates saccades, but also plays a critical role in their planning. Recordings of local field potentials from STN DBS electrodes show event related desynchronizations in the beta band immediately prior to saccades (48) that are qualitatively similar to those seen in motor planning of limb movement.

It has been proposed that the basal ganglia comprise a network that is capable of performing Bayesian statistics for movement selection (49, 50). In this scheme the STN feedback assures that increase in probability of one action is linked with reduction in the probability of other available options (51). Studies examining the effects of STN DBS on saccade generation have provided evidence for this concept. PD patients were asked to make horizontal saccades to a target that appeared either to the left or to the right. The investigators periodically changed the probability of the target appearing in each location and found that saccadic latencies shortened as the target location became more probable, or vice versa. When DBS was turned on, the latency for the more probable target location remained shortened, but the reaction time for less probable locations failed to increase. Disrupting the STN output interfered with the normalized representation of prior probabilities (7, 52).

Both STN and GPi DBS improve prosaccadic latencies. Interestingly GPi stimulation (but not STN stimulation) also reduces the AER (53). While changes in prosaccade latency could be accounted for exclusively by effects within the basal ganglia, the antisaccade task involves higher level functions including inhibition of a reflexive prosaccade and the subsequent volitional generation of a saccade in the opposite direction, both of which are functions of the prefrontal cortex. The results of this study imply that GPi DBS can improve deficits in higher control of lower motor functions (53).

EFFECTS OF DBS ON SMOOTH PURSUIT EYE MOVEMENTS

Video-oculography in 34 patients with PD revealed decreased smooth pursuit eye movement velocity compared to the velocity of a pursued target (i.e., reduced smooth pursuit gain) (54). There is conflicting literature on the effects of DBS on smooth pursuit eye movements. In one study including 14 STN DBS patients, stimulation did not affect pursuit eye movements (54), while in another study of 9 DBS patients both smooth pursuit velocity and accuracy were significantly increased with stimulation (55). Globus pallidus, via thalamic relay, projects to the smooth pursuit areas of the frontal eye fields (56, 57). It is therefore possible that basal ganglia outflow modulates the extended cortical network responsible for smooth pursuit (55).

EFFECTS OF DBS ON GAZE HOLDING

Square-wave jerks are defined by spontaneous intrusive saccades that takes the gaze away from the target followed by a return saccade within 200 ms intersaccadic interval (58). Although square-wave jerks are common in atypical parkinsonism such as multiple system atrophy and progressive supranuclear palsy; approximately 20% of patients with early idiopathic PD (10, 20, 23). Square-wave jerks in early PD are often interrupted, giving the appearance of a "staircase" [see **Figures 2A,D**; the figure reproduced with permission from (10)]. We hypothesized that enhanced inhibition of the superior colliculus in the parkinsonian state may lead to reduced inhibition of presaccadic activity FEF activity leading to its phasic increase and subsequently the square-wave jerk (10). Interruptions of the large intrusive saccades comprising the square-wave jerk, due to phasic SNr inhibition, leads to its "staircase" pattern [see **Figures 2A,D**] (10) [The figure reproduced with permission from (10)].

Pallidotomy increases the frequency of square wave jerks in patients with PD (59). As an explanation, it was proposed that the disinhibition of the ascending thalamocortical loops can reactivate the prefrontal cortex creating imbalance in the activity of the saccade-related prefrontal structures such as the frontal eye fields and supplementary motor eye fields (59). In a study examining the effects of STN DBS on square-wave jerks, the authors found reduction in the frequency of intrusive saccades after bilateral DBS (60).

SINGLE-UNIT ACTIVITY IN HUMAN BASAL GANGLIA AND EYE MOVEMENTS

The functional changes in the ocular motor system resulting from pallidal and subthalamic DBS prompt a fundamental question—is the STN or pallidum directly related to ocular motor control, i.e., do eye movement sensitive neurons exist in the STN or pallidum, or does the stimulation indirectly affect downstream ocular motor sensitive areas such as the SNr or superior colliculus to manifest its effects? Intraoperative microelectrode recordings and single channel electrooculography in 19 PD patients addressed this question. Intraoperatively, while simultaneously sampling single unit activity and oculography, the patients were asked to view a series of colored pictures and perform a visually guided saccade task (61). About one-fifth of neurons isolated from the SNr, globus pallidus, and STN had direct eye movement sensitivity (61).

DBS AND EYELID MOTOR CONTROL

DBS in a rodent model of parkinsonism was recently used to study blink hyper-reflexia, impaired reflex blink plasticity, and reduced spontaneous blink rate (62). A hyper-synchronized beta-band in the basal ganglia output was found to be associated with such blink abnormalities. High-frequency DBS of the STN affected blink hyper-reflexia and blink reflex plasticity; however there were no effects on the abnormal rate and rhythm of the spontaneous blinks (62). It is possible that that the stimulated area of STN was away from that controlling spontaneous blink rate and pattern. It is also possible that DBS parameters used in the experiments were not suitable to change the spontaneous blink abnormality. Finally it can also be speculated that DBS does not affect the discharge pattern of the basal ganglia activity, but it simply reduces the neural response gain. A clinical study showed that pallidal DBS in humans with tardive as well as axial dystonia improves forced eyelid closures (blepharospasm) (63, 64).

EFFECTS OF DBS ON THE VESTIBULAR SYSTEM

The central vestibular system facilitates stable gaze holding, the motion perception, and orientation. The brainstem, under the cerebellar guidance, modulates these functions. In support of this theory, contemporary investigations identified the disorders of human brain where motion perception is selectively affected (65–76). The discovery of non-eye movement sensitive brainstem and cerebellar vestibular neurons further supported this concept (65, 67–69, 77, 78). The non-eye movement sensitive brainstem and cerebellar neurons may have specialized role in encoding a central representation of the gravitational force (65, 67, 70), heading direction (66, 70, 79). The cerebellum sends direct projections, via the vestibulo-thalamic track (fibers that are adjacent to the medial lamniscus but medial and then dorso-medial to the STN), to the ventro-posterior and ventro-lateral thalamus (77, 78, 80). It is therefore predicted that inadvertent stimulation of the vestibulo-thalamic projections can lead to abnormal interpretation of gravitational force. A recent study investigated the effects of DBS of the nucleus ventralis intermedius of the thalamus revealed change in sense of visual verticality (subjective visual vertical) when electrical stimulation was turned on. The patients felt a tilt at 1.4 ± 0.4 degrees on the contraversive side when the stimulator was on; in contrast when stimulator was turned off, the contraversive tilt was 4.4 ± 3.0 degrees (81).

Inadvertent stimulation of medial longitudinal fasciculus or the interstitial nucleus of Cajal can lead to isolated ipsilateral head tilt (82). It is also possible that altered perception of visual vertical (orientation of self in relation to the gravity), due to inadvertent stimulation of the vestibulo-thalamic fibers, have led to reactive head tilt. Recent study investigated the effects of STN stimulation through the medial and caudal DBS electrode contact in five PD subjects (83). Imaging and electrode location from one subject is depicted in **Figure 3** [The figure modified with permission from (83)]. Perception of rotational motion in the plane of horizontal semicircular canal was most commonly reported by these patients, one patient also felt as if she was riding a swing. Latter form of complex perception could be due to the combined stimulation of the vestibulo-thalamic fibers conducting vertical semicircular canals and otolith derived signals, i.e., combination of pitch and fore-aft motion respectively. These serendipitous findings brought new insight into counter-intuitively implementing DBS for the treatment of vertigo and imbalance due to abnormal motion perception.

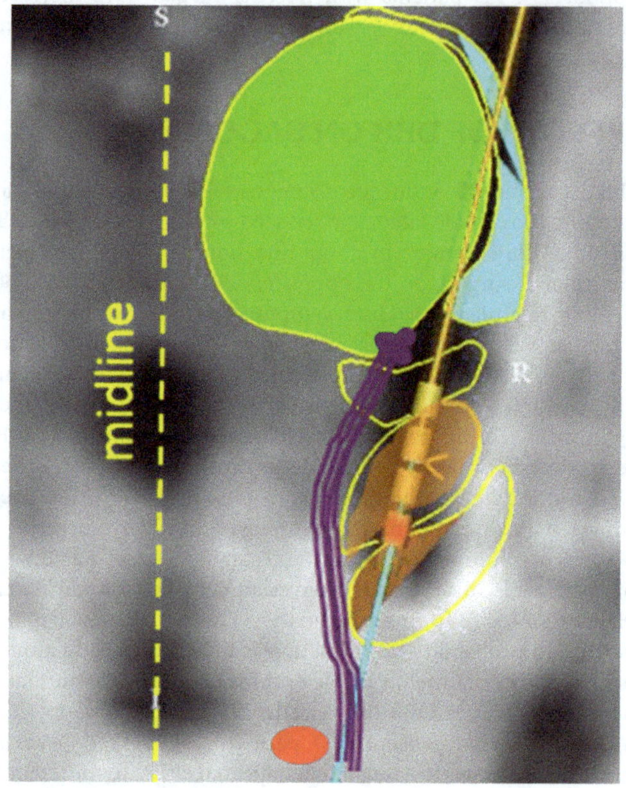

FIGURE 3 | Anatomical model that reconstructed the basal ganglia subnuclei and coordinates of DBS electrode placed in STN. The green area is the model fitted to the thalamus, orange area (yellow arrow) is fitted to STN. The red circle depicts red nucleus. Vestibulo-thalamic fibers (schematized with purple lines) are medial to the STN before they course on the medio-dorsal border of STN to enter the thalamus. DBS electrode leads are depicted with four cylinder shapes (black arrow); red colored cylinder is contact #0 on the implanted lead (Medtronic 3389). [Figure and corresponding legend modified with permission from (83)].

CONCLUSIONS

Although DBS is predominantly viewed as modulating appendicular and axial motor function, tremor, and dystonia, it also has a substantial influence on ocular motor and vestibular function. Clinically, knowledge of how these systems may be affected by stimulation, together with knowledge of the anatomical locations of motor structures relative to ocular motor regions, is critical for safe and effective programming of stimulation parameters. The underlying mechanism of action of DBS is unclear, and because the neurophysiology of eye movements is better understood, the studies of DBS on ocular motor function may offer analogies that help to interpret its effects on appendicular and axial motor function. We also acknowledge that on several occasions the DBS studies have resulted in inconsistent effects on ocular motor function. Such incoherencies could result from institutional (minor) variabilities in DBS electrode placements as well as the variabilities in tested therapeutic electrode contacts. The next generation of studies correlating the outcome of DBS on ocular motor parameters and electrical tissue activation models are desperately needed.

AUTHOR CONTRIBUTIONS

AS conceptualized the manuscript, authored manuscript. CA, JF, and FG edited manuscript.

ACKNOWLEDGMENTS

This work was supported by grants from Dystonia Coalition (AS), Dystonia Medical Research Foundation (AS), Blind Children's Foundation (FG), and RPB Unrestricted grant CCLCM-CWRU.

REFERENCES

1. FitzGerald JJ, Antoniades CA. Eye movements and deep brain stimulation. *Curr Opin Neurol.* (2016) 29:69–73. doi: 10.1097/WCO.0000000000000276
2. Benazzouz A, Hallett M. Mechanism of action of deep brain stimulation. *Neurology* (2000) 55(12 Suppl. 6):S13–6.
3. Dostrovsky JO, Levy R, Wu JP, Hutchison WD, Tasker RR, Lozano AM. Microstimulation-induced inhibition of neuronal firing in human globus pallidus. *J Neurophysiol.* (2000) 84:570–4. doi: 10.1152/jn.2000.84.1.570
4. Montgomery E. B. Jr, Gale JT. Mechanisms of action of deep brain stimulation(DBS). *Neurosci Biobehav Rev.* (2008) 32:388–407. doi: 10.1016/j.neubiorev.2007.06.003
5. Herzog J, Hamel W, Wenzelburger R, Potter M, Pinsker MO, Bartussek J, et al. Kinematic analysis of thalamic versus subthalamic neurostimulation in postural and intention tremor. *Brain* (2007) 130:1608–25. doi: 10.1093/brain/awm077
6. Groppa S, Herzog J, Falk D, Riedel C, Deuschl G, Volkmann J. Physiological and anatomical decomposition of subthalamic neurostimulation effects in essential tremor. *Brain* (2014) 137:109–21. doi: 10.1093/brain/awt304
7. Antoniades CA, Rebelo P, Kennard C, Aziz TZ, Green AL, FitzGerald JJ. Pallidal deep brain stimulation improves higher control of the oculomotor system in Parkinson's disease. *J Neurosci* (2015) 35:13043–52. doi: 10.1523/JNEUROSCI.2317-15.2015
8. Alexander GE, DeLong MR, Strick PL. Parallel organization of functionally segregated circuits linking basal ganglia and cortex. *Annu Rev Neurosci.* (1986) 9:357–81. doi: 10.1146/annurev.ne.09.030186.002041
9. Hikosaka O, Takikawa Y, Kawagoe R. Role of the basal ganglia in the control of purposive saccadic eye movements. *Physiol Rev.* (2000) 80:953–78. doi: 10.1152/physrev.2000.80.3.953
10. Shaikh AG, Xu-Wilson M, Grill S, Zee DS. 'Staircase' square-wave jerks in early Parkinson's disease. *Br J Ophthalmol.* (2011) 95:705–9. doi: 10.1136/bjo.2010.179630
11. Francois C, Percheron G, Yelnik J. Localization of nigrostriatal, nigrothalamic and nigrotectal neurons in ventricular coordinates in macaques. *Neuroscience* (1984) 13:61–76. doi: 10.1016/0306-4522(84)90259-8
12. Fisher RS, Buchwald NA, Hull CD, Levine MS. The GABAergic striatonigral neurons of the cat: demonstration by double peroxidase labeling. *Brain Res.* (1986) 398:148–56. doi: 10.1016/0006-8993(86)91260-6
13. Handel A, Glimcher PW. Quantitative analysis of substantia nigra pars reticulata activity during a visually guided saccade task. *J Neurophysiol.* (1999) 82:3458–75. doi: 10.1152/jn.1999.82.6.3458
14. Hikosaka O. GABAergic output of the basal ganglia. *Prog Brain Res.* (2007) 160:209–26. doi: 10.1016/S0079-6123(06)60012-5
15. Kato M, Miyashita N, Hikosaka O, Matsumura M, Usui S, Kori A. Eye movements in monkeys with local dopamine depletion in the caudate nucleus. I. Deficits in spontaneous saccades. *J Neurosci.* (1995) 15:912–27.
16. Wurtz RH, Hikosaka O. Role of the basal ganglia in the initiation of saccadic eye movements. *Prog Brain Res.* (1986) 64:175–90. doi: 10.1016/S0079-6123(08)63412-3
17. Basso MA, Liu P. Context-dependent effects of substantia nigra stimulation on eye movements. *J Neurophysiol.* (2007) 97:4129–42. doi: 10.1152/jn.00094.2007
18. DeJong JD, Jones GM. Akinesia, hypokinesia, and bradykinesia in the oculomotor system of patients with Parkinson's disease. *Exp Neurol.* (1971) 32:58–68. doi: 10.1016/0014-4886(71)90165-8
19. Herishanu YO, Sharpe JA. Normal square wave jerks. *Invest Ophthalmol Vis Sci.* (1981) 20:268–72.
20. Rascol O, Clanet M, Montastruc JL, Simonetta M, Soulier-Esteve MJ, Doyon B, et al. Abnormal ocular movements in Parkinson's disease. Evidence for involvement of dopaminergic systems. *Brain* (1989) 112 (Pt 5), 1193–1214. doi: 10.1093/brain/112.5.1193
21. Rottach KG, Riley DE, DiScenna AO, Zivotofsky AZ, Leigh RJ. Dynamic properties of horizontal and vertical eye movements in parkinsonian syndromes. *Ann Neurol.* (1996) 39:368–77. doi: 10.1002/ana.410390314
22. Terao Y, Fukuda H, Yugeta A, Hikosaka O, Nomura Y, Segawa M, et al. Initiation and inhibitory control of saccades with the progression of Parkinson's disease - changes in three major drives converging on the superior colliculus. *Neuropsychologia* (2011) 49:1794–806. doi: 10.1016/j.neuropsychologia.2011.03.002
23. Otero-Millan J, Schneider R, Leigh RJ, Macknik SL, Martinez-Conde S. Saccades during attempted fixation in parkinsonian disorders and recessive ataxia: from microsaccades to square-wave jerks. *PLoS ONE* (2013) 8:e58535. doi: 10.1371/journal.pone.0058535
24. Repka MX, Claro MC, Loupe DN, Reich SG. Ocular motility in Parkinson's disease. *J Pediatr Ophthalmol Strabismus* (1996) 33:144–147.
25. Nowacka B, Lubinski W, Honczarenko K, Potemkowski A, Safranow K. Ophthalmological features of Parkinson disease. *Med Sci Monit.* (2014) 20:2243–9. doi: 10.12659/MSM.890861
26. Hanuska J, Bonnet C, Rusz J, Sieger T, Jech R, Rivaud-Pechoux S, et al. Fast vergence eye movements are disrupted in Parkinson's disease: a video-oculography study. *Parkinsonism Relat Disord.* (2015) 21:797–9. doi: 10.1016/j.parkreldis.2015.04.014
27. Clark RA, Demer JL. Effect of aging on human rectus extraocular muscle paths demonstrated by magnetic resonance imaging. *Am J Ophthalmol.* (2002) 134:872–8. doi: 10.1016/S0002-9394(02)01695-1
28. White OB, Saint-Cyr JA, Tomlinson RD, Sharpe JA. Ocular motor deficits in Parkinson's disease. II. Control of the saccadic and smooth pursuit systems. *Brain* (1983) 106 (Pt 3), 571–87.
29. Abadi RV, Gowen E. Characteristics of saccadic intrusions. *Vision Res.* (2004) 44:2675–90. doi: 10.1016/j.visres.2004.05.009
30. Armstrong IT, Chan F, Riopelle RJ, Munoz DP. Control of saccades in Parkinson's disease. *Brain Cogn.* (2002) 49:198–201.
31. MacAskill MR, Anderson TJ, Jones RD. Adaptive modification of saccade amplitude in Parkinson's disease. *Brain* (2002) 125:1570–82. doi: 10.1093/brain/awf168
32. Chan F, Armstrong IT, Pari G, Riopelle RJ, Munoz DP. Deficits in saccadic eye-movement control in Parkinson's disease. *Neuropsychologia* (2005) 43:784–96. doi: 10.1016/j.neuropsychologia.2004.06.026
33. Chambers JM, Prescott TJ. Response times for visually guided saccades in persons with Parkinson's disease: a meta-analytic review. *Neuropsychologia* (2010) 48:887–99. doi: 10.1016/j.neuropsychologia.2009.11.006
34. Terao Y, Fukuda H, Ugawa Y, Hikosaka O. New perspectives on the pathophysiology of Parkinson's disease as assessed by saccade

performance: a clinical review. *Clin Neurophysiol.* (2013) 124:1491–506. doi: 10.1016/j.clinph.2013.01.021

35. Antoniades CA, Bak TH, Carpenter RH, Hodges JR, Barker RA. Diagnostic potential of saccadometry in progressive supranuclear palsy. *Biomark Med.* (2007) 1:487–90. doi: 10.2217/17520363.1.4.487
36. Hood AJ, Amador SC, Cain AE, Briand KA, Al-Refai AH, Schiess MC, et al. Levodopa slows prosaccades and improves antisaccades: an eye movement study in Parkinson's disease. *J Neurol Neurosurg Psychiatry* (2007) 78:565–70. doi: 10.1136/jnnp.2006.099754
37. Kitagawa M, Fukushima J, Tashiro K. Relationship between antisaccades and the clinical symptoms in Parkinson's disease. *Neurology* (1994) 44:2285–9. doi: 10.1212/WNL.44.12.2285
38. Rivaud-Pechoux S, Vidailhet M, Brandel JP, Gaymard B. Mixing pro- and antisaccades in patients with parkinsonian syndromes. *Brain* (2007) 130 (Pt 1):256–64. doi: 10.1093/brain/awl315
39. Choi SM, Lee SH, Choi KH, Nam TS, Kim JT, Park MS, et al. Directional asymmetries of saccadic hypometria in patients with early Parkinson's disease and unilateral symptoms. *Eur Neurol.* (2011) 66:170–4. doi: 10.1159/000330671
40. Kimmig H, Haussmann K, Mergner T, Lucking CH. What is pathological with gaze shift fragmentation in Parkinson's disease? *J Neurol.* (2002) 249:683–92. doi: 10.1007/s00415-002-0691-7
41. Blekher T, Weaver M, Rupp J, Nichols WC, Hui SL, Gray J, et al. Multiple step pattern as a biomarker in Parkinson disease. *Parkinsonism Relat Disord.* (2009) 15:506–10. doi: 10.1016/j.parkreldis.2009.01.002
42. Vidailhet M, Rivaud S, Gouider-Khouja N, Pillon B, Bonnet AM, Gaymard B, et al. Eye movements in parkinsonian syndromes. *Ann Neurol.* (1994) 35:420–6. doi: 10.1002/ana.410350408
43. Lohnes CA, Earhart GM. Saccadic eye movements are related to turning performance in Parkinson disease. *J Parkinsons Dis.* (2011) 1:109–18. doi: 10.3233/JPD-2011-11019
44. Nemanich ST, Earhart GM. Freezing of gait is associated with increased saccade latency and variability in Parkinson's disease. *Clin Neurophysiol.* (2016) 127:2394–401. doi: 10.1016/j.clinph.2016.03.017
45. Temel Y, Visser-Vandewalle V, Carpenter RHS. Saccadic latency during electrical stimulation of the human subthalamic nucleus. *Curr Biol.* (2008) 18:R412–14. doi: 10.1016/j.cub.2008.03.008
46. Yugeta A, Terao Y, Fukuda H, Hikosaka O, Yokochi F, Okiyama R, et al. Effects of STN stimulation on the initiation and inhibition of saccade in Parkinson disease. *Neurology* (2010) 74:743–748. doi: 10.1212/WNL.0b013e3181d31e0b
47. Antoniades CA, Buttery P, FitzGerald JJ, Barker RA, Carpenter RH, Watts C. Deep brain stimulation: eye movements reveal anomalous effects of electrode placement and stimulation. *PLoS ONE* (2012) 7:e32830. doi: 10.1371/journal.pone.0032830
48. Yugeta A, Hutchison WD, Hamani C, Saha U, Lozano AM, Hodaie M, et al. Modulation of Beta oscillations in the subthalamic nucleus with prosaccades and antisaccades in Parkinson's disease. *J Neurosci.* (2013) 33:6895–904. doi: 10.1523/JNEUROSCI.2564-12.2013
49. Redgrave P, Prescott TJ, Gurney K. The basal ganglia: a vertebrate solution to the selection problem? *Neuroscience* (1999) 89:1009–23.
50. Obeso JA, Rodriguez-Oroz MC, Rodriguez M, Lanciego JL, Artieda J, Gonzalo N, et al. Pathophysiology of the basal ganglia in Parkinson's disease. *Trends Neurosci.* (2000) 23:S8–19. doi: 10.1016/S1471-1931(00)00028-8
51. Mink JW. The basal ganglia: focused selection and inhibition of competing motor programs. *Prog Neurobiol.* (1996) 50:381–425. doi: 10.1016/S0301-0082(96)00042-1
52. Antoniades CA, Bogacz R, Kennard C, FitzGerald JJ, Aziz T, Green AL. Deep brain stimulation abolishes slowing of reactions to unlikely stimuli. *J Neurosci.* (2014) 34:10844–52. doi: 10.1523/JNEUROSCI.1065-14.2014
53. Straube A, Ditterich J, Oertel W, Kupsch A. Electrical stimulation of the posteroventral pallidum influences internally guided saccades in Parkinson's disease. *J Neurol.* (1998) 245:101–5. doi: 10.1007/s004150050186
54. Pinkhardt EH, Jurgens R, Lule D, Heimrath J, Ludolph AC, Becker W, et al. Eye movement impairments in Parkinson's disease: possible role of extradopaminergic mechanisms. *BMC Neurol.* (2012) 12:5. doi: 10.1186/1471-2377-12-5
55. Nilsson MH, Patel M, Rehncrona S, Magnusson M, Fransson PA. Subthalamic deep brain stimulation improves smooth pursuit and saccade performance in patients with Parkinson's disease. *J Neuroeng Rehabil.* (2013) 10:33. doi: 10.1186/1743-0003-10-33
56. Tian, Lynch JC. Subcortical input to the smooth and saccadic eye movement subregions of the frontal eye field in Cebus monkey. *J Neurosci.* (1997) 17:9233–47. doi: 10.1523/JNEUROSCI.17-23-09233.1997
57. Lynch JC, Tian JR. Cortico-cortical networks and cortico-subcortical loops for the higher control of eye movements. *Prog Brain Res.* (2006) 151:461–501. doi: 10.1016/S0079-6123(05)51015-X
58. Leigh RJ, Zee DS. *The Neurology of Eye Movements.* New York, NY; Oxford: Oxford University Press (2015).
59. Averbuch-Heller L, Stahl JS, Hlavin ML, Leigh RJ. Square-wave jerks induced by pallidotomy in parkinsonian patients. *Neurology* (1999) 52:185–8. doi: 10.1212/WNL.52.1.185
60. Wark HA, Garell PC, Walker AL, Basso MA. A case report on fixation instability in Parkinson's disease with bilateral deep brain stimulation implants. *J Neurol Neurosurg Psychiatry* (2008) 79:443–7. doi: 10.1136/jnnp.2007.117192
61. Cavanagh JF, Wiecki TV, Cohen MX, Figueroa CM, Samanta J, Sherman SJ, et al. Subthalamic nucleus stimulation reverses mediofrontal influence over decision threshold. *Nat Neurosci.* (2011) 14:1462–7. doi: 10.1038/nn.2925
62. Kaminer J, Thakur P, Evinger C. Effects of subthalamic deep brain stimulation on blink abnormalities of 6-OHDA lesioned rats. *J Neurophysiol.* (2015) 113:3038–46. doi: 10.1152/jn.01072.2014
63. Shaikh AG, Mewes K, Jinnah HA, DeLong MR, Gross RE, Triche S, et al. Globus pallidus deep brain stimulation for adult-onset axial dystonia. *Parkinsonism Relat Disord.* (2014) 20:1279–82. doi: 10.1016/j.parkreldis.2014.09.005
64. Shaikh AG, Mewes K, DeLong MR, Gross RE, Triche SD, Jinnah HA, et al. Temporal profile of improvement of tardive dystonia after globus pallidus deep brain stimulation. *Parkinsonism Relat Disord.* (2015) 21:116–9. doi: 10.1016/j.parkreldis.2014.11.013
65. Angelaki DE, Shaikh AG, Green AM, Dickman JD. Neurons compute internal models of the physical laws of motion. *Nature* (2004) 430:560–4. doi: 10.1038/nature02754
66. Shaikh AG, Meng H, Angelaki DE. Multiple reference frames for motion in the primate cerebellum. *J Neurosci.* (2004) 24:4491–7. doi: 10.1523/JNEUROSCI.0109-04.2004
67. Green AM, Shaikh AG, Angelaki DE. Sensory vestibular contributions to constructing internal models of self-motion. *J Neural Eng.* (2005) 2:S164–79. doi: 10.1088/1741-2560/2/3/S02
68. Shaikh AG, Ghasia FF, Dickman JD, Angelaki DE. Properties of cerebellar fastigial neurons during translation, rotation, and eye movements. *J Neurophysiol.* (2005) 93:853–63. doi: 10.1152/jn.00879.2004
69. Shaikh AG, Green AM, Ghasia FF, Newlands SD, Dickman JD, Angelaki DE. Sensory convergence solves a motion ambiguity problem. *Curr Biol.* (2005) 15:1657–62. doi: 10.1016/j.cub.2005.08.009
70. Yakusheva TA, Shaikh AG, Green AM, Blazquez PM, Dickman JD, Angelaki DE. Purkinje cells in posterior cerebellar vermis encode motion in an inertial reference frame. *Neuron* (2007) 54:973–85. doi: 10.1016/j.neuron.2007.06.003
71. Bertolini G, Ramat S, Laurens J, Bockisch CJ, Marti S, Straumann D, et al. Velocity storage contribution to vestibular self-motion perception in healthy human subjects. *J Neurophysiol.* (2011) 105:209–23. doi: 10.1152/jn.00154.2010
72. Bertolini G, Ramat S, Bockisch CJ, Marti S, Straumann D, Palla A. Is vestibular self-motion perception controlled by the velocity storage? Insights from patients with chronic degeneration of the vestibulo-cerebellum. *PLoS ONE* (2012) 7:e36763. doi: 10.1371/journal.pone.0036763
73. Shaikh AG, Palla A, Marti S, Olasagasti I, Optican LM, Zee DS, et al. Role of cerebellum in motion perception and vestibulo-ocular reflex-similarities and disparities. *Cerebellum* (2013) 12:97–107. doi: 10.1007/s12311-012-0401-7
74. Shaikh AG. Motion perception without Nystagmus–a novel manifestation of cerebellar stroke. *J Stroke Cerebrovasc Dis.* (2014) 23:1148–56. doi: 10.1016/j.jstrokecerebrovasdis.2013.10.005
75. Bertolini G, Wicki A, Baumann CR, Straumann D, Palla A. Impaired tilt perception in Parkinson's disease: a central

vestibular integration failure. *PLoS ONE* (2015) 10:e0124253. doi: 10.1371/journal.pone.0124253

76. Yousif N, Bhatt H, Bain PG, Nandi D, Seemungal BM. The effect of pedunculopontine nucleus deep brain stimulation on postural sway and vestibular perception. *Eur J Neurol.* (2016) 23:668–70. doi: 10.1111/ene.12947
77. Meng H, May PJ, Dickman JD, Angelaki DE. Vestibular signals in primate thalamus: properties and origins. *J Neurosci.* (2007) 27:13590–602. doi: 10.1523/JNEUROSCI.3931-07.2007
78. Meng H, Angelaki DE. Responses of ventral posterior thalamus neurons to three-dimensional vestibular and optic flow stimulation. *J Neurophysiol.* (2010) 103:817–26. doi: 10.1152/jn.00729.2009
79. Liu S, Yakusheva T, Deangelis GC, Angelaki DE. Direction discrimination thresholds of vestibular and cerebellar nuclei neurons. *J Neurosci.* (2010) 30:439–48. doi: 10.1523/JNEUROSCI.3192-09.2010
80. Hawrylyshyn PA, Rubin AM, Tasker RR, Organ LW, Fredrickson JM. Vestibulothalamic projections in man–a sixth primary sensory pathway. *J Neurophysiol.* (1978) 41:394–401. doi: 10.1152/jn.1978.41.2.394
81. Baier B, Vogt T, Rohde F, Cuvenhaus H, Conrad J, Dieterich M. (2015). Deep brain stimulation of the nucleus ventralis intermedius: a thalamic site of graviceptive modulation. *Brain Struct Funct.* 222:645–50. doi: 10.1007/s00429-015-1157-x
82. Mike A, Balas I, Varga D, Janszky J, Nagy F, Kovacs N. Subjective visual vertical may be altered by bilateral subthalamic deep brain stimulation. *Mov Disord.* (2009) 24:1556–7. doi: 10.1002/mds.22605
83. Shaikh AG, Straumann D, Palla A. Motion illusion-evidence towards human vestibulo-thalamic projections. *Cerebellum* (2017) 16:656–63. doi: 10.1007/s12311-017-0844-y

18

Modeling the Triggering of Saccades, Microsaccades and Saccadic Intrusions

Jorge Otero-Millan[1], Lance M. Optican[2], Stephen L. Macknik[3,4,5] and Susana Martinez-Conde[3,4,5]*

[1] Department of Neurology, Johns Hopkins University, Baltimore, MD, United States, [2] Laboratory of Sensorimotor Research, National Eye Institute, National Institutes of Health, Department of Health and Human Services, Bethesda, MD, United States, [3] Department of Ophthalmology, SUNY Downstate Medical Center, Brooklyn, NY, United States, [4] Department of Neurology, SUNY Downstate Medical Center, Brooklyn, NY, United States, [5] Department of Physiology and Pharmacology, SUNY Downstate Medical Center, Brooklyn, NY, United States

****Correspondence:***
Jorge Otero-Millan
jotero@jhu.edu

When we explore a static visual scene, our eyes move in a sequence of fast eye movements called saccades, which are separated by fixation periods of relative eye stability. Based on uncertain sensory and cognitive inputs, the oculomotor system must decide, at every moment, whether to initiate a saccade or to remain in the fixation state. Even when we attempt to maintain our gaze on a small spot, small saccades, called microsaccades, intrude on fixation once or twice per second. Because microsaccades occur at the boundary of the decision to maintain fixation versus starting a saccade, they offer a unique opportunity to study the mechanisms that control saccadic triggering. Abnormal saccadic intrusions can occur during attempted fixation in patients with neurodegenerative disorders. We have implemented a model of the triggering mechanism of saccades, based on known anatomy and physiology, that successfully simulates the generation of saccades of any size—including microsaccades in healthy observers, and the saccadic intrusions that interrupt attempted fixation in parkinsonian patients. The model suggests that noisy neuronal activity in the superior colliculus controls the state of a mutually inhibitory network in the brain stem formed by burst neurons and omnipause neurons. When the neuronal activity is centered at the rostral pole, the system remains at a state of fixation. When activity is perturbed away from this center, a saccade is triggered. This perturbation can be produced either by the intent to move one's gaze or by random fluctuations in activity.

Keywords: parkinsonian, progressive supranuclear palsy, square-wave jerk, saccade generation, models, theoretical

INTRODUCTION

Eye motion during exploration of a visual scene consists of a sequence of fast eye movements called saccades, which happen about three times per second, interleaved with fixation periods of relative stability (1, 2). Saccades bring objects of interest toward the high-resolution area of the retina, but have a cost which is not just energetic but also perceptual: we lose visual sensitivity briefly when saccades occur (3). The oculomotor system must decide, at any given moment, whether to initiate a saccade or to remain in the fixation state. This decision involves uncertainty, given the inherent noise in the underlying neuronal signals and cognitive processes.

If we attempt to fixate on a spot, small eye movements, called microsaccades, shift eye position one or two times per second, usually by less than 1° (4). Microsaccades share many characteristics with larger saccades and are likely generated by the same neural system (5, 6). Because microsaccades occur at the boundary of the decision to maintain fixation versus to initiate a saccade, they offer a unique opportunity to study the mechanisms that control saccadic triggering. They also show that, even when we strive to keep our eyes still, the oculomotor system will nevertheless decide, from time to time, to start a saccade (7).

Many models of the saccade generation circuit have been proposed, but they have been rarely tested with small saccades of the size of microsaccades. Indeed, many such models (8) are designed to *not* trigger saccades smaller than a given value (i.e., 2°). In addition, few studies have tested the effect of noise on the system (9–11). This is a critical limitation, in that some models would trigger saccades continuously if noise were added to their inputs. Here, we will implement a model of the saccade triggering system that can initiate both large and small (<1°) saccades and can do so in the presence of noise. We will moreover show that this noise leads to the production of spontaneous microsaccades during fixation.

Patients affected with neurological disorders can present with abnormal fixational eye movements (1). Thus, the proposed model will also explore the possible mechanisms for the generation of abnormal fixational eye movements, specifically saccadic intrusions. Saccadic intrusions, such as square-wave jerks (SWJs), macro saccadic oscillations, flutter, and opsoclonus, are common in certain neurodegenerative diseases (**Figure 1**), including progressive supranuclear palsy (PSP), spinocerebellar ataxias, Parkinson's disease (PD), and others (12, 13).

The model proposed here does not consider other types of eye movements that may affect eye position during fixation, such as drift, tremor, vestibular–ocular reflex (including quick-phases), smooth pursuit, or vergence. Also, we simplify and combine all the possible sources of noise present in the saccade triggering system. These may include inherent neural noise, sensory noise from the visual system, noise from multisensory integration processes, and/or or noise from high-level cognitive processes known to affect eye movements (14).

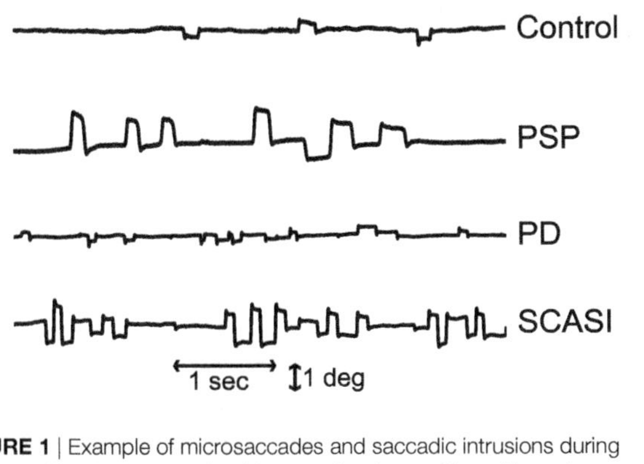

FIGURE 1 | Example of microsaccades and saccadic intrusions during attempted fixation in control subjects and patients with parkinsonian disorders: progressive supranuclear palsy (PSP), Parkinson's disease (PD), spinocerebellar ataxia with saccadic intrusions (SCASI). Figure adapted from Otero-Millan et al. (12).

Triggers

Many problems in engineering require a robust mechanism to trigger changes between two possible states depending on noisy continuous signals. One common trigger design is known as a Schmitt trigger (15) and relies on a *positive* feedback loop combined with elements with high gain and saturation. This design creates hysteresis, with the useful feature of requiring different thresholds to switch from state A to state B, and from state B to state A. Thus, a minor change in the input after a switch will not produce a switch back to the preceding state (**Figure 2**).

We propose that a similar mechanism may be used to trigger saccades. A saccade ultimately occurs when the premotor burst neurons (BNs) in the reticular formation start bursting. Another group of neurons in the reticular formation, called omnipause neurons (OPNs), fire at a fairly constant rate between saccades, and stop completely during a saccadic movement (16). These two populations of neurons are linked to each other by inhibitory connections (17). This reciprocal inhibition acts, essentially, as a positive feedback loop. During fixation, the OPNs fire and keep the BNs quiet. Before a saccade, the system switches, so the inhibition of OPNs to BNs decreases while the inhibition from BNs to OPNs increases. This positive feedback ensures that a saccade is initiated quickly and that is not interrupted easily before completion.

The signal that drives the switch between states originates in the superior colliculus (SC). Due to the SC's topographical organization, saccades of varying sizes and directions can be evoked by microstimulation of different SC locations, with caudal areas triggering large saccades, and rostral areas triggering small saccades (18). Consistent with these microstimulation findings, neuronal activity recordings in the intermediate layers of the SC established that caudal neurons fire before large saccades, and that rostral neurons fire before small saccades (19, 20). Furthermore, neurons in the SC rostral pole are active during fixation but stop during saccades (19). These combined results led to the hypothesis of two SC neuronal populations, with two distinct functions: saccade neurons and fixation neurons. More recent studies challenged this dichotomy though, by showing that rostral pole neurons fire for small microsaccades in an equivalent fashion as more caudal neurons do for larger saccades (6, 21, 22).

The SC projects to both OPNs and BNs, with stronger projections to the OPN from the SC rostral area and to the BNs from the SC caudal area (23, 24). SC projections to the BNs transform the topological coding of saccade magnitude into a rate coding, with the result that BNs fire more for larger saccades.

Here, we implement a model of the trigger mechanism formed by the SC, OPNs, and BNs, to explain how microsaccades may be triggered in the presence of both noise and a constant command to maintain a fixed eye position. We include this trigger in a distributed model of the oculomotor system, and we simulate microsaccadic generation during attempted fixation. We also reproduce some of the experimental observations from prior inactivation or stimulation experiments. Finally, we offer some

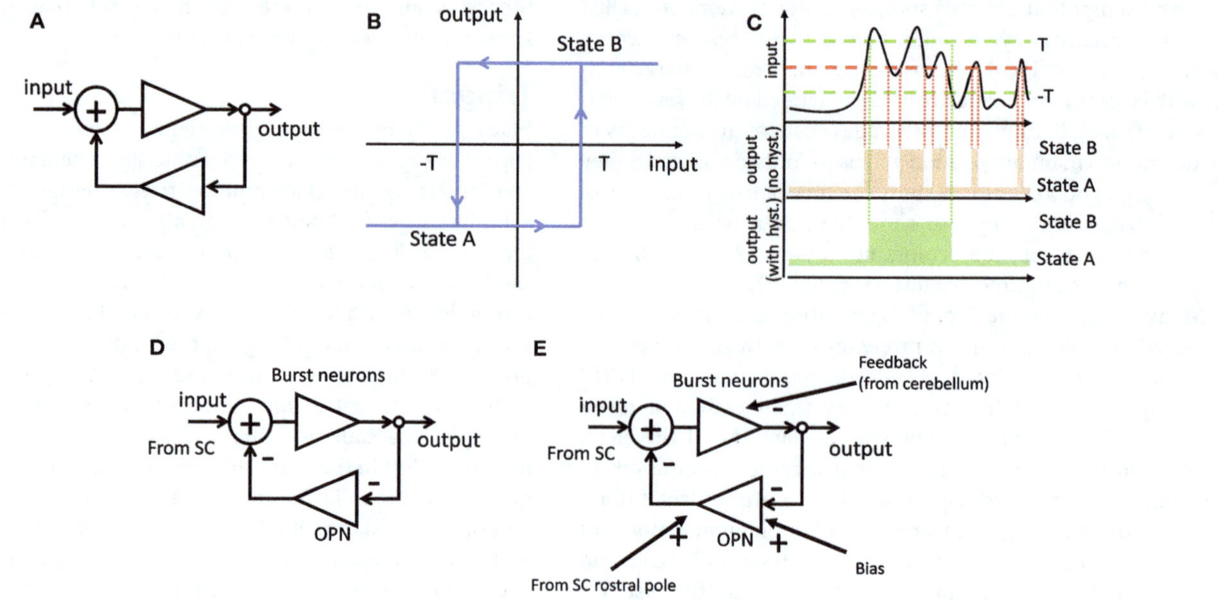

FIGURE 2 | Schmitt trigger. **(A)** Positive feedback loop. **(B)** Hysteresis function corresponding to **(A)**. When the system is in state A, the input needs to reach the value T to switch to state B. When in state B, the input needs to reach −T to switch to state A. **(C)** Effect of hysteresis. Top, example of fluctuating input. Middle, changes of state for a simple threshold (red). Bottom, unwanted switches (in middle panel) can be reduced by having hysteresis with two thresholds (green). **(D)** The same positive feedback loop as in **(A)** formed by double inhibition through brain stem neurons. Because burst neurons (BNs) inhibit omnipause neuron (OPN) which in turn inhibit BNs, the result is net positive feedback loop. **(E)** Further inputs can modulate the behavior of the system. Examples include biasing the threshold or using an additional negative feedback loop to bring the system back to the original state after a switch (that is, ending the saccade).

hypotheses regarding the mechanism that causes abnormal saccadic intrusions in certain neurological disorders.

IMPLEMENTATION OF THE MODEL

The input to the model is the desired gaze location (or location of the target), which is constant in the case of maintained fixation. This command gets updated with every eye movement after a visual feedback delay of 50 ms, to calculate the desired eye position in retinal coordinates. The frontal eye fields (FEFs) send a constant excitatory command to the SC at the corresponding location of the target, and the basal ganglia (BG) send a complementary inhibitory projection, which inhibits the entire SC map except for the location of the target. We also include a noise input to the SC, responsible for the random fluctuations that eventually trigger microsaccades during fixation. This noise input aims to represent the combination of all the potential sources of noise to the SC. The SC combines the different inputs in a map with short-range excitatory connections and long-range inhibitory connections. The SC sends the left and right motor commands to the BNs in the brain stem, as well as a signal to the OPNs, representing mostly the rostral activity. The cerebellum receives the SC command and a copy of the output of the BNs and creates a signal that feeds back to the SC and BNs to stop saccades.

The model builds on both recent and classical results on microsaccade and saccade generation. Hafed and colleagues showed that the activity in the rostral pole of the SC is related to microsaccade generation; thus the SC map can be seen as a continuum of neurons encoding the location of the intended target (22). Shinoda and colleagues showed that the inhibitory burst neurons (IBNs in the pontomedullary reticular formation) send a direct inhibitory projection to the OPNs (17), which is presumably responsible for the lack of OPN activity during saccades. The idea that IBNs inhibit OPNs is supported by results from multiple anatomical and physiological studies (25–27). Van Horn and Cullen showed that OPNs also stop during microsaccades (28), and Van Gisbergen and Robinson found previously that BNs fire for microsaccades as they do for saccades (29).

Figure 3 shows the general structure of the model with its main components. Because we aim to simulate a sequence of eye movements during attempted fixation, and not just an individual saccade, the model must close the visual loop and incorporate the effect of past eye movements. The model includes areas in the cortex, the brain stem, and the cerebellum to control saccade generation. The implementation of each participating area is described in the following sections. Finally, the model includes a final common pathway that creates the pulse-slide-step activity characteristic of the motor neurons and a motor plant that simulates the physical properties of the eye globe.

The model was implemented using Matlab-Simulink (MathWorks Natick, MA, USA) with a 1-ms fixed step for the simulations and the ode3 Bogacki–Shampine solver. **Table 1** provides the values for the parameters of the model. To optimize the parameters of the model we first tuned them to produce accurate saccades in the absence of noise. Then, we optimized the parameters of the noise and the parameters

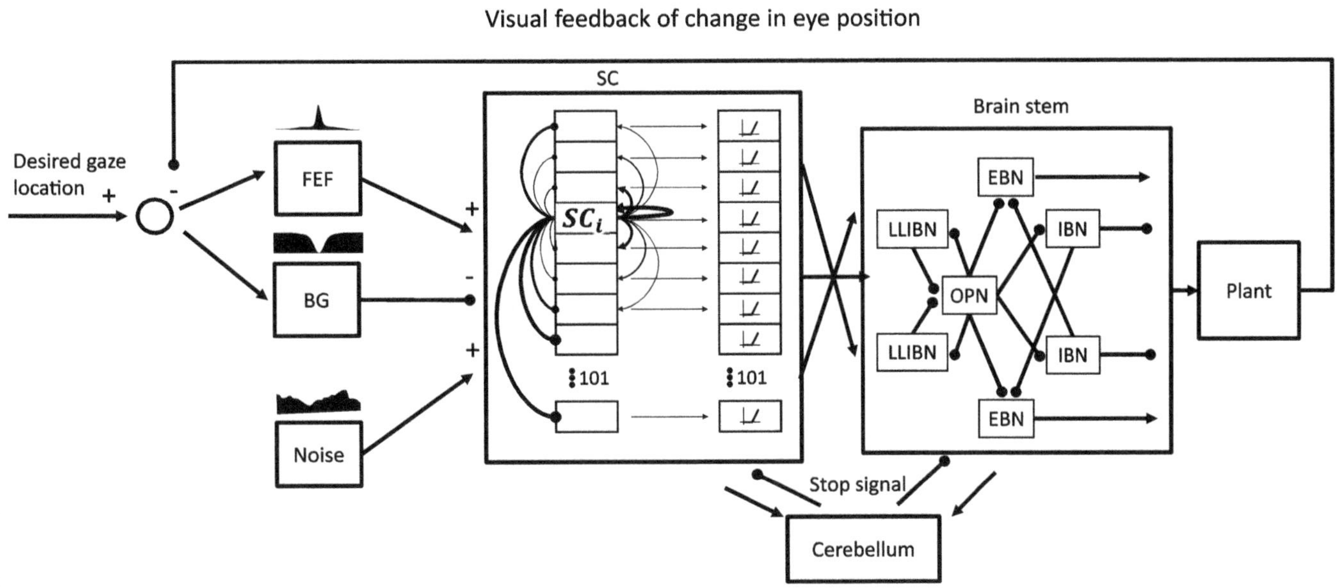

FIGURE 3 | General model structure. The focus of the model is on the network formed by the superior colliculus (SC) and the omnipause neurons (OPNs) and burst neurons (BNs) in the brain stem and how they generate microsaccades in the presence of noise. Thus, the SC and the brain stem reticular formation are the only elements modeled as a network of neurons. All the other elements are "lumped" elements that just attempt to simulate a certain transfer function. The SC receives two complementary inputs indicating the desired gaze location in retinotopic coordinates, one excitatory from frontal eye field (FEF) and one inhibitory from basal ganglia (BG). It also receives a noise input that represents all the possible sources of noise the SC may receive. The SC is a network of 101 interconnected neurons with short-range excitatory connections and long-range inhibitory connections. The output of the SC that drives the BNs includes a nonlinearity that gives more weight to neurons firing more. The SC also drives the OPNs, especially when activity is centered around the center of the SC (representing the rostral pole). The model also includes a simple model of a cerebellar circuit that would produce a stop signal to reset both the SC and the BNs after a saccade. The output of the brain stem drives the eye plant that accounts for the mechanical properties of the eye. The resulting changes in eye position are fed back to the input of the model with a delay of 50 ms.

relevant to the trigger [connections between OPNs and long lead IBNs (LLIBNs)] to produce microsaccades with comparable properties to real recordings of fixational eye movements. Finally, to simulate the different neurological disorders we only modified one or two parameters at a time to produce saccadic intrusions.

Brain Stem Reticular Formation

The reticular formation circuit we simulate is formed by one OPN, and three BNs on each side: LLIBNs, medium lead excitatory BNs (MLEBNs), and medium lead IBNs (MLIBNs). The OPN inhibits all six BNs. The IBNs inhibit the OPN and the three contralateral BNs. These inhibitory connections serve two distinct roles. First, they ensure that the BNs on only one side are active at the same time (crossing connections from IBNs to all BNs). Second, they control the switching between saccade and fixation states. In between saccades, the OPN inhibits all BNs; during saccades, the IBNs inhibit the OPN.

The connections between the OPN and the IBNs are critical for controlling the triggering of saccades. The connection between the OPN and the MLIBNs must be strong to avoid any firing during fixation; the connection between the OPN and the LLIBNs must be weak to allow for slight changes in drive from the SC to the LLBNs to trigger a saccade. At the same time, the connection between the MLIBNs and the OPN must be strong to completely inhibit it during saccades. Our LLIBNs do not show very long lead activity, but a future implementation of the model could achieve this *via* a population of neurons with variable strength of connections, rather than just a single neuron of each type (30). Similar circuits have been simulated previously to study saccades (31–33).

Every brain stem neuron in the network is modeled as a leaky integrator (time constant τ_{BN}) with an exponential output response function, modified from Zee and Robinson (34) with parameter $e_0 = 0$

$$B(x) = B_m * (1 - e^{-(x-e_0)/b}) \quad (1)$$

Superior Colliculus

We implemented the SC map following previous models (7, 35). In the model, the left and right SC correspond with a single one-dimensional structure that encodes the horizontal retinotopic space with a set of 101 neurons. The mapping between the coordinates of the retinotopic space (D) to colliculus space (d) is given by the following formula (36):

$$d(D) = B * \log((D + A) / A) \quad (2)$$

with A and B being the parameters that define the amount of retinal magnification and size, respectively.

Each neuron is characterized by a leaky integrator (with a time constant τ_{SC}) of the weighted sum of all its inputs. The output or

TABLE 1 | Model parameters.

Model parameters	
Burst neurons (BNs)	
τ_{BN}	0.001 s
b	8
B_m	800 spikes/s
Superior colliculus (SC)	
F	500
A	3°
B	1.4 mm
A_w	1
C	1
σ_{SC}	0.5 mm
τ_{SC}	0.005 s
S	5 mm
β_u	0.1
Frontal eye fields (FEFs) and basal ganglia (BG)	
σ_{FEF}	0.5 mm
σ_{BG}	1 mm
Noise	
τ_{noise}	0.02 s
σ_{noise}	0.2 mm
Brain stem	
W_{OPN_LLIBN}	0.0015
W_{OPN_BN}	0.2
W_{LLIBN_OPN}	10
W_{IBN_BN}	0.1
OPN bias	50 spikes/s
Cerebellum	
T_{cblm1}	0.02 s
T_{cblm2}	0.02 s
F_1	0.1
F_2	0.03
F_3	1
F_4	0.13

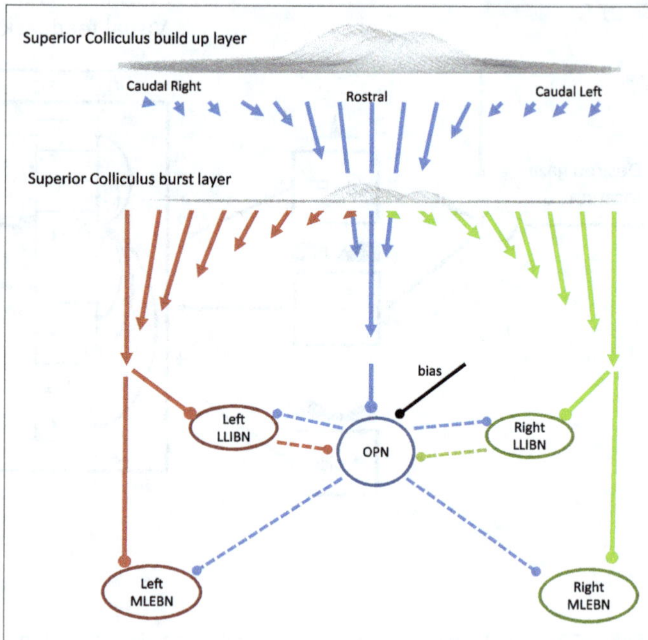

FIGURE 4 | Schematic of the projections from the superior colliculus (SC) to the reticular formation and the triggering circuit. In this model, the SC is a one-dimensional structure with 101 interconnected neurons. During fixation, the activity centers around the middle (which corresponds with the rostral area). The omnipause neuron (OPN) receives excitatory inputs from the buildup layer of the SC with stronger connections (represented as longer arrows) from the more rostral areas. The OPN inhibits all burst neurons (BNs) in the model. The BNs receive excitatory inputs from the contralateral burst layer of the SC with stronger connections from the more caudal areas so the total average input is proportional to the eccentricity of the center of mass of the SC activity. Arrows represent excitatory connections and dots represent inhibitory connections.

activation (a) of each neuron depends on a nonlinear function (with parameters β_u and F) of the output of the integrator (u) (7):

$$a(u) = F * 1/(1 + e^{-\beta_u u}) \tag{3}$$

Each neuron in the map is connected to every other neuron, and the strength and sign of the connectivity depends on the distance between the two neurons dist(i, j), which assumes equally spaced neurons along a 10 mm length (−5 to 5 mm). Neurons that are close to each other receive strong mutual excitation, and neurons that are far from each other inhibit each other. This connectivity is modeled by the synaptic weights of the connections between each neuron. The strength of the connection between neurons i and j in the map is:

$$w_{ij} = (A_w + C)e^{-(\text{dist}(i,j))^2/2\sigma_{SC}^2} - C \tag{4}$$

The maximum positive strength is defined by A_w and the maximum negative strength by C, dist(i, j) is the distance in mm between the two neurons, assuming all neurons are equally spaced and σ_{SC} defines the size of the region that receives excitatory inputs. The input to each SC neuron is defined by the sum of the weighted contributions from all other neurons in the map and the signal coming from the cortex. The cortical signal indicates the desired target location by driving a corresponding patch of SC and inhibiting the rest of the map. We also added a noise input, to simulate microsaccade generation (see following section).

Depending on the characteristics of their firing, SC neurons are typically divided into buildup neurons (if they fire long before the saccade) and BNs (if they fire only around the saccade). Here, we considered the neurons described above as buildup neurons, and we added a burst layer, which is just a thresholded version of the buildup layer. This burst layer acts essentially as a nonlinearity in the center of activity calculation that takes place from SC to BNs. Other mechanisms could achieve the same result, that is, that higher firing at a given SC location gives that location more weight. Regardless of its specific implementation, this feature ensures that the trigger does not get activated during the buildup period of large saccades, while allowing small shifts and increases of the center of activity to trigger microsaccades.

The SC sends three projections down to the reticular formation: one to the OPNs, one to the left BNs, and one to the right BNs (**Figure 4**). The OPNs receive a projection from the entire SC buildup layer, which is stronger from the rostral areas (23). Specifically, the strength of the projection decreases linearly with distance from the rostral end of each SC until it reaches zero at the extremes. That is, the more caudal the SC projection area, the weaker the connection to OPNs. The projection to contralateral BNs comes from the burst layer and is stronger from caudal than from rostral neurons. The strength of the projections from the SC map to the OPN or the BNs is given by:

$$w_{\text{SCOPN}}(i) = 1 - |\text{dist}(i,0)| / S \quad (5)$$

$$w_{\text{SCBN}}(i) = \text{dist}(i,0) \quad (6)$$

where dist(i, 0) is the distance in mm between neuron i and the neuron at the rostral pole encoding 0° eccentricity and S is the size of each SC in mm.

To make the drive from SC to BNs only dependent on the location (rather than the amount) of activity in the map, it is necessary to include a normalization mechanism that implements the center of activity calculation. In our model, we divide the total weighted drive from SC to BNs by the total activity of the SC burst layer. For stability purposes, a small fraction of the buildup activity is also included in the denominator.

FEF and BG

We have implemented a very simplified version of the outputs of the FEF and the BG that provide the drive and the inhibition that control the activity of the SC. Both outputs present Gaussian profiles (with SDs σ_{FEF} and σ_{BG}) centered at the location of the desired target. The level of activity of the FEF also depends on the eccentricity of the target. This simulates the decreased likelihood of a saccade triggered for small retinal errors (37, 38).

Random Fluctuations

To simulate the eye movements that occur during attempted fixation, we assume that the voluntary command from the cortex to the SC is constant and creates a Gaussian hill of activity centered at the location of the target. To produce microsaccades, we have introduced a noise term to the input to the colliculus. Many sources of neural noise can play a role in microsaccade generation, but here, we lump the effects of all of them into SC activity fluctuations. We have implemented a noise generator that produces noise with temporal and spatial correlations across the SC map. The temporal correlation is created by filtering white noise through leaky integrators of time constant τ_{noise}. The spatial correlation is implemented by creating one independent noise source for each neuron and combining them with weights that depend on the distance between neurons, according to a Gaussian function with an SD of σ_{noise}. To avoid the triggering of staircase saccades due to persistent noise at one location, the noise pattern is reset after each saccade. Unfortunately, no studies to date have conducted simultaneous recordings of SC neuronal populations, and so there is no good source for the estimation of the parameters of this noise component. We have used a set of values that produces realistic microsaccade distributions.

Cerebellum

We implemented a very simplified model of the cerebellum that tries to emulate the activity of the fastigial oculomotor region (FOR) related to saccades. FOR is a major cerebellar output nucleus that projects to the brain stem and is involved in saccade generation. Firing of the FOR around saccades is characterized by an early burst in the contralateral side and a late burst in the ipsilateral side (39). Inactivation of the FOR causes changes in saccadic magnitude, with saccades becoming larger or smaller than normal depending on the inactivated side (40). It has been hypothesized that the main role of the FOR could be to track the movement of the eye and send a precise command to stop the saccade on target. This command would correspond to the late burst in the ipsilateral side (41).

To achieve this behavior, our implementation of the cerebellum receives one input from the SC carrying the location of the center of activity in the activity map, and a second input from the reticular formation carrying an efference copy of the MLEBNs activity, which corresponds closely to the eye's instantaneous velocity during saccades. Though the cerebellum must integrate this efference copy, it is beyond the scope of this study to discuss the specific integration mechanism. Here, we use a second-order system as this integrator with time constants (T_{cblm1}, T_{cblm2}), but many other possible implementations would result in similar behavior. The late burst starts when the integrated efference copy (e) surpasses the input from the SC (c). The early burst corresponds to the activity coming from the SC until the efference copy reaches that point. Different gains in the four different channels [left/right SC ($c_{r/l}$) and left/right efference copy ($e_{r/l}$)] can achieve different relative timings of the early and late burst. These gains have been tuned to achieve good saccade accuracy over a range of saccade sizes

$$\text{Late burst}_{l/r} = \max((F_1 e_{r/l} - F_2 c_{l/r}), 0) \quad (7)$$

$$\text{Early burst}_{l/r} = \max((F_3 c_{r/l} - F_4 e_{l/r}), 0) \quad (8)$$

The late burst acts on the contralateral brain stem to inhibit the ipsilateral BNs. This signal has been defined as a "choke" signal, because it inhibits the BNs regardless of what input they may still receive from the SC.

The cerebellum also projects heavily to the rostral SC (42). For this reason, we have also incorporated a signal that drives the rostral SC to inhibit the caudal SC at the end of the saccade, to terminate the saccade-related burst and restart the rostral SC activity. The magnitude of this projection corresponds to the sum of the two late bursts from each side.

RESULTS

Saccades

First, we show the results of simulating a 2° saccade toward the right. **Figure 5** shows the corresponding activity in the relevant neurons and areas. The saccade starts when the LLIBN activity is enough to completely inhibit the OPN, which in turn disinhibits the EBN.

The top panels show the eye position and the eye velocity around the saccade. The other panels show the activity of the different elements of the model. The activity of the FEF and BG corresponds to the change in target position, and the activity of the SC dynamically changes toward that location. The drive to the BNs increases while the drive to the OPNs remains relatively constant. At some point, the LLIBNs inhibit the OPNs, letting the MLEBNs and MLIBNs fire and drive the saccade.

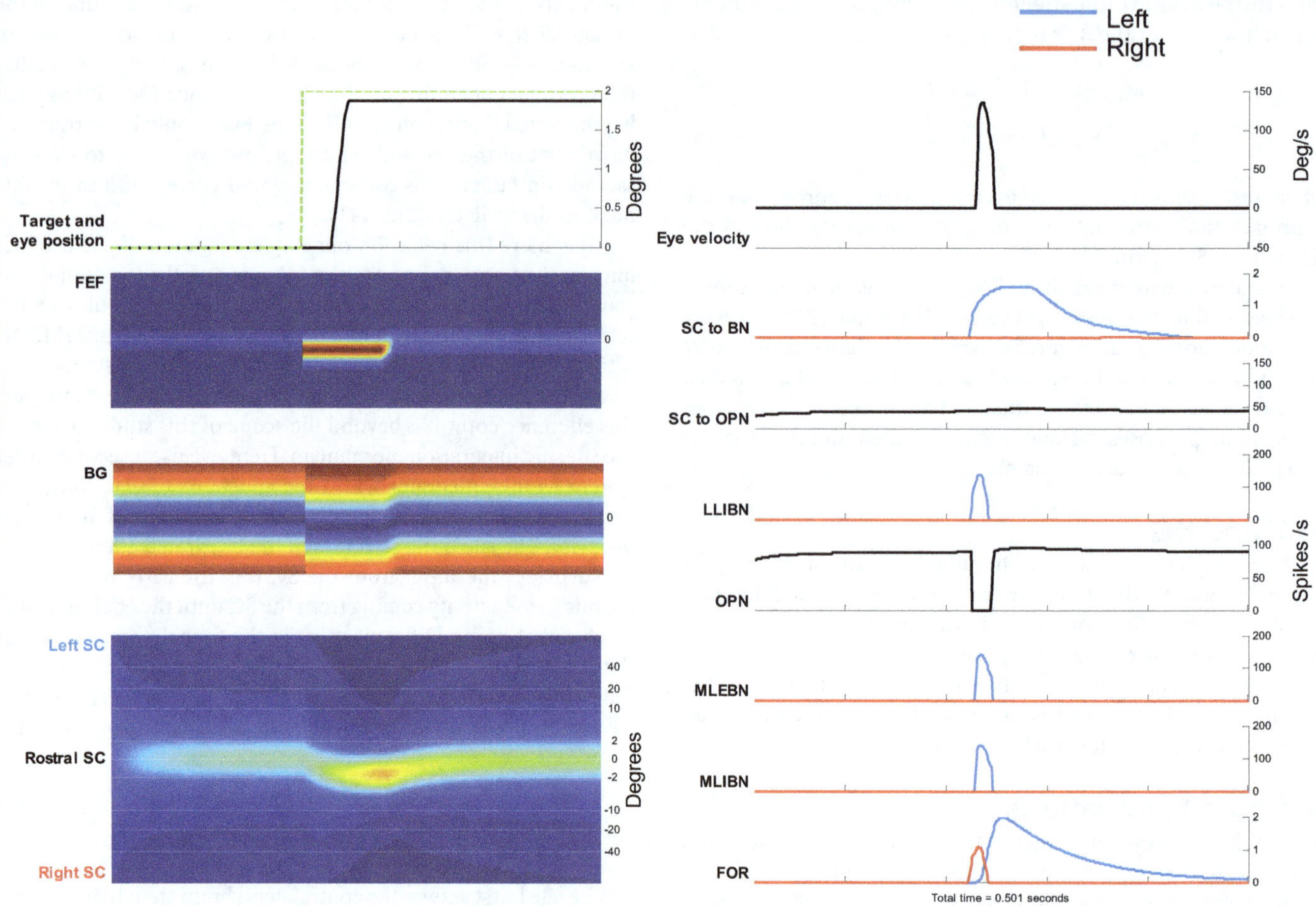

FIGURE 5 | Simulation of a 2° saccade toward the right. Left side, from top to bottom: target movement and simulated eye position. Frontal eye field (FEF) activity. Basal ganglia (BG) activity. Superior colliculus (SC) activity. Color plots show evolution of activity over time in each map. Top, neurons encoding leftward movements. Bottom, neurons encoding rightward movements. Right side, from top to bottom: eye velocity. Total projection from SC to burst neurons (BNs) (left BNs in blue and right BNs in red). Total projection from SC to omnipause neuron (OPN). Firing rate of long lead IBN (LLIBN), OPN, medium lead excitatory BN (MLEBN), medium lead IBN (MLIBN), and fastigial oculomotor region (FOR) (cerebellum).

The activity in the ipsilateral FOR inhibits the BNs, terminating the saccade.

Simulating Microsaccades During Fixation

To simulate microsaccades produced during attempted fixation, we used a constant target position and added a noise input to the SC. **Figure 6** shows the activity in the elements of the model and the resulting eye movement trace for a 5-s simulation. Every time a microsaccade is triggered, the OPN stops firing, in agreement with previous neurophysiological findings (28, 43). **Figure 6**'s panels show the activity of the different elements of the model, as in **Figure 5**. This figure also shows the noise introduced to the SC. **Figure 7** shows the distributions of various properties of microsaccades collected during a simulation of 100 s of fixation. These distributions are comparable to those obtained from actual fixation conditions (2, 44). We note that, in actual experimental scenarios, fixation periods tend to be much shorter to avoid the subject's fatigue, which is not a factor in the simulations.

SC Inactivation

Hafed and colleagues (22) found that inactivating the rostral pole of one colliculus reduces the microsaccade rate. Later, Goffart and colleagues (45) also reported a shift in fixation position following rostral SC inactivation. Here, we asked if our model could simulate those results, by comparing the output of a control setup versus an inactivation setup (**Figure 8**). We simulated the unilateral inactivation of the rostral SC by nulling the output of the neurons on one side close to the midline (**Figure 8**). This produced both a decrease in the microsaccadic rate and a shift in the eye position, consistent with the previous empirical results (22, 45). One difference between the present results and previous findings is that our simulations produced an asymmetrical distribution of microsaccade magnitudes, whereas the empirical microsaccade magnitude distributions were reported to be symmetrical. Such difference could be due to some of the simplifications that we have taken in modeling both SC as a single continuous one-dimensional structure.

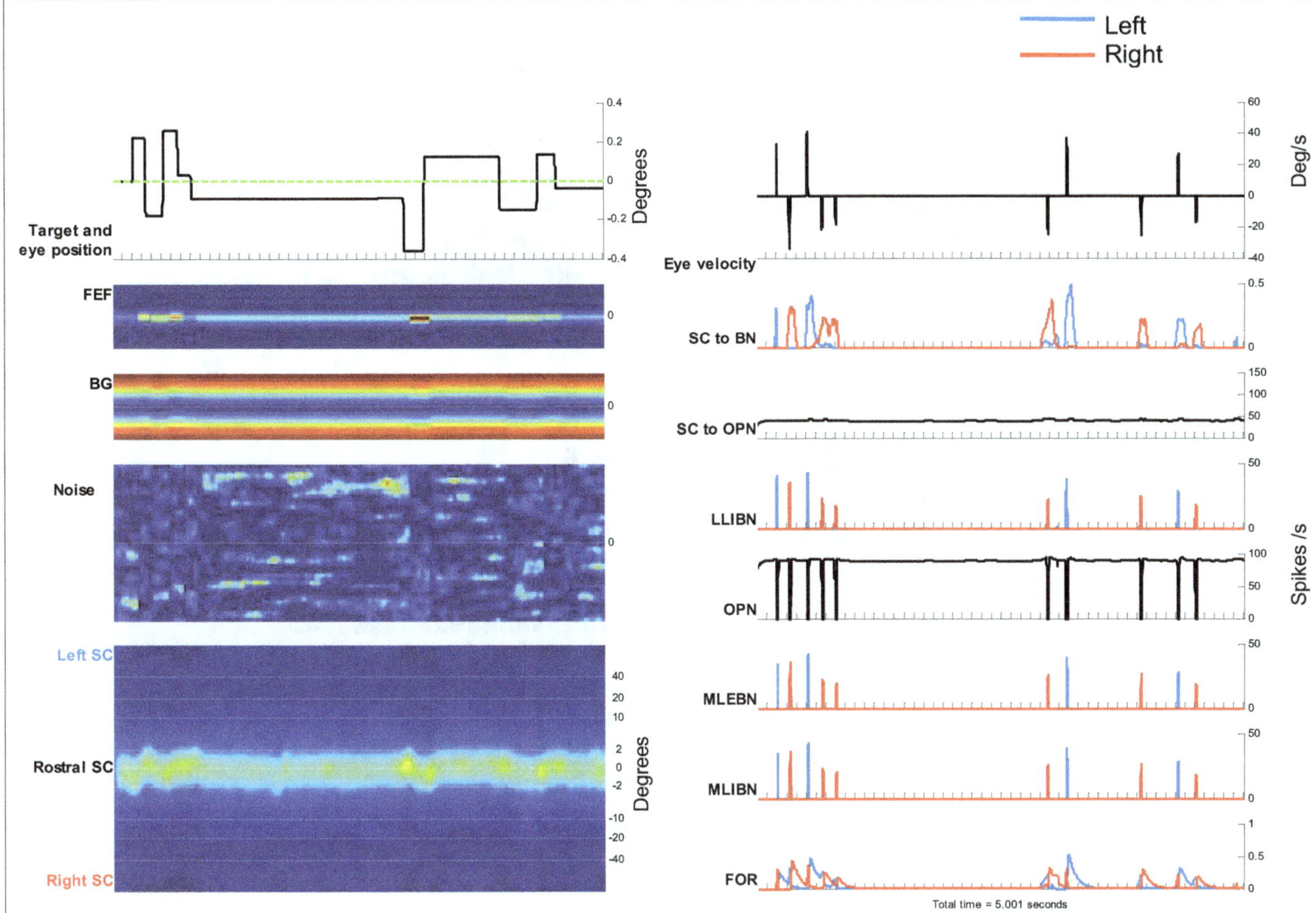

FIGURE 6 | Simulation of microsaccades during 5 s of attempted fixation. Left side, from top to bottom: target movement and simulated eye position. Frontal eye field (FEF) activity. Basal ganglia (BG) activity. Superior colliculus (SC) activity. The color plots show the evolution of activity in each map over time, with neurons encoding leftward movements on the top, and neurons encoding rightward movements on the bottom. Right side, from top to bottom: eye velocity. Total projection from SC to burst neurons (BNs) (left BNs in blue and right BNs in red). Total projection from SC to omnipause neuron (OPN). Firing rate of long lead IBN (LLIBN), OPN, medium lead excitatory BN (MLEBN), medium lead IBN (MLIBN), and fastigial oculomotor region (FOR).

Saccadic Intrusions

Saccadic intrusions are saccades that intrude accurate fixation and are prevalent in various neurodegenerative disorders. Here, we simulated the effects of damage to different areas of the oculomotor system to observe the characteristics of the corresponding saccadic intrusions.

Figure 9 shows the results of these simulations. First, we simulated the effects of BG impairment by increasing the level of noise in the SC. This resulted in more frequent microsaccades and SWJs, as observed in PD patients (12).

Next, we simulated the increased magnitude and frequency of microsaccades and SWJs in PSP (38), by raising the level of noise and lowering the gain of BNs (parameter B_m in Eq. 1). The decreased gain from BNs is consistent with slower saccades in PSP and may be a consequence of the lack of vertical BNs in PSP. Because BNs (LLIBNs) become less effective on inhibiting OPNs, they require a larger input from SC, which results in increased microsaccade magnitude together with the slower velocity.

Finally, we simulated the effect of cerebellar deficit by decreasing the gain of the stop signal coming from the cerebellum. This produced microsaccades that overshot the target, causing macrosaccadic oscillations typical of some types of spinocerebellar ataxia.

Figures 9E–H show how the simulation replicates the pattern seen in actual patient groups. Here, we model PD by just increasing noise which produces higher saccadic rate, slightly larger saccadic amplitudes, and normal saccadic velocities. We model PSP with both an increase in noise and a decrease on BN gain which produce higher saccadic rates, larger saccadic amplitudes, and lower saccadic velocities.

DISCUSSION

We have implemented a model based on known anatomy and physiology that successfully simulates the generation of saccades of any size, including the small microsaccades that occur during attempted fixation, and the saccadic intrusions that appear in patients with parkinsonian disorders. The model suggests that

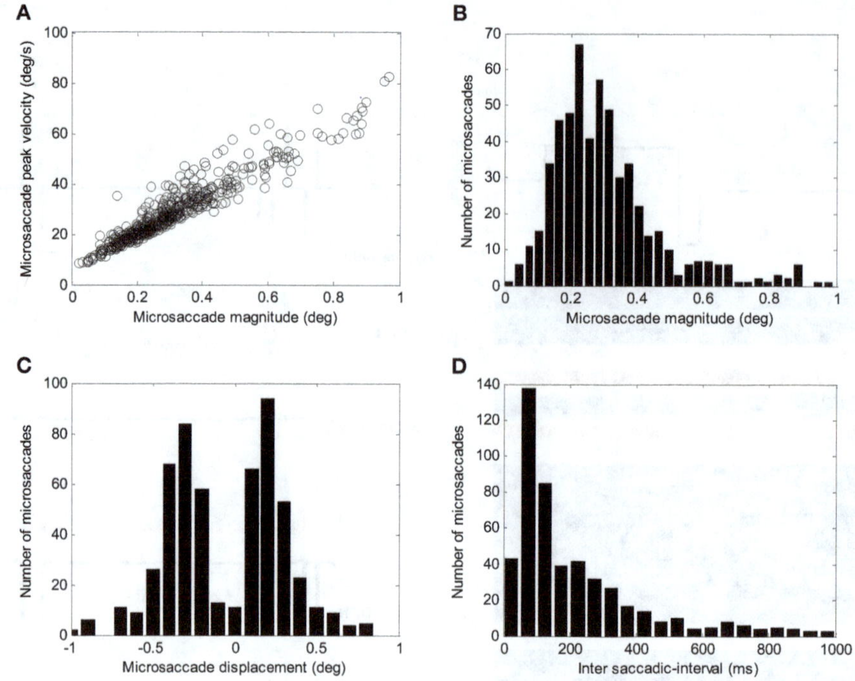

FIGURE 7 | Simulated microsaccade distributions. **(A)** Peak velocity/magnitude relationship. **(B)** Distribution of microsaccade magnitudes. **(C)** Distributions of microsaccade displacements (negative corresponds to amplitude toward the left and positive to amplitude toward the right). **(D)** Distribution of intersaccadic intervals.

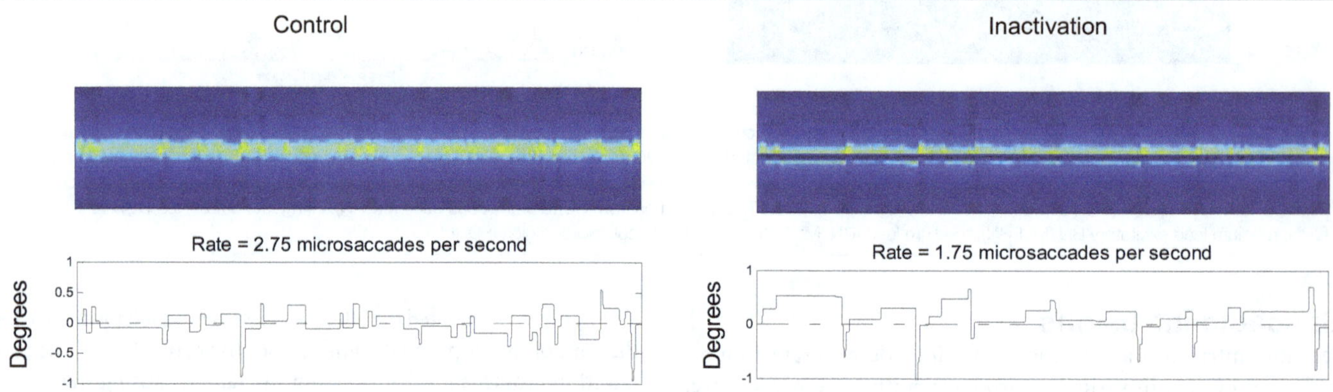

FIGURE 8 | Effects of superior colliculus (SC) inactivation. Left: 20 s of a control simulation. Right: 20 s of a simulation where the output of a set of rostral SC neurons was inactivated. The two top panels indicate the SC activity, and the two bottom panels the corresponding eye positions.

noisy activity in the SC map controls the state of a mutually inhibitory network in the brain stem formed by BNs and OPNs. When the activity is centered at the rostral pole, the system stays in a state of fixation. When activity is perturbed away from this center, a saccade is triggered. This perturbation can be produced either by the intent to move one's gaze or by random fluctuations in activity.

On the Relationship Between OPNs and SC Rostral Pole

The connectivity between the SC rostral pole and the OPNs has been proven anatomically and physiologically (23, 24). However, it is not clear whether the rostral pole controls the firing of the OPNs (46–48) or merely modulates their behavior. A main argument against the rostral pole controlling OPNs is that, during the gap paradigm, fixation neurons in the rostral pole decrease their activity, though OPN activity remains stable (46–48).

In our model, the rostral pole modulates OPN activity without the need for a one-to-one relationship between the activities of individual SC neurons and OPNs. Because the OPNs receive a projection from a large area of the colliculus (24), it could be that, even if individual neurons of the rostral pole decrease their firing, other neurons that also project to the OPNs increase their firing simultaneously. For instance,

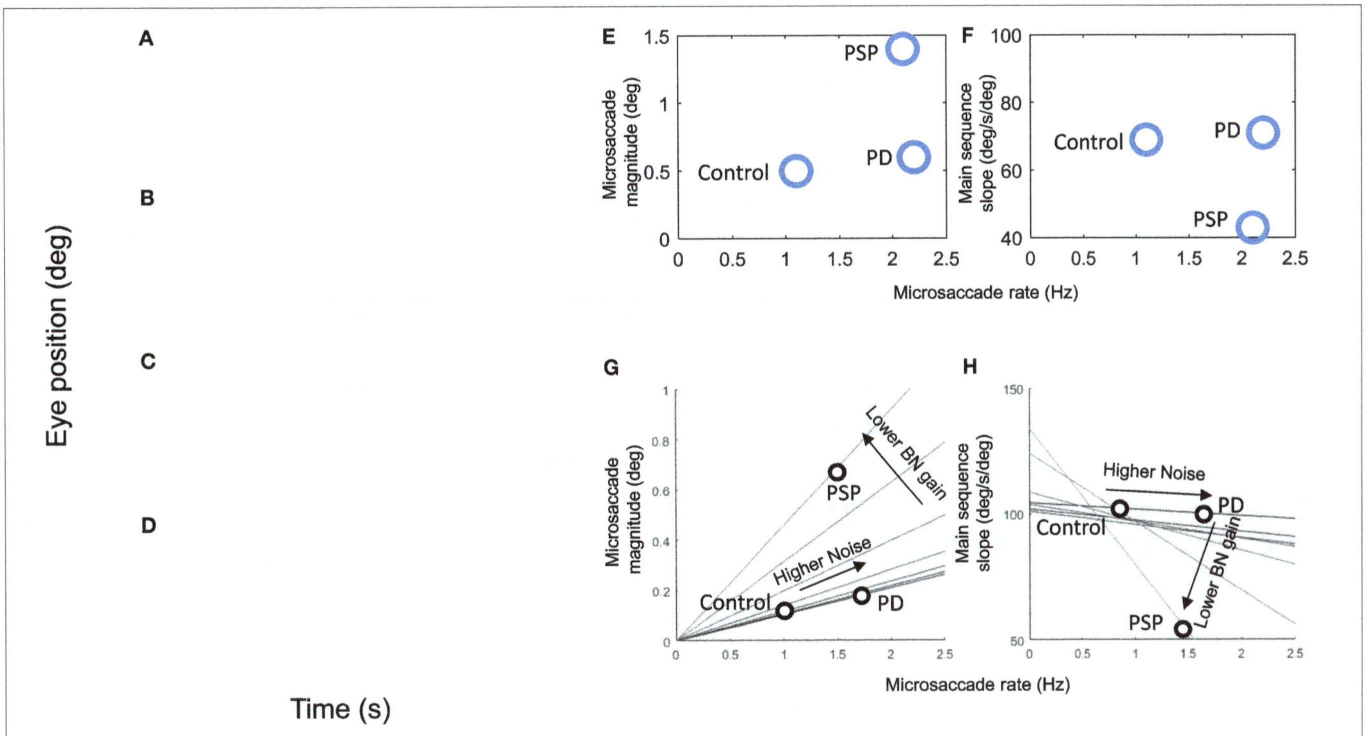

FIGURE 9 | Simulation of 5 s of fixation in **(A)** healthy observers (i.e., using normal parameters), **(B)** Parkinson's disease (PD), **(C)** progressive supranuclear palsy (PSP), and **(D)** spinocerebellar ataxia. Panels **(E,F)** show the microsaccade magnitude, rate, and velocity (main sequence slope) of three populations of healthy controls, PSP patients, and PD patients from a previous study (12). Panels **(G,H)** show the relationship between microsaccade magnitude, rate, and velocity as we vary two parameters of the simulations. Each line represents a set of simulations with the same burst neuron (BN) gain but varying amounts of noise. As noise increases, the rate (and to some extent the amplitude) of microsaccades increases. Peak velocity is not affected by the noise as long as the BN gain is normal. As we lower the BN gain, the velocity of microsaccades decreases while their amplitude increases. The microsaccade rate also decreases, but in the case of the PSP that is compensated by higher noise.

one could imagine a situation in which, during the gap period, activity in the rostral pole is lower but wider, keeping a constant drive to the OPNs.

On the Relationship Between BNs and SC Rostral Pole

Computationally, this projection has been hypothesized to perform a center of activity calculation from the spatial map in the SC to the firing rate of BNs (decomposed into vertical and horizontal components) (49).

For small saccades and microsaccades (less than 1°), the "hill" of activity in the SC may cross over toward the other side. Thus, if the center of activity is calculated only with inputs from neurons from one side, the magnitude of the desired saccade may be overestimated. Moreover, if the activity is perfectly centered at zero, BNs on both sides will receive a non-zero center of activity input. To ensure a zero input to all BNs when activity is centered at zero, there needs to be an inhibitory input to the BNs, to account for neurons encoding small saccades in the opposite direction. Those inputs could come indirectly from the opposite rostral pole as well as from the same one, since there have been reports of neurons within one rostral pole encoding saccades in both directions (6). This issue is irrelevant for larger saccades, where the "hill" of activity is contained within a single side of the colliculus.

On the Relationship Between BNs and SC Caudal Areas

Here, we set out to answer one fundamental question. Why are microsaccades not triggered by the buildup of activity in the SC caudal areas that precedes a saccade? That buildup must shift the center of activity and thus shift the OPN–BN balance. To solve this problem, we assumed that the projection from SC to BNs is nonlinear, with neurons having a larger effect when they are firing at higher rates. We simulated this by adding a second layer (BN layer) that only fires when the buildup layer reaches a certain threshold (same threshold throughout the map). That way, the brainstem BNs only receive a strong drive when some SC BNs start to fire, so increases in buildup before saccades or due to random fluctuations will not trigger a saccade. Neurons in the SC have been classified in the past as buildup or burst, but this distinction has never been reported in the rostral area. The idea of an SC burst layer is one possible solutions, but there could be other mechanisms for this type of nonlinearity, such as the enhanced synchrony of neurons firing together having a more effective drive on brain stem BNs, which could produce a similar effect. One alternative approach could be to make the connection from rostral SC to OPNs much stronger, so that a saccade is triggered only when the rostral neurons stop firing. However, microsaccades would not be triggered in such case.

What Happens First?

The nature of the neural event that initiates a saccade has been debated: do saccades start because the OPNs cease to fire, or because the BNs start to fire? Here, we have chosen to consider the system as a whole, since both structures are reciprocally connected (17) and behave as a unit. Thus, we talk about changes in the state of the system, as in going from the fixation state (OPNs fire and BNs silent) to the saccade state (OPNs silent and BNs fire). The positive feedback loop that reciprocally connects both sets of neurons ensures that when activity changes in one neuronal group it also does in the other group.

Thus, the main role of OPNs in this model is to ensure sharp changes between the two states. Without the OPNs, the circuit loses its properties of hysteresis (**Figure 1**) and any change in SC activity would be reflected directly in the BNs.

Do Other Signals Bypass the SC to Control Saccade Triggering in the Reticular Formation?

Here, we have given the role of triggering saccades exclusively to the SC and the reticular formation. In our model, all cortical influences on saccade triggering act by affecting SC activity. However, it may be the case that some cortical signals bypass the SC and affect the reticular formation directly. For instance, Valsecchi and Turatto showed that a stimulus that should be invisible to the SC affects microsaccade triggering (50). The supplementary eye fields (SEF) are a potential source for this bypassing signal: the SEF are related to the generation of antisaccades and memory-guided saccades (51), and SEF neurons project directly to the OPN area (52).

AUTHOR CONTRIBUTIONS

JO-M and LO designed the model and implemented the simulations. JO-M, LO, SM, and SM-C wrote the manuscript.

FUNDING

This work was funded by Empire Innovator Awards from the State of New York to SM-C and SM, by a National Science Foundation Award (#1523614) to SM, and by Awards from The Leon Levy Foundation, National Institutes of Health (NIH) (K99EY027846), and the Fight for Sight foundation to JO-M.

REFERENCES

1. Leigh RJ, Zee DS. *The Neurology of Eye Movements*. New York, NY: Oxford University Press (2015).
2. Otero-Millan J, Troncoso XG, Macknik SL, Serrano-Pedraza I, Martinez-Conde S. Saccades and microsaccades during visual fixation, exploration and search: foundations for a common saccadic generator. *J Vis* (2008) 8:14–21. doi:10.1167/8.14.21
3. Wurtz RH. Neuronal mechanisms of visual stability. *Vision Res* (2008) 48:2070–89. doi:10.1016/j.visres.2008.03.021
4. Martinez-Conde S, Macknik SL, Hubel DH. The role of fixational eye movements in visual perception. *Nat Rev Neurosci* (2004) 5:229–40. doi:10.1038/nrn1348
5. Otero-Millan J, Macknik SL, Serra A, Leigh RJ, Martinez-Conde S. Triggering mechanisms in microsaccade and saccade generation: a novel proposal. *Ann N Y Acad Sci* (2011) 1233:107–16. doi:10.1111/j.1749-6632.2011.06177.x
6. Hafed ZM, Krauzlis RJ. Similarity of superior colliculus involvement in microsaccade and saccade generation. *J Neurophysiol* (2012) 107(7):1904–16. doi:10.1152/jn.01125.2011
7. Martinez-Conde S, Macknik SL. Unchanging visions: the effects and limitations of ocular stillness. *Philos Trans R Soc Lond B Biol Sci* (2017) 372(1718): doi:10.1098/rstb.2016.0204
8. Trappenberg TP, Dorris MC, Munoz DP, Klein RM. A model of saccade initiation based on the competitive integration of exogenous and endogenous signals in the superior colliculus. *J Cogn Neurosci* (2001) 13:256–71. doi:10.1162/089892901564306
9. Das S, Keller EL, Arai K. A distributed model of the saccadic system: the effects of internal noise. *Neurocomputing* (1996) 11:245–69. doi:10.1016/0925-2312(95)00068-2
10. Eggert T, Robinson FR, Straube A. Modeling inter-trial variability of saccade trajectories: effects of lesions of the oculomotor part of the fastigial nucleus. *PLoS Comput Biol* (2016) 12:e1004866. doi:10.1371/journal.pcbi.1004866
11. Varsha V, Padhi R, Murthy A. A stochastic feedback model to simulate saccadic eye movement variability. *IFAC-PapersOnLine* (2017) 50(1):13521–5. doi:10.1016/j.ifacol.2017.08.2344
12. Otero-Millan J, Schneider R, Leigh RJ, Macknik SL, Martinez-Conde S. Saccades during attempted fixation in parkinsonian disorders and recessive ataxia: from microsaccades to square-wave jerks. *PLoS One* (2013) 8(3):e58535. doi:10.1371/journal.pone.0058535
13. Ramat S, Leigh RJ, Zee DS, Optican LM. What clinical disorders tell us about the neural control of saccadic eye movements. *Brain* (2007) 130:10–35. doi:10.1093/brain/awl309
14. Siegenthaler E, Costela FM, McCamy MB, Di Stasi LL, Otero-Millan J, Sonderegger A, et al. Task difficulty in mental arithmetic affects microsaccadic rates and magnitudes. *Eur J Neurosci* (2014) 39:287–94. doi:10.1111/ejn.12395
15. Schmitt OH. A thermionic trigger. *J Sci Instrum* (1938) 15:24. doi:10.1088/0950-7671/15/1/305
16. Evinger C, Kaneko CR, Fuchs AF. Activity of omnipause neurons in alert cats during saccadic eye movements and visual stimuli. *J Neurophysiol* (1982) 47:827–44. doi:10.1152/jn.1982.47.5.827
17. Shinoda Y, Sugiuchi Y, Takahashi M, Izawa Y. Neural substrate for suppression of omnipause neurons at the onset of saccades. *Ann N Y Acad Sci* (2011) 1233:100–6. doi:10.1111/j.1749-6632.2011.06171.x
18. Robinson DA. Eye movements evoked by collicular stimulation in the alert monkey. *Vision Res* (1972) 12:1795–808. doi:10.1016/0042-6989(72)90070-3
19. Munoz DP, Wurtz RH. Fixation cells in monkey superior colliculus. I. Characteristics of cell discharge. *J Neurophysiol* (1993) 70:559–75. doi:10.1152/jn.1993.70.2.576
20. Munoz DP, Wurtz RH. Saccade-related activity in monkey superior colliculus. I. Characteristics of burst and buildup cells. *J Neurophysiol* (1995) 73:2313–33. doi:10.1152/jn.1995.73.6.2334
21. Krauzlis RJ, Basso MA, Wurtz RH. Shared motor error for multiple eye movements. *Science* (1997) 276:1693–5. doi:10.1126/science.276.5319.1693
22. Hafed ZM, Goffart L, Krauzlis RJ. A neural mechanism for microsaccade generation in the primate superior colliculus. *Science* (2009) 323:940–3. doi:10.1126/science.1166112
23. Gandhi NJ, Keller EL. Spatial distribution and discharge characteristics of superior colliculus neurons antidromically activated from the omnipause region in monkey. *J Neurophysiol* (1997) 78:2221–5. doi:10.1152/jn.1997.78.4.2221
24. Büttner-Ennever JA, Horn AKE, Henn V, Cohen B. Projections from the superior colliculus motor map to omnipause neurons in monkey. *J Comp Neurol* (1999) 413:55–67. doi:10.1002/(SICI)1096-9861(19991011)413:1<55::AID-CNE3>3.0.CO;2-K
25. Raybourn MS, Keller EL. Colliculoreticular organization in primate oculomotor system. *J Neurophysiol* (1977) 40:861–78. doi:10.1152/jn.1977.40.4.861
26. Cullen KE, Guitton D. Analysis of primate IBN spike trains using system identification techniques. I. Relationship to eye movement dynamics during

head-fixed saccades. *J Neurophysiol* (1997) 78:3259–82. doi:10.1152/jn.1997.78.6.3307
27. Yoshida K, Iwamoto Y, Chimoto S, Shimazu H. Saccade-related inhibitory input to pontine omnipause neurons: an intracellular study in alert cats. *J Neurophysiol* (1999) 82:1198–208. doi:10.1152/jn.1999.82.3.1198
28. Van Horn MR, Cullen KE. Coding of microsaccades in three-dimensional space by premotor saccadic neurons. *J Neurosci* (2012) 32:1974–80. doi:10.1523/JNEUROSCI.5054-11.2012
29. Van Gisbergen JA, Robinson DA. Generation of micro- and macrosaccades by burst neurons in the monkey. In: Baker R, Berthoz A, editors. *Control of Gaze by Brain Stem Neurons*. Amsterdam/North Holland: Elsevier (1977). p. 301–8.
30. Ramat S, Leigh RJ, Zee DS, Shaikh AG, Optican LM. Applying saccade models to account for oscillations. *Using Eye Movements as an Experimental Probe of Brain function – A Symposium in Honor of Jean Büttner-Ennever* (Vol. 171). Elsevier (2008). p. 123–30. Available from: http://www.sciencedirect.com.ezproxy1.lib.asu.edu/science/article/B7CV6-4T7WBSW-P/2/a74d14d62dd9fc2cf9b20cfd5de8aa07 (Accessed: September 21, 2010).
31. Daye PM, Optican LM, Roze E, Gaymard B, Pouget P. Neuromimetic model of saccades for localizing deficits in an atypical eye-movement pathology. *J Transl Med* (2013) 11:125. doi:10.1186/1479-5876-11-125
32. Gancarz G, Grossberg S. A neural model of the saccade generator in the reticular formation. *Neural Netw* (1998) 11:1159–74. doi:10.1016/S0893-6080(98)00096-3
33. Scudder CA. A new local feedback model of the saccadic burst generator. *J Neurophysiol* (1988) 59:1455–75. doi:10.1152/jn.1988.59.5.1455
34. Zee DS, Robinson DA. A hypothetical explanation of saccadic oscillations. *Ann Neurol* (1979) 5:405–14. doi:10.1002/ana.410050502
35. Marino RA, Trappenberg TP, Dorris M, Munoz DP. Spatial interactions in the superior colliculus predict saccade behavior in a neural field model. *J Cogn Neurosci* (2011) 24:315–36. doi:10.1162/jocn_a_00139
36. Van Opstal AJ, Gisbergen JAM. A nonlinear model for collicular spatial interactions underlying the metrical properties of electrically elicited saccades. *Biol Cybern* (1989) 60:171–83. doi:10.1007/BF00207285
37. Cornsweet TN. Determination of the stimuli for involuntary drifts and saccadic eye movements. *J Opt Soc Am* (1956) 46:987–8. doi:10.1364/JOSA.46.000987
38. Otero-Millan J, Serra A, Leigh RJ, Troncoso XG, Macknik SL, Martinez-Conde S. Distinctive features of saccadic intrusions and microsaccades in progressive supranuclear palsy. *J Neurosci* (2011) 31:4379–87. doi:10.1523/JNEUROSCI.2600-10.2011
39. Ohtsuka K, Noda H. Saccadic burst neurons in the oculomotor region of the fastigial nucleus of macaque monkeys. *J Neurophysiol* (1991) 65:1422–34. doi:10.1152/jn.1991.65.6.1422
40. Goffart L, Chen LL, Sparks DL. Deficits in saccades and fixation during muscimol inactivation of the caudal fastigial nucleus in the rhesus monkey. *J Neurophysiol* (2004) 92:3351–67. doi:10.1152/jn.01199.2003
41. Lefèvre P, Quaia C, Optican LM. Distributed model of control of saccades by superior colliculus and cerebellum. *Neural Netw* (1998) 11:1175–90. doi:10.1016/S0893-6080(98)00071-9
42. Quaia C, Lefèvre P, Optican LM. Model of the control of saccades by superior colliculus and cerebellum. *J Neurophysiol* (1999) 82:999–1018. doi:10.1152/jn.1999.82.2.999
43. Brien DC, Corneil BD, Fecteau JH, Bell AH, Munoz DP. The behavioural and neurophysiological modulation of microsaccades in monkeys. *J Eye Mov Res* (2009) 3:1–12. doi:10.16910/jemr.3.2.4
44. Engbert R. Microsaccades: a microcosm for research on oculomotor control, attention, and visual perception. *Prog Brain Res* (2006) 154:177–92. doi:10.1016/S0079-6123(06)54009-9
45. Goffart L, Hafed ZM, Krauzlis RJ. Visual fixation as equilibrium: evidence from superior colliculus inactivation. *J Neurosci* (2012) 32:10627–36. doi:10.1523/JNEUROSCI.0696-12.2012
46. Everling S, Pare M, Dorris MC, Munoz DP. Comparison of the discharge characteristics of brain stem omnipause neurons and superior colliculus fixation neurons in monkey: implications for control of fixation and saccade behavior. *J Neurophysiol* (1998) 79:511. doi:10.1152/jn.1998.79.2.511
47. Bergeron A, Guitton D. In multiple-step gaze shifts: omnipause (OPNs) and collicular fixation neurons encode gaze position error; OPNs gate saccades. *J Neurophysiol* (2002) 88:1726–42. doi:10.1152/jn.2002.88.4.1726
48. Gandhi NJ, Katnani HA. Motor functions of the superior colliculus. *Annu Rev Neurosci* (2011) 34:205–31. doi:10.1146/annurev-neuro-061010-113728
49. Van Gisbergen JAM, Van Opstal AJ, Tax AAM. Collicular ensemble coding of saccades based on vector summation. *Neuroscience* (1987) 21:541–55. doi:10.1016/0306-4522(87)90140-0
50. Valsecchi M, Turatto M. Microsaccadic response to visual events that are invisible to the superior colliculus. *Behav Neurosci* (2007) 121:786–93. doi:10.1037/0735-7044.121.4.786
51. Schlag-Rey M, Amador N, Sanchez H, Schlag J. Antisaccade performance predicted by neuronal activity in the supplementary eye field. *Nature* (1997) 390:398–400. doi:10.1038/37114
52. Shook BL, Schlag-Rey M, Schlag J. Direct projection from the supplementary eye field to the nucleus raphe interpositus. *Exp Brain Res* (1988) 73:215–8. doi:10.1007/BF00279675

19

Eye Control Deficits Coupled to Hand Control Deficits: Eye–Hand Incoordination in Chronic Cerebral Injury

John-Ross Rizzo[1,2], James K. Fung[1], Maryam Hosseini[1], Azadeh Shafieesabet[1], Edmond Ahdoot[1], Rosa M. Pasculli[1], Janet C. Rucker[2,3], Preeti Raghavan[1], Michael S. Landy[4] and Todd E. Hudson[1,2]*

[1] Department of Rehabilitation Medicine, New York University Langone Medical Center, New York, NY, United States, [2] Department of Neurology, New York University Langone Medical Center, New York, NY, United States, [3] Department of Ophthalmology, New York University Langone Medical Center, New York, NY, United States, [4] Department of Psychology & Center for Neural Science, New York University, New York, NY, United States

***Correspondence:**
John-Ross Rizzo
johnross.rizzo@nyumc.org

It is widely accepted that cerebral pathology can impair ocular motor and manual motor control. This is true in indolent and chronic processes, such as neurodegeneration and in acute processes such as stroke or those secondary to neurotrauma. More recently, it has been suggested that disruptions in these control systems are useful markers for prognostication and longitudinal monitoring. The utility of examining the relationship or the coupling between these systems has yet to be determined. We measured eye and hand-movement control in chronic, middle cerebral artery stroke, relative to healthy controls, in saccade-to-reach paradigms to assess eye–hand coordination. Primary saccades were initiated significantly earlier by stroke participants relative to control participants. However, despite these extremely early initial saccades to the target, reaches were nevertheless initiated at approximately the same time as those of control participants. Control participants minimized the time period between primary saccade onset and reach initiation, demonstrating temporal coupling between eye and hand. In about 90% of all trials, control participants produced no secondary, or corrective, saccades, instead maintaining fixation in the terminal position of the primary saccade until the end of the reach. In contrast, participants with stroke increased the time period between primary saccade onset and reach initiation. During this temporal decoupling, multiple saccades were produced in about 50% of the trials with stroke participants making between one and five additional saccades. Reaches made by participants with stroke were both longer in duration and less accurate. In addition to these increases in spatial reach errors, there were significant increases in saccade endpoint errors. Overall, the magnitude of the endpoint errors for reaches and saccades were correlated across participants. These findings suggest that in individuals with otherwise intact visual function, the spatial and temporal relationships between the eye and hand are disrupted poststroke, and may need to be specifically targeted during neurorehabilitation. Eye–hand coupling may be a useful biomarker in individuals with cerebral pathology in the setting of neurovascular, neurotraumatic, and neurodegenerative pathology.

Keywords: brain injuries, eye, hand, eye movements, stroke

INTRODUCTION

It is widely accepted that cerebral pathology can impair ocular motor and manual motor control. This is true in indolent and chronic processes such as neurodegeneration and in acute processes such as stroke or those secondary to neurotrauma (1–5). More recently, it has been suggested that disruptions in these control systems are useful markers for prognostication and longitudinal monitoring (6–8). Therapeutically, neurorehabilitation strives to address these motor control deficits with approaches that restore ability at the movement level in early intervention and at the functional performance level in later intervention; however, in many cases, movement-level gains do not progress into functional performance-level improvements (9). Cerebral injuries, such as stroke, not only lead to motoric impairments but also sensory limitations; these sensorimotor deficits may compromise visual perception secondary to decreased visuomotor function and lead to difficulties with visually guided action in both the more-affected (contralateral) and less-affected (ipsilateral) hands (4, 10–16). During such experiments manual motor control is often studied objectively and typically without simultaneous eye-movement analysis. However, altered ocular motor function is a sensitive biomarker of brain injury (17, 18) in both the cognitive and motor domains (8, 19) and provides clinical insight into neurovascular, neurotraumatic, and neurodegenerative pathology.

Vision provides primary sensory information during visually guided action. Ocular motor programming controls gaze, which in turn supports the planning of hand movements. Fixations target key spatial positions and are contingent on the functional requirements of the task at hand, such as index finger placement for object manipulation or prehension (20, 21). Additionally, vision-based feedback of the hand is critical to error correction for online control, as gaze updates goal localization and spatial understanding (22). In fact, dependencies between eye and hand have been demonstrated and emphasize the concept of shared planning resources (23, 24). In acquired brain injury (ABI), motor deficits in the limb (e.g., hemiparesis) may be compounded by impairments in ocular motor control (25–33). While manual motor deficiencies are normally evident during clinical examination, ocular motor deficiencies may necessitate objective recording for detection and precise characterization (34–43). If eye and hand movements are quantified simultaneously, an improved understanding of the sensorimotor coupling between vision and eye–hand movement is achievable, and would likely be critical in providing a complete picture of the underlying neurological injury.

The complexity of the coordination between the ocular and manual motor systems is highlighted by the large cerebral network coordinating ocular and manual motor control. The neuroanatomy of human eye-movement control depends on a large interconnected system of cortical and subcortical structures, and includes the frontal eye field, the parietal eye field, the dorsolateral prefrontal cortex, the supplementary eye field, the cingulate eye field, and the basal ganglia (30, 44–58). The neuroanatomy of human reach control depends on the primary motor cortex and the premotor and supplementary cortices, relaying neural information corticofugally through the descending corticospinal tracts to orchestrate hand movements (59, 60). The somatosensory cortex, posterior parietal cortex, cerebellum, and basal ganglia further supplement reach control. The posterior parietal cortex translates visual input and information from the somatosensory cortex into motor programs (60, 61). The extensiveness of these connected networks increases the potential sensitivity of these biomarkers to cerebral damage and highlights the utility of objectifying eye–hand coordination in the setting of neurovascular, neurotraumatic, and neurodegenerative pathology.

Eye–hand coordination centers on the ability to visually encode details in the environment and direct goal-oriented hand movements, including pointing, reaching, grasping, tool use, and object manipulation, encompassing performance in many motor activities relevant to functional independence (62, 63). Precise ocular motor control, resulting in high acuity visual perception, facilitates sound manual motor control, making use of movement-relevant visual inputs (64, 65). Multimodal sensory feedback and sensory predictions in feedforward motor control are essential to visuomotor integration during task-specific movements (66). In neurological injuries, whether neurovascular, neurotraumic, or neurodegenerative, these coordinated motor programs are susceptible to a breakdown or a decoupling between effectors, as a byproduct of specific ocular motor deficits, manual motor deficits, or deficits in the temporal and spatial relationships needed for rapid and integrated motor control. In this study, we tested eye and hand-movement control in chronic, middle cerebral artery (MCA) stroke, relative to healthy controls, in both a visually guided and memory-guided saccade-to-reach paradigm to assess eye–hand coordination. To the investigators' knowledge, in the setting of ABI, this is the first investigation of objective ocular motor and somatic motor control using an unrestricted, three-dimensional (3D) eye–hand coordination task (67). We hypothesized that chronic hemispheric stroke participants without clinically diagnosed visual deficits on bedside testing would show abnormalities in saccadic and manual motor control, as compared to healthy controls.

MATERIALS AND METHODS

Participants

Thirty participants participated in the research study. There were 17 participants in the control cohort (aged 26.2 ± 4.6), and 13 participants in the stroke cohort (aged 57.4 ± 14.2). Five stroke participants had right hemispheric MCA strokes and eight had left hemispheric MCA strokes. All participants were tested for hand dominance based on the Edinburgh Handedness Inventory (68), and were right-handed. All control participants were right-handed. Two participants were unable to complete the entire protocol and were excluded from the analyses. The clinical characteristics of the stroke participants are presented in **Table 1**. All participants signed a consent form approved by the Institutional Review Board of New York University's School of Medicine. The informed consent was created and obtained as per the Declaration of Helsinki (69–71).

Inclusion Criteria

Participants with stroke met the following criteria: (1) older than 18 years, (2) brain injury in the MCA distribution at

TABLE 1 | Clinical characteristics of stroke participants.

ID	Age (years)	Sex	H/H[a]	Stroke characteristics[b]	Chronicity (years)	Fugl-Meyer Score[c]
1	78	M	R/L	R middle cerebral artery (MCA) distribution	2.0	66
2	61	F	R/L	R MCA distribution	7.0	66
3	34	M	R/R	L MCA distribution	1.7	66
4	39	F	R/R	L MCA distribution	1.4	45
5	70	M	R/R	L MCA distribution	2.8	58
6	60	F	R/L	R MCA distribution	2.6	30
7	73	M	R/L	R MCA distribution	6.0	58
8	51	F	R/L	R MCA distribution	12.2	30
9	60	M	R/R	L MCA distribution	4.4	63
10	39	M	R/L	R MCA distribution	4.7	47
11	70	M	R/L	R MCA distribution	2.0	66
12	47	F	R/R	L MCA distribution	1.5	61
13	65	F	R/R	L MCA distribution	0.7	66
Average (SD)	57.5 (14.3)				3.8 (3.2)	55.5 (13.3)

[a]*H/H, handedness/hemiparesis: handedness (as assessed by Edinburgh)/hemiparesis laterality.*
[b]*Stroke characteristics, lesion location obtained from medical history with participant and/or family members serving as historian; region and laterality cross-validated for consistency with examination findings.*
[c]*Fugl-Meyer Score, a summation of the Upper Extremity Score (out of 66), which reflects the extent of poststroke motor impairment.*

least 4 months prior to enrollment, (3) ability to complete the Fugl-Meyer Scale to define arm motor impairment (72), (4) a full range of eye movements in horizontal and vertical directions, as assessed by the experimenter, (5) ability to perform pointing tasks as assessed by a clinician, (6) willingness to complete all clinical assessments, and (7) an ability to give informed consent and HIPPA certifications.

Exclusion Criteria

Participants were excluded for: (1) cognitive dysfunction less than 24 on the Folstein Mini–Mental Status Exam (73), (2) significant injury to the eye, weakness in extraocular muscles or presence of visual field cuts, (3) hemi-spatial neglect, (4) major disability, as determined by a score greater than 4 on the modified Rankin scale (74), (5) previous neurological illness, confounding medical conditions or significant injury to the upper extremity, (6) significant depression determined by a score less than 11 on the Geriatric Depression scale (75), (7) pregnancy, and (8) electrical implant devices, e.g., pacemakers or defibrillators.

A focused stroke history and neurological and musculoskeletal examinations were performed on all participants. Visual impairments were assessed by the Beery-Buktenica Developmental Test of Visual-Motor Integration (Beery VMI) (76–78), by standard clinical tests for visual acuity (Snellen chart) (79) and visual fields (confrontation and if in question, Goldman or Humphrey visual field testing) (80). Participants were also assessed for hemi-spatial neglect *via* the Schenkenberg's line bisection test (81) and the single-letter cancelation test (82). Lastly, the 25-item National Eye Institute Visual Functioning Questionnaire and a 10-item supplement survey were completed to quantify the extent of disability due to perceived visual deficits (83).

Apparatus

Monitor and Physical Configuration of the Rig

Participants sat at a table with a computer display (19.5″ Dell D2015H LED monitor, resolution 1,920 × 1,080) 60 cm away. A 43.5 cm × 23.5 cm rectangle, identical in size to the computer monitor, was outlined on the table surface between the participant and the display. Participants sat centered to the horizontal length of the screen in a height-adjustable chair. Participants were seated approximately 60 cm from the screen and 40 cm from the table-mounted eye tracker. This physical configuration of the table surface and monitor allowed participants to simultaneously view the screen and make point-to-point reaches on the tabletop (**Figure 1A**).

Computer and Software Program

An ASUS ROG G750JM 17-Inch Gaming Laptop (AsusTek Computer Inc., Taipei, Taiwan) was utilized for this experiment. Custom Matlab (MathWorks, Inc., Natick, MA, USA) scripts, making use of additional functions from the Psychophysics Toolbox (84), were used to display visual stimuli and perform real-time integration of data acquired from the Tobii eyetracker and Polhemus limb tracker.

Eye and Limb Trackers

The Tobii X120 eyetracker (Tobii, Danderyd, Sweden) was used to record gaze position (120 Hz, 0.5° accuracy). Kinematics of the finger were measured using a Polhemus Liberty™ 240/16 (Polhemus, Colchester, VT, USA), and Polhemus MicroSensor 1.8 (240 Hz, 0.08 cm accuracy). The motion sensor was affixed to the distal aspect of the index finger of the hand on the to-be-tested arm (the dominant arm for controls, and both arms in participants with stroke). The Polhemus sensor was affixed to the finger by first placing it on the finger and securing it at three locations (proximal and distal phalanx and wrist), using soft flexible neoprene mini-sleeves that were affixed with Velcro and custom fit to each participant.

Procedure

Calibration

The Polhemus output was calibrated to the space occupied by the virtual screen represented on the tabletop using a 9-point calibration. The fingertip location was found relative to the sensor by

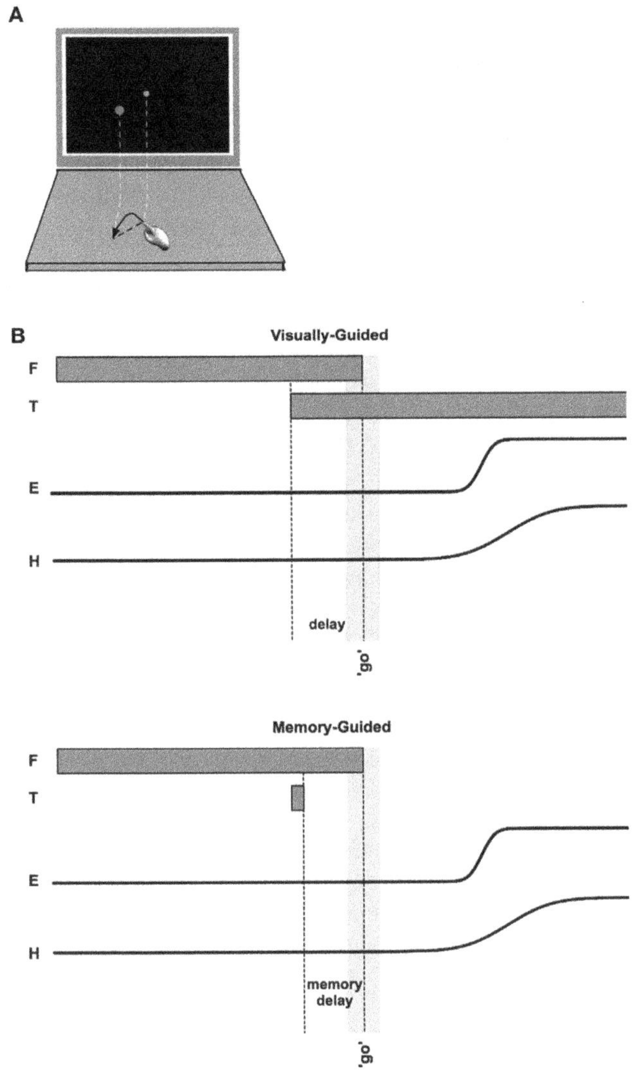

FIGURE 1 | (A) Schematic of monitor and tabletop during a reach. **(B)** Sequencing of events within visually guided (upper) and memory-guided (lower) trials. Fixation (F) appears first. After an unpredictable length of time, the target (T) appears. The "go" signal (simultaneous offset of F and an auditory beep) occurs after a variable time interval following target onset (indicated by the light gray vertical bar). Eye (E) and hand (H) movements follow the go signal.

asking participants to place their fingertip at a known tabletop location (relative to the calibrated "virtual screen" coordinate system).

An authentication procedure verified that the distance from the screen to the participants' eyes was 60 cm, and an 11-point spatial calibration of the eyetracker was completed (1 center point and 10 equidistant points around a 7.62-cm virtual circle were fixated in random order). The eyetracker calibration was performed twice per session, at the start of the experiment and at its halfway-point.

Experiment

After completion of the inclusion/exclusion questionnaires and consent forms, participants were instructed to: "touch a series of tabletop locations as displayed on the computer screen, performing combined look-and-point movements as accurately as possible within the allotted time." Participants were also instructed to make a "true" pointing movement from the start position to the target (lifting the hand and finger in the process), rather than dragging the fingertip across the surface (as if drawing). Participants initiated the task only after the experimenter confirmed that they understood the task and the 1:1 relationship between the computer screen and tabletop.

Participants performed either center-in or center-out reaches on the tabletop as instructed by the visual display. Start points and targets were chosen from a set of six locations: one at the screen center, and the remaining five located on a circle of diameter 7.6 cm. Starting points (gray) and targets (blue) were displayed as circles of 1 cm radius. The position of the finger was represented on screen as a red dot of 4 mm radius. Finger position was displayed in real-time starting 500 ms after the last reach ended, until the following target was displayed.

At the beginning of each trial, participants moved their finger onto the start position, covering the start circle on the screen with the finger-indicator dot. Maintaining finger position, participants were required to fixate the start position on the screen. If at any time the finger or eye left the start position before the go signal, the screen flashed red (50 ms) and the trial restarted. Once the fingertip indicator and fixation were maintained at the start position for 150 ms, a target appeared. There were two conditions (**Figure 1**). In the memory-guided condition, the target was flashed for 100 ms. In the visually guided condition, the target was displayed prior to the go signal and remained illuminated until the end of the trial (i.e., a delayed-saccade task) (85) (note that the pattern of results reported below was the same in these two conditions, and were combined). These two saccade-to-reach paradigms were utilized in this experimental setting to increase exploration of the neuroanatomical saccade network during objective testing.

For both paradigms, participants were required to continue fixating the start position (not the blue target) until a "go" beep sounded and the start position disappeared, and then to move both their eyes and fingertip quickly and accurately to the designated target. To prevent anticipation of the go signal, the duration of the delay between presentation of the target and the go signal was unpredictable, ranging from 250 to 750 ms. The end location of the reach was determined by a combined low-velocity (<5% peak) and 3 mm *z*-plane threshold and was displayed as a white dot.

Prior to starting data acquisition, a series of familiarization trials was performed. The familiarization period ended when participants successfully touched 5 of the 10 most recent targets. This performance criterion was meant to insure that all participants understood the procedure and were able to complete the required reaches and eye movements. Following familiarization there were two halves to the experiment (76 look-and-points in each). In one half, reaches all began at the central position and targets were chosen randomly from the five peripheral locations. In the other half, start positions were chosen randomly from the five peripheral locations and the target was always the central position. The order of the two halves of the experiment was randomized across participants.

Whenever possible, participants with stroke performed the experiment with both the more-affected and less-affected arms. Participants who did not feel capable of performing the experiment with the more-affected arm participated with the less-affected arm only. One participant completed the more-affected side session and did not return for the scheduled less-affected side session; three participants completed the less-affected side session and did not return for the scheduled more-affected-side session. Two participants dropped out and two participants were unable to complete the entire protocol for a given session and related data were excluded.

Statistical Analysis

Raw eye- and hand-position data were initially filtered by a 3-point median filter to remove outliers. Kinematic data traces were then obtained by first aligning data to the time of reach onset. Velocity traces were unremarkable, and are not explored further.

Two-sample *t*-tests were used to determine whether pairs of means or variances differed. Our results were unchanged if comparisons were made using Welch's *t*-test, which makes use of equations designed to account for possible heteroscedasticity and unequal sample sizes (the Welch-Satterthwaite equation for degrees of freedom). As a complement to traditional *t*-tests, we have plotted Bayesian 95% confidence regions around all computed estimates in the figures; as can be seen graphically in the corresponding figures by comparing confidence bounds, Bayesian analogs of the reported *t*-tests confirm our statistical analyses. Single proportions were compared via the *z*-test for equality of proportions (S_1 of N_1 vs. S_2 of N_2), where z is

$$z = \frac{S_1/N_1 - S_2/N_2}{\sqrt{\left(\frac{S_1+S_2}{N_1+N_2}\right)\left(1-\frac{S_1+S_2}{N_1+N_2}\right)\left(\frac{1}{N_1}+\frac{1}{N_2}\right)}}.$$

Finally, we note that separating temporal and spatial errors by target directions either toward or away from the more-affected side (i.e., away or toward the affected hemisphere) did not affect the pattern of results described below.

RESULTS

Demographics and Questionnaire Assessments

The clinical characteristics of the participants with stroke are presented in **Table 1**. The ABI cohort had a mean unweighted VFQ score of 91.33 ± 13.01 vs. 94.87 ± 4.87 in healthy controls ($p = 0.203$, ns). For the 10-item supplement, the ABI cohort had a mean score of 95 ± 11.57 vs. 96.27 ± 6.64 in controls ($p = 0.375$, ns). For the composite and 10-item supplement, the ABI cohort had a mean score of 92.36 ± 12.18 vs. 95.12 ± 4.65 in controls ($p = 0.244$, ns). In the ABI cohort, the mean Fugl-Meyer Score was 55.54 ± 13.33, with a range of 30–66.

Latencies and Durations of Eye and Hand Movements

Saccade and reach latencies are plotted in **Figure 2** relative to the go signal. Note that the initial (primary) saccades made by participants with stroke are significantly earlier ($p < 0.05$, comparing controls to both less-affected and more-affected sides) than those of control participants [control saccade onsets: 0.529 s, CI: (0.514, 0.543); less-affected arm: 0.106 s, CI: (0.08 0.132); more-affected arm: 0.082 s, CI: (0.052 0.112)]. However, despite the extremely early initial saccades to the target by participants with stroke, reaches were initiated at approximately the same time [no significant differences between control and either less-affected or more-affected reach onsets: control reach onsets: 0.556 s, CI: (0.544 0.568); less-affected arm: 0.545 s, CI: (0.521 0.568); more-affected arm: 0.60 s, CI: (0.567 0.632)].

The temporal decoupling, defined as the interval between the primary saccade and reach onset, is clearly increased in stroke. The coupling between eye and fingertip onsets in controls was 27 ms [CI: (8.5 45)], whereas there was a 439 ms [CI: (404 474)] separation for the less-affected side in stroke, and a 519-ms [CI: (476 562)] separation for the more-affected side in stroke (differences between pairs of coupling times were all significant, all $p < 0.05$). Thus, there was a decrease in coupling with reduction in arm motor capacity or an increase in arm motor impairment (from control

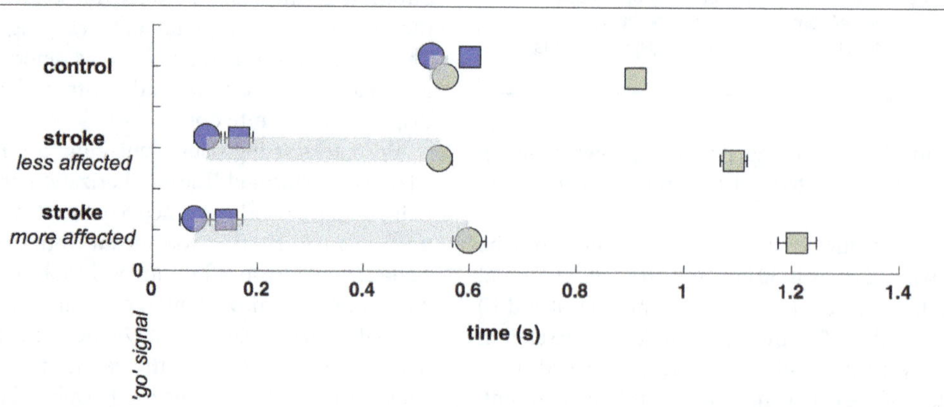

FIGURE 2 | Saccade and Reach Latencies (onsets: circles, terminations: squares). Saccade onsets (blue circles) occur substantially earlier in the stroke cohort, although reach onsets (green circles) are nearly the same across participants regardless of cohort or laterality (with a small delay on the more-affected side). Time between saccade and reach onsets is shown with a light gray bar.

to less-affected and less- to more-affected limb reaches in stroke). While it is not surprising that reaches made by the more-affected arm in stroke were prolonged relative to controls [604 ms, CI: (587 622) vs. 352 ms, CI: (348 356)], reaches made with the less-affected arm were also significantly prolonged relative to controls [546 ms, CI: (537 555) vs. 352 ms]. In addition, more-affected-side reaches were prolonged relative to less-affected side reaches (all $p < 0.05$).

Frequency of Eye Movements

The significant delay between initial saccade and reach onset in both the more- and less-affected sides of stroke participants relative to a minimal saccade-reach temporal separation in control participants suggests that an important temporal decoupling has occurred. Therefore, we examined the time period between the primary saccade and initiation of reach. Participants with stroke frequently made multiple saccades between the start and target positions (this pattern was the same in more- and less-affected arm reaches, and these are combined here), rather than a single saccade as seen in control trials. **Figure 3** displays histograms of the number of additional saccades (past the initial, or primary saccade) that were made by each group. Note that control participants overwhelmingly produced a single (primary) saccade to the target and maintained fixation in the terminal position of the primary saccade until the end of the reach in approximately 90% of all trials. In stark contrast, stroke participants generated this pattern in only about half of trials ($z = 32.2$, $p < 0.05$); these participants commonly produced from one to five additional saccades (**Figure 3**). Example saccade traces illustrating this phenomenon are shown in **Figure 4**.

Spatial Errors of the Eye and Hand Movements

Despite the increased duration of reaches in the less- and more-affected arm trials relative to control trials (allowing for a greater degree of feedback control), spatial errors (reach endpoint distance from the target) increased in stroke participants [control: 9.3 mm, CI: (9.0 9.5); less-affected arm: 19.2 mm, CI: (18.4 20.0); more-affected arm: 21.4 mm, CI: (20.5 21.4)] rather than decreased (**Figure 5**; all $p < 0.05$). In addition to these increases in reach error, **Figure 5** shows even larger increases in saccade endpoint error [control: 18.3 mm, CI: (17.9 18.7); less-affected arm: 36.4 mm, CI: (35.2 37.6); more-affected arm: 41.6 mm, CI: (40.3 43.0); all $p < 0.05$]. **Figure 6** shows the correlation between gaze and reach endpoint errors across subjects. Saccade and reach errors are correlated ($r = 0.76$, $p < 0.05$) across participants and levels of arm motor impairment.

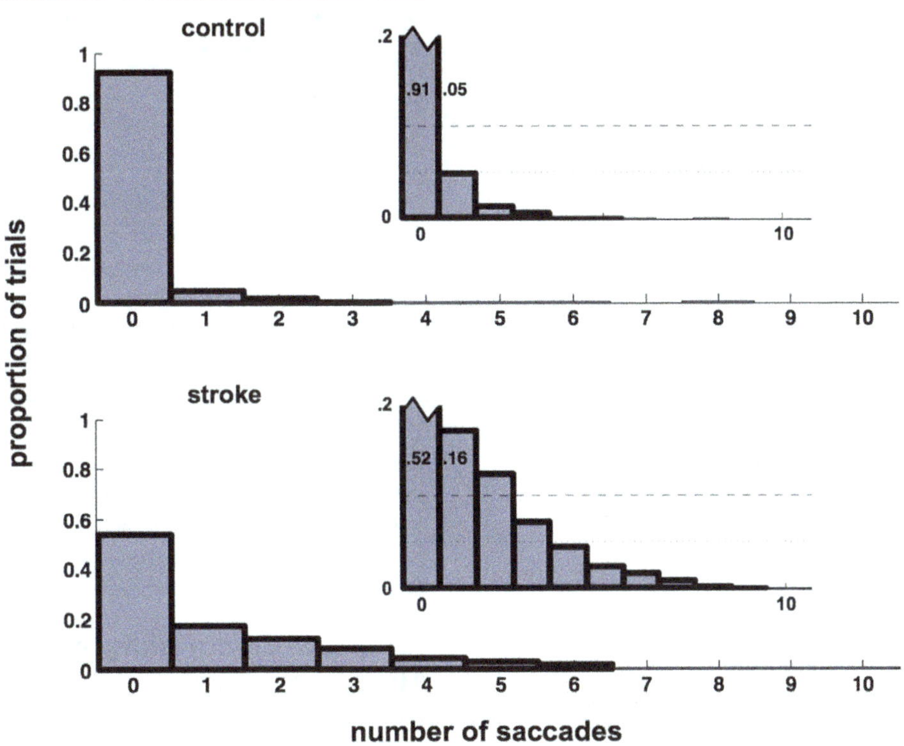

FIGURE 3 | Histograms of the number of saccades in addition to the primary saccade. Control participants (upper histograms) overwhelmingly produce a primary saccade only (91% of trials). About 96% of trials contain either no additional saccades beyond the primary saccade, or contain a single secondary saccade (see inset). For stroke participants (lower histogram), the same 96% of trials contains up to five secondary saccades (see inset). Insets show the same histograms with re-scaled axes to highlight histogram heights for non-primary saccades. This re-scaling truncates the ordinate at $p = 0.2$, which allows the pattern in the smaller-height histogram bars (those corresponding to trials that included non-primary saccades) to be seen. Heights of the first two bars in each inset are labeled to help emphasize the re-scaling.

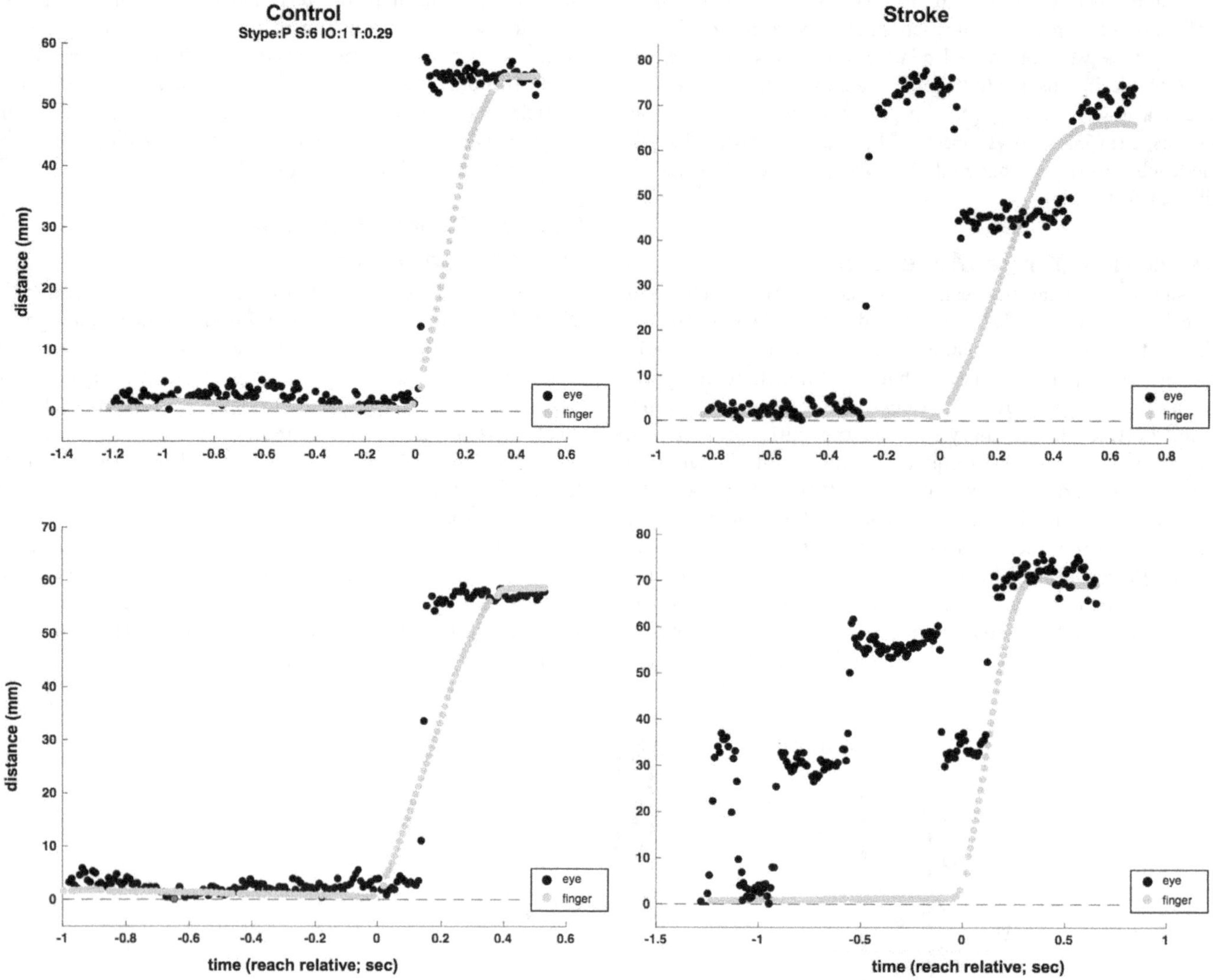

FIGURE 4 | Two-sample (raw, unfiltered) eye (black) and hand (gray) traces from control (left column) and stroke (right column) participants (plotted in screen mm to allow for simultaneous plotting of eye and hand traces). Multiple eye movements are evident in the time before reach completion in the two stroke trials, as opposed to single saccades at or near the time of the reach in control trials.

Correlation between Arm Motor Impairment and Eye–Hand Latency Decoupling

We then asked if the extent of eye–hand decoupling was larger in participants with greater arm motor impairment (lower scores) as assessed by the Fugl-Meyer Score. Although the predicted trend is in fact observed, it is not statistically significant for the less-affected ($r = -0.64$, ns) or more-affected ($r = -0.34$, ns) arms.

DISCUSSION

We have demonstrated a number of findings in eye–hand coordination after stroke in individuals with otherwise intact visual function. Most important among these results is the temporal decoupling between the primary saccade onset and the reach onset in the saccade-to-reach tasks. Saccades and reaches in stroke participants were also less accurate regardless of reaching limb (more- or less-affected side), as compared to controls. We discuss each of these findings in turn, paying particular attention to the clinical implications these results may have on eye–hand coordination in the setting of neurovascular, neurotraumatic, and neurodegenerative pathology.

Temporal Decoupling and Latency Abnormalities

The temporal decoupling between eye and hand is clearly noted in the latency differences for both the less-affected and more-affected reaches poststroke. While there are several important elements to extract from the timing data, the most substantial finding was that saccades made by stroke participants occurred significantly earlier in both the less-affected and more-affected arms, as compared to the saccade onsets of control participants (**Figure 2**). This is consistent with earlier reports

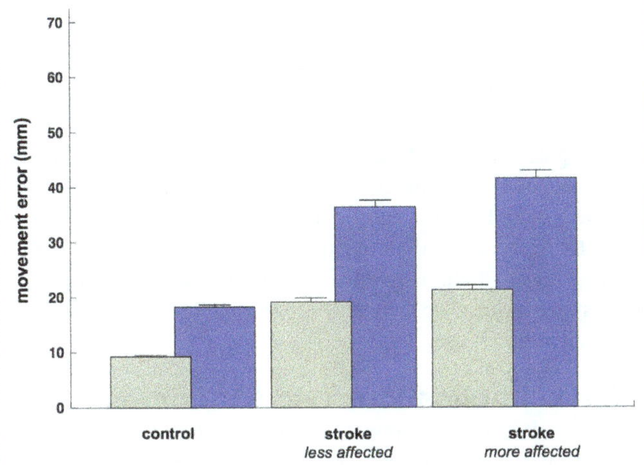

FIGURE 5 | Average endpoint error by participant grouping and/or arm (mm at the screen). Green bars show average reach error, and blue bars show average (primary) saccade error.

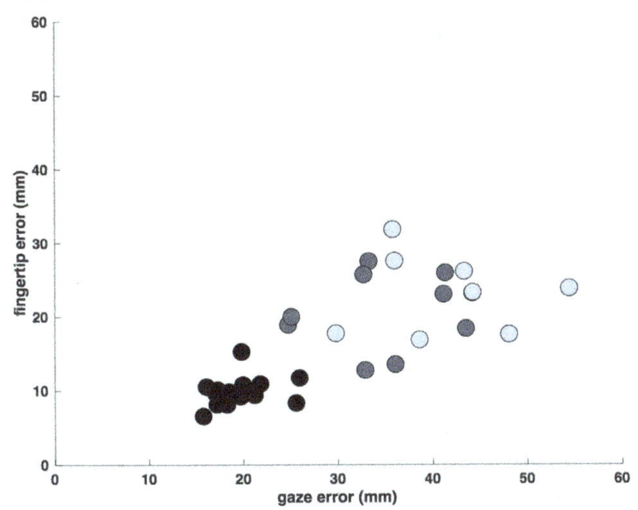

FIGURE 6 | Average saccade vs. reach endpoint error (mm at the screen). Each data point is the average error for a single participant/arm (control movements: black, less-affected arm: gray, more-affected arm: blue). Errors display a dependence on arm motor impairment, generally increasing across participants from control to stroke, and from less- to more-affected limbs ($r = 0.76$, $p < 0.05$).

of an upper-motor-neuron-like disinhibition phenomenon, in which participants with cerebrovascular damage anticipate the movement go signal, notwithstanding instructions to the contrary (86). Despite extremely early primary saccades to the target, reaches by stroke participants were initiated at roughly the same time as those of control participants, yielding the temporal decoupling that distinguished our cohorts (**Figure 2**). Thus, temporal decoupling appears to be a result of the unusually early onset of initial saccades, rather than due to the late onset of arm movements.

The eyes frequently fixate an object of interest before starting a manual motor movement (87); though, a more invariant feature is that gaze is spatially directed to the target prior to the arrival of the hand (88), typically close to the peak acceleration of the reach (89–91). The ocular motor system controls the gaze that then provides the needed visual information to optimally direct the hand; this is performed so fixations are "just in time," providing information at a critical moment, during which additional fovea-based fine detail is required for the task (92). Additionally, the short-term memory limitations of visual features are well known aspects of visual function and further support the idea that information acquired during prior fixations factors marginally into the computations necessary for ongoing fine motor control (93, 94). The information that is used across fixations within a visual scene is principally semantic in nature: for example, the memory of a global environment but not specific details (95, 96). Consequently, eye movements are intimately coupled in time and space to the motor action of the hand (97).

Vision may be best understood through action production, as sensorimotor coupling involves the distillation of visual perception into defined benefits for the planning and execution of somatic behavior (98, 99). As previously detailed, gaze is often directed at environmental objects with relevance to future action; in particular, during object manipulation the line of sight is directed at spatial targets upon which manual interactions may subsequently be focused (20, 100, 101). Complex, manual interactions with an object have multiple stages (e.g., stage 1: reach for the object; stage 2: grasp it; stage 3: lift and maneuver it), such as might occur when one reaches for a bottle of water lying on its side, then lifts it from the table and finally re-orients it for ease of grasp by a colleague. All stages of such a complex task have significance not only for the planning and motor control of the hand position but also for the planning of gaze, suggesting that manual activity "stages" can differentially affect eye position (59). For example, adding weight to the hand during a visually guided reach (in an effort to up-regulate the motor command and efference copy) modulates saccadic output (102).

These examples illustrate a two-way flow of information between eye–hand and hand–eye, which may be particularly relevant in pathology with arm motor impairments. This may be compounded, as demonstrated here, when visual information is not timed correctly and is decoupled from manual motor activity, limiting the opportunity for relevant visual information to support the evolving manual motor planning necessary for accurate reaching. However, to understand the full progression of reaches (and reach errors) generated in the present experiments, one must understand the planning deficits and errors generated. These spatial accuracy compromises may be a byproduct of impaired planning, feedback, and/or online (feedforward) corrective mechanisms.

Spatial Errors and Predictive Control

Despite increasing reach duration in the less- and more-affected arm trials relative to controls, theoretically allowing additional time for feedback control mechanisms to take effect, spatial errors increased. The fact that there was an increased opportunity for feedback mechanisms to reduce reach errors and yet these errors increased may indicate that feedback mechanisms produced inappropriate trajectory "corrections" and caused increased errors, or inappropriate plans were activated for a given reach while feedback mechanisms were suppressed, or poor estimates of reach errors were generated, or a combination thereof. In addition to increased reach error in stroke, there was an even larger increase in saccade endpoint error from controls to less-affected and then more-affected limbs in stroke.

It is particularly interesting that there was such a large decrement in saccade accuracy between the control and less-/more-affected arm reaches. This increase in endpoint error may have been a byproduct of the increased frequency of saccades, as stroke participants were found to elicit multiple saccades between the start and target position, rather than a single saccade as was found in control trials. In fact, stroke participants commonly produced between one and five additional saccades relative to controls in the time period before reach termination (**Figures 3** and **4**). This behavior is akin to what might be seen under "normal" conditions when one, given some degree of uncertainty, attempts to visually estimate the length of an object or distance. Although saccadic dysmetria has been documented and ascribed to lesions involving the cortex, pretectum, thalamus, superior colliculus, and cerebellum (103–105), we are unaware of any previous example in the literature of the above ocular–manual behavior occurring under experimental conditions, nor any report of it arising in a participant population with ABI undergoing an investigation of eye–hand coordination.

Prediction is an essential component of goal-oriented somatic action; the physical world is constantly changing and consequently an important aspect of eye–hand control. Grasping a cup being given to you requires both anticipating the object's direction and motion, and planning a motor response that predicts the trajectory to successfully intersect with it. If visual perception were merely used to generate 3D cues for eye–hand coordination, our fingers would regularly miss their spatial goal due to poor predictions of objects and/or hand motion. Prediction is required for optimized motor control, which translates into functional performance (106). These principles are most clearly highlighted in sports, where athletes of higher skill demonstrate finely tuned ocular motor control with predictive capacity, driving superior, complex, somatic motor control (107–111). For instance, expert-level soccer goalkeepers can more accurately predict soccer ball trajectories during anticipation tasks and leverage more efficient and effective strategies during visual search when compared to novices (112, 113).

As a pathologic illustration, optic ataxia manifests with an inability to efficiently adjust online hand trajectories targeted at moving spatial targets or to properly reach for/grasp objects under visual control. These deficits in rapid error corrections and their mechanistic underpinnings shed light on the coupling required between eye and hand during visually led function (114). In ABI, impairments are prominent during dynamic eye–hand coordination tasks, emphasizing potential difficulties in rapidly processing sensory information, sensorimotor integration and planning, in addition to motor execution. Inefficiently handling sensory information may lead to difficulties in predicting target motion, a deficit in feedforward mechanisms, and in the integration of sensory feedback toward error correction (3, 115). In fact, predictive control is vital to optimized visuomotor planning (116). It is presently accepted that impaired planning is a result of an inability to program motor action sequences in space and time (10, 117–120), and, that post-ABI there are deficits in the motor programming necessary to plan for static or dynamically moving targets (121–124). We believe our findings to be consistent with these prior results and may suggest why these deficits are apparent in both the less- and more-affected sides.

Clinical Implications and Outcomes

Here, we describe a pattern of abnormalities following MCA stroke that affects both eye–hand coupling and sensory-motor performance, where the strength of the deficit increases for reaches made with the less-affected to reaches made with the more-affected arms of stroke participants relative to the baseline performance in control participants. These findings suggest that in individuals with otherwise intact visual function, the spatial and temporal relationships between the eye and hand are disrupted poststroke, and may need to be specifically targeted during neurorehabilitation. Eye–hand coupling may be a useful biomarker in individuals with cerebral pathology in the setting of neurovascular, neurotraumatic, and neurodegenerative pathology.

Quantitative eye-movement analysis has proven to be a high-value research tool within ABI (49, 125, 126); objective ocular motor recordings have even been used for screening in a diagnostic capacity (127–130). In a broader scope, eye movements and the upper limb have been sensitive markers of cerebral injury when examining visuomotor skill (131). Additionally, function of the eye and arm following acute ABI can predict outcomes in the subacute and chronic stages following injury, with greater performance when compared to self-reported health status or neuropsychologic assessment (3, 132, 133). These prognostic capabilities extend to the identification of individuals who may require more comprehensive intervention or who are poor responders (6, 7). In fact, eye-movement findings have even been shown to be a biomarker of cognitive recovery beyond the times at which presumed full recovery had been reached, as assessed by established metrics (8). While the evidence is greater for neurotraumatic and neurovascular etiologies, the literature base also includes neurodegeneration, in which eye movements may be a biomarker of progression and useful in clinical trials of pharmacological agents to slow disease advancement (134–137). At the bedside, regardless of whether a clinical assessment of visual function is found to be remarkable or unremarkable, as was the case in our pathologic cohort following stroke, disruption of the normal coordination between ocular and manual motor control may lead to maladaptive compensation strategies. This dysfunctional, compensatory behavior, which may require objective screening, and be evidenced by increased saccade frequency during temporal decoupling, may lead to problems in either motor planning and/or control systems and have untoward consequences on function.

It is paramount to remember that sensorimotor control strategies are critical for skilled somatic behavior in humans and that disruptions leading to incoordination may ultimately hamper recovery following ABI. Visuomotor integration is characterized by temporal and spatial relationships between the ocular and manual motor systems (138, 139); small abnormalities in eye-movement timing relative to hand-movement timing, irregularities that could go undetected, may disrupt the framework on which combined movement plans are constructed (140). Moreover, eye-movement execution for visually guided reaches may occur concurrently with motor planning for limb movement (141, 142). This could add in a compound fashion to the already known motor planning deficits in chronic stroke (123), generating computational delays and providing a potential explanation for stifled rehabilitation progress and recovery plateaus. As ocular motor control precedes and is an integral component of visually guided limb control (138, 139, 143, 144), eye–hand coordination is critical to function. Understanding the synchronous and interdependent control systems that direct the eye and hand will likely be important to restoring upper extremity function poststroke. Within neurorehabilitation, one must remember that there is a key difference between gross motor ability and functional motor control. The distinction between these two sides of recovery is not the simple capacity to move the limb but rather the character and efficiency of that control.

CONCLUSION

Despite the robust opportunities within ocular–manual motor investigations in the setting of ABI, examination with quantitative dual-effector recordings in 3D has not been formally tested. We report on a number of findings in chronic, MCA stroke, relative to healthy controls, in visually guided (delayed) and memory-guided saccade-to-reach paradigms to assess eye–hand coordination. As compared to healthy controls, stroke participants demonstrated significant temporal decoupling between primary saccade and reach onsets, greater endpoint errors in both effector systems (poorer spatial performance), and an increased frequency of saccades during the temporal decoupling. Future studies that further characterize coupling objectively in unconstrained and naturalistic tasks with ecological validity may produce high-yield results for neurorehabilitation in the setting of neurovascular, neurotraumatic, and neurodegenerative pathology.

AUTHOR CONTRIBUTIONS

Conception and design of the study and substantial manuscript drafting: J-RR, JF, MH, AS, EA, RP, AA, PR, JR, ML, and TH. Acquisition and analysis of data: J-RR, JF, EA, MH, RP, AS, and TH.

ACKNOWLEDGMENTS

We would like to thank Dr. Tamara Bushnik and the NYULMC Rusk Research Team for their thoughts, suggestions, and contributions. This research was supported in part by National Institutes of Health Grants EY08266 (to ML), HD071978 (to PR), TR000038 (to J-RR), UL1TR001445 (to J-RR, ML, and PR), and 5K12 HD001097 (to J-RR, ML, and PR).

REFERENCES

1. Tippett WJ, Krajewski A, Sergio LE. Visuomotor integration is compromised in Alzheimer's disease patients reaching for remembered targets. *Eur Neurol* (2007) 58:1–11. doi:10.1159/000102160
2. Verheij S, Muilwijk D, Pel JJ, van der Cammen TJ, Mattace-Raso FU, van der Steen J. Visuomotor impairment in early-stage Alzheimer's disease: changes in relative timing of eye and hand movements. *J Alzheimers Dis* (2012) 30:131–43. doi:10.3233/JAD-2012-111883
3. Caeyenberghs K, van Roon D, van Aken K, De Cock P, Linden CV, Swinnen SP, et al. Static and dynamic visuomotor task performance in children with acquired brain injury: predictive control deficits under increased temporal pressure. *J Head Trauma Rehabil* (2009) 24:363–73. doi:10.1097/HTR.0b013e3181af0810
4. Gao KL, Ng SS, Kwok JW, Chow RT, Tsang WW. Eye-hand coordination and its relationship with sensori-motor impairments in stroke survivors. *J Rehabil Med* (2010) 42:368–73. doi:10.2340/16501977-0520
5. Procacci NM, Stanford TR, Wittenberg GF. The relationship between visual orienting and interlimb synchrony in a patient with a superior parietal infarction: a case study. *Neurocase* (2009) 15:73–88. doi:10.1080/13554790802620558
6. Heitger MH, Jones RD, Anderson TJ. A new approach to predicting post-concussion syndrome after mild traumatic brain injury based upon eye movement function. *Conf Proc IEEE Eng Med Biol Soc* (2008) 2008:3570–3. doi:10.1109/IEMBS.2008.4649977
7. Heitger MH, Jones RD, Macleod AD, Snell DL, Frampton CM, Anderson TJ. Impaired eye movements in post-concussion syndrome indicate suboptimal brain function beyond the influence of depression, malingering or intellectual ability. *Brain* (2009) 132:2850–70. doi:10.1093/brain/awp181
8. Dong W, Yan B, Johnson BP, Millist L, Davis S, Fielding J, et al. Ischaemic stroke: the ocular motor system as a sensitive marker for motor and cognitive recovery. *J Neurol Neurosurg Psychiatry* (2013) 84:337–41. doi:10.1136/jnnp-2012-303926
9. O'Dell MW, Lin CC, Harrison V. Stroke rehabilitation: strategies to enhance motor recovery. *Annu Rev Med* (2009) 60:55–68. doi:10.1146/annurev.med.60.042707.104248
10. Beer RF, Dewald JP, Rymer WZ. Deficits in the coordination of multijoint arm movements in patients with hemiparesis: evidence for disturbed control of limb dynamics. *Exp Brain Res* (2000) 131:305–19. doi:10.1007/s002219900275
11. Fisher BE, Winstein CJ, Velicki MR. Deficits in compensatory trajectory adjustments after unilateral sensorimotor stroke. *Exp Brain Res* (2000) 132:328–44. doi:10.1007/s002219900316
12. McCrea PH, Eng JJ. Consequences of increased neuromotor noise for reaching movements in persons with stroke. *Exp Brain Res* (2005) 162:70–7. doi:10.1007/s00221-004-2106-8
13. Tsang WW, Ng SS, Lee MW, Tse SP, Yip EW, Yuen JK. Does postural stability affect the performance of eye-hand coordination in stroke survivors? *Am J Phys Med Rehabil* (2013) 92:781–8. doi:10.1097/PHM.0b013e3182876adb
14. Velicki MR, Winstein CJ, Pohl PS. Impaired direction and extent specification of aimed arm movements in humans with stroke-related brain damage. *Exp Brain Res* (2000) 130:362–74. doi:10.1007/s002219900262

15. Wenzelburger R, Kopper F, Frenzel A, Stolze H, Klebe S, Brossmann A, et al. Hand coordination following capsular stroke. *Brain* (2005) 128:64–74. doi:10.1093/brain/awh317
16. Zackowski KM, Dromerick AW, Sahrmann SA, Thach WT, Bastian AJ. How do strength, sensation, spasticity and joint individuation relate to the reaching deficits of people with chronic hemiparesis? *Brain* (2004) 127:1035–46. doi:10.1093/brain/awh116
17. Leigh RJ, Kennard C. Using saccades as a research tool in the clinical neurosciences. *Brain* (2004) 127:460–77. doi:10.1093/brain/awh035
18. White OB, Fielding J. Cognition and eye movements: assessment of cerebral dysfunction. *J Neuroophthalmol* (2012) 32:266–73. doi:10.1097/WNO.0b013e3182688230
19. Anderson T. Could saccadic function be a useful marker of stroke recovery? *J Neurol Neurosurg Psychiatry* (2013) 84:242. doi:10.1136/jnnp-2012-304481
20. Johansson RS, Westling G, Backstrom A, Flanagan JR. Eye-hand coordination in object manipulation. *J Neurosci* (2001) 21:6917–32.
21. Flanagan JR, Bowman MC, Johansson RS. Control strategies in object manipulation tasks. *Curr Opin Neurobiol* (2006) 16:650–9. doi:10.1016/j.conb.2006.10.005
22. Gaveau V, Pisella L, Priot AE, Fukui T, Rossetti Y, Pelisson D, et al. Automatic online control of motor adjustments in reaching and grasping. *Neuropsychologia* (2014) 55:25–40. doi:10.1016/j.neuropsychologia.2013.12.005
23. Prablanc C, Echallier JE, Jeannerod M, Komilis E. Optimal response of eye and hand motor systems in pointing at a visual target. II. Static and dynamic visual cues in the control of hand movement. *Biol Cybern* (1979) 35:183–7. doi:10.1007/BF00337063
24. Prablanc C, Echallier JF, Komilis E, Jeannerod M. Optimal response of eye and hand motor systems in pointing at a visual target. I. Spatio-temporal characteristics of eye and hand movements and their relationships when varying the amount of visual information. *Biol Cybern* (1979) 35:113–24. doi:10.1007/BF00337063
25. Bogousslavsky J. Impairment of visually evoked eye movements with a unilateral parieto-occipital lesion. *J Neurol* (1987) 234:160–2. doi:10.1007/BF00314136
26. Bogousslavsky J, Meienberg O. Eye-movement disorders in brainstem and cerebellar stroke. *Arch Neurol* (1987) 44:141–8. doi:10.1001/archneur.1987.00520140013011
27. Catz A, Ron S, Solzi P, Korczyn AD. Saccade characteristics in patients with hemispheric stroke. *J Neurol Rehabil* (1997) 11:175–80.
28. Colombo A, Gibertoni M, Sorgato P. [Clinical study of disorders of eye movements (voluntary and following) after acute vascular accidents involving the cerebral hemispheres (author's transl)]. *Riv Patol Nerv Ment* (1981) 102:38–46.
29. Lekwuwa GU, Barnes GR. Cerebral control of eye movements. II. Timing of anticipatory eye movements, predictive pursuit and phase errors in focal cerebral lesions. *Brain* (1996) 119(Pt 2):491–505. doi:10.1093/brain/119.2.491
30. Pierrot-Deseilligny C, Ploner CJ, Muri RM, Gaymard B, Rivaud-Pechoux S. Effects of cortical lesions on saccadic eye movements in humans. *Ann N Y Acad Sci* (2002) 956:216–29. doi:10.1111/j.1749-6632.2002.tb02821.x
31. Waespe W, Baumgartner R. Enduring dysmetria and impaired gain adaptivity of saccadic eye movements in Wallenberg's lateral medullary syndrome. *Brain* (1992) 115(Pt 4):1123–46. doi:10.1093/brain/115.4.1125
32. Rivaud S, Muri RM, Gaymard B, Vermersch AI, Pierrot-Deseilligny C. Eye movement disorders after frontal eye field lesions in humans. *Exp Brain Res* (1994) 102:110–20. doi:10.1007/BF00232443
33. Pierrot-Deseilligny C, Rivaud S, Gaymard B, Agid Y. Cortical control of reflexive visually-guided saccades. *Brain* (1991) 114(Pt 3):1473–85. doi:10.1093/brain/114.3.1473
34. Agrawal Y, Schubert MC, Migliaccio AA, Zee DS, Schneider E, Lehnen N, et al. Evaluation of quantitative head impulse testing using search coils versus video-oculography in older individuals. *Otol Neurotol* (2014) 35:283–8. doi:10.1097/MAO.0b013e3182995227
35. Eggert T. Eye movement recordings: methods. *Dev Ophthalmol* (2007) 40:15–34. doi:10.1159/000100347
36. Houben MM, Goumans J, van der Steen J. Recording three-dimensional eye movements: scleral search coils versus video oculography. *Invest Ophthalmol Vis Sci* (2006) 47:179–87. doi:10.1167/iovs.05-0234
37. Imai T, Sekine K, Hattori K, Takeda N, Koizuka I, Nakamae K, et al. Comparing the accuracy of video-oculography and the scleral search coil system in human eye movement analysis. *Auris Nasus Larynx* (2005) 32:3–9. doi:10.1016/j.anl.2004.11.009
38. Kimmel DL, Mammo D, Newsome WT. Tracking the eye non-invasively: simultaneous comparison of the scleral search coil and optical tracking techniques in the macaque monkey. *Front Behav Neurosci* (2012) 6:49. doi:10.3389/fnbeh.2012.00049
39. McCamy MB, Otero-Millan J, Leigh RJ, King SA, Schneider RM, Macknik SL, et al. Simultaneous recordings of human microsaccades and drifts with a contemporary video eye tracker and the search coil technique. *PLoS One* (2015) 10:e0128428. doi:10.1371/journal.pone.0128428
40. Stahl JS, van Alphen AM, De Zeeuw CI. A comparison of video and magnetic search coil recordings of mouse eye movements. *J Neurosci Methods* (2000) 99:101–10. doi:10.1016/S0165-0270(00)00218-1
41. van der Geest JN, Frens MA. Recording eye movements with video-oculography and scleral search coils: a direct comparison of two methods. *J Neurosci Methods* (2002) 114:185–95. doi:10.1016/S0165-0270(01)00527-1
42. Yee RD, Schiller VL, Lim V, Baloh FG, Baloh RW, Honrubia V. Velocities of vertical saccades with different eye movement recording methods. *Invest Ophthalmol Vis Sci* (1985) 26:938–44.
43. Machado L, Rafal RD. Control of fixation and saccades in humans with chronic lesions of oculomotor cortex. *Neuropsychology* (2004) 18:115–23. doi:10.1037/0894-4105.18.1.115
44. Noudoost B, Clark KL, Moore T. A distinct contribution of the frontal eye field to the visual representation of saccadic targets. *J Neurosci* (2014) 34:3687–98. doi:10.1523/JNEUROSCI.3824-13.2014
45. Schall S, Schmidt A. [Dental assistants-continuing education in Munich (7)]. *Quintessenz J* (1991) 21:611–3.
46. Louie K, Grattan LE, Glimcher PW. Reward value-based gain control: divisive normalization in parietal cortex. *J Neurosci* (2011) 31:10627–39. doi:10.1523/JNEUROSCI.1237-11.2011
47. Stuphorn V, Brown JW, Schall JD. Role of supplementary eye field in saccade initiation: executive, not direct, control. *J Neurophysiol* (2010) 103:801–16. doi:10.1152/jn.00221.2009
48. Stuphorn V, Bauswein E, Hoffmann KP. Neurons in the primate superior colliculus coding for arm movements in gaze-related coordinates. *J Neurophysiol* (2000) 83:1283–99.
49. Hutton SB. Cognitive control of saccadic eye movements. *Brain Cogn* (2008) 68:327–40. doi:10.1016/j.bandc.2008.08.021
50. Histed MH, Pasupathy A, Miller EK. Learning substrates in the primate prefrontal cortex and striatum: sustained activity related to successful actions. *Neuron* (2009) 63:244–53. doi:10.1016/j.neuron.2009.06.019
51. Pasupathy A, Miller EK. Different time courses of learning-related activity in the prefrontal cortex and striatum. *Nature* (2005) 433:873–6. doi:10.1038/nature03287
52. Thakkar KN, van den Heiligenberg FM, Kahn RS, Neggers SF. Frontal-subcortical circuits involved in reactive control and monitoring of gaze. *J Neurosci* (2014) 34:8918–29. doi:10.1523/JNEUROSCI.0732-14.2014
53. Mahamed S, Garrison TJ, Shires J, Basso MA. Stimulation of the substantia nigra influences the specification of memory-guided saccades. *J Neurophysiol* (2014) 111:804–16. doi:10.1152/jn.00002.2013
54. Watanabe M, Munoz DP. Effects of caudate microstimulation on spontaneous and purposive saccades. *J Neurophysiol* (2013) 110:334–43. doi:10.1152/jn.00046.2013
55. Gaymard B. Cortical and sub-cortical control of saccades and clinical application. *Rev Neurol (Paris)* (2012) 168:734–40. doi:10.1016/j.neurol.2012.07.016
56. Shires J, Joshi S, Basso MA. Shedding new light on the role of the basal ganglia-superior colliculus pathway in eye movements. *Curr Opin Neurobiol* (2010) 20:717–25. doi:10.1016/j.conb.2010.08.008
57. Hikosaka O, Takikawa Y, Kawagoe R. Role of the basal ganglia in the control of purposive saccadic eye movements. *Physiol Rev* (2000) 80:953–78.
58. Gaymard B, Rivaud S, Cassarini JF, Dubard T, Rancurel G, Agid Y, et al. Effects of anterior cingulate cortex lesions on ocular saccades in humans. *Exp Brain Res* (1998) 120:173–83. doi:10.1007/s002210050391
59. Belardinelli A, Stepper MY, Butz MV. It's in the eyes: planning precise manual actions before execution. *J Vis* (2016) 16:18. doi:10.1167/16.1.18
60. Hall J, Guyton A. *Textbook of Medical Physiology*. Philadelphia: W.B. Saunders (2005).

61. Rathelot JA, Strick PL. Muscle representation in the macaque motor cortex: an anatomical perspective. *Proc Natl Acad Sci U S A* (2006) 103:8257–62. doi:10.1073/pnas.0602933103
62. Bard C, Fleury M, Hay L. *Development of Eye Hand Coordination Across the Lifespan*. Columbia, SC: University of South Carolina Press (1990).
63. Crawford JD, Medendorp WP, Marotta JJ. Spatial transformations for eye-hand coordination. *J Neurophysiol* (2004) 92:10–9. doi:10.1152/jn.00117.2004
64. Farber SD. *Assessing Neuromotor Performance Enablers*. Thorofare, NJ: Slack (1991).
65. Zoltan B, Pedretti LW. *Evaluation of Muscle Tone and Coordination*. St. Louis: C.V. Mosby (1990).
66. Desrosiers J, Hebert R, Bravo G, Dutil E. Upper-extremity motor co-ordination of healthy elderly people. *Age Ageing* (1995) 24:108–12. doi:10.1093/ageing/24.2.108
67. Rizzo JR, Hosseini M, Wong EA, Mackey WE, Fung JK, Ahdoot E, et al. The intersection between ocular and manual motor control: eye-hand coordination in acquired brain injury. *Front Neurol* (2017) 8:227. doi:10.3389/fneur.2017.00227
68. Edlin JM, Leppanen ML, Fain RJ, Hacklander RP, Hanaver-Torrez SD, Lyle KB. On the use (and misuse?) of the Edinburgh Handedness Inventory. *Brain Cogn* (2015) 94:44–51. doi:10.1016/j.bandc.2015.01.003
69. Carlson RV, Boyd KM, Webb DJ. The revision of the declaration of Helsinki: past, present and future. *Br J Clin Pharmacol* (2004) 57:695–713. doi:10.1111/j.1365-2125.2004.02103.x
70. Eckenwiler LA, Ells C, Feinholz D, Schonfeld T. Hopes for Helsinki: reconsidering "vulnerability". *J Med Ethics* (2008) 34:765–6. doi:10.1136/jme.2007.023481
71. Schmidt H, Mehring S, McMillan J. Interpreting the declaration of Helsinki (2008): "must", "should" and different kinds of obligation. *Med Law* (2010) 29:565–91.
72. Fugl-Meyer AR, Jaasko L, Leyman I, Olsson S, Steglind S. The post-stroke hemiplegic patient. 1. A method for evaluation of physical performance. *Scand J Rehabil Med* (1975) 7:13–31.
73. Srivastava A, Rapoport MJ, Leach L, Phillips A, Shammi P, Feinstein A. The utility of the mini-mental status exam in older adults with traumatic brain injury. *Brain Inj* (2006) 20:1377–82. doi:10.1080/02699050601111385
74. Rankin J. Cerebral vascular accidents in patients over the age of 60. I. General considerations. *Scott Med J* (1957) 2:127–36. doi:10.1177/003693305700200401
75. Volz M, Mobus J, Letsch C, Werheid K. The influence of early depressive symptoms, social support and decreasing self-efficacy on depression 6 months post-stroke. *J Affect Disord* (2016) 206:252–5. doi:10.1016/j.jad.2016.07.041
76. Zagar R, Mead JD. Analysis of a short test battery for children. *J Clin Psychol* (1983) 39:590–7. doi:10.1002/1097-4679(198307)39:4<590::AID-JCLP2270390422>3.0.CO;2-B
77. Malloy P, Belanger H, Hall S, Aloia M, Salloway S. Assessing visuoconstructional performance in AD, MCI and normal elderly using the Beery Visual-Motor Integration Test. *Clin Neuropsychol* (2003) 17:544–50. doi:10.1076/clin.17.4.544.27947
78. Temple V, Drummond C, Valiquette S, Jozsvai E. A comparison of intellectual assessments over video conferencing and in-person for individuals with ID: preliminary data. *J Intellect Disabil Res* (2010) 54:573–7. doi:10.1111/j.1365-2788.2010.01282.x
79. Tannenbaum S. The eye chart and Dr. Snellen. *J Am Optom Assoc* (1971) 42:89–90.
80. Beck RW, Bergstrom TJ, Lichter PR. A clinical comparison of visual field testing with a new automated perimeter, the Humphrey Field Analyzer, and the Goldmann perimeter. *Ophthalmology* (1985) 92:77–82. doi:10.1016/S0161-6420(85)34065-4
81. Schenkenberg T, Bradford DC, Ajax ET. Line bisection and unilateral visual neglect in patients with neurologic impairment. *Neurology* (1980) 30:509–17. doi:10.1212/WNL.30.5.509
82. Johnston CW, Diller L. Exploratory eye movements and visual hemi-neglect. *J Clin Exp Neuropsychol* (1986) 8:93–101. doi:10.1080/01688638608401299
83. Mangione CM, Lee PP, Gutierrez PR, Spritzer K, Berry S, Hays RD, et al. Development of the 25-item National Eye Institute Visual Function Questionnaire. *Arch Ophthalmol* (2001) 119:1050–8. doi:10.1001/archopht.119.7.1050
84. van Boxtel JJ, Lu H. A biological motion toolbox for reading, displaying, and manipulating motion capture data in research settings. *J Vis* (2013) 13:7. doi:10.1167/13.12.7
85. LeVasseur AL, Flanagan JR, Riopelle RJ, Munoz DP. Control of volitional and reflexive saccades in Tourette's syndrome. *Brain* (2001) 124:2045–58. doi:10.1093/brain/124.10.2045
86. Rizzo J-R, Hudson TE, Abdou A, Lui YW, Rucker JC, Raghavan P, et al. Disrupted saccade control in chronic cerebral injury: upper motor neuron-like disinhibition in the ocular motor system. *Front Neurol* (2017) 8:12. doi:10.3389/fneur.2017.00012
87. Carlton LG. Visual information: the control of aiming movements. *Q J Exp Psychol* (1981) 33:87–93. doi:10.1080/14640748108400771
88. Binsted G, Elliott D. Ocular perturbations and retinal/extraretinal information: the coordination of saccadic and manual movements. *Exp Brain Res* (1999) 127:193–206. doi:10.1007/s002210050789
89. Helsen WF, Elliott D, Starkes JL, Ricker KL. Temporal and spatial coupling of point of gaze and hand movements in aiming. *J Mot Behav* (1998) 30:249–59. doi:10.1080/00222899809601340
90. Helsen WF, Elliott D, Starkes JL, Ricker KL. Coupling of eye, finger, elbow, and shoulder movements during manual aiming. *J Mot Behav* (2000) 32:241–8. doi:10.1080/00222890009601375
91. Starkes J, Helsen W, Elliott D. A menage a trois: the eye, the hand and on-line processing. *J Sports Sci* (2002) 20:217–24. doi:10.1080/026404102317284772
92. Hayhoe MM, Shrivastava A, Mruczek R, Pelz JB. Visual memory and motor planning in a natural task. *J Vis* (2003) 3:49–63. doi:10.1167/3.1.6
93. Irwin DE. Information integration across saccadic eye movements. *Cogn Psychol* (1991) 23:420–56. doi:10.1016/0010-0285(91)90015-G
94. Ballard DH, Hayhoe MM, Pelz JB. Memory representations in natural tasks. *J Cogn Neurosci* (1995) 7:66–80. doi:10.1162/jocn.1995.7.1.66
95. Irwin DE. Integrating information across saccadic eye movements. *Curr Dir Psychol Sci* (1996) 5:94–100. doi:10.1111/1467-8721.ep10772833
96. O'Regan JK. Solving the "real" mysteries of visual perception: the world as an outside memory. *Can J Psychol* (1992) 46:461–88. doi:10.1037/h0084327
97. Land M, Mennie N, Rusted J. The roles of vision and eye movements in the control of activities of daily living. *Perception* (1999) 28:1311–28. doi:10.1068/p2935
98. Ballard DH. Animate vision. *Artif Intell* (1991) 48:57–86. doi:10.1016/0004-3702(91)90080-4
99. Cilo M, Politzer T, Ripley DL, Weintraub A. Vision examination of TBI patients in an acute rehabilitation hospital. *NeuroRehabilitation* (2010) 27:237–42. doi:10.3233/NRE-2010-0603
100. Brouwer AM, Franz VH, Gegenfurtner KR. Differences in fixations between grasping and viewing objects. *J Vis* (2009) 9:18.1–24. doi:10.1167/9.1.18
101. Cavina-Pratesi C, Hesse C. Why do the eyes prefer the index finger? Simultaneous recording of eye and hand movements during precision grasping. *J Vis* (2013) 13:15. doi:10.1167/13.5.15
102. van Donkelaar P, Siu KC, Walterschied J. Saccadic output is influenced by limb kinetics during eye-hand coordination. *J Mot Behav* (2004) 36:245–52. doi:10.3200/JMBR.36.3.245-252
103. Ohtsuka K, Noda H. The effect of microstimulation of the oculomotor vermis on discharges of fastigial neurons and visually-directed saccades in macaques. *Neurosci Res* (1991) 10(4):290–5. doi:10.1016/0168-0102(91)90086-E
104. Keating EF, Kenney DV, Gooley SG, Pratt SE, McGillis SL. Targeting errors and reduced oculomotor range following ablations of the superior colliculus or pretectum/thalamus. *Behav Brain Res* (1986) 22:191–210. doi:10.1016/0166-4328(86)90064-1
105. Pierrot-Deseilligny C, Rosa A, Masmoudi K, Rivaud S, Gaymard B. Saccade deficits after a unilateral lesion affecting the superior colliculus. *J Neurol Neurosurg Psychiatry* (1991) 54(12):1106–9. doi:10.1136/jnnp.54.12.1106
106. Hudson TE, Maloney LT, Landy MS. Movement planning with probabilistic target information. *J Neurophysiol* (2007) 98:3034–46. doi:10.1152/jn.00858.2007
107. Mann DT, Williams AM, Ward P, Janelle CM. Perceptual-cognitive expertise in sport: a meta-analysis. *J Sport Exerc Psychol* (2007) 29:457–78. doi:10.1123/jsep.29.4.457

108. McRobert AP, Williams AM, Ward P, Eccles DW. Tracing the process of expertise in a simulated anticipation task. *Ergonomics* (2009) 52:474–83. doi:10.1080/00140130802707824
109. Piras A, Lobietti R, Squatrito S. A study of saccadic eye movement dynamics in volleyball: comparison between athletes and non-athletes. *J Sports Med Phys Fitness* (2010) 50:99–108.
110. Willams AM, Hodges NJ, North JS, Barton G. Perceiving patterns of play in dynamic sport tasks: investigating the essential information underlying skilled performance. *Perception* (2006) 35:317–32. doi:10.1068/p5310
111. Williams AM. Perceptual skill in soccer: implications for talent identification and development. *J Sports Sci* (2000) 18:737–50. doi:10.1080/02640410050120041
112. Savelsbergh GJ, Williams AM, Van der Kamp J, Ward P. Visual search, anticipation and expertise in soccer goalkeepers. *J Sports Sci* (2002) 20:279–87. doi:10.1080/026404102317284826
113. Savelsbergh GJ, Van der Kamp J, Williams AM, Ward P. Anticipation and visual search behaviour in expert soccer goalkeepers. *Ergonomics* (2005) 48:1686–97. doi:10.1080/00140130500101346
114. Battaglia-Mayer A, Archambault PS, Caminiti R. The cortical network for eye-hand coordination and its relevance to understanding motor disorders of parietal patients. *Neuropsychologia* (2006) 44:2607–20. doi:10.1016/j.neuropsychologia.2005.11.021
115. Caeyenberghs K, Leemans A, Geurts M, Taymans T, Vander Linden C, Smits-Engelsman BC, et al. Brain-behavior relationships in young traumatic brain injury patients: fractional anisotropy measures are highly correlated with dynamic visuomotor tracking performance. *Neuropsychologia* (2010) 48:1472–82. doi:10.1016/j.neuropsychologia.2010.01.017
116. Hudson TE, Maloney LT, Landy MS. Optimal compensation for temporal uncertainty in movement planning. *PLoS Comput Biol* (2008) 4:e1000130. doi:10.1371/journal.pcbi.1000130
117. Cirstea MC, Levin MF. Compensatory strategies for reaching in stroke. *Brain* (2000) 123(Pt 5):940–53. doi:10.1093/brain/123.5.940
118. Ketcham CJ, Rodriguez TM, Zihlman KA. Targeted aiming movements are compromised in nonaffected limb of persons with stroke. *Neurorehabil Neural Repair* (2007) 21:388–97. doi:10.1177/1545968306297872
119. Kusoffsky A, Apel I, Hirschfeld H. Reaching-lifting-placing task during standing after stroke: coordination among ground forces, ankle muscle activity, and hand movement. *Arch Phys Med Rehabil* (2001) 82:650–60. doi:10.1053/apmr.2001.22611
120. Takahashi CD, Reinkensmeyer DJ. Hemiparetic stroke impairs anticipatory control of arm movement. *Exp Brain Res* (2003) 149:131–40. doi:10.1007/s00221-002-1340-1
121. Beer R, Dewald J, Rymer Z. Disturbances of voluntary movement coordination in stroke: problems of planning or execution? *Prog Brain Res* (1999) 123:455–60. doi:10.1016/S0079-6123(08)62881-2
122. Rizzo JR, Hudson TE, Abdou A, Rashbaum IG, George AE, Raghavan P, et al. Motor planning poststroke: impairment in vector-coded reach plans. *Physiol Rep* (2015) 3:e12650. doi:10.14814/phy2.12650
123. Raghavan P, Krakauer JW, Gordon AM. Impaired anticipatory control of fingertip forces in patients with a pure motor or sensorimotor lacunar syndrome. *Brain* (2006) 129:1415–25. doi:10.1093/brain/awl070
124. Raghavan P, Santello M, Gordon AM, Krakauer JW. Compensatory motor control after stroke: an alternative joint strategy for object-dependent shaping of hand posture. *J Neurophysiol* (2010) 103:3034–43. doi:10.1152/jn.00936.2009
125. Rizzo JR, Hudson TE, Dai W, Birkemeier J, Pasculli RM, Selesnick I, et al. Rapid number naming in chronic concussion: eye movements in the King-Devick test. *Ann Clin Transl Neurol* (2016) 3(10):801–11. doi:10.1002/acn3.345
126. Rizzo JR, Hudson TE, Dai W, Desai N, Yousefi A, Palsana D, et al. Objectifying eye movements during rapid number naming: methodology for assessment of normative data for the King-Devick test. *J Neurol Sci* (2016) 362:232–9. doi:10.1016/j.jns.2016.01.045
127. Contreras R, Ghajar J, Bahar S, Suh M. Effect of cognitive load on eye-target synchronization during smooth pursuit eye movement. *Brain Res* (2011) 1398:55–63. doi:10.1016/j.brainres.2011.05.004
128. Maruta J, Suh M, Niogi SN, Mukherjee P, Ghajar J. Visual tracking synchronization as a metric for concussion screening. *J Head Trauma Rehabil* (2010) 25:293–305. doi:10.1097/HTR.0b013e3181e67936
129. Suh M, Basu S, Kolster R, Sarkar R, McCandliss B, Ghajar J, et al. Increased oculomotor deficits during target blanking as an indicator of mild traumatic brain injury. *Neurosci Lett* (2006) 410:203–7. doi:10.1016/j.neulet.2006.10.001
130. Suh M, Kolster R, Sarkar R, McCandliss B, Ghajar J; Cognitive and Neurobiological Research Consortium. Deficits in predictive smooth pursuit after mild traumatic brain injury. *Neurosci Lett* (2006) 401:108–13. doi:10.1016/j.neulet.2006.02.074
131. Heitger MH, Anderson TJ, Jones RD, Dalrymple-Alford JC, Frampton CM, Ardagh MW. Eye movement and visuomotor arm movement deficits following mild closed head injury. *Brain* (2004) 127:575–90. doi:10.1093/brain/awh066
132. Heitger MH, Jones RD, Dalrymple-Alford JC, Frampton CM, Ardagh MW, Anderson TJ. Mild head injury – a close relationship between motor function at 1 week post-injury and overall recovery at 3 and 6 months. *J Neurol Sci* (2007) 253:34–47. doi:10.1016/j.jns.2006.11.007
133. Heitger MH, Jones RD, Dalrymple-Alford JC, Frampton CM, Ardagh MW, Anderson TJ. Motor deficits and recovery during the first year following mild closed head injury. *Brain Inj* (2006) 20:807–24. doi:10.1080/02699050600676354
134. Galetta KM, Chapman KR, Essis MD, Alosco ML, Gillard D, Steinberg E, et al. Screening utility of the King-Devick test in mild cognitive impairment and Alzheimer disease dementia. *Alzheimer Dis Assoc Disord* (2016) 31(2):152–8. doi:10.1097/WAD.0000000000000157
135. Boxer AL, Garbutt S, Seeley WW, Jafari A, Heuer HW, Mirsky J, et al. Saccade abnormalities in autopsy-confirmed frontotemporal lobar degeneration and Alzheimer disease. *Arch Neurol* (2012) 69:509–17. doi:10.1001/archneurol.2011.1021
136. Garbutt S, Matlin A, Hellmuth J, Schenk AK, Johnson JK, Rosen H, et al. Oculomotor function in frontotemporal lobar degeneration, related disorders and Alzheimer's disease. *Brain* (2008) 131:1268–81. doi:10.1093/brain/awn047
137. Heuer HW, Mirsky JB, Kong EL, Dickerson BC, Miller BL, Kramer JH, et al. Antisaccade task reflects cortical involvement in mild cognitive impairment. *Neurology* (2013) 81:1235–43. doi:10.1212/WNL.0b013e3182a6cbfe
138. Lee D, Poizner H, Corcos DM, Henriques DY. Unconstrained reaching modulates eye-hand coupling. *Exp Brain Res* (2014) 232:211–23. doi:10.1007/s00221-013-3732-9
139. Gorbet DJ, Sergio LE. The behavioural consequences of dissociating the spatial directions of eye and arm movements. *Brain Res* (2009) 1284:77–88. doi:10.1016/j.brainres.2009.05.057
140. Kaplan J, Hier DB. Visuospatial deficits after right hemisphere stroke. *Am J Occup Ther* (1982) 36:314–21. doi:10.5014/ajot.36.5.314
141. Coutte A, Olivier G, Faure S, Baccino T. Preparation of forefinger's sequence on keyboard orients ocular fixations on computer screen. *Cogn Process* (2014) 15:415–22. doi:10.1007/s10339-014-0612-6
142. Rand MK, Stelmach GE. Effects of hand termination and accuracy requirements on eye-hand coordination in older adults. *Behav Brain Res* (2011) 219:39–46. doi:10.1016/j.bbr.2010.12.008
143. Khan A, Song J, McPeek R. The eye dominates in guiding attention during simultaneous eye and hand movements. *J Vis* (2011) 11:9. doi:10.1167/11.1.9
144. Song JH, McPeek RM. Eye-hand coordination during target selection in a pop-out visual search. *J Neurophysiol* (2009) 102:2681–92. doi:10.1152/jn.91352.2008

20

A GABAergic Dysfunction in the Olivary–Cerebellar–Brainstem Network may Cause Eye Oscillations and Body Tremor. II. Model Simulations of Saccadic Eye Oscillations

Lance M. Optican and Elena Pretegiani*

Laboratory of Sensorimotor Research, IRP, National Eye Institute, National Institutes of Health, Bethesda, MD, United States

Correspondence:
Lance M. Optican
lanceoptican@nih.gov

Eye and body oscillations are shared features of several neurological diseases, yet their pathophysiology remains unclear. Recently, we published a report on two tennis players with a novel presentation of eye and body oscillations following self-administration of performance-enhancing substances. Opsoclonus/flutter and limb tremor were diagnosed in both patients. Common causes of opsoclonus/flutter were excluded. High-resolution eye movement recordings from one patient showed novel spindle-shaped, asymmetric saccadic oscillations (at ~3.6 Hz) and ocular tremor (~40–60 Hz). Based on these findings, we proposed that the oscillations are the result of increased $GABA_A$ receptor sensitivity in a circuit involving the cerebellum (vermis and fastigial nuclei), the inferior olives, and the brainstem saccade premotor neurons (excitatory and inhibitory burst neurons, and omnipause neurons). We present a mathematical model of the saccadic system, showing that the proposed dysfunction in the network can reproduce the types of saccadic oscillations seen in these patients.

Keywords: saccade, vermis, fastigial nuclei, inferior olive, omnipause neurons, eye movement, flutter, opsoclonus

INTRODUCTION

Oscillations of the head, body, limbs, or eyes characterize several neurological conditions. Nevertheless, their underlying mechanisms are not understood well enough to guide therapy (1). Oculo- and somatomotor systems are similarly organized, and some disorders involve both eye and body oscillations. The anatomy and physiology of the oculomotor system have been studied more than that of other systems. If we could understand ocular oscillations, it might provide insights into

---

Abbreviations: BN, SC burst neurons; BUN, SC buildup neurons; CB, cerebellum; cFN, caudal fastigial nucleus; cSC, caudal SC; EBN, excitatory burst neurons; GABA, γ-aminobutyric acid; PuC, Purkinje cells (vermis); Glu, glutamate; Gly, glycine; IBN, inhibitory burst neurons; IO, inferior olive; LIBN, long-lead inhibitory burst neurons; NRTP, nucleus reticularis tegmenti pontis; NRTPc, NRTP → contra OMV; NRTPi, NRTP → ipsi OMV; PF, parallel fiber; OMV, oculomotor vermis; OPN, omnipause neurons; PIR, post-inhibitory rebound; rSC, rostral SC; SC, superior colliculus; SWMSO, square-wave macrosaccadic oscillations; FOR, fastigial oculomotor region.

the pathophysiology of oscillatory dysfunctions of somatomotor circuits. Here, we present a mathematical model of the saccadic system that has sufficient anatomical and physiological detail to simulate saccadic eye oscillations in patients with opsoclonus. A model of ocular and limb tremor will be presented in a companion paper.

Previously, we studied two patients with a novel presentation of eye and body oscillations following self-administration of performance-enhancing substances (2). Opsoclonus consists of large saccadic oscillations lasting a few or many cycles, without intersaccadic intervals, around all three axes (3–6). If oscillations occur only in the horizontal plane it is called flutter. Opsoclonus can be triggered by both saccadic and non-saccadic eye movements, by eye closure, and can persist in the dark (7). How neural circuits generate these oscillations is not clear. Note that in our patient, there is a diverse range of waveforms, including opsoclonus (quasi-sinusoidal movements), square-wave oscillations, and square-pulse oscillations (**Figure 1**). Such a diversity of waveforms has been seen before, and it has been proposed that a common mechanism accounts for all the waveforms (8), but no mechanism has yet been proposed that can do so.

Opsoclonus arises in various diseases [including paraneoplastic, parainfectious, toxic-metabolic, and idiopathic causes (9)], thus one mechanism may not explain all forms of opsoclonus. Nonetheless, opsoclonus is often associated with cerebellar disease (10, 11). Saccades are generated by high-gain burst neurons that are gated by dominant, inhibitory neurons in the brainstem, which pause during saccades [omnipause neurons (OPN)]. Thus, Zee and Robinson (12) proposed that any saccadic oscillations without an intervening interval would require that the OPN be shut off.

Autopsy of one of Cogan's patients with opsoclonus found encephalitis with lymphocytic infiltration chiefly in the hypothalamus, midbrain, and pons (3). However, studies have shown no consistent pathology in the raphe interpositus (site of the OPN) in patients with opsoclonus (13). Although structural

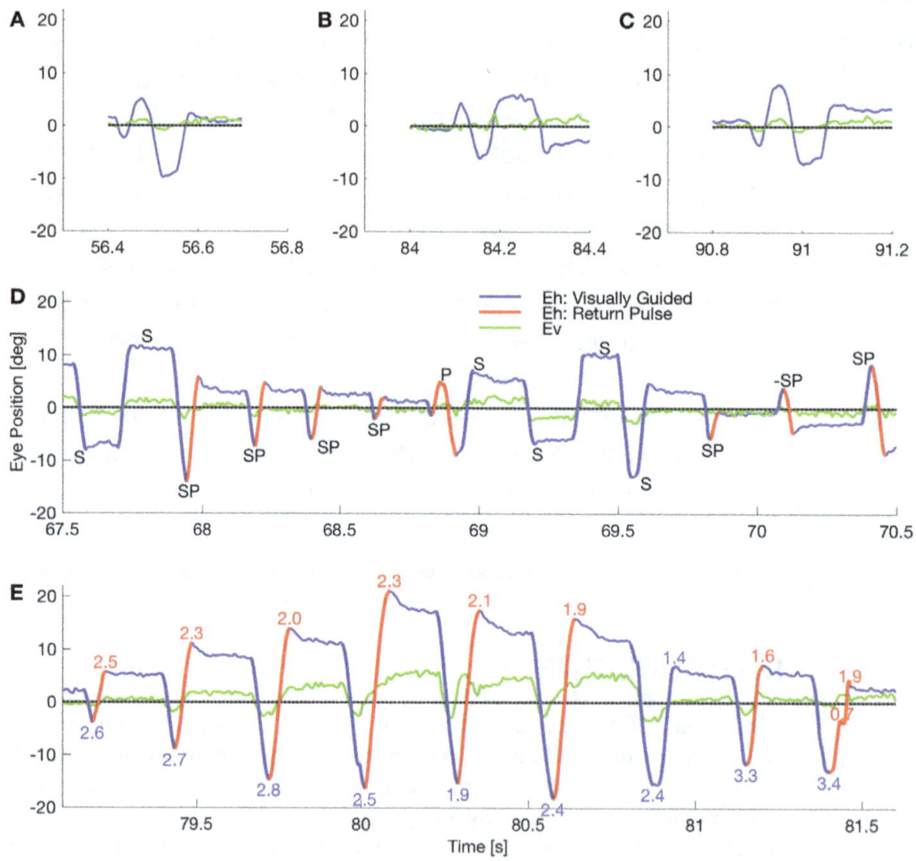

FIGURE 1 | Waveforms in a patient with opsoclonus. **(A–C)** The subject made few of the sinusoidal movements that classically define opsoclonus. There were occasional movements with 0.5–1.5 cycles, but these three movements were the longest oscillations in a fixation record that lasted 156 s. **(D)** The subject mostly made macrosaccadic square-wave oscillations (marked S), back-to-back oscillations with no intersaccadic intervals (pulses, marked P), and a combined half-square wave and pulse waveform (square-pulse, marked SP). Note that all these waveforms occurred within a 3 s window. The direction of the square-pulse oscillation suddenly reversed at about 70.15 s (marked −SP). Finally, the duration of a square-wave half-cycle can vary (e.g., the short cycle at ~69.6 s), suggesting that there is a spectrum from opsoclonus to square-pulse to square-wave oscillations. **(E)** The subject made several series of square-pulse oscillations with an increasing gain followed by a decreasing gain (indicated by the numbers at the extreme positions). This type of movement is called a *spindle*. Square-wave spindles are common in cerebellar disease, but this is the first square-pulse spindle to be reported. By comparing the timing of the horizontal and vertical eye movements in these panels, it is evident that the macroscopic movements are coupled.

imaging of the brain of opsoclonus patients has not shown any consistent abnormalities, functional imaging has been linked to increased activity in the fastigial nuclei (14). Oguro et al. (15) recorded SPECT images in two patients with opsoclonus and found hyperperfusion in the midline cerebellum (CB) in one, and hypoperfusion in the other patient.

At least three hypotheses for the pathomechanism of opsoclonus/flutter have been proposed, based on different clinical and experimental observations. One line of evidence would suggest a dysfunction of the cerebellar Purkinje cells (PuC). Mutant mice with a modified glutamate receptor on PuC show clustered PuC action potentials, likely induced by climbing fiber activation, and opsoclonus-like eye movements (16). Jen et al. (17) found antibodies to PuC in patients with opsoclonus. They proposed that those antibodies blocked the parallel fiber (PF) input to PuC, allowing spontaneous oscillations generated in the inferior olives (IO) to be passed to the oculomotor vermis through the flocculus.

Alternatively, disinhibition of caudal fastigial nuclei (cFN) might induce unwanted saccades through excitatory projections to brainstem burst neurons (6, 14). Wong et al. (6) modified a lumped model of the saccadic system by adding a negative feedback path from a high pass filtered efference copy of eye position, through the ipsilateral cFN, to the motor error comparator. When the delay and the gain of this feedback pathway were increased (to 20 ms and ~8.5, respectively) to simulate disinhibition of the cFN, ~15 Hz sinusoidal oscillations occurred. However, this mechanism cannot explain how the brain generates non-sinusoidal saccadic oscillations, such as square waves, square pulses, and spindles. This mechanism also does not suggest how a disease process could change the loop's delay by 20 ms, or raise its gain from normal (~0.7) to ~8, or how it could hold off the OPN, which prevent saccades. Furthermore, lesions of the vermis that disinhibit the cFN cause hypometric saccades, not oscillations (18, 19).

A third idea is that reduction of glycinergic inhibition generates oscillations in the positive feedback loop between left and right saccadic brainstem inhibitory burst neurons (20). This gives rise to small, sinusoidal oscillations, but alone would not be enough to simulate all the waveforms seen in opsoclonus. Thus, none of these theories have been fully supported by lesion studies in animals, clinical findings, or model simulations (21).

Unfortunately, high temporal resolution recordings of eye movements from patients with opsoclonus/flutter, analysis of which could clarify the underlying mechanisms, are extremely rare, because of the difficulty in recording them (given the severity of the clinical symptoms and/or the inability to calibrate the recordings). In our previous study (2), a detailed analysis of one patient's movements (**Figure 1**) suggested that ocular oscillations might be generated by a dysfunction of the cerebellar–olivary–brainstem network.

That patient had taken anabolic–androgenic steroids (AAS), which are allosteric modulators of $GABA_A$ receptors ($GABA_AR$), with both acute and chronic effects. These effects can enhance or diminish the sensitivity of the chloride channel to γ-aminobutyric acid (GABA), depending on the receptor's subunit composition and the GABA concentration at the synaptic level (22, 23). We shall assume that in our patient, the AAS increased the gain of the chloride current in the $GABA_AR$ (24). Indeed, the key point of our model is that opsoclonus requires increased inhibition of oculomotor vermis (OMV), cFN, and OPN. Increased inhibition of cFN is not necessarily incompatible with the finding of increased BOLD or fMRI signal of cFN during opsoclonus (14). Increasing cFN inhibition does not necessarily mean that they fire less. As we will see below, in our model the main effect of increasing cFN inhibition is to delay its burst onset, which could be tested in animal models. Thus, even if cFN excitability were significantly reduced, the intense saccadic activity during opsoclonus oscillations (averaged over time) would increase the blood flow and oxygen consumption of the cFN. Our hypothesis of inhibitory receptor dysfunction is very different from prior models, wherein the hypothesis was either damage to the OPN, or damage to the CB causing hyperactivation of the cFN. This is also consistent with the lack of evidence of damage to the CB and pons in opsoclonus. Here, we present model simulations of the cerebellar–olivary–brainstem network that support our hypothesis.

SUBJECTS AND METHODS

Two patients described in our previous article (2) developed opsoclonus/flutter after self-administration of performance-enhancing substances. This study was carried out in accordance with the recommendations of the ethics committee of the University of Siena, Italy. All subjects gave written informed consent in accordance with the Declaration of Helsinki. The ethics committee of the University of Siena, Italy, approved this study. Briefly, neuro-ophthalmological examinations revealed horizontal saccadic intrusions and intermittent ocular flutter. Both patients' brain MRI were normal. CSF showed few oligoclonal bands. Common infectious, toxic, paraneoplastic, and metabolic causes of opsoclonus/flutter were excluded by negative blood and CSF exams. No tumors were found.

Both patients reported a few months of abuse of substances to improve performance. Patients stopped using the drugs after the symptoms began. Patient 1 provided a sample of the compound for testing, which led to the identification of the AAS nandrolone, stanozolol, and testosterone propionate. Treatment with intravenous IgG and benzodiazepine led to recovery in 3–4 weeks in both patients.

Eye Movement Recording

Eye movement recording during fixation, horizontal (10 and 18° amplitudes), and vertical (8°) saccades was possible in patient 2 because he had inter-oscillatory intervals of steady fixation that allowed a satisfactory calibration. Eye position was recorded at 240 Hz with an ASL 504 eye-tracker device (Applied Science Laboratories, Bedford, MA, USA). All analyses were performed with custom Matlab (The Mathworks, Natick, MA, USA) scripts.

Model

A new model was created by extending the saccadic system model used to simulate eye movement disorders in a cerebellar patient (25). The basic architecture is an *adaptive, velocity feedback, integral controller, but without a motor error comparator*

(**Figure 2**). For simplicity, only the horizontal direction of saccades is modeled. Both the superior colliculi (SCs) and the caudal fastigial nuclei (cFN) drive the brainstem premotor burst neurons [PBN; consisting of the short-lead excitatory burst neurons (EBN), inhibitory burst neurons (IBN), and long-lead inhibitory burst neurons (LIBN)]. An efference copy of eye velocity (from the EBN) is fed back to the OMV, which projects to the fastigial oculomotor region in the cFN, closing the loop. A pause in activity starts at a locus in the contraversive (with respect to the saccade direction, e.g., left side for a rightward saccade) OMV corresponding to the amount of drive that the cFN should provide for an individual saccade, based on the context of the movement. If the saccade does not get on target, the CB learns to initiate the pause at a different locus under the same context the next time (26–28). At saccade start, the OMV activity at the initial locus pauses, releasing the contraversive cFN from inhibition. The cFN then fires, exciting the ipsiversive EBN and IBN. During the saccade, a wave of inhibition (driven by feedback of a velocity efference copy from the EBN) spreads across the OMV. Thus, the OMV acts as a spatial integrator of eye velocity. When the inhibition spreads to the ipsiversive OMV, it disinhibits the ipsiversive cFN, which activates the contraversive IBN. The contraversive IBN then inhibits the ipsiversive EBN and IBN. This stops the movement. At this point, the excitation from the ipsiversive cFN also reactivates the OPN. The EBN and IBN have a very high gain, thus, without OPN reactivation the saccade would be followed by an oscillation of back-to-back saccades with no intersaccadic interval. The caption to **Figure 2** gives a color-coded explanation of how the model makes a saccade. Details of the model are given in the Appendix in Supplementary Material.

Although our main hypothesis is that opsoclonus results from an increased sensitivity of $GABA_AR$, here we simulate a lumped model. This is necessary for two reasons. First, we think that the opsoclonus is caused by abnormal levels of activity in a large network, encompassing the CB, IO, and brainstem. Second, to understand the effects of the $GABA_AR$ dysfunction at the biophysical level, we would need to know the types of subunits that make up the receptor in the diverse types of neurons in the circuit, in particular, their gains and time constants. Unfortunately, these values are unknown. Thus, we implement the suspected changes in $GABA_AR$ function simply by changing various gains in a lumped model. Details of which gains are changed are given with each of the simulations in the Section "Results." Model parameters are given in **Table 1**, and parameters for the different neuron types are given in **Table 2**.

RESULTS

Normal Saccades

This model assumes that microsaccades (<2°) and macrosaccades (≥2°) are made by the same circuit (29–32). It can simulate

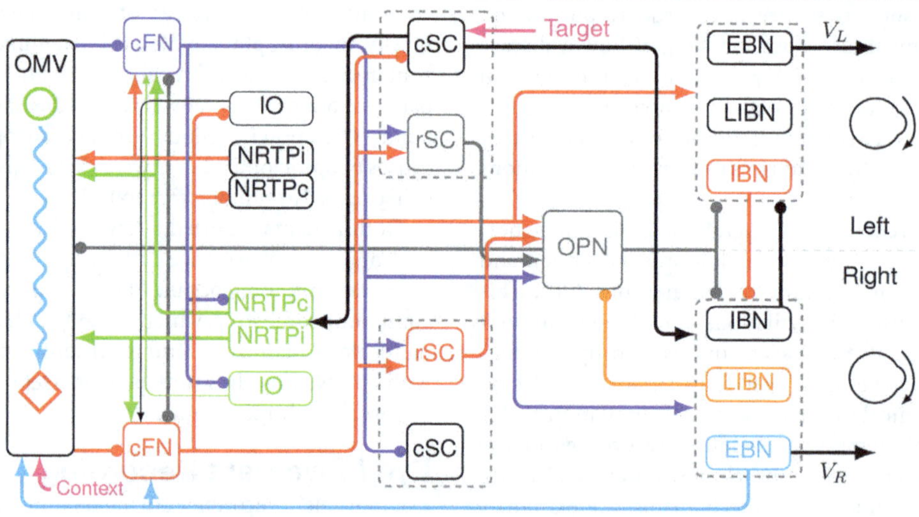

FIGURE 2 | Schematic of a neuromimetic model of the saccadic system, showing the connections needed to make a rightward eye movement. Before the movement, the oculomotor vermis (OMV), the cFN, both rostral SC (rSC) and omnipause neurons (OPN) are on (gray lines), and the premotor burst neurons (PBN) are off. At the start of a rightward saccade, cerebral cortex sends target information to the left caudal SC (cSC) (magenta arrow). The left cSC begins to fire (black line), which inhibits the rSC and excites the right excitatory burst neurons (EBN), inhibitory burst neurons (IBN), and long-lead inhibitory burst neurons (LIBN). However, the OPN are holding the EBN and IBN off. The right LIBN, however, are not held off, and they inhibit the OPN (orange line), allowing the right EBN and IBN to fire, which starts the movement. The left cSC also drives the right nucleus reticularis tegmenti pontis (NRTP), which inhibits the left OMV (at a locus determined by context, magenta arrow) and excites both cFN (green lines). The left cFN begins driving the right PBN (blue lines). As the movement proceeds, an efference copy of eye velocity is fed back from the right EBN to the OMV (cyan line). This causes a wave of inhibition to spread to the right across the OMV (cyan wavy line). Connectivity in the vermis must be left–right symmetric, because it must make saccades in both directions. The spread is not symmetric because the feedback signal is a rightward velocity, which causes the spread to be to the right only. When the wave of inhibition reaches the location corresponding to the ending point of the saccade on the right side of the OMV (red diamond), the right cFN is disinhibited (red line). The right cFN excites the left PBN overcoming the inhibition by the right PBN. The left IBN comes on and inhibits the right PBN, choking off the drive to the right motor neurons and stopping the movement. The OPN and rSC reactivate, because of the right cFN input, preventing saccadic oscillations and holding the eyes on target.

TABLE 1 | Important model parameters.

Parameter	Value	Function (units)	Parameter	Value	Function (units)
SynDel	0.0008	Synaptic delay (s)	NI G	20	Neural integrator gain
VisDelay	0.05	Visual delay (s)	NI Tc	20	Neural integrator time constant (s)
Refrac	0.2	Refractory disable (s)	Plant Te	0.008	Small plant time constant (s)
ErrThr	0.5	Retinal error threshold (°)	SC Gdisfa	2	Disfacilitation gain from cFN
MaxDis	800	Maximum discharge rate (sp/s)	SC Tdisfa	0.025	cFN disfacilitation time constant (s)
BrstDel	0.05	SC burst delay (s)	SC Gx	1	cSC cross-inhibitory gain
IO G_l	1	IO low pass gain	SC Tx	0.01	cSC cross-inhibitory time constant (s)
IO Tc	0.1	IO low pass time constant (s)	rSC Delay	0.05	Delay time before burst (s)
IO I_u	5	IO output upper limit	OMV Gp	1	Cerebellar plant model gain
IO I_l	0.1	IO output lower limit	OMV Tp	0.008	Cerebellar plant model time constant (s)
IO P_W	0 or 1	IO noise power	OMV T_f	0.25	OMV fatigue time constant (s)
IO G_W	1	IO noise gain	OMV G_l	0.5	OMV fatigue low pass gain
IO T_W	0.002	IO noise time constant (s)	OMV T_l	1.5	OMV fatigue low pass time constant (s)
IO F_{io}	30	IO sine frequency (Hz)	OMV C_l	0.5	OMV fatigue clip low
IO G_{io}	0.35	IO sine gain	OMV C_u	1	OMV fatigue clip high
OMV G_f	0.34	OMV fatigue gain	OMV G_{lk}	0.5	OMV leaky integrator gain
LIBN G_{rsc}	6	Inhibitory gain from rSC to LIBN	OMV T_{lk}	0.5	OMV leaky integrator time constant (s)
OPN G_{rsc}	3	Excitatory gain from rSC to OPN	IBN2EBN	1.2	Gain from IBN to EBN
OPN Tone	200	Bias on OPN	IBN2IBN	0.3	Gain from IBN to contra IBN
cFN2EBN	0.5	Gain from cFN to contra EBN	IBN2LIBN	200	Gain from IBN to LIBN
cFN2IBN	50	Gain from cFN to contra IBN	EBN2IBN	0.01	Gain from EBN to ipsi IBN

LIBN, long-lead inhibitory burst neurons; EBN, excitatory burst neurons; IBN, inhibitory burst neurons; OPN, omnipause neurons; IO, inferior olive; SC, superior colliculus; OMV, oculomotor vermis; cSC, caudal SC; rSC, rostral SC.

TABLE 2 | Model parameters for different neuron types.

Parameter	EBN	IBN	LIBN	OPN	cFN	rSC	cSC
Gain	1.000	1.000	1.000	1.000	1.000	1.000	1.000
Time constant (s)	0.002	0.002	0.003	0.002	0.003	0.010	0.010
Adaptation gain	0.050	0.050	0.000	0.010	0.000	1.000	1.000
Adaptation TC (s)	0.100	0.100	0.010	0.006	0.003	0.006	0.006
Inhibitory gain	4.000	12.000	0.015	1.000	2.000	0.100	15.000
Excitatory gain	1.000	0.800	1.000	1.000	1.000	1.000	3.100
OPN gain	10.000	100.00	0.000	0.000	0.000	1.000	1.000

EBN, excitatory burst neurons; IBN, inhibitory burst neurons; LIBN, long-lead inhibitory burst neurons; OPN, omnipause neurons; cSC, caudal SC; rSC, rostral SC.

amplitudes from 0.5 to 50° in both leftward and rightward directions (Figure S1 in Supplementary Material). For amplitudes above 10°, the cortical circuit assumes that the actual goal of the saccade is only 90% of the target jump. Thus, for large saccades, the model undershoots the target but automatically makes corrective saccades to get on target.

A simulated eye movement and the activity in major model neurons are shown in **Figure 3**. In this highly simplified, one-dimensional, model of the CB, we can see the latency differences between contra- and ipsiversive OMV and cFN bursts (33–35). Indeed, it is our central hypothesis of saccadic system function that the role of the oculomotor vermis is to create this timing difference (26–28). To simulate all three dimensions of opsoclonus (horizontal, vertical, and torsional), the model presented here would have to be duplicated, once for each axis.

Opsoclonus/Flutter

Opsoclonus/flutter oscillations can exhibit many waveforms. For example, **Figure 1** shows eye movements recorded in one session while patient 2 was fixating (abscissa shows time in seconds from the beginning of a single record). **Figures 1A–C** show examples of the quasi-sinusoidal movements that define classic opsoclonus. Examples of largely horizontal square-wave macrosaccadic oscillations (SWMSO, half-cycles in blue, marked S), a pulse saccadic oscillation without an intersaccadic interval (red, P), and combined half-cycles of SWMSO followed without an intersaccadic interval by a return saccade, which we call a square-pulse oscillation (SP), are shown in **Figure 1D**. These different waveforms occurred over an interval of just 3 s. We also see an example where the square-pulse changes direction from rightward to leftward (marked −SP). Note that there seems to be a continuum of intersaccadic interval durations (e.g., saccade marked S at about 69.55 s), thus the difference between opsoclonus, square-wave and square-pulse oscillations may only be due to a small change in a few parameters. The vertical component of the eye movement (green) is small but is phase-locked to the horizontal movement. This phase locking is characteristic of opsoclonus. Square-pulse oscillations have been recorded before in patients with opsoclonus, although not commented upon (6, 14).

Figure 1E shows a 2.5 s example of a square-pulse oscillation that grows in amplitude for about 1 s, and then decreases in amplitude [numbers at each extremum indicate gain of the movement, assuming that the eye is trying to get back to the central fixation target (gray line)]. As in **Figure 1D**, the vertical eye movement is phase locked to the horizontal eye movement. Because of the shape of the movement envelope, these types of oscillations are called *spindles*.

Figure 1 also reveals an asymmetry in the oscillations. In **Figures 1D,E**, we see that the saccades to the left usually have higher gains than those to the right. We infer from this that the left cFN projections to the right IBN and OPN are weaker than the right cFN projections to the left IBN and OPN, causing a delay in stopping the leftward saccade.

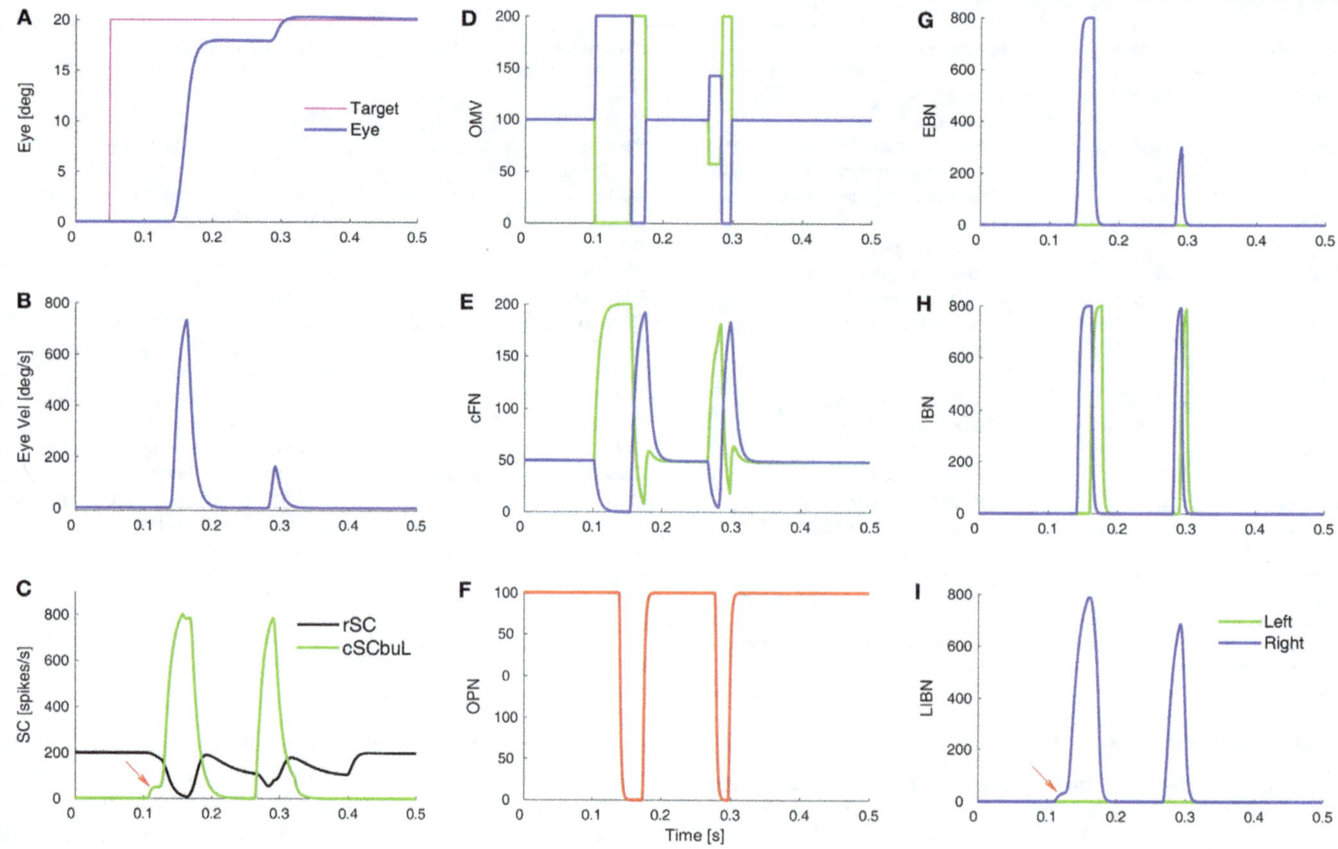

FIGURE 3 | Simulation of a normal saccade to target at 20°, showing time courses of activity in different model areas. **(A,B)** The eye position and velocity traces. **(C)** The activity of burst neurons (BN) in the rostral SC (rSC) and buildup neurons (BUN) in the left caudal SC (cSC). Red arrow indicates the small pre-saccadic buildup of activity (cSC burst neurons are not shown, as they are the same as the buildup neurons, but without the small buildup). **(D)** The activity of the lumped oculomotor vermis (OMV). For a rightward saccade, the left OMV (green) pauses first, followed by the right OMV (blue). **(E)** Activity in the contraversive (green) and ipsiversive (blue) cFN, which are inhibited by their respective OMV. The critical point is that when the ipsiversive cFN (blue) turns on it drives the contraversive inhibitory burst neurons (IBN) on **(H)**. The left IBN's reactivation stops the saccade. **(F)** Activity of the omnipause neurons (OPN). **(G)** Activity of the excitatory burst neurons (EBN). **(H)** Activity of the IBN. **(I)** The long-lead inhibitory burst neurons (LIBN) are turned on when the cSC BUN activity begins building up (red arrow), because they are not inhibited by the OPN, but the LIBN inhibit the OPN. Ordinate scale for neuronal activity is simulated spikes per second.

Tests of Two Prior Hypotheses

Here, we use the new model to test the hypothesis that fastigial disinhibition by Purkinje cell malfunction results in saccadic oscillations, as in the Wong et al. (6) model. In their model, the role of the CB is like that of most models, in that it accelerates the saccade and stops it on target (26, 27, 36). In their simulations, macrosaccadic flutter (back-to-back saccades with no intersaccadic interval) occurs when the loss of OMV inhibition of the cFN increases the gain and the delay in the feedback loop around the brainstem and through the cFN. Their model cannot make other types of oscillations, such as SWMSO, tremor, or square-pulse oscillations. It also faces problems pointed out with the similar Zee and Robinson model (12), in that to make oscillations requires a change in the loop delay that must be set according to the patient's oscillation frequency, which can cover a very wide range (37).

In the present model, the CB helps accelerate and steer the saccade, and then stops it on target, but it is an adaptive, velocity feedback, integral controller, and not a motor error controller (i.e., its goal is not to reduce the motor error to 0). However, oscillations are controlled by membrane properties of neurons, and not loop delays (37, 38). Our model behaves differently from that of Wong et al. because its OMV and cFN essentially act as a switching network to control the timing of when the ipsiversive and contraversive EBN and IBN turn on and off. Intuition can help us understand a linear feedback controller, but intuition is not helpful in a switching/timing model. Thus, we need simulations to understand the effects of $GABA_A$R dysfunction in these models.

Before a saccade starts, the locus of initial inhibition in the OMV must be determined (**Figure 2**, green circle). As the saccade progresses, a wave of inhibition must spread across the OMV (cyan wavy line) until it reaches the ipsiversive side (**Figure 2**, red diamond), disinhibiting the ipsiversive cFN. **Figure 4** shows the effect of making the OMV less active than normal. This will cause the ipsiversive cFN to restart too soon, and the saccade (**Figure 4B**) will be smaller than normal (**Figure 4A**). This result contradicts the hypothesis of Wong et al. but is consistent with

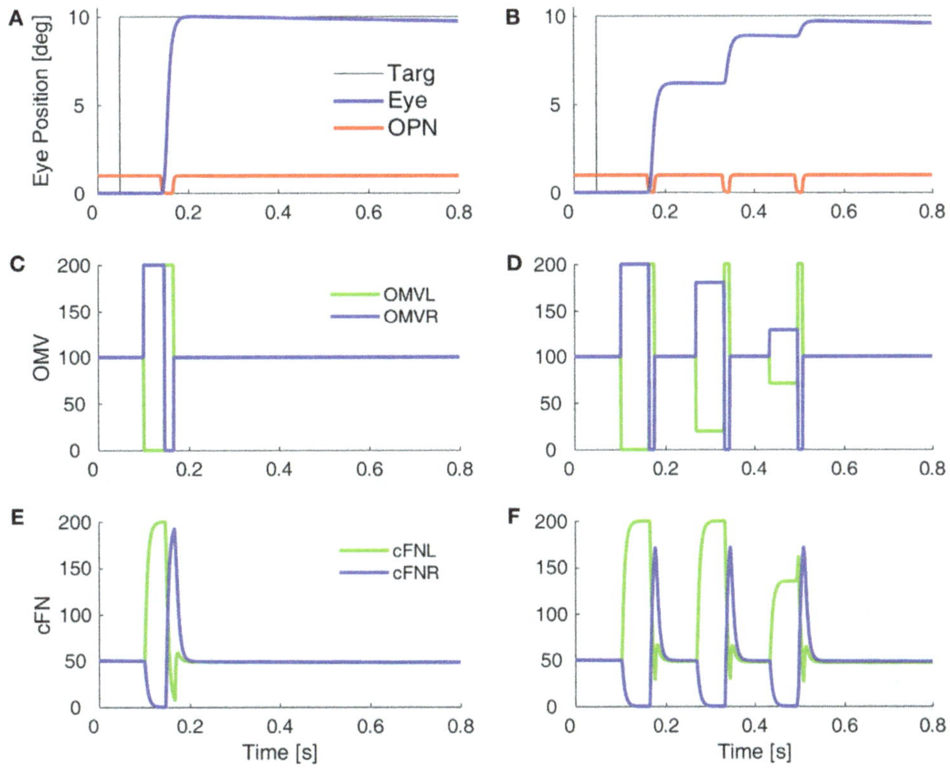

FIGURE 4 | Simulation of loss of vermal inhibition onto fastigial nuclei, i.e., the hypothesis of Wong et al. (6). In our model, loss of oculomotor vermis (OMV) inhibition will cause the ipsiversive cFN to turn on too soon. In the simulation, to get the ipsiversive cFN to start too soon, we increased the gain of the forward model of the plant in the OMV (from 1 to 300), which caused a rapid spread of inhibition from contraversive to ipsiversive, so that the ipsiversive OMV turn off too soon. One might expect this to result in hypermetric saccades, or even oscillations. However, in our model, the OMV play a very different role than in Wong et al.'s model. Importantly, the ipsiversive OMV determines the duration of the saccade. **(A)** Saccade with normal OMV activity. **(B)** Saccade with reduced OMV activity. The saccades are hypometric, because the right cFN is not adequately inhibited and thus reactivates too soon. The OMV activity **(C,D)** and the cFN activity **(E,F)** on the left and right sides.

neurophysiological results, which found that cerebellar vermis lesions result in hypometria, not opsoclonus or sinusoidal oscillations (18, 19).

Another hypothesis of how opsoclonus might be generated suggests that antibodies block PF to PuC synapses, thus reducing inhibition on the flocculus. This allows spontaneous oscillatory activity in the IOs to be passed to the ocular motor nuclei (17). This hypothesis has already been tested in the context of oculopalatal tremor (OPT) (39, 40). OPT has waveforms that look like large, random oscillations, but the movements around each axis are independent. These studies showed that if oscillatory activity from a normal IO projected through the flocculus to the brainstem, the resulting eye movements were very small and had pulsatile waveforms. The development of OPT required a pulsatile oscillator (caused by abnormally tight electrotonic coupling in the IO), and a learned response from the cerebellar cortex to enhance the movement's gain. Thus, these results suggest that IO oscillations would not, alone, be enough to cause saccadic oscillations in opsoclonus.

Square-Wave Macrosaccadic Oscillations

Figure 1D shows an example of SWMSO in our patient (marked S). SWMSO and spindles also occur in cerebellar disorders (41). Thus, we look for the effects of an increased gain of $GABA_AR$ in the CB as the mechanism for causing SWMSO. In the Wong et al. (6) model, the cFN, but not the OMV, is inside the feedback loop, so loss of OMV inhibition to the cFN causes the loop gain to increase. They also had to significantly increase the loop delay (no mechanism for which was proposed). In our model, the behavior is very different, because both the cFN and the OMV are inside the feedback loop and the $GABA_AR$ dysfunction results in an increased inhibition in both structures.

Purkinje cells are GABAergic, and we assume that increasing the gain of $GABA_AR$ in the OMV would mitigate the loss of GABA from the PuC when they become inhibited at saccade start. This would have the effect of slowing the spread of inhibition during the saccade. Thus, to simulate SWMSO, we reduced the gain of the feedback integration within the OMV (**Figure 5A**). Here, the saccade gains are less than twice normal size, so they decay in size as the oscillation progresses. Also shown is the gain of the fatigue circuit in the CB, which reduces the gain if neuronal activity is too high for too long. In this case, the fatigue gain declines only slightly during the oscillation (green line).

Figure 5B shows the effect of lowering the OMV feedback gain further, which makes the saccade gain higher, and the circuit unstable. The saccade gain is more than twice normal size, and

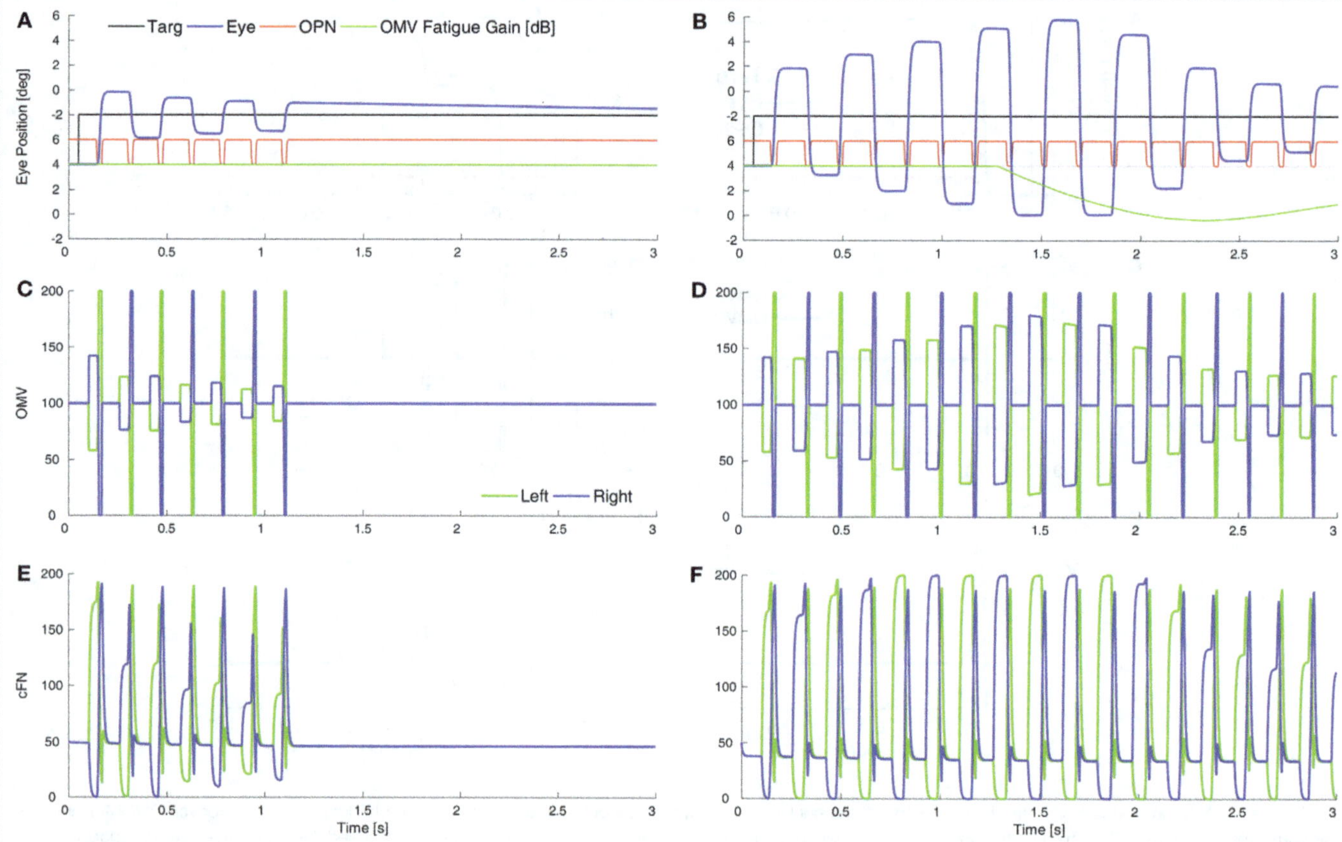

FIGURE 5 | Simulation of square-wave macrosaccadic oscillations (SWMSO). **(A)** A saccade to a 2° target jump. To simulate an increase of inhibition at the $GABA_A$ receptors ($GABA_AR$) in the oculomotor vermis (OMV), the cerebellar forward plant model gain was reduced from 1 to 0.075, as if the reduction in γ-aminobutyric acid (GABA) inhibition of Purkinje cells was less pronounced, and thus the spread of inhibition across the OMV was slower than normal. The inhibitory gain from the OMV to the cFN was increased from 2.0 to 2.01. The gain of the resultant saccade's amplitude is almost twice the target amplitude, causing SWMSO. During the oscillation, the gain of the cerebellar fatigue circuit drops very slightly (green line). The oscillations decay because the loop gain is less than 2.0. **(B)** The OMV and cFN $GABA_AR$ gains are increased even more (represented as a forward plant gain of 0.025, and a cFN inhibitory gain of 2.12), so that the saccadic gain becomes greater than 2. This results in growing oscillations. However, neuronal fatigue (green line) decreases the gain, damping the oscillation, resulting in an SWMSO spindle. **(C,D)** The activity in the simulated OMV and **(E,F)** the activity in the cFN.

the oscillations grow for a few saccades. However, the high rate of firing and high frequency of saccades result in marked fatigue of the cerebellar activity (green line), and the saccades begin to shrink. The envelope of the oscillation looks like a spindle.

Although the cFN activity is delayed relative to normal during each saccade, the cFN activity over the whole oscillation is very high. This is consistent with findings from imaging studies that the midline CB (**Figures 5C,D**) and deep cerebellar nuclei (**Figures 5E,F**) are strongly activated during opsoclonus (14, 15).

It is important to note the difference between the results in **Figure 4** (hypometria) and **Figure 5** (hypermetria). In **Figure 4**, we *increased* the gain of the OMV's forward model of the plant (from 1 to 300), which caused a rapid spread of inhibition from contraversive to ipsiversive. This caused the ipsiversive OMV to turn off too soon (removal of OMV inhibition is Wong et al.'s hypothesis), allowing the ipsiversive cFN to turn on too soon, resulting in hypometria. In **Figure 5**, we *decreased* the forward model's gain to represent increased $GABA_AR$ activity in OMV, thus slowing the spread of inhibition across the OMV and resulting in hypermetria.

Square-Pulse Macrosaccadic Oscillations and Ocular Flutter

One of the unusual waveforms found in our patient is the square-pulse oscillation (SP in **Figure 1D**). To simulate this waveform requires two sets of changes. First, the saccades must be hypermetric (as in **Figure 5**). In addition, it is necessary to delay the onset of the OPN in one direction (here, after leftward saccades). Thus, a rightward movement results in a hypermetric saccade that is followed by a hypermetric leftward saccade. However, after the leftward saccade, the OPN reactivation is delayed, resulting in a return movement with no intersaccadic interval, driven by post-inhibitory rebound (PIR) in the brainstem EBN. Importantly, PIR of the EBN must last at least as long as the return pulse, making the adaptation time constant, T_a, an important parameter (Figure S2 in Supplementary Material). A short delay of OPN reactivation (magenta) allows for a half-cycle (tick marks and red part of trace) of ocular flutter (**Figure 6A**). If the reactivation of the OPN is further delayed, three half-cycles of flutter can be obtained (**Figure 6B**). In addition, if the CB does not shut down after the saccade to the left, the OMV and

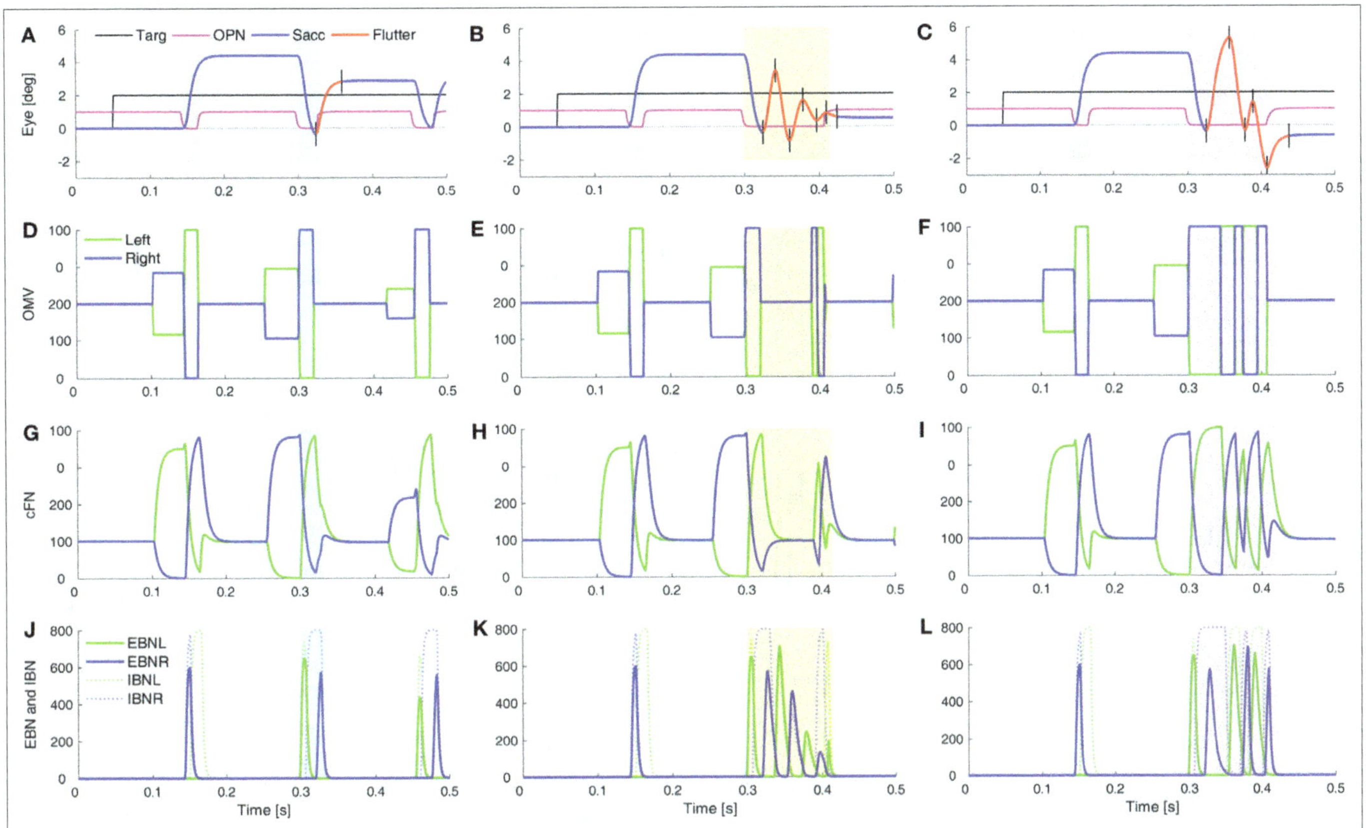

FIGURE 6 | Simulation of post-saccadic oscillations (flutter). Saccades were made hypermetric by changes as in **Figure 5**. In addition, the reactivation of omnipause neurons (OPN) (magenta) was delayed for leftward saccades (blue rectangles), but not rightward saccades (green rectangles). **(A)** The effect of a slower reactivation of OPN (magenta, delay increased from 10 to 22 ms) resulted in a half-cycle of large amplitude ocular flutter (back-to-back saccades with no intersaccadic intervals) after the leftward saccade (black tick marks and red trace). **(B)** If the reactivation of OPN is delayed even more (to 100 ms), more cycles (here, three half-cycles) of ocular flutter occur. The cerebellum (CB) has become quiescent, so the flutter is driven only by post-inhibitory rebound in the brainstem. **(C)** Similar to panel **(B)**, but the CB was not inhibited during the oscillations, so the oculomotor vermis (OMV) and cFN also contributed to the flutter, making it larger than the flutter in panel **(B)**. **(D–F)** The activity in the simulated OMV, **(G–I)** the activity in the cFN, and **(J–L)** the activity in the excitatory burst neurons (EBN) and inhibitory burst neurons (IBN).

cFN can participate in the oscillation, increasing its amplitude (**Figure 6C** and compare **Figures 6E,F**). Thus, random fluctuations in the delay until reactivation of the OPN, and whether or not there is cerebellar involvement, can account for the varying size and number of saccadic pulse waveforms in opsoclonus. Experimental studies will be needed to determine whether EBN PIR and oscillations in the CB contribute to ocular flutter.

What might cause the delay of the OPN reactivation? Under our hypothesis, the opsoclonus is caused by an abnormally high GABA$_A$R gain. If the cFN were abnormally inhibited, saccades would be hypermetric, because the ipsiversive cFN would not turn on in time to stop the saccade on target. They might also be too weak to turn the OPN back on at the end of the saccade. OPN receive both GABA and Gly inhibitory transmitters (42). If their GABA$_A$R currents were also enhanced, it might take more excitation to reactivate the OPN, causing them to turn on late. This is consistent with the inference from **Figure 1** that the left cFN is weaker than the right cFN.

If the OPN reactivation is delayed even more, as may happen during blinks or large off-vertical saccades (37), ocular flutter (back-to-back saccades with no intersaccadic interval) occurs (as in **Figure 6B**). Pathological flutter has been associated with lesions in the region of the OPN, and with lesions of the projection from cFN to the brainstem (43, 44). Here, we see that the functional effect that causes flutter is the delay in reactivation of the OPN.

Figure 7 shows a combination of the effect of lowering cerebellar feedback gain and fatigue (as in **Figure 5**) and slowing OPN reactivation (as in **Figure 6**). This results in a square-pulse oscillation spindle (**Figure 7A**, like the one in **Figure 1E**). Here, the OPN are only delayed after leftward saccades. In **Figure 7B**, we simulate a classic opsoclonus oscillation by delaying OPN after both leftward and rightward saccades. This simulation looks very much like the patient's eye movement in **Figure 1B**. The patient's quasi-sinusoidal oscillations were usually short (0.5–2.5 cycles), with amplitude about 5–10°. There were very few of these movements, compared to square-pulse oscillations. Importantly, these waveforms are not pure sinusoids. They appear to be back-to-back saccades, which is how they were simulated.

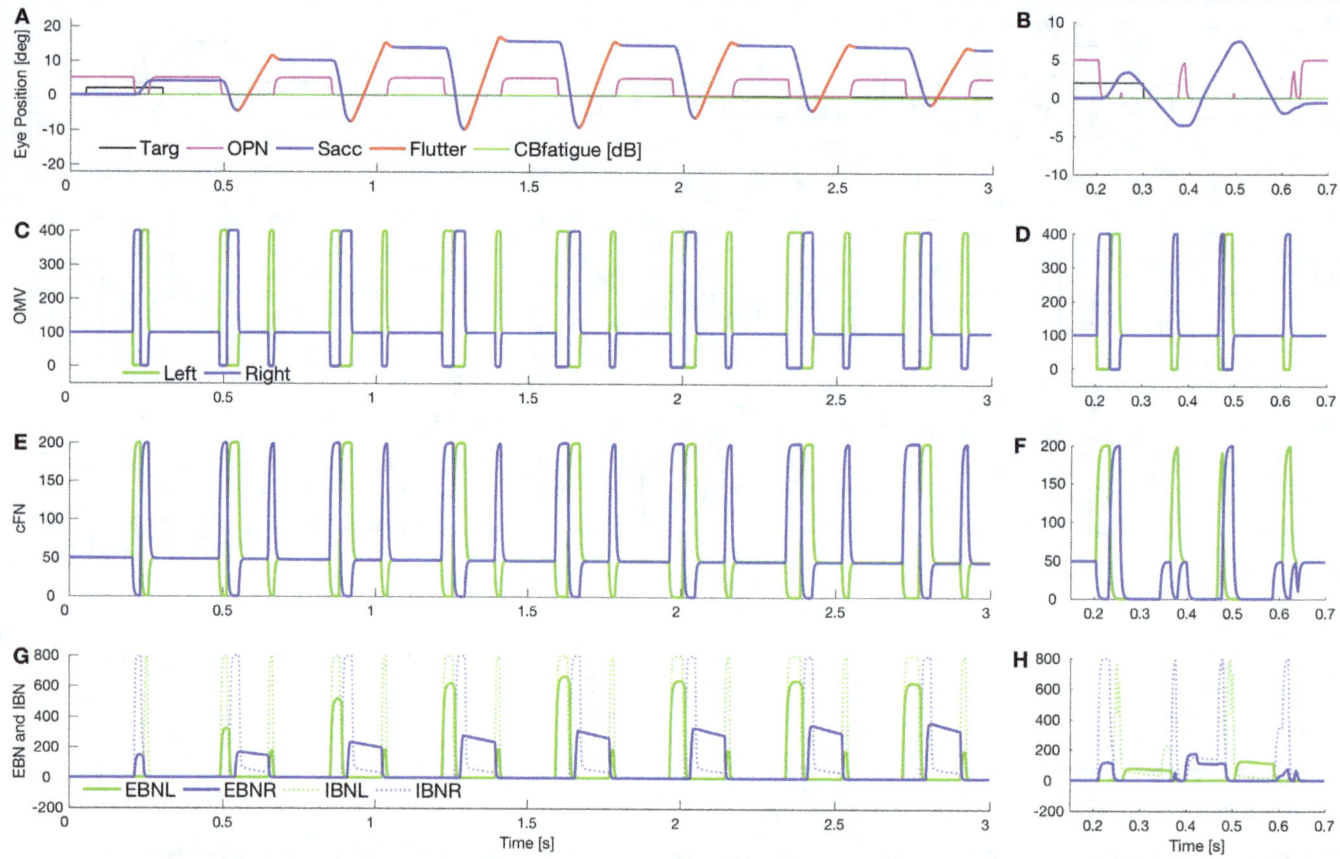

FIGURE 7 | Simulation of square-pulse spindle and opsoclonus. **(A)** Increasing omnipause neurons (OPN) (magenta) reactivation time (to 134 ms) after leftward saccades, and increasing the excitatory burst neurons (EBN) adaptation gain (from 0.05 to 0.01) and time constant (from 100 to 500 ms) gives a spindle-shaped square-pulse waveform with a small dynamic overshoot, like the movement in **Figure 1E**. The first rightward saccade and all the leftward saccades were visually guided (blue), but with a higher than normal gain [oculomotor vermis (OMV) feedback gain reduced from 1.0 to 0.5, making saccadic gain about 2.2]. After each leftward saccade, a half-cycle of flutter to the right (red) brought the eye back but ended beyond the target. The effect combination of higher gain and fatigue (as in **Figure 5B**) causes the spindle shape. **(B)** Simulation of a true opsoclonus waveform, similar to that in **Figure 1B**. The delay of OPN reactivation was increased to 100 ms after both leftward and rightward saccades. Note that neither in the patient nor in the simulation is the waveform a pure sinusoid. This suggests that opsoclonus is actually caused by a series of back-to-back saccades. As OPN recovery time varies, the exact shape of the waveform will vary from quasi-sinusoidal to square wave. **(C,D)** Activity in the simulated OMV. **(E,F)** Activity in the cFN. **(G,H)** Activity in the EBN and inhibitory burst neurons (IBN). Note the pulse part of the waveform is caused by post-inhibitory rebound of the EBN [right only in panel **(G)**, both left and right in panel **(H)**].

DISCUSSION

The purpose of this model is to show the possible interactions between brain circuits that determine eye movement waveforms. We found that it is not the absolute level of activity, but the relative timing of different areas in the brain, which is important. Here, although the activities in the lumped neurons have highly simplified waveforms, they have the correct timing.

The main predictions of this model are that opsoclonus saccadic waveforms can result from increased GABA inhibition of neurons in the vermis, fastigial nuclei, and brainstem (omnipause and burst neurons), due to increased sensitivity of $GABA_AR$.

$GABA_AR$ Mechanisms

The $GABA_AR$ consists of five subunits with many subtypes (α_{1-6}, β_{1-3}, γ_{1-3}, δ, ε, π, θ, and ρ_{1-3}) providing diverse receptor functions (45, 46). AAS are allosteric modulators of the $GABA_AR$. Their modulatory activity depends upon which steroid is administered and the $GABA_AR$ subunit composition, being greater for the α_2 than the α_1 subunit, but also acting through the δ and ε subunits (22, 24, 47). Subunit expression is different in different brain areas but is poorly defined because of the lack of specificity of markers and the inattention to cell types important for eye movements, e.g., OPN. IO dendrites contain the α_2 subunit, but their somas contain α_3 subunits (23, 48, 49). The α_2 subunit is more prominent than the α_1 subunit in the cerebellar granule cell and molecular layers (50). Purkinje cells and brainstem reticular formation express the α_1 subunit, and deep cerebellar nuclei express both subunits (45, 51). We assume that increasing $GABA_AR$ modulation and decreasing excitation from cFN to OPN would delay OPN reactivation. Despite these speculations, exactly how AAS affected the $GABA_AR$ in our patients cannot be known. A more detailed biophysical model of opsoclonus awaits further experiments on the effects of $GABA_AR$ dysfunction in identified cell types.

We have shown how our hypothesis that $GABA_AR$ are dysfunctional in a cerebellar–olivary–brainstem network (2) can be implemented by varying parameters in the model. Here, we focused on dysfunction that resulted in a higher gain of $GABA_AR$. Opsoclonus has many causes, and so other mechanisms besides $GABA_AR$ modulation may also cause the diverse types of opsoclonus seen in other patients. Whatever the underlying biophysical mechanism, our model allows us to hypothesize how different regions in the brain must be affected to obtain the various waveforms observed in opsoclonus.

Opsoclonus and Oscillatory Eye Movements

Given the large differences in waveforms seen in patients with opsoclonus, including quasi-sinusoidal, square-wave and square-pulse waveforms, it is not surprising that they have been regarded as different types of movements. However, we have shown that a single model can simulate all of these types of movements, simply by changing a few parameters. Thus, we agree with the hypothesis of Ellenberger et al. (8), who emphasized that these waveforms occur together in the same patients, and thus might be unified as dyskinesias of the saccadic system. Furthermore, although the classic waveform for opsoclonus is a large, sinusoidal oscillation, these may, in fact, simply be back-to-back saccades with no intervening interval, i.e., quasi-sinusoidal oscillations. With low bandwidth recordings (e.g., from electroculograms) these waveforms would be low pass filtered and thus would look sinusoidal. However, higher quality recordings from video or eye coil systems reveal their quasi-sinusoidal nature.

These waveforms can all be obtained from a model of the saccadic system by making appropriate parameter changes in both cerebellar and brainstem circuits, but not by making changes in either alone. We infer from our model that the *mixture* of opsoclonus (quasi-sinusoidal), square-wave and square-pulse oscillations resulting from cerebellar/brainstem dysfunction may commonly co-occur in patients with opsoclonus. Thus, as earlier studies have argued, opsoclonus is not caused by a cerebellar deficit alone. Nor is it caused by lesions of the OPN region. Instead, we hypothesize that opsoclonus occurs when neuronal activity in the CB and brainstem are mistimed.

subjects gave written informed consent in accordance with the Declaration of Helsinki. The ethics committee of the University of Siena, Italy, approved this study.

AUTHOR CONTRIBUTIONS

EP proposed the underlying theory. LO implemented the model and ran the simulations. Both authors wrote the manuscript.

FUNDING

This research was supported by the Intramural Research Program of the National Eye Institute, NIH.

SUPPLEMENTARY MATERIAL

FIGURE S1 | Family of saccades simulated with normal parameter values. **(A)** Saccades from −50 to +50°. Note that saccades larger than 10° undershoot the target by 10%. The model automatically makes a corrective saccade that gets on target (gray lines). **(B)** Inset magnifies saccades to left and right 0.5 and 2° targets. **(C)** Velocity traces for saccades in panels **(A,B)**. Peak speeds were approximately matched to those found by Clark and Stark (52) in normal human subjects.

FIGURE S2 | Simulation of post-inhibitory rebound (PIR) in a model neuron (Eq. 1). PIR depends heavily on three parameters: the gain and time constant of the adaptation element, and the amount of hyperpolarization before the rebound. Here, the excitatory input was set to 0. The neuron has two inhibitory inputs, one for γ-aminobutyric acid (GABA) and one for glycine [NB: the omnipause neurons (OPN) and the IBN are glycinergic, and some LIBN are GABAergic]. The total inhibition to the neuron is thus the sum of the GABA and Gly inputs. For convenience, the sum is set to 1. GABAergic inhibitory input changed briefly from 0.8 to 0. Glycinergic OPN inhibition changed briefly from 0.2 to 0. Thus, the total inhibition to the cell changed from 1.0 to 0. **(A)** Effect of changing the adaptation gain (G_a) on the peak of the rebound activity (adaptive time constant was set to 6 ms). **(B)** Effect of changing the adaptive time constant (T_a, with adaptive gain set to 1.0). Other parameters for the neuron were: $G_I = 1$, $T_I = 2$ ms, $G_o = 1.0$, $\delta = 0.8$ ms. As the time constant increases from 2 to 21 ms, the amplitude and width of the rebound activity increase. Above 21 ms, however, the amplitude begins to decrease. The duration of the rebound is truncated when the OPN resume firing. **(C)** Effect of reducing γ-aminobutyric acid (GABA) inhibition on rebound amplitude. The maximum amount of GABA ranged from 0.0 to 0.8 (accounting for from 0 to 80% of the inhibition on the neuron). As the proportion of GABA was reduced, the hyperpolarization decreased, and the rebound amplitude decreased.

REFERENCES

1. Hallett M. Tremor: pathophysiology. *Parkinsonism Relat Disord* (2014) 20(Suppl 1):S118–22. doi:10.1016/S1353-8020(13)70029-4
2. Pretegiani E, Rosini F, Rocchi R, Ginanneschi F, Vinciguerra C, Optican LM, et al. GABAAergic dysfunction in the olivary-cerebellar-brainstem network may cause eye oscillations and body tremor. *Clin Neurophysiol* (2017) 128(3):408–10. doi:10.1016/j.clinph.2016.12.014
3. Cogan DG. Ocular dysmetria; flutter-like oscillations of the eyes, and opsoclonus. *AMA Arch Ophthalmol* (1954) 51(3):318–35. doi:10.1001/archopht.1954.00920040324006
4. Cogan DG. Opsoclonus, body tremulousness, and benign encephalitis. *Arch Ophthalmol* (1968) 79(5):545–51. doi:10.1001/archopht.1968.03850040547009
5. Averbuch-Heller L, Remler B. Opsoclonus. *Semin Neurol* (1996) 16(1):21–6. doi:10.1055/s-2008-1040955
6. Wong AM, Musallam S, Tomlinson RD, Shannon P, Sharpe JA. Opsoclonus in three dimensions: oculographic, neuropathologic and modelling correlates. *J Neurol Sci* (2001) 189(1–2):71–81. doi:10.1016/S0022-510X(01)00564-0
7. Zangemeister WH, Muller-Jensen A, Zschocke S. Benign encephalitis: electro-oculographic analysis of opsoclonus. *J Neurol* (1979) 222(2):95–108. doi:10.1007/BF00313003

8. Ellenberger C Jr, Keltner JL, Stroud MH. Ocular dyskinesia in cerebellar disease. Evidence for the similarity of opsoclonus, ocular dysmetria and flutter-like oscillations. *Brain* (1972) 95(4):685–92. doi:10.1093/brain/95.4.685
9. Wong A. An update on opsoclonus. *Curr Opin Neurol* (2007) 20(1):25–31. doi:10.1097/WCO.0b013e3280126b51
10. Ross AT, Zeman W. Opsoclonus, occult carcinoma, and chemical pathology in dentate nuclei. *Arch Neurol* (1967) 17(5):546–51. doi:10.1001/archneur.1967.00470290100013
11. Ellenberger C Jr, Campa JF, Netsky MG. Opsoclonus and parenchymatous degeneration of the cerebellum. The cerebellar origin of an abnormal ocular movement. *Neurology* (1968) 18(11):1041–6. doi:10.1212/WNL.18.11.1041
12. Zee DS, Robinson DA. A hypothetical explanation of saccadic oscillations. *Ann Neurol* (1979) 5(5):405–14. doi:10.1002/ana.410050502
13. Ridley A, Kennard C, Scholtz CL, Buttner-Ennever JA, Summers B, Turnbull A. Omnipause neurons in two cases of opsoclonus associated with oat cell carcinoma of the lung. *Brain* (1987) 110(Pt 6):1699–709. doi:10.1093/brain/110.6.1699
14. Helmchen C, Rambold H, Sprenger A, Erdmann C, Binkofski F, fMRI study. Cerebellar activation in opsoclonus: an fMRI study. *Neurology* (2003) 61(3):412–5. doi:10.1212/01.WNL.0000073271.66866.51
15. Oguro K, Kobayashi J, Aiba H, Hojo H. Opsoclonus-myoclonus syndrome with abnormal single photon emission computed tomography imaging. *Pediatr Neurol* (1997) 16(4):334–6. doi:10.1016/S0887-8994(97)00031-3
16. Yoshida T, Katoh A, Ohtsuki G, Mishina M, Hirano T. Oscillating Purkinje neuron activity causing involuntary eye movement in a mutant mouse deficient in the glutamate receptor delta2 subunit. *J Neurosci* (2004) 24(10):2440–8. doi:10.1523/JNEUROSCI.0783-03.2004
17. Jen JC, Lopez I, Baloh RW. Opsoclonus: clinical and immunological features. *J Neurol Sci* (2012) 320(1–2):61–5. doi:10.1016/j.jns.2012.06.017
18. Takagi M, Zee DS, Tamargo RJ. Effects of lesions of the oculomotor vermis on eye movements in primate: saccades. *J Neurophysiol* (1998) 80(4):1911–31.
19. Barash S, Melikyan A, Sivakov A, Zhang M, Glickstein M, Thier P. Saccadic dysmetria and adaptation after lesions of the cerebellar cortex. *J Neurosci* (1999) 19(24):10931–9.
20. Shaikh AG, Miura K, Optican LM, Ramat S, Leigh RJ, Zee DS. A new familial disease of saccadic oscillations and limb tremor provides clues to mechanisms of common tremor disorders. *Brain* (2007) 130(Pt 11):3020–31. doi:10.1093/brain/awm240
21. Lemos J, Eggenberger E. Saccadic intrusions: review and update. *Curr Opin Neurol* (2013) 26(1):59–66. doi:10.1097/WCO.0b013e32835c5e1d
22. Yang P, Jones BL, Henderson LP. Role of the alpha subunit in the modulation of GABA(A) receptors by anabolic androgenic steroids. *Neuropharmacology* (2005) 49(3):300–16. doi:10.1016/j.neuropharm.2005.03.017
23. Oberlander JG, Penatti CA, Porter DM, Henderson LP. The Buzz about anabolic androgenic steroids: electrophysiological effects in excitable tissues. *Neuroendocrinology* (2012) 96(2):141–51. doi:10.1159/000339123
24. Bitran D, Hilvers RJ, Frye CA, Erskine MS. Chronic anabolic-androgenic steroid treatment affects brain GABA(A) receptor-gated chloride ion transport. *Life Sci* (1996) 58(7):573–83. doi:10.1016/0024-3205(95)02326-7
25. Daye PM, Optican LM, Roze E, Gaymard B, Pouget P. Neuromimetic model of saccades for localizing deficits in an atypical eye-movement pathology. *J Transl Med* (2013) 11:125. doi:10.1186/1479-5876-11-125
26. Lefevre P, Quaia C, Optican LM. Distributed model of control of saccades by superior colliculus and cerebellum. *Neural Netw* (1998) 11(7–8):1175–90. doi:10.1016/S0893-6080(98)00071-9
27. Quaia C, Lefevre P, Optican LM. Model of the control of saccades by superior colliculus and cerebellum. *J Neurophysiol* (1999) 82(2):999–1018.
28. Optican LM, Quaia C. Distributed model of collicular and cerebellar function during saccades. *Ann N Y Acad Sci* (2002) 956:164–77. doi:10.1111/j.1749-6632.2002.tb02817.x
29. Otero-Millan J, Troncoso XG, Macknik SL, Serrano-Pedraza I, Martinez-Conde S. Saccades and microsaccades during visual fixation, exploration, and search: foundations for a common saccadic generator. *J Vis* (2008) 8(14):1–18. doi:10.1167/8.14.21
30. Hafed ZM, Goffart L, Krauzlis RJ. A neural mechanism for microsaccade generation in the primate superior colliculus. *Science* (2009) 323(5916):940–3. doi:10.1126/science.1166112
31. Otero-Millan J, Macknik SL, Serra A, Leigh RJ, Martinez-Conde S. Triggering mechanisms in microsaccade and saccade generation: a novel proposal. *Ann N Y Acad Sci* (2011) 1233:107–16. doi:10.1111/j.1749-6632.2011.06177.x
32. Sun Z, Junker M, Dicke PW, Thier P. Individual neurons in the caudal fastigial oculomotor region convey information on both macro- and microsaccades. *Eur J Neurosci* (2016) 44(8):2531–42. doi:10.1111/ejn.13289
33. Ohtsuka K, Noda H. Saccadic burst neurons in the oculomotor region of the fastigial nucleus of macaque monkeys. *J Neurophysiol* (1991) 65(6):1422–34.
34. Fuchs AF, Robinson FR, Straube A. Role of the caudal fastigial nucleus in saccade generation. I. Neuronal discharge pattern. *J Neurophysiol* (1993) 70(5):1723–40.
35. Ohtsuka K, Noda H. Discharge properties of Purkinje cells in the oculomotor vermis during visually guided saccades in the macaque monkey. *J Neurophysiol* (1995) 74(5):1828–40.
36. Dean P. Modelling the role of the cerebellar fastigial nuclei in producing accurate saccades: the importance of burst timing. *Neuroscience* (1995) 68(4):1059–77. doi:10.1016/0306-4522(95)00239-F
37. Ramat S, Leigh RJ, Zee DS, Optican LM. Ocular oscillations generated by coupling of brainstem excitatory and inhibitory saccadic burst neurons. *Exp Brain Res* (2005) 160(1):89–106. doi:10.1007/s00221-004-1989-8
38. Ramat S, Leigh RJ, Zee DS, Shaikh AG, Optican LM. Applying saccade models to account for oscillations. *Prog Brain Res* (2008) 171:123–30. doi:10.1016/S0079-6123(08)00616-X
39. Hong S, Leigh RJ, Zee DS, Optican LM. Inferior olive hypertrophy and cerebellar learning are both needed to explain ocular oscillations in oculopalatal tremor. *Prog Brain Res* (2008) 171:219–26. doi:10.1016/S0079-6123(08)00631-6
40. Shaikh AG, Hong S, Liao K, Tian J, Solomon D, Zee DS, et al. Oculopalatal tremor explained by a model of inferior olivary hypertrophy and cerebellar plasticity. *Brain* (2010) 133(Pt 3):923–40. doi:10.1093/brain/awp323
41. Selhorst JB, Stark L, Ochs AL, Hoyt WF. Disorders in cerebellar ocular motor control. II. Macrosaccadic oscillation. An oculographic, control system and clinico-anatomical analysis. *Brain* (1976) 99(3):509–22. doi:10.1093/brain/99.3.509
42. Horn AK, Buttner-Ennever JA, Wahle P, Reichenberger I. Neurotransmitter profile of saccadic omnipause neurons in nucleus raphe interpositus. *J Neurosci* (1994) 14(4):2032–46.
43. Ashe J, Hain TC, Zee DS, Schatz NJ. Microsaccadic flutter. *Brain* (1991) 114 (Pt 1B):461–72. doi:10.1093/brain/114.1.461
44. Tsutsumi T, Murakami M, Kawaishi J, Chida W, Watanabe K. Ocular flutter associated with a lesion of the right upper pontine tegmentum. *Auris Nasus Larynx* (2009) 36(6):695–7. doi:10.1016/j.anl.2009.02.007
45. Fritschy JM, Benke D, Mertens S, Oertel WH, Bachi T, Mohler H. Five subtypes of type A gamma-aminobutyric acid receptors identified in neurons by double and triple immunofluorescence staining with subunit-specific antibodies. *Proc Natl Acad Sci U S A* (1992) 89(15):6726–30. doi:10.1073/pnas.89.15.6726
46. Sieghart W. Structure, pharmacology, and function of GABAA receptor subtypes. *Adv Pharmacol* (2006) 54:231–63. doi:10.1016/S1054-3589(06)54010-4
47. Jones BL, Whiting PJ, Henderson LP. Mechanisms of anabolic androgenic steroid inhibition of mammalian epsilon-subunit-containing GABAA receptors. *J Physiol* (2006) 573(Pt 3):571–93. doi:10.1113/jphysiol.2006.106534
48. Laurie DJ, Seeburg PH, Wisden W. The distribution of 13 GABAA receptor subunit mRNAs in the rat brain. II. Olfactory bulb and cerebellum. *J Neurosci* (1992) 12(3):1063–76.
49. Devor A, Fritschy JM, Yarom Y. Spatial distribution and subunit composition of GABA(A) receptors in the inferior olivary nucleus. *J Neurophysiol* (2001) 85(4):1686–96.
50. Sieghart W, Sperk G. Subunit composition, distribution and function of GABA(A) receptor subtypes. *Curr Top Med Chem* (2002) 2(8):795–816. doi:10.2174/1568026023393507
51. Pirker S, Schwarzer C, Wieselthaler A, Sieghart W, Sperk G. GABA(A) receptors: immunocytochemical distribution of 13 subunits in the adult rat brain. *Neuroscience* (2000) 101(4):815–50. doi:10.1016/S0306-4522(00)00442-5
52. Clark MR, Stark L. Control of human eye movements: III. Dynamic characteristics of the eye tracking mechanism. *Math Biosci* (1974) 20(3–4):239–65. doi:10.1016/0025-5564(74)90003-0

21

Eye Movements in Parkinson's Disease and Inherited Parkinsonian Syndromes

Elena Pretegiani and Lance M. Optican*

Laboratory of Sensorimotor Research, National Eye Institute, NIH, Bethesda, MD, United States

***Correspondence:**
Elena Pretegiani
elena.pretegiani@nih.gov

Despite extensive research, the functions of the basal ganglia (BG) in movement control have not been fully understood. Eye movements, particularly saccades, are convenient indicators of BG function. Here, we review the main oculomotor findings reported in Parkinson's disease (PD) and genetic parkinsonian syndromes. PD is a progressive, neurodegenerative disorder caused by dopaminergic cell loss within the substantia nigra pars compacta, resulting in depletion of striatal dopamine and subsequent increased inhibitory BG output from the internal globus pallidus and the substantia nigra pars reticulata. Eye movement abnormalities are common in PD: anomalies are more evident in voluntary than reflexive saccades in the initial stages, but visually guided saccades may also be involved at later stages. Saccadic hypometria (including abnormally fragmented saccades), reduced accuracy, and increased latency are among the most prominent deficits. PD patients show also unusually frequent and large square wave jerks and impaired inhibition of reflexive saccades when voluntary mirror saccades are required. Poor convergence ability and altered pursuit are common. Inherited parkinsonisms are a heterogeneous group of rare syndromes due to gene mutations causing symptoms resembling those of PD. Eye movement characteristics of some parkinsonisms have been studied. While sharing some PD features, each syndrome has a distinctive profile that could contribute to better define the clinical phenotype of parkinsonian disorders. Moreover, because the pathogenesis and the underlying neural circuit failure of inherited parkinsonisms are often well defined, they might offer a better prospect than idiopathic PD to understand the BG function.

Keywords: saccades, basal ganglia, α-synuclein, PARK, manganese, Gaucher disease, brain iron accumulation, parkinsonism

INTRODUCTION

The basal ganglia (BG) are subcortical nuclei located at the base of the forebrain and extensively connected directly and indirectly with all cortical and subcortical structures. The BG promote the initiation of goal-directed movement by removing sustained inhibition of the desired movement and suppressing unwanted movements. Despite considerable advancements in understanding the BG anatomy and function, their complex role in modulating motor behavior, remains far from fully elucidated. The saccadic system offers unique advantages in studying the BG because the neural circuits underlying it are relatively well understood and their functional corticobasal loops are likely similar to those involved in regulating other movements (1). Moreover, saccades can be easily and accurately measured.

Eye movements, and particularly the saccadic system, allow to test a distributed network involving cortical (mainly frontal and parietal) and subcortical (BG, midbrain, brain stem, thalamus, and cerebellum) structures. Other than clinically assessed, eye movements can be quantified through electro-oculography, scleral search coil system, and video-oculography. While electrooculography is the only system allowing recording of eye movement with closed eyes, and search coil contact lenses provide the best temporal and spatial resolution, video-oculography is the most used technique given its non-invasiveness (2).

The saccadic system is usually explored by testing reflexive saccades (pro-saccades) toward a visual stimulus that suddenly appears simultaneously, after (gap paradigm), or overlapping (overlap paradigm), the offset of a fixation point exposure. With respect to the simultaneous condition, latency is usually shorter with a gap and longer with an overlap (3). The antisaccade paradigm, in which the saccade is directed to the opposite direction than the stimulus, is used to test voluntary eye movements and inhibition of reflexive movements. The dorsolateral prefrontal cortex is supposed to be involved in the suppression of the unwanted reflexive movement and, with the posterior-parietal cortex, in the generation of the correct mirror movement, while the frontal eye field (FEF) is associated with antisaccade latency (4). Fixation, memory guided saccades toward previously briefly exposed stimuli, and smooth pursuits are also commonly applied to the evaluation of BG function.

Specific eye movement abnormalities follow BG dysfunction (5, 6). Therefore, eye movements are often analyzed to differentiate Parkinson's disease (PD) from other parkinsonian syndromes. Indeed, ocular motor abnormalities of idiopathic neurodegenerative parkinsonisms such as progressive supranuclear palsy, multisystem atrophy, corticobasal syndrome, and dementia with Lewy bodies, have been extensively studied and are well known by clinicians (2, 6). Yet, eye movements in genetic parkinsonisms are seldom investigated. Nonetheless, eye movement features might support the differential diagnosis of genetic syndromes. Moreover, inherited diseases with known pathogenesis and neurodegenerative progression might offer a better prospect than idiopathic PD to delineate the neural circuits underlying specific failures of the BG.

Here, we report the main findings of oculomotor studies in PD and genetic parkinsonian syndromes (**Table 1**).

Parkinson's Disease

Parkinson's disease is a progressive, neurodegenerative disorder. Classic clinical manifestations are tremor at rest, muscular rigidity, akinesia (or bradykinesia), and postural instability (7, 8). Included in the typical features of PD are flexed posture and freezing of gait. Non-motor symptoms such as cognitive impairment, apathy, depression, anosmia, dysautonomia, and sleep disorder are also common.

Parkinson's disease motor manifestations are caused by dopaminergic cell loss within the substantia nigra pars compacta (SNc), resulting in dysfunction of the BG. A cardinal neuropathological feature is the development of intracytoplasmic aggregates of α-synuclein, termed Lewy bodies. Because the dopaminergic neurons in SNc project to the striatum (caudate and putamen), SNc cell loss results in depletion of striatal dopamine (9). PD motor symptoms are recognized when 60% of SNc cells are lost, corresponding to 80% depletion of striatal dopamine.

While partly challenged by more recent findings, the classical model depicts two parallel pathways connecting the BG nuclei (**Figure 1**) (10). The striatum receives input from the FEF, supplementary eye field, DLPFC, and the parietal eye field (PEF). In the direct pathway, dopaminergic projections from the SNc target striatal neurons expressing D1 receptors; D1 neurons send direct inhibitory projections to the BG output nuclei: the

TABLE 1 | Main saccadic features in PD and genetic parkinsonisms.

	PD	PARK1	PARK2	PARK6	PARK9	HMNDYT1	NBI	Gaucher disease
Horizontal saccades								
Latency	Norm/↑	↑	Norm	↑	Norm/↑	↑	NA	↑
Gain	↓	Norm	↓	Norm	↓	Norm	Norm	↓
Precision	↓	Norm	NA	NA	↓	↓	NA	↓
Velocity	Norm	Norm	Norm	Norm	↓	Norm	Norm	↓
Vertical saccades								
Latency	Norm/↑	↑	Norm	NA	↑	↑	NA	Norm
Gain	↓	Norm/↓	↓	NA	↓	Norm	↓	↓
Precision	↓	Norm/↓	NA	NA	↓	↓	↓	↓
Velocity	Norm	Norm	Norm	NA	↓	Norm	↓	↓
Multistep frequency	↑	↑	NA	↑	↑	↑	NA	NA
Antisaccades								
Latency	↑	↑	Norm	Norm	↑	↑	NA	NA
Errors	↑	↑	↑	Norm	↑	↑	NA	NA
Corrections	NA	Norm	NA	NA	↓	Norm	NA	NA

PD, Parkinson's disease; PARK, Parkinson's disease-related locus; HMNDYT1, hypermanganesemia with dystonia, polycythemia, and cirrhosis; NBI, neurodegeneration with brain iron accumulation.

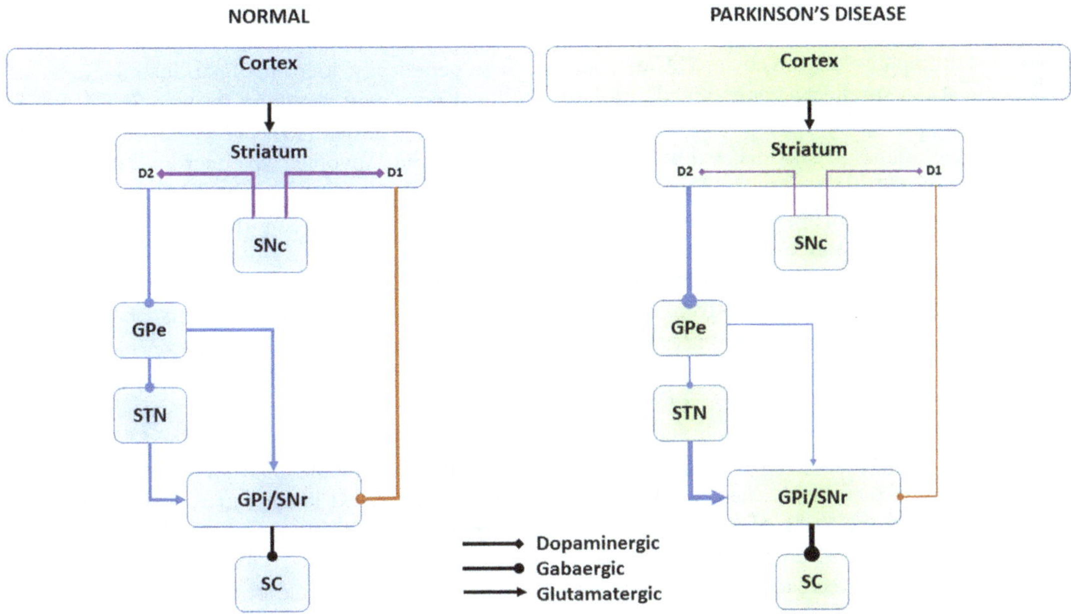

FIGURE 1 | Direct and indirect basal ganglia pathways. The cerebral cortex sends input to the striatum. Dopaminergic projections from the SNc (violet connectors) target striatal neurons expressing D1 or D2 receptors. Direct pathway (orange connectors): D1 neurons send direct inhibitory projections to the SNr/GPi. Indirect pathway (blue connectors): D2 neurons connect indirectly to the GPi/SNr through the GPe and STN. The SNr inhibits the SC. In Parkinson's disease, dopaminergic depletion leads to reduced inhibitory direct pathway output (thin lines) and increased excitatory indirect pathway output (thick lines) onto the GPi/SNr and, consequently, increased SNr inhibition onto the SC as net effect. SNc, substantia nigra pars compacta; GPe, external globus pallidus; STN, subthalamic nucleus; GPi, internal globus pallidus; SNr, substantia nigra pars reticulata; SC, superior colliculus.

internal globus pallidus (GPi) and the substantia nigra pars reticulata (SNr). In the indirect pathway, D2 expressing neurons receive projections from the SNc and connect indirectly to the GPi/SNr through the external globus pallidus (GPe) and the subthalamic nucleus (STN) (11). The SNr inhibits the superior colliculus (SC). The SC is a crucial structure for both voluntary and reflexive saccades. The SC, indeed, integrates visual, somato-sensory, and auditory stimuli in a spatial map and produces a motor saccade command that is sent to the brain stem saccade generators. The cortical-BG-SC pathway is supposed to be particularly important in selecting the most appropriate or most rewarding movement when multiple internal and/or external inputs compete to orient the body, or the eyes, to different locations (12, 13).

In PD, dopaminergic depletion leads to reduced inhibitory direct pathway output and increased excitatory indirect pathway output onto the GPi/SNr (8, 14). The hyperactivated SNr induces excessive inhibition of the SC, which is considered to be responsible for the typical eye movement abnormalities in PD (15).

However, voluntary saccade generation involves a cortex-BG-SC pathway, whereas reflexive saccades can be generated by direct projections from the parietal cortex onto saccade-related neurons in the intermediate layer of the SC (16). This processing is supposed to largely bypass the BG circuit and it is considered the reason why reflexive saccades are mostly preserved in PD, particularly at early stages of the disease, while voluntary saccades are more severely affected (15, 17). According to this picture, a recent fMRI study, while failing to find differences in saccadic metrics between PD patients and controls, found that PD showed left frontal underactivation during horizontal prosaccades and right parietal overactivation during horizontal and vertical prosaccades and horizontal antisaccades (18).

One of the most prominent features of eye movement abnormality in PD is saccade hypometria (15, 19). As expected, hypometria is more severe in voluntary saccades, particularly in memory-guided saccades, where a subject is required to make a saccade to a remembered target location. Reflexive saccades, usually preserved in the initial stages of PD, can become hypometric in later stages (2). Reflexive saccade hypometria is thought to result solely from excessive SC inhibition, compared to hypometric voluntary saccades that are supposed to be caused by both increased SC inhibition and reduced pre-oculomotor drive due to dysfunctional frontal cortex-BG-SC circuit (20). An alternative explanation for hypometria in PD involves a dysfunction of the cerebellum which is hyperactivated in PD (21). However, a fundamentally preserved saccadic adaptive ability in PD suggests normal cerebellar function, at least during the early stage of the disease (22).

Abnormally fragmented saccades, called multistep or staircase saccades, have been described in PD. These movements, where the target is reached by several hypometric saccades, are observed also in normal subjects (23), but they are more frequent when PD patients execute memory-guided or self-paced saccades (24). Their exact mechanism is still not understood. Gaze fragmentation is supposed to reflect an inappropriate inhibition of the saccade generator (25, 26). Therefore, multistep saccades in PD might be an expression of saccadic hypometria or improper reactivation of omnipause neurons due to SC dysfunction (27), but they could also just reflect a general facilitation in the execution of small saccades (20).

Latency of voluntary saccades is usually delayed in PD, indicating difficulty in initiating volitional eye movements. Latency of reflexive saccades can be spared during the early stages of the disease, when PD patients may produce saccades even faster than normal (express saccades), particularly for small target eccentricities. This facilitation disappears at advanced stages when latency of reflexive saccades also increases, particularly for large target eccentricities (20).

Parkinson's disease patients show also impairment of inhibition of reflexive saccades to a visual cue when a voluntary mirror saccade is required (so-called antisaccades) (28). Dysfunction of the suppression of unwanted saccades in the DLPFC following dopaminergic depletion in the prefrontal cortex, "leaky" suppression of the SC from the BG, and cognitive impairment have all been associated with impaired saccadic inhibition and "hyper-reflexivity" in PD (4, 15, 29). Antisaccades can reveal deficits of executive functions even in early stages of PD (30). Recently, antisaccade errors have been related to freezing of gait, and increased antisaccade latency in PD has been correlated with impaired postural control (31, 32).

Square wave jerks are saccadic intrusions (usually 0.5–5°) that move the eye from and back to the fixation point with an intersaccadic interval of about 200 ms. Abnormally frequent and large square wave jerks in PD patients have been ascribed to compensatory increased activity in the FEF (19, 26). PD patients show other abnormal eye movements such as poor convergence ability and altered pursuit (33). Pursuit is often saccadic in PD patients who can also show increased pursuit latency and reduced gain and impaired preparation and execution of cue-dependent memory-based smooth-pursuits (34, 35).

A long debate has characterized the finding of ocular tremor in PD patients (36–38). Indeed, while some researchers support the presence of pervasive ocular tremor in PD (39, 40), others consider it the simple consequence of the vestibulo-ocular reflex induced by head movement (41, 42).

Eye movement abnormalities are supposed to impair some behaviors of PD patients. Deficient generation of voluntary saccades, for example, might explain the visual search pattern of PD: patients scan smaller areas than normal with fewer, hypometric saccades, which could lead to a mild degree of visuospatial neglect in PD patients (43). Facilitation of small saccades might underlie reading difficulties (44). Impairment in the generation of voluntary saccades can also affect stability and walking (6).

While impaired oculomotor performance is attributed to dopamine depletion, studies on the effect of dopaminergic treatment on eye movement have given inconsistent results (45, 46).

Finally, PD patients show several oculo-visual dysfunctions (i.e., hallucinations and impairment of visual acuity, color and contrast sensitivity, motion perception, stereopsis), but whether and how they impact eye movement is difficult to establish (47, 48).

Parkinson Disease 1 (*PARK1*)

Parkinson disease 1 (*PARK1*, OMIM number #168601) is the first genetically identified parkinsonism. Its associated autosomal dominant mutation in gene *SNCA* was initially isolated in Italian families (49). *SNCA* encodes a presynaptic protein, α-synuclein, involved in neuronal plasticity. Intra-neuronal aggregates of α-synuclein are the hallmark of neurodegenerative synucleinopathies, being the major component of Lewy bodies in PD and Lewy body dementia. Tau-inclusions may be also frequent. Neuronal loss is more severe in the brain stem, hippocampus, dorsal motor nucleus of the vagus, SNc, nucleus basalis of Meynert, and locus coeruleus, but it involves also cortical areas (49, 50). The clinical phenotype of patients with mutations in *PARK1* resembles typical sporadic PD, except for earlier onset, rapid progression, and frequent cognitive decline. Eye movement recording from two patients with mutated *PARK1* showed increased latency of reflexive and voluntary saccades, more frequent multistep saccades, but normal average gain and precision, and normal saccade velocity and duration; patients made more directional errors at the antisaccade task, but corrected as frequently as normal (51).

Parkinson Disease 2 (*PARK2*)

Parkinson disease 2 (*PARK2*, #60016) is due to homozygous and compound heterozygous mutations in *Parkin (PRKN)* and it is the most common genetic parkinsonism. Parkin defects interfere with the ubiquitin-mediated proteolytic pathway and cause accumulation of 22-kD glycosylated α-synuclein leading to neurodegeneration with more involvement of the SNc than the locus coeruleus with respect to idiopathic PD (50). Phenotype is similar to that of sporadic PD.

Recording of eye movements in symptomatic patients with *PARK2* mutations showed hypometric saccades with normal latency, antisaccades with normal latency but increased error rate, and reduced gain of smooth pursuit (52, 53).

Parkinson Disease 6 (*PARK6*)

Parkinson disease 6 (*PARK6*, #605909) results from mutations in *PINK1* coding a mitochondrial protein (PTEN-induced putative kinase 1), causing increased susceptibility to cellular stress and apoptosis (54). Neurodegeneration affects the SNc, brain stem reticular formation, and nucleus basalis of Meynert and it is associated with cortical and brain stem Lewy bodies (50). Patients present with parkinsonism, gait disturbances, and psychosis. A cohort of *PINK1* mutation carriers showed increased latency of horizontal prosaccades with normal gain and velocity, higher rate of multistep saccades, normal error rate in the antisaccade task; homozygous (but not heterozygous) patients showed also hypometric memory guided saccades (55).

Parkinson Disease 9 (*PARK9*)

Parkinson disease 9 (*PARK9* or Kufor-Rakeb syndrome, #606693) is a rare autosomal recessive juvenile-onset levodopa-responsive parkinsonism due to mutations in *ATP13A2* (*PARK9*) encoding a lysosomal P-type ATP-ase (56). Mutation of *PARK9* leads to α-synuclein accumulation and increased manganese toxicity (57), causing cortical and subcortical neurodegeneration. Beside progressive parkinsonism patients present also with pyramidal signs, facial-faucial-finger mini-myoclonus, and cognitive decline (58).

Neuroimaging shows reduced dopamine transporter activity and reduced gray matter in the motor cortex, prefrontal cortex, somatosensory association cortex, cingulate, caudate, thalamus, and cerebellum. Accumulation of iron in the BG has been detected in some cases.

Typical eye movement abnormalities are vertical supranuclear gaze palsy, slowing of vertical and horizontal saccades, and saccadic pursuit (58, 59). Eye movement recordings from three patients showed hypometric and slow saccades with worse precision, increased or normal latency of horizontal saccades and increased latency of vertical saccades (51, 60). Target was often reached by multistep saccades. Antisaccades directional error rate was increased and patients never corrected the errors (51).

Hypermanganesemia with Dystonia, Polycythemia, and Cirrhosis (HMNDYT1)

Hypermanganesemia with dystonia, polycythemia, and cirrhosis (HMNDYT1, #613280) is a parkinsonism due to recessive mutations in *SLC30A10* (61). Loss of function of the encoded manganese transporter leads to a primary metabolic disorder causing hypermanganesemia. Manganese accumulation induces cell toxicity in the liver, bone marrow, and nervous system. Brain MRI T1 hyperintense lesions are present in the caudate and lentiform nuclei, thalamus, corticospinal tract, substantia nigra, posterior pons, and bulbar olives, cerebellum and cerebello-rubro-thalamic pathways.

Eye movement recording from two affected patients showed increased latency of reflexive and voluntary saccades, normal gain and velocity, but worse precision, and increased frequency of multistep saccades. Antisaccade errors were increased, but they were corrected as frequently as normal (51).

Manganese is also a known cause of environmental intoxication upon overexposure in workers and drug abusers (62, 63). In these cases, manganese accumulates in the globus pallidus more than in other brain structures, causing parkinsonism and oculomotor abnormalities. A detailed description of the oculomotor abnormalities is available only for subjects with ephedrone-induced parkinsonism (62). Ephedrone (also called methcathinone or α-methylamino-propiophenone) is a home-made drug obtained by oxidation of ephedrine or pseudoephedrine with potassium permanganate and acetic acid (62). Ephedrone addicts can face manganese intoxication leading to severe, rapidly progressive, non-levodopa responsive parkinsonism and dystonia. Patients showed hypometric and slow horizontal saccades with normal latency, and increased latency of vertical saccades; antisaccades showed normal latency, but increased error rate with normal correction frequency. These findings differ with respect to those shown by subjects with genetic hypermanganesemia, perhaps indicating that the slow manganese accumulation in HMNDYT1 might allow for some adaptation.

Neurodegeneration with Brain Iron Accumulation

Neurodegeneration with brain iron accumulation is a genetically heterogenous disorder causing progressive accumulation of iron in the BG and other brain regions, most cases being associated with mutations in *PANK2* and *PLA2G6*. Pantothenate kinase-associated neurodegeneration (PKAN, formerly Hallervorden-Spatz syndrome, #234200) is a recessive disease associated with mutations in *PANK2*. Patients present with cognitive dysfunction and extrapyramidal features such as parkinsonism and dystonia. Eye movement abnormalities include hypometric and slow vertical saccades, normal horizontal saccades, saccadic pursuit, impaired vestibulo-ocular reflex suppression, poor convergence, square-wave jerk saccadic intrusions, and abnormal vertical optokinetic reflex (64). Patients with *PLA2G6* mutations (#603604) can present with up gaze palsy, poor convergence, saccadic intrusions, and saccadic pursuit (65).

Gaucher Disease

Gaucher disease (#230800, #230900, #231000) is the most common autosomal recessive lysosomal storage disorder and it is due to mutations in *GBA* leading to deficit of glucocerebrosidase and intracellular accumulation of glucosylceramide. Typical features are hepatosplenomegaly and pancytopenia. Several patients with Gaucher disease presented with parkinsonism. In these patients, neuronal loss occurred in SNc, hippocampus, and cortex (50). Ocular motor abnormalities have been proposed as an early marker to detect neurological impairment in type 3 Gaucher disease, distinguishing it from the subtype without neurological involvement (type1) (66, 67).

Patients affected by type 3 Gaucher disease showed slow velocity (affecting horizontal more than vertical saccades), saccadic hypometria, and increased horizontal saccade latency (68). Saccadic pursuit and oculomotor apraxia were also reported.

Recently, heterozygous *GBA* mutation carriers have been found to be at higher risk to develop PD and Lewy body dementia (69, 70). The phenotype of these patients can be indistinguishable from that of idiopathic PD.

CONCLUSION

Studies of eye movements in inherited parkinsonian syndromes are often limited by small sample sizes and by inconsistent examination techniques and paradigms. Nevertheless, these reports support distinct pictures of eye movement disorders for each genetic syndrome, highlighting some features as possible markers for differential diagnosis and for evaluation of disease extension and progression. Still, some characteristics tend to recur across syndromes and could be more informative about BG functions: saccades with increased latency but normal velocity suggest a role of BG in motor initiation rather than execution, so that bradykinesia in parkinsonism should be interpreted more as a delayed motor onset than a slow movement. Also, increased error rate in the antisaccade task, with often normal frequency of correction, might indicate that BG participate more in selecting than planning the proper movement among competitive movements. Other less frequent features are usually associated with more severe phenotypes, possibly indicating more profound BG damage or degenerative involvement of other brain structures.

More studies, applying the same saccadic paradigms and integrating clinical, genetic, neuroimaging, and neuropathological data, are needed for better picturing the oculomotor features associated with BG dysfunctions in PD and parkinsonisms and their relationship with other motor and non-motor symptoms. Clarifying these aspects might provide clinical/diagnostic indications to guide the evaluation of patients with parkinsonism, including its genetic variants. Also, it will help in understanding the modulatory role of BG in behavior.

AUTHOR CONTRIBUTIONS

EP and LO: design of the work, acquisition and interpretation of data for the work, drafting the work, and final approval of the article.

FUNDING

Study funded by the Intramural Research Programs of NEI.

REFERENCES

1. Watanabe M, Munoz DP. Probing basal ganglia functions by saccade eye movements. *Eur J Neurosci* (2011) 33(11):2070–90. doi:10.1111/j.1460-9568.2011.07691.x
2. Gorges M, Pinkhardt EH, Kassubek J. Alterations of eye movement control in neurodegenerative movement disorders. *J Ophthalmol* (2014) 2014:658243. doi:10.1155/2014/658243
3. Saslow MG. Latency for saccadic eye movement. *J Opt Soc Am* (1967) 57(8):1030–3. doi:10.1364/JOSA.57.001024
4. Crawford TJ, Bennett D, Lekwuwa G, Shaunak S, Deakin JF. Cognition and the inhibitory control of saccades in schizophrenia and Parkinson's disease. *Prog Brain Res* (2002) 140:449–66. doi:10.1016/S0079-6123(02)40068-4
5. Kennard C, Lueck CJ. Oculomotor abnormalities in diseases of the basal ganglia. *Rev Neurol (Paris)* (1989) 145(8–9):587–95.
6. Anderson TJ, MacAskill MR. Eye movements in patients with neurodegenerative disorders. *Nat Rev Neurol* (2013) 9(2):74–85. doi:10.1038/nrneurol.2012.273
7. Jankovic J. Parkinson's disease: clinical features and diagnosis. *J Neurol Neurosurg Psychiatry* (2008) 79(4):368–76. doi:10.1136/jnnp.2007.131045
8. Rodriguez-Oroz MC, Jahanshahi M, Krack P, Litvan I, Macias R, Bezard E, et al. Initial clinical manifestations of Parkinson's disease: features and pathophysiological mechanisms. *Lancet Neurol* (2009) 8(12):1128–39. doi:10.1016/S1474-4422(09)70293-5
9. Shulman JM, De Jager PL, Feany MB. Parkinson's disease: genetics and pathogenesis. *Annu Rev Pathol* (2011) 6:193–222. doi:10.1146/annurev-pathol-011110-130242
10. Calabresi P, Picconi B, Tozzi A, Ghiglieri V, Di Filippo M. Direct and indirect pathways of basal ganglia: a critical reappraisal. *Nat Neurosci* (2014) 17(8):1022–30. doi:10.1038/nn.3743
11. DeLong MR, Wichmann T. Circuits and circuit disorders of the basal ganglia. *Arch Neurol* (2007) 64(1):20–4. doi:10.1001/archneur.64.1.20
12. Hikosaka O, Takikawa Y, Kawagoe R. Role of the basal ganglia in the control of purposive saccadic eye movements. *Physiol Rev* (2000) 80(3):953–78.
13. Hikosaka O. Basal ganglia mechanisms of reward-oriented eye movement. *Ann N Y Acad Sci* (2007) 1104:229–49. doi:10.1196/annals.1390.012
14. DeLong M, Wichmann T. Update on models of basal ganglia function and dysfunction. *Parkinsonism Relat Disord* (2009) 15(Suppl 3):S237–40. doi:10.1016/S1353-8020(09)70822-3
15. Terao Y, Fukuda H, Ugawa Y, Hikosaka O. New perspectives on the pathophysiology of Parkinson's disease as assessed by saccade performance: a clinical review. *Clin Neurophysiol* (2013) 124(8):1491–506. doi:10.1016/j.clinph.2013.01.021
16. May PJ. The mammalian superior colliculus: laminar structure and connections. *Prog Brain Res* (2006) 151:321–78. doi:10.1016/S0079-6123(05)51011-2
17. Gaymard B. Cortical and sub-cortical control of saccades and clinical application. *Rev Neurol (Paris)* (2012) 168(10):734–40. doi:10.1016/j.neurol.2012.07.016
18. Lemos J, Pereira D, Almendra L, Rebelo D, Patricio M, Castelhano J, et al. Distinct functional properties of the vertical and horizontal saccadic network in Health and Parkinson's disease: an eye-tracking and fMRI study. *Brain Res* (2016) 1648(Pt A):469–84. doi:10.1016/j.brainres.2016.07.037
19. White OB, Saint-Cyr JA, Tomlinson RD, Sharpe JA. Ocular motor deficits in Parkinson's disease. II. Control of the saccadic and smooth pursuit systems. *Brain* (1983) 106(Pt 3):571–87. doi:10.1093/brain/106.3.571
20. Terao Y, Fukuda H, Yugeta A, Hikosaka O, Nomura Y, Segawa M, et al. Initiation and inhibitory control of saccades with the progression of Parkinson's disease – changes in three major drives converging on the superior colliculus. *Neuropsychologia* (2011) 49(7):1794–806. doi:10.1016/j.neuropsychologia.2011.03.002
21. Wu T, Hallett M. The cerebellum in Parkinson's disease. *Brain* (2013) 136 (Pt 3):696–709. doi:10.1093/brain/aws360
22. MacAskill MR, Anderson TJ, Jones RD. Adaptive modification of saccade amplitude in Parkinson's disease. *Brain* (2002) 125(Pt 7):1570–82. doi:10.1093/brain/awf168
23. Kimmig H, Haussmann K, Mergner T, Lucking CH. What is pathological with gaze shift fragmentation in Parkinson's disease? *J Neurol* (2002) 249(6):683–92. doi:10.1007/s00415-002-0691-7
24. Blekher T, Weaver M, Rupp J, Nichols WC, Hui SL, Gray J, et al. Multiple step pattern as a biomarker in Parkinson disease. *Parkinsonism Relat Disord* (2009) 15(7):506–10. doi:10.1016/j.parkreldis.2009.01.002
25. Optican LM, Rucker JC, Keller EL, Leigh RJ. Mechanism of interrupted saccades in patients with late-onset Tay–Sachs disease. *Prog Brain Res* (2008) 171(5):567–70. doi:10.1016/S0079-6123(08)00681-X
26. Shaikh AG, Xu-Wilson M, Grill S, Zee DS. 'Staircase' square-wave jerks in early Parkinson's disease. *Br J Ophthalmol* (2011) 95(5):705–9. doi:10.1136/bjo.2010.179630
27. Paul K, Gnadt JW. Activity of omnipause neurons during "staircase saccades" elicited by persistent microstimulation of the superior colliculus. *Vision Res* (2006) 46(20):3430–42. doi:10.1016/j.visres.2006.05.014
28. Rivaud-Pechoux S, Vidailhet M, Brandel JP, Gaymard B. Mixing pro- and antisaccades in patients with parkinsonian syndromes. *Brain* (2007) 130 (Pt 1):256–64. doi:10.1093/brain/awl315
29. van Stockum S, MacAskill M, Anderson T, Dalrymple-Alford J. Don't look now or look away: two sources of saccadic disinhibition in Parkinson's disease? *Neuropsychologia* (2008) 46(13):3108–15. doi:10.1016/j.neuropsychologia.2008.07.002
30. Antoniades CA, Demeyere N, Kennard C, Humphreys GW, Hu MT. Antisaccades and executive dysfunction in early drug-naive Parkinson's disease: the discovery study. *Mov Disord* (2015) 30(6):843–7. doi:10.1002/mds.26134
31. Walton CC, O'Callaghan C, Hall JM, Gilat M, Mowszowski L, Naismith SL, et al. Antisaccade errors reveal cognitive control deficits in Parkinson's disease with freezing of gait. *J Neurol* (2015) 262(12):2745–54. doi:10.1007/s00415-015-7910-5
32. Ewenczyk C, Mesmoudi S, Gallea C, Welter ML, Gaymard B, Demain A, et al. Antisaccades in Parkinson disease: a new marker of postural control? *Neurology* (2017) 88(9):853–61. doi:10.1212/WNL.0000000000003658
33. Almer Z, Klein KS, Marsh L, Gerstenhaber M, Repka MX. Ocular motor and sensory function in Parkinson's disease. *Ophthalmology* (2012) 119(1):178–82. doi:10.1016/j.ophtha.2011.06.040
34. Shibasaki H, Tsuji S, Kuroiwa Y. Oculomotor abnormalities in Parkinson's disease. *Arch Neurol* (1979) 36(6):360–4. doi:10.1001/archneur.1979.00500420070009

35. Fukushima K, Fukushima J, Barnes GR. Clinical application of eye movement tasks as an aid to understanding Parkinson's disease pathophysiology. *Exp Brain Res* (2017) 235(5):1309–21. doi:10.1007/s00221-017-4916-5
36. Duval C, Beuter A, Gauthier S. Fluctuations in tremor at rest and saccadic eye movements in subjects with Parkinsons disease. *Parkinsonism Relat Disord* (1997) 3(4):195–205. doi:10.1016/S1353-8020(97)00019-9
37. Duval C, Beuter A. Fluctuations in tremor at rest and eye movements during ocular fixation in subjects with Parkinson's disease. *Parkinsonism Relat Disord* (1998) 4(2):91–7. doi:10.1016/S1353-8020(98)00023-6
38. Duval C. Ocular tremor in Parkinson's disease: the debate is not over. *Mov Disord* (2013) 28(6):713–4. doi:10.1002/mds.25514
39. Gitchel GT, Wetzel PA, Baron MS. Pervasive ocular tremor in patients with Parkinson disease. *Arch Neurol* (2012) 69(8):1011–7. doi:10.1001/archneurol.2012.70
40. Baron MS, Gitchel GT, Wetzel PA. Scientific data support that ocular tremor is genuine and unrelated to head movement. *Parkinsonism Relat Disord* (2014) 20(12):1449–50. doi:10.1016/j.parkreldis.2014.09.032
41. Kaski D, Saifee TA, Buckwell D, Bronstein AM. Ocular tremor in Parkinson's disease is due to head oscillation. *Mov Disord* (2013) 28(4):534–7. doi:10.1002/mds.25342
42. Leigh RJ, Martinez-Conde S. Tremor of the eyes, or of the head, in Parkinson's disease? *Mov Disord* (2013) 28(6):691–3. doi:10.1002/mds.25478
43. Matsumoto H, Terao Y, Furubayashi T, Yugeta A, Fukuda H, Emoto M, et al. Small saccades restrict visual scanning area in Parkinson's disease. *Mov Disord* (2011) 26(9):1619–26. doi:10.1002/mds.23683
44. Yu CY, Lee T, Shariati MA, Santini V, Poston K, Liao YJ. Abnormal eye movement behavior during reading in Parkinson's disease. *Parkinsonism Relat Disord* (2016) 32:130–2. doi:10.1016/j.parkreldis.2016.08.008
45. Reilly JL, Lencer R, Bishop JR, Keedy S, Sweeney JA. Pharmacological treatment effects on eye movement control. *Brain Cogn* (2008) 68(3):415–35. doi:10.1016/j.bandc.2008.08.026
46. Srivastava A, Sharma R, Sood SK, Shukla G, Goyal V, Behari M. Saccadic eye movements in Parkinson's disease. *Indian J Ophthalmol* (2014) 62(5):538–44. doi:10.4103/0301-4738.133482
47. Armstrong RA. Oculo-visual dysfunction in Parkinson's disease. *J Parkinsons Dis* (2015) 5(4):715–26. doi:10.3233/JPD-150686
48. Weil RS, Schrag AE, Warren JD, Crutch SJ, Lees AJ, Morris HR. Visual dysfunction in Parkinson's disease. *Brain* (2016) 139(11):2827–43. doi:10.1093/brain/aww175
49. Golbe LI, Di Iorio G, Bonavita V, Miller DC, Duvoisin RC. A large kindred with autosomal dominant Parkinson's disease. *Ann Neurol* (1990) 27(3):276–82. doi:10.1002/ana.410270309
50. Poulopoulos M, Levy OA, Alcalay RN. The neuropathology of genetic Parkinson's disease. *Mov Disord* (2012) 27(7):831–42. doi:10.1002/mds.24962
51. Pretegiani E, Rosini F, Federico A, Optican LM, Rufa A. Eye movements in genetic parkinsonisms affecting the α-synuclein, PARK9, and manganese network. *Clin Neurophysiol* (2017). doi:10.1016/j.clinph.2017.09.107
52. Helmchen C, Schwekendiek A, Pramstaller PP, Hedrich K, Klein C, Rambold H. Blink amplitude but not saccadic hypometria indicates carriers of Parkin mutations. *J Neurol* (2006) 253(8):1071–5. doi:10.1007/s00415-006-0168-1
53. Machner B, Klein C, Sprenger A, Baumbach P, Pramstaller PP, Helmchen C, et al. Eye movement disorders are different in Parkin-linked and idiopathic early-onset PD. *Neurology* (2010) 75(2):125–8. doi:10.1212/WNL.0b013e3181e7ca6d
54. Valente EM, Abou-Sleiman PM, Caputo V, Muqit MM, Harvey K, Gispert S, et al. Hereditary early-onset Parkinson's disease caused by mutations in PINK1. *Science* (2004) 304(5674):1158–60. doi:10.1126/science.1096284
55. Hertel S, Sprenger A, Klein C, Kompf D, Helmchen C, Kimmig H. Different saccadic abnormalities in PINK1 mutation carriers and in patients with non-genetic Parkinson's disease. *J Neurol* (2009) 256(7):1192–4. doi:10.1007/s00415-009-5092-8
56. Ramirez A, Heimbach A, Grundemann J, Stiller B, Hampshire D, Cid LP, et al. Hereditary parkinsonism with dementia is caused by mutations in ATP13A2, encoding a lysosomal type 5 P-type ATPase. *Nat Genet* (2006) 38(10):1184–91. doi:10.1038/ng1884
57. Gitler AD, Chesi A, Geddie ML, Strathearn KE, Hamamichi S, Hill KJ, et al. Alpha-synuclein is part of a diverse and highly conserved interaction network that includes PARK9 and manganese toxicity. *Nat Genet* (2009) 41(3):308–15. doi:10.1038/ng.300
58. Williams DR, Hadeed A, al-Din AS, Wreikat AL, Lees AJ. Kufor Rakeb disease: autosomal recessive, levodopa-responsive parkinsonism with pyramidal degeneration, supranuclear gaze palsy, and dementia. *Mov Disord* (2005) 20(10):1264–71. doi:10.1002/mds.20511
59. Behrens MI, Bruggemann N, Chana P, Venegas P, Kagi M, Parrao T, et al. Clinical spectrum of Kufor-Rakeb syndrome in the Chilean kindred with ATP13A2 mutations. *Mov Disord* (2010) 25(12):1929–37. doi:10.1002/mds.22996
60. Machner B, Sprenger A, Behrens MI, Ramirez A, Bruggemann N, Klein C, et al. Eye movement disorders in ATP13A2 mutation carriers (PARK9). *Mov Disord* (2010) 25(15):2687–9. doi:10.1002/mds.23352
61. Quadri M, Federico A, Zhao T, Breedveld GJ, Battisti C, Delnooz C, et al. Mutations in SLC30A10 cause parkinsonism and dystonia with hypermanganesemia, polycythemia, and chronic liver disease. *Am J Hum Genet* (2012) 90(3):467–77. doi:10.1016/j.ajhg.2012.01.017
62. Bonnet C, Rusz J, Megrelishvili M, Sieger T, Matouskova O, Okujava M, et al. Eye movements in ephedrone-induced parkinsonism. *PLoS One* (2014) 9(8):e104784. doi:10.1371/journal.pone.0104784
63. O'Neal SL, Zheng W. Manganese toxicity upon overexposure: a decade in review. *Curr Environ Health Rep* (2015) 2(3):315–28. doi:10.1007/s40572-015-0056-x
64. Egan RA, Weleber RG, Hogarth P, Gregory A, Coryell J, Westaway SK, et al. Neuro-ophthalmologic and electroretinographic findings in pantothenate kinase-associated neurodegeneration (formerly Hallervorden-Spatz syndrome). *Am J Ophthalmol* (2005) 140(2):267–74. doi:10.1016/j.ajo.2005.03.024
65. Khan AO, AlDrees A, Elmalik SA, Hassan HH, Michel M, Stevanin G, et al. Ophthalmic features of PLA2G6-related paediatric neurodegeneration with brain iron accumulation. *Br J Ophthalmol* (2014) 98(7):889–93. doi:10.1136/bjophthalmol-2013-304527
66. Harris CM, Taylor DS, Vellodi A. Ocular motor abnormalities in Gaucher disease. *Neuropediatrics* (1999) 30(6):289–93. doi:10.1055/s-2007-973507
67. Capablo JL, Saenz de Cabezon A, Fraile J, Alfonso P, Pocovi M, Giraldo P, et al. Neurological evaluation of patients with Gaucher disease diagnosed as type 1. *J Neurol Neurosurg Psychiatry* (2008) 79(2):219–22. doi:10.1136/jnnp.2006.111518
68. Benko W, Ries M, Wiggs EA, Brady RO, Schiffmann R, Fitzgibbon EJ. The saccadic and neurological deficits in type 3 Gaucher disease. *PLoS One* (2011) 6(7):e22410. doi:10.1371/journal.pone.0022410
69. Clark LN, Ross BM, Wang Y, Mejia-Santana H, Harris J, Louis ED, et al. Mutations in the glucocerebrosidase gene are associated with early-onset Parkinson disease. *Neurology* (2007) 69(12):1270–7. doi:10.1212/01.wnl.0000276989.17578.02
70. Clark LN, Kartsaklis LA, Wolf Gilbert R, Dorado B, Ross BM, Kisselev S, et al. Association of glucocerebrosidase mutations with dementia with Lewy bodies. *Arch Neurol* (2009) 66(5):578–83. doi:10.1001/archneurol.2009.54

Permissions

 Every chapter published in this book has been scrutinized by our experts. Their significance has been extensively debated. The topics covered herein carry significant findings which will fuel the growth of the discipline. They may even be implemented as practical applications or may be referred to as a beginning point for another development.

The contributors of this book come from diverse backgrounds, making this book a truly international effort. This book will bring forth new frontiers with its revolutionizing research information and detailed analysis of the nascent developments around the world.

We would like to thank all the contributing authors for lending their expertise to make the book truly unique. They have played a crucial role in the development of this book. Without their invaluable contributions this book wouldn't have been possible. They have made vital efforts to compile up to date information on the varied aspects of this subject to make this book a valuable addition to the collection of many professionals and students.

This book was conceptualized with the vision of imparting up-to-date information and advanced data in this field. To ensure the same, a matchless editorial board was set up. Every individual on the board went through rigorous rounds of assessment to prove their worth. After which they invested a large part of their time researching and compiling the most relevant data for our readers.

The editorial board has been involved in producing this book since its inception. They have spent rigorous hours researching and exploring the diverse topics which have resulted in the successful publishing of this book. They have passed on their knowledge of decades through this book. To expedite this challenging task, the publisher supported the team at every step. A small team of assistant editors was also appointed to further simplify the editing procedure and attain best results for the readers.

Apart from the editorial board, the designing team has also invested a significant amount of their time in understanding the subject and creating the most relevant covers. They scrutinized every image to scout for the most suitable representation of the subject and create an appropriate cover for the book.

The publishing team has been an ardent support to the editorial, designing and production team. Their endless efforts to recruit the best for this project, has resulted in the accomplishment of this book. They are a veteran in the field of academics and their pool of knowledge is as vast as their experience in printing. Their expertise and guidance has proved useful at every step. Their uncompromising quality standards have made this book an exceptional effort. Their encouragement from time to time has been an inspiration for everyone.

The publisher and the editorial board hope that this book will prove to be a valuable piece of knowledge for researchers, students, practitioners and scholars across the globe.

List of Contributors

Silvia Colnaghi
Laboratory of Neuro-otology and Neuro-ophtalmology, Fondazione Istituto Neurologico Nazionale Casimiro Mondino (IRCCS), Pavia, Italy
Department of Public Health, Experimental and Forensic Medicine, University of Pavia, Pavia, Italy

Giorgio Beltrami
Department of Electrical, Computer and Biomedical Engineering, University of Pavia, Pavia, Italy

Guy Poloni and Anna Pichiecchio
Neuroradiology Department, Fondazione Istituto Neurologico Nazionale Casimiro Mondino (IRCCS), Pavia, Italy

Stefano Bastianello
Neuroradiology Department, Fondazione Istituto Neurologico Nazionale Casimiro Mondino (IRCCS), Pavia, Italy
Department of Brain and Behavioral Sciences, University of Pavia, Pavia, Italy

Maurizio Versino
Laboratory of Neuro-otology and Neuro ophtalmology, Fondazione Istituto Neurologico Nazionale Casimiro Mondino (IRCCS), Pavia, Italy
Department of Brain and Behavioral Sciences, University of Pavia, Pavia, Italy

Carlo Andrea Galimberti
Epilepsy Centre, Fondazione Istituto Neurologico Nazionale Casimiro Mondino (IRCCS), Pavia, Italy

Pamela Federighi, Francesca Rosini and Alessandra Rufa
Eye Tracking and Visual Application Lab (EVA Lab), Department of Medicine, Surgery and Neuroscience, University of Siena, Siena, Italy

Stefano Ramat
Department of Electrical, Computer and Biomedical Engineering, University of Pavia, Pavia, Italy

Elena Pretegiani
Laboratory of Sensorimotor Research, National Eye Institute, National Institutes of Health, Bethesda, MD, United States

Antonio Federico
UOC Neurology and Neurometabolic Diseases, Department of Medicine, Surgery and Neuroscience, University of Siena, Siena, Italy

Ivanna M. Pavisic, Timothy J. Shakespeare, Keir X. X. Yong, Catherine F. Slattery, Ross W. Paterson, Alexander J. M. Foulkes, Kirsty Macpherson, Amelia M. Carton, Nick C. Fox, Jonathan M. Schott, Sebastian J. Crutch and Silvia Primativo
Dementia Research Centre, Department of Neurodegenerative Diseases, Institute of Neurology, University College London, London, United Kingdom

Nicholas C. Firth and Daniel C. Alexander
Centre for Medical Image Computing, Department of Computer Science, University College London, London, United Kingdom

Samuel Parsons, David Martinez Rego and John Shawe-Taylor
Centre for Computational Statistics and Machine Learning, Faculty of Engineering Science, Department of Computer Science, University College London, London, United Kingdom

Ting-Feng Lin, Dominik Straumann and Melody Ying-Yu Huang
Department of Neurology, University Hospital Zurich, University of Zurich, Zurich, Switzerland
Neuroscience Center Zurich (ZNZ), University of Zurich and ETH Zurich, Zurich, Switzerland

Christina Gerth-Kahlert
Department of Ophthalmology, University Hospital Zurich, Zurich, Switzerland University Langone Medical Center, New York,

James V. M. Hanson
Department of Ophthalmology, University Hospital Zurich, Zurich, Switzerland
Neuroimmunology and Multiple Sclerosis Research, Clinic for Neurology, University Hospital Zurich, University of Zurich, Zurich, Switzerland

John-Ross Rizzo
Department of Neurology, New York University School of Medicine, New York, NY, United States
Department of Physical Medicine and Rehabilitation, New York University School of Medicine, New York, NY, United States
Department of Rehabilitation Medicine, New York University Langone Medical Center, New York, USA
Department of Neurology, New York University Langone Medical Center, New York, USA

Maryam Hosseini, Eric A. Wong, James K. Fung, Edmond Ahdoot, Preeti Raghavan, Azadeh Shafieesabet and Rosa M. Pasculli
Department of Rehabilitation Medicine, New York United States

Wayne E. Mackey and Michael S. Landy
Department of Psychology and Center for Neural Science, New York University, New York, USA

Janet C. Rucker
Department of Neurology, New York University School of Medicine, New York, United States
Department of Neurology, New York University Langone Medical Center, New York, United States
Department of Ophthalmology, New York University Langone Medical Center, New York, United States

Todd E. Hudson
Department of Rehabilitation Medicine, New York University Langone Medical Center, New York, USA
Department of Neurology, New York University Langone Medical Center, New York, USA

Robert G. Alexander, Stephen L. Macknik and Susana Martinez-Conde
State University of New York (SUNY) Downstate Medical Center, Brooklyn, NY, United States

Andrew Abdou
Rutgers School of Biomedical and Health Sciences, New Brunswick, NJ, USA

Yvonne W. Lui
Department of Radiology, New York University Langone Medical Center, New York, USA

Ariel Winnick
Department of Neurology, The Johns Hopkins University School of Medicine, Baltimore, MD, United States

Amir Kheradmand
Department of Neurology, The Johns Hopkins University School of Medicine, Baltimore, MD, United States
Department of Otolaryngology - Head and Neck Surgery, The Johns Hopkins University School of Medicine, Baltimore, MD, United States

Alexandra Lloyd-Smith Sequeira
Department of Neurology, New York University School of Medicine, New York, NY, United States

Ali G. Hamedani
Department of Neurology, Hospital of the University of Pennsylvania, Philadelphia, PA, United States

Daniel R. Gold
Department of Neurology, Johns Hopkins Hospital, Baltimore, MD, United States
Department of Ophthalmology, Johns Hopkins Hospital, Baltimore, MD, United States
Department of Neurosurgery, Johns Hopkins Hospital, Baltimore, MD, United States
Department of Otolaryngology - Head and Neck Surgery, Johns Hopkins Hospital, Baltimore, MD, United States

Diego Kaski and Adolfo M. Bronstein
Division of Brain Sciences, Department of Neuro-Otology, Imperial College London, London, UK
Department of Neuro-Otology, University College London, National Hospital for Neurology and Neurosurgery, London, UK

Aasef G. Shaikh
Department of Neurology, Case Western Reserve University, Cleveland, OH, United States
Neurological Institute, University Hospitals, Cleveland, OH, United States
Neurology Service, Louis Stokes, Cleveland, VA, United States

Fatema F. Ghasia
Daroff-Dell'Osso Ocular Motility Laboratory, Louis Stokes Cleveland VA Medical Center, Cleveland, OH, United States
Cole Eye Institute, Cleveland Clinic, Cleveland, OH, United States

Alessandro Serra
Neurology, Louis Stokes VA Medical Center, University Hospitals and Case Western Reserve School of Medicine, Cleveland, OH, United States

Clara G. Chisari
Neurology, University of Catania, Catania, Italy

Manuela Matta
Neurology, Ospedale San Luigi Gonzaga, Orbassano, Italy

Caroline Tilikete
Neuro-Ophthalmology and Neurocognition, Hôpital Neurologique Pierre Wertheimer, Hospices Civils de Lyon, Bron, France
Lyon I University, Lyon, France
ImpAct Team, CRNL INSERM U1028 CNRS UMR5292, Bron, France

Virginie Desestret
Neuro-Ophthalmology and Neurocognition, Hôpital Neurologique Pierre Wertheimer, Hospices Civils de Lyon, Bron, France
Lyon I University, Lyon, France
SynatAc Team, Institut NeuroMyogène INSERM U1217/UMR CRS 5310, Lyon, France

Thomas Cronin, Qadeer Arshad and Barry M. Seemungal
Division of Brain Sciences, Department of Medicine, Charing Cross Hospital, London, United Kingdom

Josefine Blume, Stanislav Beniaminov and Per Svenningsson
Section of Neurology, Department of Clinical Neuroscience, Center for Molecular Medicine, Karolinska Institute, Stockholm, Sweden

Cecilia Kämpe Björkvall
Hematology Center Karolinska, Department of Medicine at Huddinge, Karolinska Institutet, Karolinska University Hospital Huddinge, Stockholm, Sweden

Maciej Machaczka
Department of Medicine, Sunderby Regional Hospital of Norrbotten County, Luleå, Sweden

Chrystalina Antoniades
NeuroMetrology Lab, Nuffield Department of Clinical Neurosciences, University of Oxford, Oxford, United Kingdom

James Fitzgerald
NeuroMetrology Lab, Nuffield Department of Clinical Neurosciences, University of Oxford, Oxford, United Kingdom
Nuffield Department of Surgical Sciences, University of Oxford, Oxford, United Kingdom

Jorge Otero-Millan
Department of Neurology, Johns Hopkins University, Baltimore, MD, United States

Lance M. Optican
Laboratory of Sensorimotor Research, National Eye Institute, National Institutes of Health, Department of Health and Human Services, Bethesda, MD, United States

Stephen L. Macknik and Susana Martinez-Conde
Department of Ophthalmology, SUNY Downstate Medical Center, Brooklyn, NY, United States
Department of Neurology, SUNY Downstate Medical Center, Brooklyn, NY, United States
Department of Physiology and Pharmacology, SUNY Downstate Medical Center, Brooklyn, NY, United States

Lance M. Optican
Laboratory of Sensorimotor Research, National Eye Institute, National Institutes of Health, Department of Health and Human Services, Bethesda, MD, United States

Sarah L. Kang
Case Western Reserve University School of Medicine, Cleveland, OH, United States

Index